MasterMinding Wounds

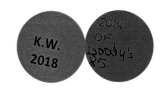

MasterMinding Wounds

Author
Michael B. Strauss, M.D.

Co-Authors
Igor V. Aksenov, M.D., Ph.D.
Stuart S. Miller, M.D.

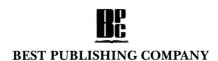

BEST PUBLISHING COMPANY

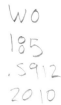

Cover Design: Travis Moore
Text Layout and Design: Travis Moore
Editing: Catherine Morris and Linda Locklear

No responsibility is assumed by the Publisher or Editors for any injury and/or damage to persons or property as a matter of product liability, negligence, or otherwise, or from any use or operation of any methods, product, instructions, or ideas contained in the material herein. No suggested test or procedure should be carried out unless, in the reader's judgment, its risk is justified. Because of rapid advances in the medical sciences, we recommend that the independent verification of diagnoses and drug dosages should be made.

International Standard Book Number: 978-1-930536-52-4
Library of Congress catalog card number: 2009925160

For more information contact:
Best Publishing Company
Flagstaff, AZ 86003-0100, USA
Telephone: 928.527.1055
Fax: 928.526.0370
E-mail: divebooks@bestpub.com
Website: www.bestpub.com

CONTENTS

PREFACE VII
INTRODUCTION IX
ACKNOWLEDGEMENTS XI

PART I
SETTING THE STAGE 1

CHAPTER 1 PUTTING PROBLEM WOUNDS INTO PERSPECTIVE 5
CHAPTER 2 PROBLEM WOUND PRESENTATIONS 25

PART II
EVALUATION OF WOUNDS 53

CHAPTER 3 CLASSIFICATION SYSTEMS FOR THE
DIABETIC FOOT WOUND............................ 57
CHAPTER 4 CLASSIFICATION SYSTEMS FOR
PRESSURE ULCERS/INDOLENT WOUNDS 85
CHAPTER 5 THE WOUND SCORE - A SOLUTION FOR THE
WOUND CLASSIFICATION DILEMMA 109

PART III
THE STRATEGIC MANAGEMENT OF PROBLEM WOUNDS............. 129

CHAPTER 6 MEDICAL MANAGEMENT STRATEGIES................ 133
CHAPTER 7 PREPARATION OF THE WOUND BASE................ 165
CHAPTER 8 PROTECTION AND STABILIZATION OF THE WOUND 193
CHAPTER 9 SELECTION OF WOUND DRESSING AGENTS 219
CHAPTER 10 WOUND OXYGENATION AND
HYPERBARIC OXYGEN THERAPY 253

PART IV
IDENTIFICATION AND MANAGEMENT OF THE "END-STAGE" WOUND . 287

CHAPTER 11 THE "END-STAGE" HYPOXIC WOUND 293
CHAPTER 12 OTHER "END-STAGE" WOUNDS 331

PART V
PREVENTION OF NEW AND RECURRENT WOUNDS **369**

CHAPTER 13   WOUND PREVENTION THROUGH PATIENT
     EDUCATION 379
CHAPTER 14   SKIN CARE AND TOENAIL MANAGEMENT 399
CHAPTER 15   PROTECTIVE FOOTWEAR 419
CHAPTER 16   MINIMALLY INVASIVE PROACTIVE SURGERIES 445

APPENDICES

A. MASTERMINDING WOUNDS FROM A TO Z 483
B. AIDS FOR MASTERMINDING WOUNDS 491
C. ADDITIONAL SOURCES OF INFORMATION ON PROBLEM
     WOUNDS AND RELATED SUBJECTS 507
D. WOUND CARE ORGANIZATIONS, SOCIETIES, AND ASSOCIATIONS . . . 539
E. PARTING COMMENTARIES 545
F. INDEX 561

PREFACE

The precursors of *MasterMinding Wounds* began a dozen years ago when I generated a simplified **Wound Score** to quantify the seriousness of wounds. As the score was refined, it became a core ingredient of a **Master Algorithm**. The **Master Algorithm** offers a strategic approach to evaluation, management, and prevention (EMP) of wounds. With the evolution of the **Master Algorithm**, it became apparent that wound management decisions needed to be based on more than the **Wound Score**, especially in the most challenging situations where patient survival and limb salvage become considerations. As a result, the **Host-Function Score** and **Goal-Aspiration Score** were integrated into the **Master Algorithm** to objectify decision making for these difficult situations.

In the interim, a number of high caliber guidelines, reviews, position papers, and wound care texts have been published (Appendix C-1 and C-2). Although they represent a wealth of wound care information, it is not always easy to determine the best management for a particular patient from the information they contain. Furthermore, the information in the guidelines tends to be highly focused and limited to a specific topic, while many of the textbooks were collections of chapters written by multiple authors without transitions or uniting features between the chapters. The result is that, for the most part, these sources fail to provide a strategic approach for the comprehensive EMP (evaluation, management, and prevention) of challenging wounds. It was our goal to generate a practical, "user-friendly," fully integrated, highly visual approach to wound management which, we believe, *MasterMinding Wounds* achieves.

Another noteworthy event in the genesis of this book occurred with my appointment to the Diabetic Foot Committee of the American Foot and Ankle Society in 2000. While serving on the committee I was able to orchestrate the generation of four exhibits over a five year period on diabetic foot problems that were presented at successive American Academy of Orthopaedic Surgeons meetings from 2001-2005. Michael Pinzur, M.D. and Naomi Fields, M.D., chairpersons of the foot committee, collaborated with me on the projects. The exhibit subjects were based on topics from the **Master Algorithm**. Production of the exhibits was an exercise in refinement of ideas and the concise expression of concepts. Information from these exhibits as well as elements of over 70 of our papers and poster presentations generated during the past dozen years became integral components of *MasterMinding Wounds* (Appendix C-4 and C-5) and provide the tactics (that is, the specific interventions) for the EMP of problem wounds found in many of the chapters of our text.

INTRODUCTION

Several features make *MasterMinding Wounds* unique and special. The first of these is the "Power of Ten" (J. Poniewozik, *Time* [Essay], 24 Dec 2007, p-96). Ten point evaluation systems using five assessments, each graded 2 points (best) to 0 points (worst) a la the Apgar score (Apgar, V., *Curr Res Anesth Anal*, 1953, 32(4):260-267), provide an ideal format for listing and grading information. With a little ingenuity they can be readily adapted to almost any situation. The "Power of Ten" is intuitively obvious in that high scores are good and low scores are bad. By grouping the points comprising the scores as high, medium, and low, appropriate decisions or interventions are apparent for a particular scoring group. Five new and unique 0 to 10 point scores each consisting of five assessments plus an additional three stand alone 0 to 2 point assessments are introduced in *MasterMinding Wounds* (duplicated in Appendix B). Although at first inspection the multiple scores and assessments may seem "overkill," their integration into the **Master Algorithm** results in an objective, comprehensive, almost seamless approach to the EMP of wounds—something that makes our text different than all the other texts we reviewed.

Another unique feature of *MasterMinding Wounds* is its consistency, something that is facilitated by the writing of a text by a single set of authors. Commencing with Chapter 5, the information in this text provides a chapter full of information for almost every heading in the **Master Algorithm**. To facilitate understanding, tables, unique and original illustrations, clinical photos, text boxes, and clinical scenarios are employed throughout the text. We have utilized an ample amount of tables since they allow us to summarize large amounts of information, yet do not detract from the flow of the text. For example, by grouping the indications and mechanisms of several thousand wound care dressing agents into categories, four basic options become apparent. Other examples and unique features are the tables used to summarize over 20 bioengineered wound dressing agents and over a dozen negative pressure wound therapy options.

To assure patient anonymity, the clinical scenarios and photos have been modified, usually by combining information from several sources to illustrate principles, but not reveal patient identities. Additional features include subject outlines to introduce the major sections of each chapter, discussion questions at the end of each chapter, and a comprehensive appendix. The appendix, consisting of five sections, is a special creation in itself. Appendix A includes wound subject topics A through Z with chapter references for each. Appendix B is a readily accessible recapitulation of the **Master Algorithm**, scores, and assessments we have generated for *MasterMinding Wounds*. Appendix C consists of five reference sources, each with brief editorial comments for each citation including 1) guidelines and position papers, 2) wound texts, 3) wound journals, 4) our wound-related publications, and 5) our exhibit, podium, and poster presentations.

Appendix D is a listing of wound societies and organizations with their focus of interest and contact information. Finally, Appendix E is a parting point essay on the integration of wound care in hospital and wound clinic settings and how hyperbaric oxygen therapy, when indicated, is a useful adjunct and a continuity of care measure for both.

Although the "perfect" wound text has yet to be written, we feel strongly that there are features of *MasterMinding Wounds* that have applications to every level of wound caregiver, from the surgeon who directs his/her attention to the wound base, to the patient or family member who provides the day-to-day care, and every level of wound caregiver in between. For those clinicians who find no practical purposes for grading systems, *MasterMinding Wounds* provides the essential and uncontestable strategies for managing "problem" and "end-stage" wounds (Parts III and IV). For those who find comfort in quantifying observations and using grades and scores to make decisions, *MasterMinding Wounds* provides a consistent, intuitive approach based on 0 to 10 point scores and 0 to 2 point assessments. With applications of the "Power of Ten," severities, progress (or deterioration), and patient factors become objective and quantifiable. In addition, the grading systems are useful tools to compare efficacies of interventions through the use of comparative scores for studying a wound care product or wound management technique. Improvements/deteriorations and outcomes likewise are quantified and easily determined using the objective "Power of Ten" **Wound Score**. We feel that these user-friendly devices add a new dimension in the EMP (evaluation, management and prevention) of wounds.

ACKNOWLEDGEMENTS

We are proud of our open-minded approach to wound management. None of us have been influenced by vendors of wound care products and/or been provided industry supported grants or other incentives to utilize any specific agent, instrument, or technique. Whenever possible and/or feasible, listings of agents, chapter orders, etc., were done either alphabetically or chronologically (as done for scoring systems in Chapters 3 and 4) to avoid showing preferences to others' works. Our opinions have arisen from the best possible source of information, the "laboratory of experiences and observations." This has been gained though management of thousands of wounds in every conceivable setting from surgical procedures in the operating room, in-hospital, outpatient and skilled nursing facility wound care, and home care management. On this behalf, we are indebted to our colleagues (see Appendix E) including physicians, nurses, and allied health care providers. Their dedicated care, keen observations, and provocative inquiries have helped us formulate the approach we use for the EMP of wounds and the practical information that is such an important ingredient of *MasterMinding Wounds*. A couple of special acknowledgements go to Rebecca Albert, R.D., who edited our nutrition section (in Chapter 6) into a very concise and precise section on this critical aspect of wound management, and Rodger Dierker, Pharm.D., who helped us make sense out of all of the wound dressing agents (in Chapter 9) and determine the appropriate terminology for each.

Our next goals are to further validate our scores and assessments to the point that they meet all the requirements of evidence-based medicine and satisfy the complaints of even our most harsh critics. At the same time, our sincerest intentions are that others incorporate the information in this text to make their wound (and hyperbaric medicine) programs the highest quality possible through the use of objective assessments and standardized outcome measures as the **Wound Score** so facilitates. The ultimate achievement will be when we read others' works using our algorithms and scoring systems and validate additionally (or even reject) our observations.

This section would not be complete without an expression of appreciation to my co-authors, our publisher, and my wife. Not only did my co-authors keep me "on task," but also when really challenging problems needed to be solved or specific references were required, they were always quick to find the solutions. Their fine-tuning of the scores and assessments, editing of less than clear concepts, and contributions in their specialties of pulmonary/critical care medicine and hyperbaric medicine by Dr. Aksenov, and emergency medicine and hyperbaric medicine by Dr. Miller added scholarship and accuracy to the text. We are grateful to our publisher, Best Publishing Company, for repeatedly granting us extensions on our deadlines with words of encouragement rather than threats of breach of contract. Feedback of our preliminary drafts was a source of encouragement and drove us to make *MasterMinding Wounds* an extraordinary text. I am extremely grateful to my wife, Wendy Strauss, Pharm.D., an editor extraordinaire who was both a terrible nuisance and an invaluable asset—always looking over my shoulder to make suggestions about my word choices and syntax, then re-reviewing the editing once the appropriate changes were made. If there is clarity to the text, she certainly deserves significant credit for it. In addition, she contributed her pharmacy expertise to help me generate multiple unique and innovative tables. Lastly, thank you to all of my friends, family, and co-workers who were supportive and tolerant of the enormous time required to put together this comprehensive text.

Michael B. Strauss, M.D.
F.A.C.S., A.A.O.S

PART I

SETTING THE STAGE

CHAPTER	TITLE	PAGE
1	PUTTING PROBLEM WOUNDS INTO PERSPECTIVE	5
2	PROBLEM WOUND PRESENTATIONS	25

INTRODUCTION TO PART I

Although the readers of *MasterMinding Wounds* may want to proceed directly to the evaluation, management, and prevention sections of this text, selected background information is helpful in putting problem wounds into focus as well as in defining the magnitude of this important problem. The subsequent two chapters, "Putting Problem Wounds into Perspective" and "Problem Wound Presentations," help achieve these two goals. "Putting Problem Wounds into Perspective" deals with the magnitude of problem wounds, the assessment of new products, and the extent of the problem in overall numbers and costs. "Problem Wound Presentations" is provided to demonstrate the variety of presentations of problem wounds. The nomenclature used in this section includes the common and lay terms which patients, families, and most non-experts in wound management use to describe wounds. Chapter 1 introduces the concept of **strategic management**, which is fundamental to management of problem wounds and becomes the core information for Part III, "The Strategic Management of Problem Wounds." An additional concept introduced in Chapter 1 is that of quantifying the patient's goals and potential for following instructions to achieve healing of challenging wounds. This is achieved by generating a **Goal-Aspiration Score**, one of several unique tools and highly practical scoring systems we present in *MasterMinding Wounds*. Finally, whereas most other textbooks on wound care narrow their scope to dealing only with foot and/or diabetic wounds, our wound evaluation, management, and prevention approach is generic and applicable to wounds of almost all types and in any anatomical location (Part I, Figure 1).

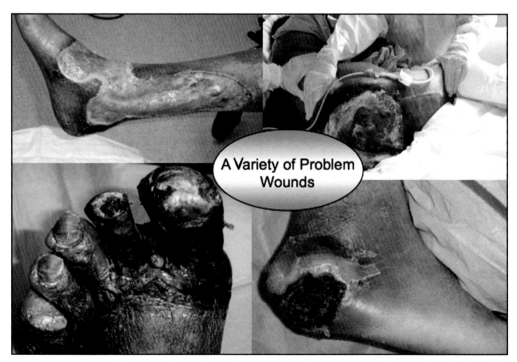

Part I, Figure 1. Problem wounds are observed in a variety of circumstances. They need not be limited to the foot nor restricted to diabetic patients, as so many classification systems are. The wound evaluation, management, and prevention system that emerges in this text is universally applicable to almost every wound situation and type of patient.

<u>NOTES</u>

PUTTING PROBLEM
WOUNDS INTO PERSPECTIVE

CHAPTER ONE OVERVIEW

INTRODUCTION 7
THE CONCEPT OF MOIST WOUND HEALING. 8
MAKING SENSE OF THE DATA 9
A RATIONAL APPROACH FOR MAKING MANAGEMENT DECISIONS 11
THE GOAL-ASPIRATION SCORE. 14
MAGNITUDE AND COSTS OF THE PROBLEM WOUND 17
THE STRATEGIC APPROACH TO WOUND MANAGEMENT 19
CONCLUSIONS 19
QUESTIONS 21
REFERENCES. 22

"Not every wound is a problem."

INTRODUCTION

Putting Wounds into Perspective – Recently, the management of wounds has garnered extensive attention. This is reflected in the proliferation of wound healing centers, health care professionals devoted to wound management, and a plethora of wound care products[1-3] (Figure 1-1). Not all wounds require special attention. Every day thousands, perhaps hundreds of thousands, of surgical wounds are created in operating rooms, surgical centers, and physicians' offices throughout the world. Over 99.9 percent of wounds heal without incident. Another group of wounds such as cuts and scrapes are not serious enough to even require professional attention; these occur almost too frequently to be counted. In both of these situations, wound healing invariably proceeds uneventfully. Only very rarely do wounds fail to heal primarily. When they do not, it is described as a wound complication—or if the problem does not improve with the initial interventions, a "problem" wound. To define a problem wound may be easy, if using the criterion of whether or not healing is proceeding as expected. To use objective criteria and grade a problem wound is more of a challenge. More than a dozen grading systems for problem wounds exist.[4-15] In Chapters 3 and 4, these and other published wound grading systems are described and analyzed. From this information, including their merits and their deficiencies, we have generated a wound scoring system for defining problem wounds objectively (Chapter 5).

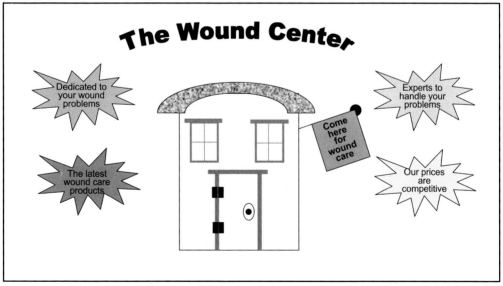

Figure 1-1. Not all wound care facilities are the same. The patient and family should ascertain that the facility 1) has affiliations with a hospital for expedient transfer of life or limb threatening problems, 2) has surgeons on the staff are accessible to perform definitive surgeries, 3) hyperbaric oxygen therapy is available, and 4) personnel are dedicated to the multidisciplinary approach to wound management.

Obviously, "Not every wound is a problem." In the total perspective, only a very small percentage fails to heal as expected. Size, infection, depth, and other factors (as will be defined in Chapter 5) determine whether a wound will heal without incident.

This objective scoring system is multifunctional. It is not only useful for the evaluation of wounds, but also for selecting which interventions are needed for management, quantitatively measuring progress in healing, for defining outcomes, and assisting in research purposes.

THE CONCEPT OF MOIST WOUND HEALING

Challenges and Moist Wound Healing – Many challenges become evident when dealing with problem wounds. These include the reliability of the data on the usefulness of wound care products, time lags for new developments to become accepted as standards of practice, and making decisions for wound management on evidence-based information as compared to experience. The concept of "moist wound healing" is a major development in wound management that has become almost universally accepted in the wound healing community during the past decade.[16] Moist wound healing implies that dressing materials and wound covering agents should be designed and selected to keep the wound base moist. This is logical and sensible, since the environment of the wound base should be maintained as close to the internal environment of the body as possible.

The concept of the body tissues functioning in a "sea of fluid" is basic to the biology of all living things and a fundamental component of the evolutionary concept that ontogeny (development of the living organism) recapitulates phylogeny (evolution of the species).

In the wound healing situation, it is logical that the environment of the wound should be maintained as physiological as possible—and as close to normal tissue fluids as feasible.

When the wound is not healthy enough to maintain the optimal physiological environment, wound covering dressing agents are selected to compensate for the deficiencies (Chapter 9).

Tissue Fluids – All internal tissues in the body are "bathed" in tissue fluids.[17-20] The body fluids surrounding these tissues provide an optimal physiological environment for the tissues, comprised of the cells which are needed to survive, properly function, and reproduce. Additionally, body fluids provide an interface for oxygen, nutrients, and wastes to enter and leave the tissues and a conduit for their transfer to and from the adjacent capillaries.

Capillaries and Wounds that are Too Moist – Capillaries, in turn, are the exchange portions of the circulatory system. They are the sites where nutrients transported from other parts of the body diffuse into tissue fluids, where waste products from the tissues diffuse out and are subsequently carried to other portions of the body for detoxification, elimination, or both (Figure 1-2). However, in certain situations such as in wounds that

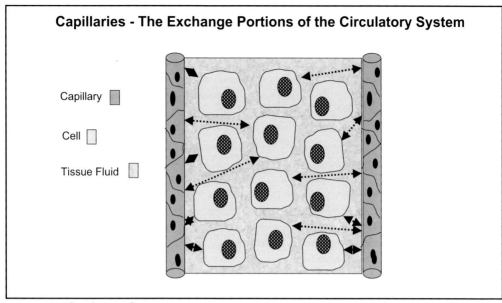

Capillaries - The Exchange Portions of the Circulatory System

Capillary

Cell

Tissue Fluid

Figure 1-2. All exchange of oxygen, nutrients, waste products, etc., occur at the capillary. The products diffuse through the tissue fluids to reach the cell (←→). All cells are bathed in tissue fluid. Therefore, it makes sense to make the environment around the wound healing tissues as similar to tissue fluids as possible.

leak a large volume of tissue fluids (e.g. the patient with severe chronic venous insufficiency of the lower extremities), wounds that have macerated skin edges, wounds which are highly exudative or are covered with thin-dry eschars, the choice of a moist dressing—or maintaining the moist wound environment may not be the optimal management for wound healing.

MAKING SENSE OF THE DATA

Dealing with New Problems – A relevant question is, how does the wound care practitioner assess the enormous amount of information that is generated about wounds and make decisions about the proliferation of new products for wound management that become available at ever increasing rates? There is no simple answer to this question. Our observations suggest that many products on initial introduction to the wound care market are heralded as the answer to problem wound management. Seemingly, initial good data validates their effectiveness. However, with time and experience, usually after a couple of years of the product being on the market, the outcomes when using these products do not meet expectations. Recent examples include the use of various agents with growth factors incorporated into the product and multiple bioengineered dressing materials. In fact, recently the Center for Medicare-Medicaid Services (CMS) has issued a directive that it no longer authorizes reimbursements for the use of agents with growth factors in them that are targeted as an adjunct to wound healing.[21, 22] Private carriers of medical insurance typically impose stringent restrictions on use of new, costly wound care products. The answer to the dilemma in making decisions about using new products should be based on fundamentals. What is the wound problem and what are the proposed mechanisms of action of the new product? Without attention to other wound healing strategies such as removing infected bone, maximizing nutrition, perfusion status,

Often, petitions and other attestations are required to use new, expensive wound care products. Statements that nothing else will work and the patient is at risk of losing life or limb if the product is not used are often used in these requests.

When such products are used in lieu of integrating all the **Strategic Management** elements (Part III), failure is likely and the wound care product quickly loses its attractiveness.

etc., the new product may unjustifiably be doomed to failure. Thus, the use and evaluation of a new product must be done in the context of best practice management of the wound. Incredible as it seems, according to the Institute of Medicine, the time it takes for a new medical product or management approach to be conceived, tested, utilized, and then become a standard of practice can be as much as 15-20 years[23, 24] (Figure 1-3). This is termed the information "lag time." This suggests that many new products and techniques for wound management, as in almost all other areas of medicine, are in various stages of development and can be expected to become available to our armamentarium of wound care management in the future.

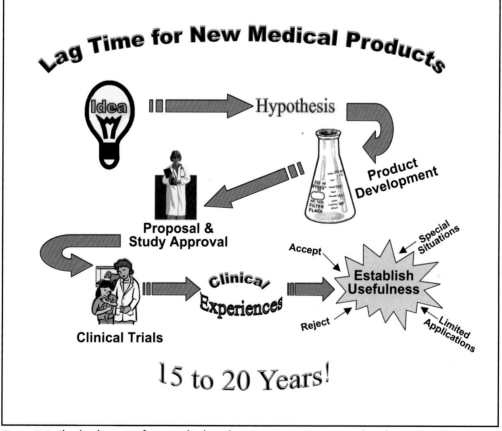

Figure 1-3. The development of new medical products is a time-consuming and costly process. For truly new products, the time for gestation of the idea to acceptance in clinical practice can be 15 years or longer. For most wound care products, the lag time is much shorter because the products are variations, refinements, or modifications of products that are already in use.

A RATIONAL APPROACH FOR MAKING MANAGEMENT DECISIONS

Evidence-based Information – The "gold standard" for use of procedures and products in medicine is the evidence-based indication. Evidence is provided by studies. The most convincing studies are randomized control trials (RCT), especially if the

> The strongest level of evidence is provided by a meta-analysis of RCT's using "Odds Ratios" (number of those NOT developing the problem by the new treatment divided by the number developing the problem in the control group—if this scheme fits the model).
>
> The odds ratio (usually with 95% confidence intervals) for each RCT in the meta-analysis is then plotted on a 0.01 to 100 horizontal scale. In the situation above, odds ratios less than 1 favor the treatment, whereas odds numbers greater than 1 favor the controls.
>
> The sum of the individual odds ratios divided by the number of studies provides the summated odds ratio for the treatment intervention. The "weighted" summated odds ratio takes into consideration sample size and variance for each study.

treating physicians are blinded as to whether their patients are in the control or treatment arm of the study. If the RCT shows a benefit with the treatment arm, then there is justification for using the intervention. If several RCTs are available, it is desirable to compare them using a meta-analysis. There is a hierarchy of the quality of evidence with

> Information based on evidenced-based indications is more applicable for medical problems than for surgical procedures. This is because it is easier to set up blinded RCT's for medications where either placebos or currently available medications are compared with a new product rather than to compare surgical procedures.
>
> For surgical procedures, setting up RCT's are challenging. Standards of practice dictate that outcomes meet community expectations. Where outcomes are highly predictable, as they are for most surgical procedures, RCT's border on being unethical, especially if the only thing the patient has to show for the trial is a scar on the skin. Surgical RCT's are almost cost prohibitive for the placebo arm since several thousand dollars of cost are associated with any visit to the operating room. Finally, in order to gather sufficient data in a reasonable time frame, multi-center studies may be the only option. Their validity for surgical procedures, as compared to medication trials, can be questioned due to differences in surgical training, skills, personal preferences and variations in techniques. With medication RCT's, these differences are generally not a factor in assessing the validity of the study.
>
> The use of evidence-based indications for wound management has both surgical and medical perspectives. Certainly product selection lends itself to evidence-based information. However, since the healing responses of every complicated wound (especially in patients with compromised recuperative abilities) are different, the use of evidence-based information to select wound care products has to be balanced with the practitioner's experiences. Likewise, surgical interventions for these problems often need to be unique and innovative such that logic and experience are far more important in deciding what to do than information from RCT's.

TABLE 1-1. EXAMPLES OF SYSTEMS USED TO RANK LEVEL OF EVIDENCE

American Heart Association	National Cancer Institute	McMaster's Group (Canada)	US Preventative Services Task Force	New Zealand Guidelines Group	Journal of Bone & Joint Surgery*
Level 1 SS RCT's -1A Meta-analysis of + RCT's -1B One or more + RCT's -1C Meta-analysis with inconsistent, but significant results Level 2 Statistically insignificant RCT's Level 3 Prospective, controlled, but not randomized cohort studies Level 4 Historic, non-randomized cohort or case control studies Level 5 Human case series Level 6 Animal or mechanical model Level 7 Reasonable extrapolations from existing data Level 8 Rational conjecture; Historical acceptance	Level 1 Evidence supported by RCT -1i Double blinded RCT -1ii Non blinded RCT Level 2 Evidence supported by controlled but non-randomized trials Level 3 Evidence supported by case studies -3i Population based and consecutive -3ii Consecutive; not population based -3iii Neither population nor consecutive	Level 1 -Systemic reviews w/homogeneity of RCT's Individual high-quality RCT's Level 2 - Lower quality RCT's - Cohort studies Level 3 -Case controlled studies Level 4 -Case series Level 5 - Expert opinion; physiology, bench research	I: Evidence obtained from 1 well designed RCT II-1: Evidence obtained from well-designed controlled trials without randomization II-2 Evidence obtained from well-designed cohort or case control analytic studies, preferably more than 1 center or research group II-3: Evidence obtained from multiple time series with or without the intervention. Dramatic results in uncontrolled experiments (e.g.. drug results, histology information) III. Opinions of respected authorities based on clinical experience; reports of expert committees; descriptive studies and case reports	1.Randomized controlled trials 2. Non-randomized controlled studies 3. Non-experimental designs: - Cohort studies - Case control studies 4. Case Series 5 Expert Opinion	Level 1 - High quality RCT trial with SS difference or no SS difference, but narrow CI's -Systematic review of Level-1 RCT's -Level II --Lesser quality RCT --Prospective comparative study --Systematic review of Level II studies or Level I studies with inconsistent results Level III -Case control study -Retrospective comparative study -Systematic review of Level III studies Level IV Case Series Level V Expert Opinion -** Each level of evidence is paired with 4 domains-see notes

*The Journal of Bone and Joint Surgery is adapted from material from the Centre for Evidence-Based Medicine, Oxford, UK. **Each level of evidence is paired with 4 domains (1. Therapeutic studies, 2. Prognostic studies, 3. Diagnostic studies, and 4. Economic and decision analyses to give over 20 permutations)

Blue font indicates "Level of Evidence" based on clinical observations, outcomes, lab studies, expert opinion, etc.

Key: CI = confidence interval, RCT = randomized control trial and SS = statistically significant

randomized control studies at the top of the list and expert opinions generally at the bottom of the list. The dilemma is that there is no unified hierarchy; different organizations devise their own rankings, although all have comparable features and rate RCTs as the highest level of evidence and opinions as the lowest level of evidence (Table 1-1).

Putting RCTs into Perspective – Most evaluation and management therapeutic decisions are based on the lower levels of evidence in the "Level of Evidence" hierarchy (see blue font area of Table 1-1) or on no accepted evidence-based information at all. The Office of Technology Assessment estimated that efficacy based on clinical RCTs was used in less than 20% of medical practice.[25,26] There are several reasons for this statement. First, decisions made in selecting procedures and surgical treatments, especially for wound problems where almost every situation is a unique problem of its own, do not have evidence-based indications at any level to justify their use. Second, even though RCTs may show statistically significant benefits of a treatment intervention, the results in the clinical setting may not be same as the results found in the RCTs. Additionally, statistical significance does not always translate into real clinical significance. This seems to be a frequent occurrence with agents used for managing the wound base. Third, inter-rater reliability of some assessments reveal lack of uniform consistency among experts. In the problem wound literature there are few studies that validate the use of a particular intervention or demonstrate the reliability of a wound grading system. Parts II and III present the available evidence for using a particular intervention or wound grading system. The majority of these interventions or wound grading systems have no validating or reliability information to justify their use.

A Rational Approach to Decision Making – Evidence-based indications based on RCTs are the "gold standard," yet, as discussed above, most decisions made in medicine and surgery, in general, and in wound management, in particular, are not made on

TABLE 1-2. A RATIONAL APPROACH FOR MAKING MANAGEMENT DECISIONS

ELEMENTS	COMMENTS, FURTHER ELABORATION	GRADING CRITERIA (For each element)
Clinical Judgment	Based on personal experiences, reports of others' experiences and review studies	**2 Points** Overwhelming information or experiences support the element
Pathophysiologic Mechanisms	How the mechanisms of the intervention modify the pathophysiology of the condition	
Laboratory Studies	Provides objective indications, e.g. selection of antibiotics from C & S's and use of HBO based on $P_{tc}O_2$ studies	**1 Point** Information is consistent with the element
Need for other Treatment Options	Failure to improve and/or poor outcomes with current or usual management(s)	**0 Points** No data, no benefit or possible harm from information regarding the element
Evidence-based Clinical Reports	Randomized control trial(s) and/or other high quality studies, e.g. cohort, head-to-head, etc.	

Treatment Choice: Summate the grades for each of the five elements and if equal to (Rational Approach) or greater than 6, justification exists for the treatment choice

Notes: *Use half points if the information is mixed or intermediate between two of the grading criteria.
C & S's = Culture and Sensitivities, e.g. = For example, HBO = Hyperbaric oxygen, $P_{tc}O_2$ = Transcutaneous oxygen measurement.

evidence-based indications. How then should treatment decisions for problem wounds be made? The following is suggested: **A Rational Approach to Making Management Decisions** based on the use of five elements[27-30] (Table 1-2). The elements include: 1) Clinical Judgment, 2) Pathophysiologic Mechanisms, 3) Laboratory Studies, 4) Need for other Treatment Options and 5) Evidence-based Clinical Reports. In order to quantify the decision making process, each element is graded on a 2 to 0 point scale with "2" indicating that the information is conclusive for the criteria, "1" the information is consistent with the criteria, and "0" the information does not support the criteria or is contraindicated for the condition. The grades for each element are summated and, if over six points, the treatment choice is justified (Table 1-2).

> The rational approach for making management decisions in selecting a treatment choice is the first example of the use of five elements or assessments (each assessment graded from 0 to 2) to generate a score. All scores range from 0 (worst possible situation) to 10 (best possible situation). The scores provide a quantitative basis for evaluating wounds and making rational decisions about their management. Other 0 to 10 scores, which will be introduced, include the **Goal-Aspiration Score**, the **Host-Function Score** and The **Wound Score**.

TABLE 1-3. THE GOAL-ASPIRATION SCORE

ASSESSMENTS	COMMENTS, FURTHER ELABORATION	FULL	SOME	NONE
		Use half points if the information is mixed or intermediate between 2 of the grading criteria		
Comprehension	Awareness of the problems and the options for management	2 Point	1 Point	0 Point
Motivation	To heal the wounds and/or avoid lower limb amputations			
Compliance	Attention to diabetes management, weight control, skin and nail care, diet, non-smoking, etc.			
Support	Degree and quality of care provided			
Independence	Ability for patient to perform			

Goal-Aspiration Score: Summate the points for each of the five assessments.

Interpretation: Scores of 4 or greater support the decision for limb salvage and/or surgeries to facilitate wound healing such as contracture releases and major debridements. This score (4 or greater) indicates the patient and/or family are able and willing to take an active part in wound care.

THE GOAL-ASPIRATION SCORE
Role of the Goal-Aspiration Score – Regardless of the evidence that exists to justify a management intervention, the patient and/or the family must actively participate in the decision. This is especially imperative when dealing with the "end stage" wound

(Chapter 11) where a decision to do everything possible to salvage the limb versus proceeding directly to a lower limb amputation needs to be made. For these reasons, the **Goal-Aspiration Score** was generated (Table 1-3). The **Goal-Aspiration Score** is another 0 to 10 point score based on five assessments, grading 0 to 2 points. It serves three purposes. First, it complements the rational approach for making management decisions. Without the patient's and/or family's contributions to the decision-making process and their cooperation in optimizing the healing process, outcomes are likely to be poor,

> The patient's level of function is another important consideration in making life or limb saving decisions. The **Host-Function Score** is a third tool that aids in this process. It will be further discussed in the next chapter.

even if the decisions for management are rational and evidence-based. Second, it helps to objectify the decision making process for salvage attempts versus amputation options, as just mentioned above. Third, the **Goal-Aspiration Score** serves as a guideline for gauging the frequency of follow-up visits during the wound healing process and after healing has been achieved (Chapter 13).

Assessments of the Goal-Aspiration Score – Like the other scores, the **Goal-Aspiration Score** consists of five assessments with each assessment graded 0 (none) to 2 (full) (Table 1-3). The summation of the five assessments results in a 0 to 10 point score which quantifies the patient's (or caregiver's) desires and predicts the cooperation likely to be

Clinical Correlation:
An 80-year-old female had severe lower extremity flexion contractures and secondary residual deficits from a cerebral vascular accident. Multiple non-healing pressures sores were present over bony prominences including the pre-sacral region, the hip trochanters, and the lateral aspects of the feet and ankles due to inability to off-load these sites because of the contractures. In addition, the patient's nutrition status was so poor that wound healing was unlikely to occur.

The family decided they wanted everything possible to be done to heal the patient's wounds and were willing to take full responsible for their mother's care. The **Goal-Aspiration Score**, taking fully into consideration the family's role, was 6 ½ (Patient comprehension = 0, Family motivation = 2, Family compliance with management = 2, family support = 2, and patient's ability to do activities of daily living = ½.

This justified the insertion of a percutaneous endoscopic gastrostomy (PEG) tube for feeding and subsequent surgical release of contractures after the patient's nutritional status improved. Once the contractures were released, the wound sites could be effectively off-loaded and over a period of months, with the family as the caregivers, all wounds healed.

Comment:
The **Goal-Aspiration Score** facilitated the decision making process and provided quantifiable justification (Table 1-3) to proceed with the PEG and subsequent surgical releases of the contractures. Although most of the assessments were not based on the patient's input, the family served as an appropriate surrogate.

received from them during the wound healing process. The five assessments used to generate the **Goal-Aspiration Score** include: 1) **Comprehension**, 2) **Motivation**, 3) **Compliance**, 4) **Family and/or caregivers' support,** and 5) **Independence**. Each component of the **Goal-Aspiration Score** provides information as to the patient's (or his/her family's) expectations and ability to provide the care needed to achieve a successful outcome.

Comprehension – This assessment is a reflection of the patient's intellectual capacities. Important components of this assessment are whether the patient is able to appreciate the seriousness of the wound healing problem, what the treatment options are and what will be required in terms of wound care measures both in extent and duration. Full comprehension (2 points on the assessment grade) implies that the patient is fully cognizant of the above information; some comprehension (1 point) that the patient partially understands what is involved; and none (0 points) the patient is oblivious to the above. Consequences of strokes, Alzheimer's disease, mental retardation, and transient encephalopathies, for example, those associated with sepsis or liver and renal failure, are the major reasons patients score low on this assessment. In this latter situation, surrogates such as family members or those with Health Care Proxy or Durable Power of Attorney assume the responsibility for understanding the comprehension assessment.

Motivation – Reflects the patient's desires to achieve a successful outcome for his/her wound problem. Many times seemingly strong motivation is observed in the patient's refusal to accept a lower limb amputation when no other alternatives exist. The reasons may be preservation of body image, religious issues, or the inability to appreciate the seriousness of the problem. Consequently, comprehension of the problem is an important ingredient of motivation. Problems sometimes arise regarding motivation when the patient or surrogates do not comprehend the seriousness of the problem and that alternates such as major limb amputation or initiation of comfort measures only (in the case of the need for artificial life support) is in the best interests of the patient. Although the adage that something can always be done for the patient, healing of the problem may not be one of them and patient comfort needs to become the highest management priority.

Compliance – Is an essential requirement for successful healing of challenging wounds. Compliance is not only reflected in attention to wound care, but also in a number of indirect observations such as attention to diabetes management (reflected in hemoglobin A1c levels), weight control, non-smoking, appropriate activity, maintenance of healthy skin, and toenail care. Compliance is integrally related to the first two **Goal-Aspiration Score** assessments, namely comprehension and motivation. Without understanding of the requirements for care of the wound and the time for healing, as well as the motivation to continue with often repetitive and tedious wound care measures, wound healing success may not occur. Attention to compliance may largely rest with the patient's family or other caregivers, as will be discussed in the next assessment.

Family/Caregiver Support – May be the crucial link between the physicians or other health care providers who direct the management of the patient and the patients themselves. Often patients are unable to manage their wound care problems because of the location of the wound, mobility problems, casting or other orthotics, contractures or inability to comprehend what needs to be done. Wound care management may then need to be provided by home health care services or personnel in skilled nursing/assisted living care facilities. The best possible results, however, seem to occur when the family members learn how to care for the wound and take full responsibility for this activity.

Consequently, we always encourage the family to become involved in the wound care of their family member after providing appropriate instruction in how to do so appropriately.

Independence – A patient's independence may not seem pertinent to generating the **Goal-Aspiration Score**, but this assessment serves several purposes. First, it is an indication of the patient's potential to do their own wound care, as well as follow other compliance issues. Also, it complements the information obtained from the comprehension, motivation and support assessments. When the patient is limited in their ability or unable to do their activities of daily living, others must provide this care. When questions arise regarding resolving a serious wound problem with a lower limb amputation versus extensive, prolonged wound care with questionable potential for healing, the importance of this assessment is appreciated. The third reason for including this assessment as a component of the **Goal-Aspiration Score** is for consistency purposes. By including this assessment, it becomes the fifth component of the **Goal-Aspiration Score** and makes it possible to generate a range of scores from 0 to 10, as in the other scores used in this text.

Clinical Correlation:

An active overweight 50-year-old male was at risk of lower limb amputation due to refractory osteomyelitis associated with ulcerations and deformities caused by a severe Charcot arthropathy of the midfoot.

After careful deliberation with due consideration to patient comprehension, motivation, and compliance, the patient elected to undergo measures to salvage the foot including antibiotics, hyperbaric oxygen therapy, debridement surgery, stabilization with external fixation, casting, and convalescence, which would take a year's time, the patient and his wife decided to proceed with the salvage option.

After some reluctance, the patient's wife agreed to learn wound care measures and pin tract care of the external fixator. She mastered the techniques and provided exquisite care for husband—eventually persuading him to lose weight and become compliant with his diabetes management.

The wounds healed, the foot was stabilized, and the patient resumed community ambulatory activity.

Comment:

Although the surgeon and other health care providers would like to take credit for the successful outcome, it was in no small measure due to the wound care the patient's wife provided after hospital discharge following the surgical interventions and eleven months of care she provided during the convalescence period.

MAGNITUDE AND COSTS OF THE PROBLEM WOUND

Cost Considerations – Although reliable data about the extent and costs of all problem wounds does not exist, extrapolations can be made from the information available about diabetic lower limb wounds. In observations, about 85% of problem wounds are associated with diabetes mellitus. Seven percent of the population of the United States (USA) has diabetes.[31] This equates to approximately 21 million people with

Clinical Correlation:

A spry, but frail 86-year-old female lived alone, managing all of her activities of daily living. Family members' visits were done several times a week to attend to shopping and cleaning needs. The patient was a limited community ambulator and attended almost all family functions including church and traveling to other cities.

A limb threatening bunion wound complicated by peripheral neuropathy, diabetes, peripheral artery disease, and chronic venous insufficiency developed.

Amputation was not considered an option by the patient and her family because of the likelihood of losing her independence and need for assisted living care for the remainder of her life.

Excision of the bunion wound and metatarsalphalangeal joint arthroplasty (Keller bunionectomy) was done with antibiotic coverage, cast protection, and adjunctive hyperbaric oxygen treatments were provided. Even with these precautions the wound dehisced, but eventually healed by secondary intention, allowing the patient to resume the level of activity that existed prior to surgery.

Comment:

Although all assessments of the **Goal-Aspiration Score** were important considerations in making a decision to avoid a lower limb amputation in this patient, the patient's ability to live alone and do all her activities of daily living was of paramount importance. Had she undergone a lower limb amputation, it is doubtful in her frail state, that she could have successfully used a prosthesis, most likely becoming a wheelchair ambulator with the need for assistance to don and remove the prosthesis and make transfers. The costs of an assisted living facility or live-in attendants to meet these needs could have become an insurmountable financial burden for the patient and her family.

The other important consideration in this scenario is that the loss of independence strongly contributes to depression and would possibly accelerate the decline of this previously spry patient's cognitive functions.

diabetes in the USA. It is estimated that lower-extremity ulcers are responsible for 20% of the hospital admissions of diabetic patients.[32] Expenditures for diabetic management amount to about $132 billion dollars a year and of these, $18.7 billion dollars a year are for chronic complications[33] Chronic wounds of all types represent an $11 billion drain on our health care system.[34] The annual cost for chronic diabetic wounds is estimated to be about $5-7 billion dollars in the U.S.[35] The U.S. expenditure for wound care products alone is estimated to be greater than $4 billion a year.[36] As population ages, the prevalence of lower extremity amputations in patients with diabetes continues to increase, accounting for nearly $2 billion and an estimated 2,600 patient-years of hospital stay annually in the United States alone.[37] In a recent analysis, which is approximately 10 years old, it was determined that the overall economic impact attributable to a newly diagnosed diabetic foot ulcer was $28,000 for a 40 to 65-year-old man the first 2 years after diagnosis.[38] Management of diabetic ulcers of the lower extremity in inpatients cost Medicare an average of $14,400 per episode in 1996.[39] The cost for pedal amputation ranged from $19,000 to more than $40,000.[40-42] These figures do not include rehabilitation expenses, which range from an additional $40,000 to $50,000.[43] Again, much of these costs will be significantly higher in 2008 dollars.

Realized vs. Unrealized Costs – These dollar amounts are considered to be "realized costs." Realized costs are those that can be accounted for from the collection of billing data and include such items as hospital charges, surgery charges, physician charges, medications, wound dressing materials, special shoe needs, and rehabilitation. Perhaps even more important to the patient with a limb threatening wound and his or her family are the unrealized costs of care for the rest of the patient's life, especially if a lower limb amputation becomes necessary. Unrealized costs include those resulting from loss of income from interrupted employment and the loss of the ability to live independently. This latter problem can be very devastating for the patient who has impairments from wounds, but has been able to remain independent with two intact lower limbs. The loss of a lower limb may signal the end of an independent existence and the need for assistance with activities of daily living, transportation for medical appointments, as well as social activities, and placement in an assisted living or skilled nursing facility.

Prosthesis Challenges – Although successful prosthetic wear and independent ambulation without walking aids is expected to be the rule with young amputees, the prosthesis in the older patient may come to be used only as a pivot for transfers to and from a wheelchair. If the patient is obese, impaired mentally, and/or arthritic, donning of the prosthesis may not even be realistic.

THE STRATEGIC APPROACH TO WOUND MANAGEMENT

Considerations for Managing Wounds – As the complexity of wounds increases, interventions for their successful management become more challenging. As the challenges increase, it becomes increasingly important to involve the most expert persons possible for each aspect of wound management. This defines the strategic approach and, in essence, it is the integration of multiple disciplines with precisely timed interventions to optimize outcomes. Five components comprise the strategic management of the problem wound (Part III). These include: 1) **Medical management strategies**, 2) **Preparation of the wound base**, 3) **Protection and stabilization of the wound environment**, 4) **Selection of agents to cover and dress the wound base** and 5) **Wound oxygenation**. To borrow from the lexicon of military parlance, tactics are the specific interventions used for each strategy management component. Often many tactics are available. For example, for selection of agents to cover and dress the wound, there are several hundred different choices (tactics) from which to choose. Other aspects of problem wound management require similar degrees of knowledge about the available options. Three additional considerations also help to define the strategic approach to wound management. They include: 1) **Logical decision making based on an objective scoring system** (that is, the **Wound Score**, to be presented in Chapter 5), 2) **Appreciation that the healing of the problem wound represents a continuum of responses** and 3) **The use of objective parameters to measure outcomes**.

CONCLUSIONS

Features of *Masterminding Wounds* – Although this text is dedicated to wound solutions by providing tools for the care of serious wounds, it should be realized that "not every wound is a problem." In fact, problem wounds comprise only a small fraction of the wound spectrum. This chapter has provided the background to assess information to justify decision making for managing problem wounds, both from treatment intervention and patient goal perspectives. Finally, it shows the costs, both tangible and intangible of problem wounds, with particular reference to patients with diabetes and our health care system. This alone justifies another text to provide solutions for problem wounds. Finally, the concept of the strategy management of problem wounds is introduced, which will be comprehensively described in Part III. Our text is differentiated, as the remaining chapters will show, by providing the tools (two of which have already been introduced, namely the rational approach to making management decisions and the **Goal-Aspiration Score)** to objectively and logically evaluate, manage and prevent problem wounds.

QUESTIONS

1. Why have problem wounds garnered so much attention recently?

2. What are some of the limitations for making treatment decisions based only on evidence-based indications?

3. How can wound care products show statistically significant benefits in randomized controlled trials but not be efficacious in the clinical setting?

4. What factors other than evidence-based indications deserve consideration when making decisions about treatment interventions for problem wounds?

5. How do realized costs differ from unrealized costs when dealing with problem wounds and amputations?

6. How does the **Goal-Aspiration Score** assist in making decisions about managing problem wounds?

7. What are the components of the strategic approach to wound management?

REFERENCES

1. Ovington, L. Hanging wet-to-dry dressing out to dry. Advances in Skin & Wound Care, 2002 Mar/Apr; 15(2):79-86

2. Cuzzell J. Choosing a wound dressing. Geriatr Nurs. 1997 Nov/Dec; 18(6):260-5

3. Calianno C. How to choose the right treatment and dressing for the wound. Nursing Management. 2003 Oct; 34(10):6-14

4. Bates-Jensen B, McNees P. The Wound Intelligence System: early issues and findings from multi-site tests. Ostomy Wound Manage. 1996 Nov-Dec;42(10A Suppl):53S-61S

5. Coerper S, Wicke C, Pfeffer F, Koveker G, Becker HD. Documentation of 7051 chronic wounds using a new computerized system within a network of wound care centers. Arch Surg. 2004 Mar;139(3):251-8

6. Ferrell BA. Pressure ulcers. Assessment of healing. Clin Geriatr Med. 1997 Aug;13(3):575-86.

7. Goldman RJ, Salcido R. More than one way to measure a wound: an overview of tools and techniques. Adv Skin Wound Care. 2002 Sep-Oct;15(5):236-43

8. Houghton PE, Kincaid CB, Campbell KE, Woodbury MG, Keast DH. Photographic assessment of the appearance of chronic pressure and leg ulcers. Ostomy Wound Manage. 2000 Apr;46(4):20-6, 28-30

9. Johnson M, Miller R. Measuring healing in leg ulcers: practice considerations. Appl Nurs Res. 1996 Nov;9(4):204-8

10. Langemo DK, Melland H, Hanson D, Olson B, Hunter S, Henly SJ. Two-dimensional wound measurement: comparison of 4 techniques. Adv Wound Care. 1998 Nov-Dec;11(7):337-43

11. Lavery LA, Armstrong DG, Harkless LB. Classification of diabetic foot wounds. J Foot Ankle Surg. 1996 Nov-Dec;35(6):528-31

12. Oyibo SO, Jude EB, Tarawneh I, Nguyen HC, Harkless LB, Boulton AJ. A comparison of two diabetic foot ulcer classification systems: the Wagner and the University of Texas wound classification systems. Diabetes Care. 2001 Jan;24(1):84-8

13. Sharp A. Pressure ulcer grading tools: how reliable are they? J Wound Care. 2004 Feb;13(2):75-7

14. Shea JD. Pressure sores: classification and management. Clin Orthop. 1975 Oct;(112):89-100

15. Wagner FW Jr. The dysvascular foot: a system for diagnosis and treatment. Foot Ankle. 1981 Sep;2(2):64-122

16. Field C, Kerstein M. Overview of wound healing in a moist environment. American Journal of Surgery. 1994;167(Suppl 1-A):2S-5S

17. Bolton L. Operational definition of moist wound healing. J Wound Ostomy Continence Nurs. 2007 Jan-Feb;34(1):23-9

18. Chang H. Wind S, Kerstein MD. Moist wound healing. Dermatol Nurs. 1996 Jun;8(3):174-6, 204

19. Kerstein MD. Moist wound healing: the clinical perspective. Ostomy Wound Manage. 1995 Aug;41(7A Suppl):37S-44S; discussion 45S

20. Kerstein MD. The scientific basis of healing. Adv Wound Care. 1997 May-Jun;10(3):30-6

21. Changes to the Hospital Outpatient Prospective Payment System and Calendar Year 2006 Payment Rates, CMS Rules, Federal Register: CMS-1501-FC: Sections 1-3

22. Centers for Medicare & Medicaid Services. Decision Memo for Autologous Blood-Derived Products for Chronic Non-Healing Wounds (CAG-00190N), December 15, 2003

23. Lenfant C. Clinical research to clinical practice – lost in translation? New England Journal of Medicine 2003; 349(9):868-874

24. Heilman RD. Drug development history, "overview," and what are GCPs? Qual Assur. 1995 Mar;4(1):75-9

25. Berwick DM. Health services research and quality of care assignments for the 1990's, Medical Care. 1989; 27(8):763-771

26. Naylor CD. Grey zones of clinical practice: some limits to evidence-based medicine. Lancet. 1995 Apr 1;345(8953):840-2

27. Strauss MB, Miller SM. The role of hyperbaric oxygen in the management of chronic refractory osteomyelitis. In: Kindwall, EP, ed. Hyperbaric Medicine Practice, Third Edition, Flagstaff, AZ Best Publishing Co. 2008

28. Strauss MB, Miller SM. The role of hyperbaric oxygen in crush injury, skeletal muscle-compartment syndrome, and other acute traumatic ischemias. In: Kindwall, EP, ed. Hyperbaric Medicine Practice, Third Edition, Flagstaff, AZ Best Publishing Co. 2008

29. Strauss MB. Hyperbaric oxygen for crush injuries and compartment syndromes: Surgical considerations. In: Bakker DJ. Cramer FS, eds. Hyperbaric Surgery, Perioperative Care, Flagstaff, AZ Best Publishing Co., 2002;341-359

30. Strauss MB. Evidence review of HBO for crush injury, compartment syndrome and other traumatic ischemias, Undersea and Hyperbaric Medicine, 2001; 28(Suppl):35-36

31. Centers for Disease Control and Prevention (CDC) website. http://www.cdc.gov/diabetes/pubs/estimates05.htm National Diabetes Fact Sheet. National Estimates on Diabetes, 2005

32. Bouter KP, Storm AJ, de Groot RR, et al. The diabetic foot in Dutch hospitals: epidemiological features and clinical outcome. Eur J Med. 1993 Apr;2(4):215-8

33. Hogan P, Dall T, Nikolov P. Economic costs of diabetes in the US in 2002. Diabetes Care. 2003 Mar;26(3):917-32

34. Frykberg RG. The Diabetic Foot. 61st Scientific Sessions of the American Diabetes Association, June 22 - 26, 2001, Philadelphia, Pennsylvania

35. Pecoraro RE, Ahroni JH, Boyko EJ, et al. Chronology and determinants of tissue repair in diabetic lower extremity ulcers. Diabetes. 1991

36. Jackson S, Stevens J. Market analysis: The future of wound care. Business Strategies for Medical Technology Executives Jan/Feb 2006

37. Armstrong DG. Is diabetic foot care efficacious or cost effective? Ostomy Wound Manage. April 2001;47:28–32

38. Ramsey SD, Newton K, Blough D, et al. Incidence, outcomes, and cost of foot ulcers in patients with diabetes. Diabetes Care. 1999;22:382–387

39. Harrington C, Zagari MJ, Corea J, Klitenic J. A cost analysis of diabetic lower-extremity ulcers. Diabetes Care. 2000;23: 1333–1338

40. Tennvall GR, Apelqvist J, Eneroth M. Costs of deep foot infections in patients with diabetes mellitus. Pharmacoeconomics. 2000;18:225–238

41. Cianci P, Petrone G, Drager S, et al. Salvage of the problem wound and potential amputation with wound care and adjunctive hyperbaric oxygen therapy: an economic analysis. J Hyperb Med. 1988; 3:127–141

42. Mackey WC, McCullough JL, Conlon TP, et al. The costs of surgery for limb- threatening ischemia. Surgery. 1986;99: 26–35

43. Cianci P. Adjunctive hyperbaric oxygen therapy in the treatment of the diabetic foot. J Am Podiatr Med Assoc. 1994;84:448–455

CHAPTER

2

PROBLEM WOUND PRESENTATIONS

CHAPTER TWO OVERVIEW

INTRODUCTION 27

WOUND ISCHEMIA/HYPOXIA. 28

UNCONTROLLED INFECTION 37

DEFORMITIES. 39

POST-TRAUMATIC WOUNDS 42

NEUROPATHY AND WOUNDS. 45

RISK FACTORS FOR DEVELOPING WOUNDS 46

CONCLUSIONS 48

QUESTIONS. 49

REFERENCES. 50

"A wound by any other name…"

INTRODUCTION

Classification of wounds can be challenging and confusing. The distinction between various causes of the wound, that is wound etiologies, descriptive features of the wound and wound scoring systems need to be appreciated (Figure 2-1). This chapter discusses etiological-associated reasons in which wounds do not heal as expected. The failure of wounds to heal is the generic explanation provided in Chapter 1 used to describe a problem wound. There are many etiological-associated reasons wounds do not heal as expected. Some are obvious, such as insufficient perfusion or post-traumatic tissue damaged beyond all repair. Other etiologies are more subtle, such as malnutrition or other medically related considerations. Neuropathy, which is so often implicated in wound problems, is invariably associated with other etiological-associated reasons that lead to wound healing challenges. Most often, there are several etiological factors that contribute to wound healing problems.

Three generic conditions explain, for the majority of circumstances, why wound healing does not progress as expected and the wound becomes a non-healing or problem type (Figure 2-2). The three conditions are: 1) **Wound ischemia/hypoxia**, 2) **Uncontrolled infection, and 3) Persistence of deformities**. Each condition is associated with underlying etiological factors and/or comorbidities. Peripheral arterial disease is

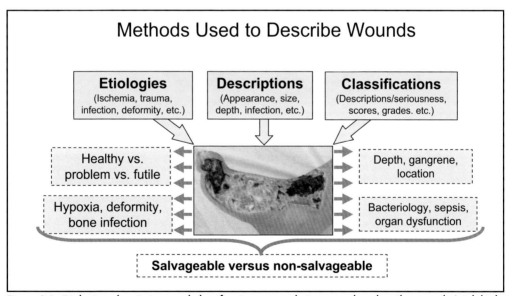

Figure 2-1. Etiologies, descriptions and classifications are techniques used to describe wounds (pink highlights). From this information, criteria can be used to make decisions for management (gray highlights). Of course, the fundamental question to answer is whether or not the wound is salvageable. Assessment of the patient's function (Host-Function Score) is crucial for making decisions whether to salvage, amputate, or provide comfort care measures only.

the most frequent cause of wound ischemia/hypoxia; however, other conditions can also contribute to this cause. Osteomyelitis and avascular soft tissues are the main reasons infected wounds do not respond to management. Deformity, as the reason for non-healing of wounds, is most frequently a consequence of neuropathy, but genetic factors, inherited physical abnormalities, and trauma are other causes of deformity. Any comprehensive management program for non-healing wounds must address these three generic conditions. We offer a five-part "Strategic Management" approach (Part III) to meet this goal. The remainder of this chapter focuses on the three generic reasons wounds fail to heal as expected, the role of neuropathy, and other risk factors that can lead to problem wounds.

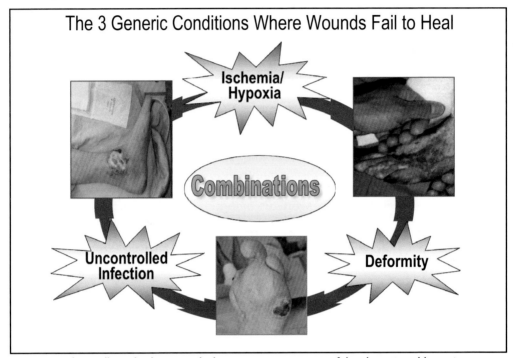

Figure 2-2. Almost all non-healing wounds demonstrate one or more of the above 3 problems. Appropriate management requires a strategic management approach (Part III) to address all these problems.

WOUND ISCHEMIA/HYPOXIA

Metabolic Demands for Healing

There are many reasons why wounds do not heal. The most important of these is the lack of an adequate blood supply. Ordinarily, non-critical tissues such as skin, subcutaneous tissues, skeletal muscle, and connective tissues have minimal metabolic requirements and therefore require minimal perfusion when at rest. However, with activity for wound healing and control of infection, many-fold increases in blood supply are required. Blood supply to muscle can increase as much as 40-fold between rest and activity.[1] For neutrophils to kill bacteria, the oxidative burst in the cell requires 20-60 fold increases in oxygen uptake.[2] During fracture healing, blood supplies are noted to increase 6-fold at the fracture site.[3] Additionally, in a recent animal model study, a high rate of energy metabolism as reflected in adenosine triphosphate (ATP) content of the callus in the early phase of fracture healing noted a 224-fold increase at the fracture site.[4] From this information, we estimate that for wound healing to occur, the increase in blood supply must be sufficient to meet at least a 20-fold increase in metabolic activity. If these requirements are not met, the wound will fail to heal and would be labeled as a non-healing wound.

Oxygen Reserves

Where do the increased blood supply, oxygen delivery, and metabolic substrates come from? They come from the body's ability to regulate blood flow to tissues where it is needed. In an average sized human, the blood volume is approximately 5 liters. If every blood vessel were maximally dilated, every sinusoid and venous reservoir filled to capacity, and every arteriovenous shunt wide open, the estimated blood volume to fill the vascular system would be over one hundred liters.[1] The regional control of blood flow to non-critical tissues is reduced through the sympathetic nervous system. Obviously non-critical tissues at rest require and receive very little blood flow. However, there is the potential for the marked augmentation of blood flow (at least 20-fold) to them when the tissues' metabolic demands require it.[1]

Loss of sympathetic control of blood flow is observed clinically with postural hypotension (atherosclerotic blood vessels that can no longer vasodilate to increase flow) in diabetic patients secondary to neuropathy (auto sympathectomy), septic shock, and in the extremely rare condition of erthomelagia.

The admonishment to not swim after eating a large meal has a good physiological basis. Because of a finite blood volume, the sympathetic nervous system has to direct where the blood flow to non-critical tissues goes—the so-called "Rob Peter to pay Paul" principle. If the blood flow is directed to the gut, the muscles in the extremities are at risk of cramping secondary to ischemia and vice versa if the swimming muscles "rob" the gut of its blood supply.

Tissue Oxygen Tensions and Wound Healing

Measurements of tissue and transcutaneous oxygen tensions help to substantiate the above information. In the normal situation, oxygen tensions decrease from 160 mmHg in inspired air to <0.5 mmHg in the mitochondria (Table 2-1). If the oxygen tensions in the tissue fluids are in the 30-40 mmHg range, healing is expected to occur (in the absence of other factors that can interfere with wound healing, as will be discussed shortly).[5,6,7] This physiological range of oxygen tensions predicts that the metabolic activity required in the wound and peri-wound areas has the potential to increase by "the magic" 20-fold factor (Figure 2-3). If the juxta-wound transcutaneous oxygen tensions are in the 10-30 mmHg range, this predicts that there may not be sufficient ability to increase metabolic activity enough for wound healing to occur. In this situation, tissues will remain alive, but wound healing is not likely to occur; the wound will appear to be in a state of suspended animation. Finally, if the juxta-wound transcutaneous oxygen tensions are less than 10 mmHg, wounds will deteriorate because there is not enough metabolic activity to maintain even the steady state situation. Since the blood supply is responsible for the delivery of oxygen to the wound as well as the other factors required for healing, such as substrates and nutrients, juxta-wound transcutaneous oxygen tensions are a good indirect measurement of blood flow and the potential to increase metabolic activity. Transcutaneous oximetry and hyperbaric oxygen, as well as their roles in predicting wound healing, will be discussed in the wound oxygenation chapter (Chapter 10).

TABLE 2-1. THE GRADIENT OF OXYGEN TENSIONS FROM INSPIRED AIR TO THE MITOCHONDRIA

Level	O_2 tensions in mmHg	Comment
Inspired air	160	
Pulmonary vein	100	
Aorta	85	
Arterioles	70	
Capillary	50	Gas exchange and other agents in the blood at this level
Tissue fluids	30-40	Tensions necessary for cell functions to occur
Cell	10	Repair, secretion production, and disease control functions
Mitochondria	<0.5	Energy production for all cell activity

(320-fold decrease)

Comment: Although O_2 tensions decrease by 320-fold from inspired air to the mitochondria, for wound healing to occur, tissue fluid O_2 tensions in the 30-40 mmHg range are required. Levels below this will not provide sufficient O_2 tensions to the mitochondria so organelles can carry out their energy generating mechanisms and allow cells to do their repair (wound healing), secretory production and disease control functions.

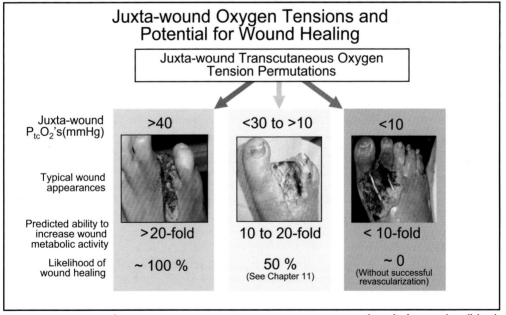

Juxta-wound Oxygen Tensions and Potential for Wound Healing

Juxta-wound Transcutaneous Oxygen Tension Permutations

Juxta-wound $P_{tc}O_2$'s(mmHg)	>40	<30 to >10	<10
Typical wound appearances			
Predicted ability to increase wound metabolic activity	>20-fold	10 to 20-fold	< 10-fold
Likelihood of wound healing	~ 100 %	50 % (See Chapter 11)	~ 0 (Without successful revascularization)

Figure 2-3. Juxta-wound transcutaneous oxygen ($P_{tc}O_2$s) measurements predict which wounds will heal. Hyperbaric oxygen (Chapter 10) adds another dimension to both predicting which wounds will heal and promoting wound healing. The ability to increase metabolic activity in the wound is a direct consequence of the juxta-wound $P_{tc}O_2$s.

Healing Stages

Much is known about the science of wound healing. In normal healing, the wound evolves through three stages from the time of injury until healing is completed. Oxygen requirements are different for each stage of healing (Figure 2-4).[8-11] The greatest oxygen requirements for healing occur during the first stage, the inflammatory stage. During this period the substances required to initiate the wound healing cascade must be brought to the wound. These substances include growth factors, cytokines, fibroblasts, and leukocytes. During the inflammatory stage, the metabolic demands of the wound increase greatly, perhaps 20-fold or more as discussed previously. Many of the inflammatory mediators have vasoactive properties, which initiate vasodilation, thereby increasing the blood flow to the wound site. The clinical consequences of the inflammatory response and increased blood flow are warmth, swelling, redness, and pain at the wound site, the four cardinal signs of inflammation.

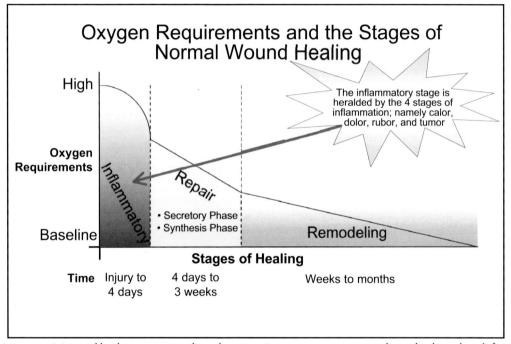

Figure 2-4. Normal healing progresses through stages. Oxygen requirements to achieve the desired goals for each stage decrease as wound healing progresses. If oxygen tensions are too low, healing will not proceed from one stage to another, leading to wound healing problems.

The rhyming Latin terms for the inflammatory response namely, calor, dolor, rubor, and tumor were described by Aulus Cornelius Celsus (to be differentiated from the 18th century Swedish astronomer Anders Celsius) in the first century AD. Celsus earned the distinction of being acknowledged as the "Cicero of physicians" and the "Hippocrates of the Romans."

Fibroblast Activity and Angiogenesis

Adequate oxygen tensions are not only required for the tissues in the wound to remain viable, but also for them to initiate their reparative processes. Oxygen has also been ascribed to be a cell signaling, up-regulator agent akin to other growth factors that are mobilized to the wound.[12-13] The fibroblast is the cell type that is ultimately responsible for wound healing (Figure 2-5). Its oxygen requirements for migration to the wound site, replication, and secretory activities are recognized.[5, 6] The fibroblast will lie dormant unless the wound's margins have 30-40 mmHg oxygen tensions. Angiogenesis occurs as a consequence of fibroblast activity in an adequately oxygenated environment. The functioning fibroblast, as part of its secretory activity, lays down a matrix for angiogenesis to proceed from the intact blood supply to the depths of the wound.

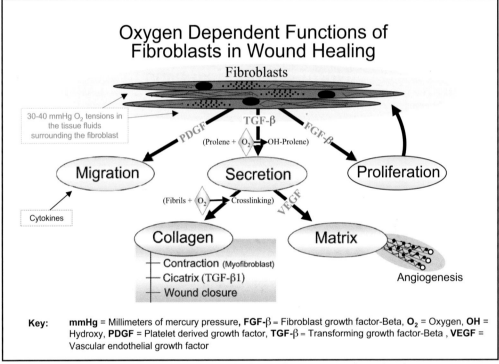

Figure 2-5. The fibroblast is the key cell in wound healing. It has 3 oxygen-dependent functions. Angiogenesis and wound closure are consequences of its secretory activity. Growth factors act as signaling devices to initiate the different functions of the fibroblast. Oxygen roles are highlighted in green.

Repair Stage

Fibroblast activity predominates in this, the second stage of wound healing. Initially in this stage the fibroblast has secretory functions, which later on transition to synthesis functions. During the secretory stage, the fibroblast secretes a matrix that becomes the precursor for angiogenesis, as mentioned above, collagen formation and ultimately wound healing. Angiogenesis generates a blood supply to the hypoxic/anoxic central portions of the wound so healing can proceed to this level. Collagen formation and maturation are a function of the synthesis phase of repair. As collagen forms, the wound closes, partly by collagen maturation (scar) formation and partly by wound contraction due to the contractile properties of the myofibroblast. Although an oxygen gradient is required for wound healing, if the tissue fluids adjacent to the margins of the wound do not have an adequate oxygen supply, fibroblast activity and angiogenesis will not proceed due to insufficient oxygen tensions.[14] The result would be a non-healing wound.

Remodeling Stage

The third stage of wound healing is the remodeling stage. The oxygen requirements for this stage are the lowest of any of the three stages. Eventually, the oxygen requirements decrease to the levels that existed prior to development of the wound, which signals the end of wound healing. The remodeling stage lasts for months and includes the maturation of collagen into a fibrous tissue scar to increase the tensile strength of the wound. Once sutures are removed from a wound, at approximately two weeks after its closure, the tensile strength of the wound is only 10 percent of what it was before the wound occurred.[15] By six weeks, the tensile strength increases to about 50 percent of normal. Clinical signs that indicate completion of the remodeling phase include normalization of color, swelling, and temperature. Remodeling in a wound may continue for a year or more. This is why plastic surgeons are reluctant to do scar revisions, or orthopaedic surgeons are reluctant to remove hardware from healing fractures (the stages of bone healing are essentially analogous to those of soft tissue healing) before this time.

TABLE 2-2. CONDITIONS WHICH INTERFERE WITH PERFUSION

Condition	Effects, Comments, Causes
Peripheral artery disease	Decreased flow; inability to increase flow for the demands of wound healing, infection control or activity
Trauma	Physical disruption and/or injury to the vessel
Outflow obstruction	Venous stasis disease, external compression (casts/tourniquets), fluid retention, and compartment syndromes
Vasculitis, Raynauds	Associated with collagen vascular diseases; sympathetic (vasoconstriction) over activity may be a component
Thromboembolism	Associated with hypercoaguable conditions
Hypotension	Cardiac, hypovolemia, anemia, and septic causes
Vasospasm	Associated with trauma, hypothermia, and surgery
Medication induced	Ergotamine, alpha adrenergic agents, medication infiltrations and nicotine (smoking)

Conditions that Interfere with Perfusion

Many conditions can interfere with the blood supply to a wound (Table 2-2). The most common cause is peripheral artery disease. Patients with diabetes are especially prone to develop this problem.[16] One can often find atherosclerosis and calcification of arterial walls leading to a pipe stem appearance to their vessels on radiographic imaging studies. It has been demonstrated that the prevalence of arterial disease in the limbs of persons with diabetes is approximately twenty times higher than in comparable age and sex-matched persons without diabetes.[17] Arteries that have their lumens narrowed by arteriosclerosis can no longer dilate to increase their blood flow when needed for wound healing, repair and infection control (Figure 2-6). Although discrete lesions of large or medium sized vessels may be amendable to angioplasty, endarterectomy, or revascularization, frequently the arterial disease is so diffuse, the runoff so poor or the vessels so small that revascularization is not feasible for the limb with an ischemic wound.

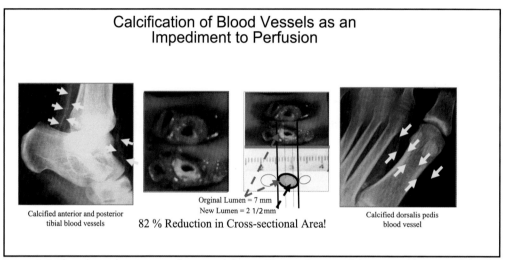

Figure 2-6. The atherosclerotic artery loses its ability to dilate to the size of the original lumen and thereby does not allow the increase in the blood flow required for wound healing and control of infection. The 82% reduction in cross-sectional area translates to an ~80% decrease in blood flow. The 20% (of maximal potential blood transport in a non-atherosclotic blood vessel) flow may be sufficient for the "steady state," but insufficient for the increased metabolic demands of wound healing.

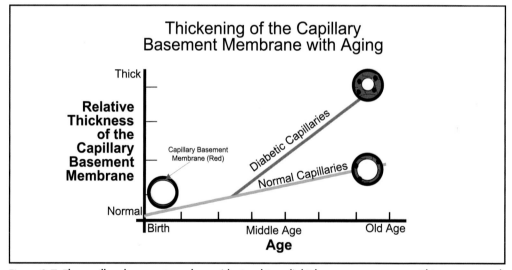

Figure 2-7. The capillary basement membrane (depicted in red) thickens as a person ages. This process accelerates in diabetic patients. The thickened basement membrane becomes a diffusion barrier to oxygen and other substances that must move from the capillary to the cell and vice versa. The thickened capillary meets the definition of microangiopathy.

Thickening of the capillary basement membrane, an age-related occurrence, may contribute to declining aerobic performances in athletes and others as they age. Since the thickening acts as a diffusion barrier to oxygen, carbon dioxide, nutrients, etc., it may become a limiting factor for exchange of these substances and set the limits for an individual's maximal athletic performance.

Microangiopathy

Is vessel disease at the microscopic level, so called microangiopathy, a definable entity? We are convinced that it is. First, if runoff as demonstrated by an angiogram is poor, it is logical to conclude that the disease is at the very small and microscopic vessel level. Second, thickening of the capillary basement membrane occurs prematurely in diabetic blood vessels[18, 19] (Figure 2-7). This acts as a diffusion barrier for both oxygen and nutrients, which of course occurs at the microscopic level of the vascular tree. Third is the trash syndrome, microemboli occlude end arteries. The results are manifested as necrosis of tissue distal to the occluded vessels. Fourth, in conditions where outflow is obstructed and/or perfusion at the capillary level is compromised, such as in venous stasis disease and compartment syndromes respectively, the pathophysiology of the problem occurs at the microscopic level, which could be considered a manifestation, albeit remedial, of a microangiopathy. Other conditions that interfere with perfusion, either directly or indirectly include: vasculitities, thrombotic events, post-infection or post-traumatic cicatrix formation, Raynaud's phenomenon, Buerger's disease, smoking, ergotamine poisoning, hypercholesterolemia, and edema (Table 2-2).

Edema

The significance of edema as a factor that contributes to circulation and wound oxygenation problems must be appreciated. Directly, edema in closed, un-yielding spaces such as myofascial compartments, casts, tight bandages, and/or wounds encased with cicatrix can lead to collapse of the microcirculation. When flow is blocked at this level, it is tantamount to application of a tourniquet to the microcirculation. The result is arrest of blood flow at the capillary level where oxygen, nutrients, and waste products of metabolism exchange occur. This, in fact, defines a compartment syndrome. While this problem is not usually associated with chronic, non-healing problem wounds, it is associated with problem wounds from trauma and after prolonged ischemia times to tissues (see next section). This latter problem is especially associated with acute thrombo-occlusive events where revascularization is performed, but the tissue ischemia time is prolonged.

Indirect Effects of Edema

Edema can also lead to two indirect causes of wound ischemia and hypoxia. First, edema increases the diffusion distance of oxygen and nutrients from the capillary to the target cell (Figure 2-8). Oxygen diffuses relatively poorly through tissue fluids, especially as compared to carbon dioxide, which has 20 times the diffusing capacity in fluids as oxygen does.[20] Oxygen tensions in tissue fluids decrease rapidly as the distance it diffuses increases. The fall off is calculated to be proportional to the square root of the oxygen concentration in the tissue fluids adjacent to the capillary.[21] Consequently, edema can be very detrimental to wound healing. A second effect of edema is that of its conversion from soft, pitting, to brawny, to dense cicatrix with chronicity. Fibrosis occurs in response to the growth factor TGF-1 (transforming growth factor-1) expression in prolonged, presumably hypoxia environments.[22] Cicatrix is even a greater barrier to oxygen diffusion than edema. More importantly, when a wound arises, the cicatrix becomes an obstruction to angiogenesis and an important reason why wounds do not heal in these situations.

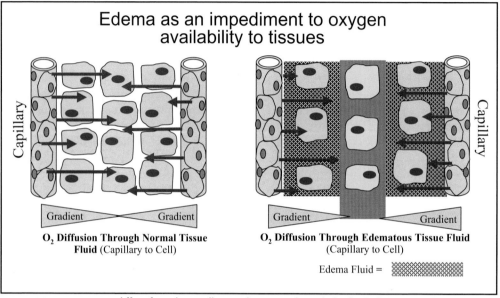

Figure 2-8. Oxygen must diffuse from the capillary to the tissues through the fluids that surround each internal cell in the body. Oxygen diffusion distance is proportional to the square root of the plasma oxygen content.[21] Consequently, a small increment in edema fluid can have a geometrical decrease on oxygen availability to the cell.

Clinical Correlation:
A 64-year-old male developed a large, non-healing wound over the anterior lateral aspect of the left lower extremity after radiation treatment of a squamous cell carcinoma (Figure 2-9). All treatment interventions were ineffective. Biopsies did not show recurrent tumor.

Options were discussed with the patient and he agreed to staged debridement and subsequent skin grafting. At surgery, a dense plate mass of cicatrix, about 11 mm thick, was excised. Subsequently, a healthy granulating wound base amendable to skin grafting developed.

Comment:
The thick, dense cicatrix was an impenetrable physical barrier, acting like an embedded foreign object, to oxygenation of the wound base, angiogenesis and epithelialization. No interventions less than surgical excision would produce a favorable outcome.

Edema as an impediment to oxygen availability to tissues

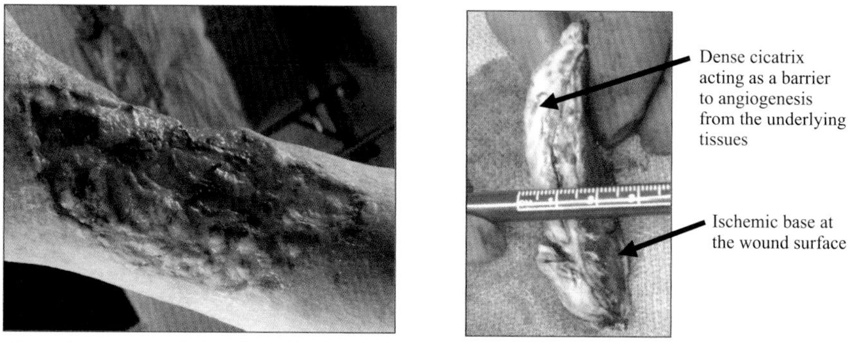

Avascular and necrotic-based, non-healing wound after radiation treatment of skin cancer

11 mm thick "plate" of cicatrix making wound base essentially avascular

Figure 2-9. Hypoxia is one of the three primary reasons (in addition to deformity and bone infection) that wounds fail to heal. The dense cicatrix that formed in the hypoxic wound base thwarted angiogenesis from the vascularized underlying tissues. Surgical removal (debridement) in these situations is the first step for achieving wound healing.

UNCONTROLLED INFECTION

Infected Bone

The presence of infected bone or avascular, infected soft tissues in the wound base is a second reason for non-healing of various wounds. Infected bone in the problem wound is very frequently avascular. This means it is dead and for all practical purposes antibiotics and white blood cells do not reach the bacteria to control the infection. The result is that the wound persists even with optimal antibiotic and wound care measures. The lack of blood supply explains, from a microscopic perspective, why the infection does not respond to interventions. Osteomyelitis is usually present in non-healing wounds that are associated with tracts from the skin surface to underlying bone.[23, 24, 25]

The Interface

Cicatrix, a dense, almost avascular fibrous scar tissue, is generated around the infected bone. Teleologically, this represents the body's attempts to isolate the infected bone from surrounding non-infected tissues. Cicatrix forms in hypoxic environments, is poorly, if at all, vascularized, and acts as a barrier for oxygen, leukocytes, nutrients and antibiotic diffusion into the wound site. Occasionally calcifications or cartilage fragments develop in the hypoxic cicatrix. This becomes an interface (Figure 2-10). On the infection side of the interface, organisms are protected from the host's infection fighting responses and the delivery of antibiotics. On the other side of the interface, healthy host tissues are present, but are unable to penetrate the interface to "fight" the infection. The extent of dead bone and the amount of the interface varies in each case where infected bone contributes to a non-healing wound. This complicates the comparison of management interventions and is a reason we advocate an inclusive wound evaluation system (Chapter 5) that relies on more than the wound depth alone, as is typically used to describe pressure sores, to help make management decisions.

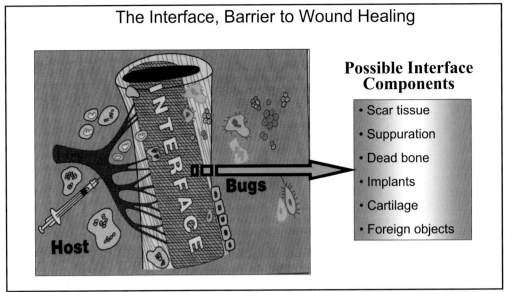

The Interface, Barrier to Wound Healing

Possible Interface Components

- Scar tissue
- Suppuration
- Dead bone
- Implants
- Cartilage
- Foreign objects

Figure 2-10. The interface represents an attempt by the body to isolate the focus of infection from the rest of the body. It consists of dense scar tissue that acts as a barrier between the intact host factors and the focus of infection. Eradication of infection requires the removal of infected bone and/or other interface components as well as the interface. Scar tissue (cicatrix) is the main component of the interface.

Other Soft Tissue Barriers

Although infected, avascular bone is the most common cause of uncontrolled infection in problem wounds, other tissues can also be the cause. Bursae over bony prominences are probably the second most common cause of these problems and should always be suspected when a non-healing wound persists and bone biopsy cultures are negative for osteomyelitis. The bursae serve as pads over bony prominences in association with gliding surfaces, such as the overlying skin. They consist of a closed sac lined with synovial membrane to facilitate gliding between the underlying bone and the overlying soft tissues. In problem wounds, they frequently become avascular and through metaplasia convert to avascular scar tissue. Once infected, they essentially become an infected interface. Other relative avascular connective tissues such as ligaments, joint capsules, tendons and fascia, as well as cartilage, can undergo similar metaplastic changes to become an avascular infection focus. Radiation injury of soft tissues can have analogous effects (Figure 2-9). In such situations, debridement of the avascular tissue must be an integral part of wound management. The consequences of failing to recognize and manage this problem are persistence of the non-healing wound.

Aggravated Infections

Aggravated infections as a cause of uncontrolled infection differ from chronic non-healing wounds because they require immediate medical and surgical interventions to prevent loss of life or limb (Chapter 12). These infections tend to advance quickly with rapid deterioration progressing to severe sepsis. Usually they occur in patients who have underlying host comorbidities such as diabetes, peripheral artery disease, chronic kidney disease, collagen vascular disease, etc. Aggravated infections include gas gangrene, necrotizing fasciitis, closed spaced abscesses, and/or tenosynovitis. Each of these condi-

Clinical Correlation:

A 50-year-old female patient with diabetes with previous partial toe amputations and profound sensory neuropathy developed a small wound under the first metatarsal head of the right foot. This arose as a consequence of hallux rigidus and sesmoid resections to manage a malperforans ulcer. Management consisted of monthly callus debridements and the use of antibiotic ointments. No significant bunion deformity was present.

The patient was admitted on an emergency basis with a septic foot after completing a cruise. The skin over the medial aspect of the first metatarsal head was necrotic. Nuclear medicine imaging did not demonstrate osteomyelitis of the metatarsal head. The skin and an infected, avascular bursa were debrided on the ward to the joint capsule level. Subsequently, the patient underwent a partial first ray amputation, the choice she preferred to skin grafting or healing by secondary intention.

Comment:

The increased walking activity associated with the cruise presumably inoculated the bursa via the small plantar wound. Infection was not controlled with oral antibiotics started on the cruise due to the poor vascularity of the bursa.

Infection progressed rapidly to the point of sepsis and any management short of excision of the bursa would probably have been unsuccessful.

tions has special features, such as their pathophysiology, specific bacterial flora, locations, and management issues (Chapter 12). The fulminating course and resulting wounds present very challenging problems, which typically require interdisciplinary management with primary care physicians, medical intensive care specialists, surgeons, infection disease consultants, hyperbaric medicine physicians, nurse wound specialists, physical therapists and clinical nutritionists.

DEFORMITIES

Static Problems

Mechanical problems that manifest themselves as deformities are the third major reason that problem wounds do not heal. These problems may be of static, dynamic or combination types. Static mechanical problems are wounds associated with underlying bony deformities that do not heal because of the size of the deformity even when the wound site is off-loaded by orthotics or strict non-weight bearing. Deformities may be associated with bone spurs, contractures, heredity factors, joint collapse (Charcot arthropathy), muscle imbalances, neuropathy, tendon and/or ligament insufficiency, trauma, or combinations of these (Table 2-3). Usually, the deformity problems are complicated by the formation of callus and bursa over the deformities. Calluses (hyperkeratosis) form externally, while bursae form between the deformity and the skin surfaces. Again, teleologically speaking, these are frustrated attempts by the body to protect its skin integrity by generating these responses to stresses. When they occur as physiological responses, they are desirable, such as the normal bursae found between the skin and bony protuberances of joints, such as the elbow, shoulder and knee or the thickening of skin over the palms of the hand associated with manual labor.

TABLE 2-3. STATIC DEFORMITIES AS PRECURSORS TO PROBLEM WOUNDS

Condition	Common Locations	Causes, Pathophysiology
Bone Spurs	Juxta-articlular; muscle origin & insertion sites	Abnormal stresses; "wear and tear"
Contractures	Joints of appendicular skeleton	Residuals of strokes, multiple sclerosis, Parkinsonism, spinal cord injury, etc.
Charcot arthropathy	Feet & ankles	Bone resorption & collapse secondary to trauma & hyperemia
Hereditary conditions	Near ends of long bones	Osteochondromas, Ollier's disease
Ligament/tendon insufficiency	Feet & ankles	Posterior tibial tendon insufficiency/rupture, collateral ligament/plantar fascia deficiency
Neuropathy induced	Lower extremities, hands	Diabetes mellitus, alcoholism, vitamin deficiency, Charcot Marie Tooth, etc.
Post-traumatic	Any fracture site	Healing with malalignment and/or deformities
Combinations	Especially lower extremities	e.g. neuropathy + trauma + deformity contributes to Charcot arthropathy

Pathological Calluses

Calluses and bursae become pathological when they begin to magnify the deformity. At this point they are vulnerable to ulcer formation. The ulcer may arise from within, that is the bony deformity leads to erosion through the skin or from without, or externally (Figure 2-11). Ulcers that arise externally from calluses do so because of moisture formation under the callus. This leads to maceration and erosion through the skin and underlying soft tissues to the bony deformity. The next step is the introduction of bacteria. Bacteria may be introduced through fissures in the firm, dry callus overlying the moist callus, propagation of the maceration into the firm callus, or iatrogenic causes. Iatrogenic causes include the patients themselves or members of the wound team debriding the firm hard callus to the macerated and/or ulcerated tissues. Even if sterile instruments are used, the ulcer base will become colonized with bacteria. A more serious complication is the sealing-off of the ulcer once it has been colonized.

The bacteria will begin to multiply leading to an abscess. Dissection of the infection along tissue planes can lead to ascending sepsis including cellulitis, panniculitis, tenosynovitis, and/or necrotizing fasciitis. This can all occur from the seemingly innocent appearing ulceration that develops under a callus.

Sensory neuropathy all too frequently contributes to the progression of this problem. In the absence of pain perception, the neuropathic patient typically continues to ignore or be oblivious to the callus. In contrast, a patient with normal sensation readily complains of the callus often using the analogy of "feeling like I'm walking with a stone in my shoe" and seeks immediate attention for it.

Many times the callus problem in the neuropathic patient does not receive attention until the patient (or family member) notes staining of the sock, odor or the foot becomes red and swollen.

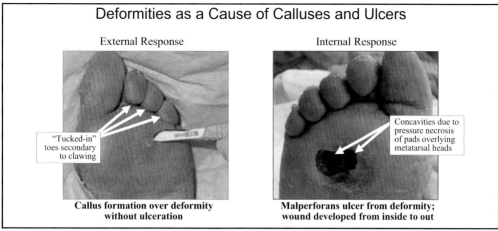

Figure 2-11. Depressed metatarsal (MT) heads secondary to clawing of the toes (note that the toes are "tucked" in to the forefoot) cause increased contact stresses to the soft tissues under the MT heads. The body's initial reaction is callus formation, which represents an attempt to protect the skin from ulceration. With increasing stresses, an ulcer develops from inside to out due to the pressure exerted by the depressed MT heads on the underlying soft tissues.

Pathological Bursae

What occurs externally with the callus has counterparts in the bursae. Like cicatrix, bursae are relatively avascular structures, lined with a synovial membrane. Once infected in the problem wound, they are not likely to heal without removal of the underlying bony deformity and the entire bursa with the scar tissue that replaces the physiologically active synovial membrane. If the tract over the infected bursae becomes sealed off, the progression of infection to limb and life threatening consequences can occur, as previously described for the callus. The hypertropic bursa is invariably a sign that underlying bone deformity exists (Figure 2-12). Massive bursa formation is especially likely to be found at the apex of rocker bottom foot deformities, with or without associated open wounds, and in patients with Charcot arthropathy of their feet.

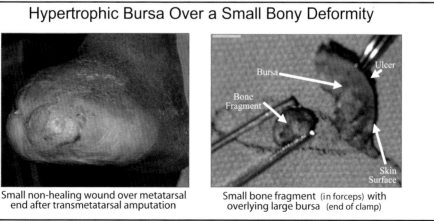

Figure 2-12. A large essentially avascular bursa developed over the bone fragment at the end of the metatarsal. The ulceration developed and failed to heal with dressing agents and immobilization (removable walker boot) due to the deformity. Whereas the bursa at the base of the tract cultured bacteria, the bone did not. After removal of the underlying deformity and the infected bursa, the operative site healed primarily and remained healed.

Dynamic Problems

Repetitive mechanical stresses, especially if associated with altered mechanics of weight bearing secondary to deformities, cause wounds. If the stresses are not allayed, non-healing, problem wounds result. A blister is an example of a wound generated by mechanical stresses. It invariably arises from rubbing of the skin, a shear stress, against an unyielding object. Healing is not likely to occur unless the underlying pressure area is relieved; failure to do so will lead to progression of the blister to an ulcer and then to a deep penetrating wound. If a profound sensory neuropathy is present, the patient is likely not to appreciate the injury while it is occurring. Hence, by the time the blister is noted by the appearance of drainage, stains on clothing and/or odor, it may have progressed to an ulcer.

Static plus Dynamic Problems

Non-healing wounds from combinations of static deformities and dynamic stresses are the types that usually heal with off-loading the wound site. Most pressure sores, especially those that develop in the feet of ambulatory patients, are of this type. Wounds associated with minimal underlying deformities also fit into this group. These differ from purely static or dynamic wounds in three aspects. First, these wounds may occur in the presence of minimal deformities where neither the size of the deformity nor the amount of shear stresses alone could account for the wound. A blister that develops over the heel (a bony prominence) of a hiker who donned inadequate footwear could be ascribed to this cause. Second, the dynamic, shear component of these wounds, especially those associated with walking in patients who have neurological impairments, may be very difficult to control in contrast to the first cause described above. Third, the static plus dynamic type of wound can usually be controlled with minimally invasive surgical techniques such as tenotomies and minimal corrections of deformities (Chapters 8 and 16) in contrast to the purely static underlying deformity induced wound, where excision of ulcers and extensive debridements of underlying cicatrix, bursa, and bone are required.

POST-TRAUMATIC WOUNDS

Gradient of Injury

Wounds that occur as a consequence of trauma may not heal for any of the reasons just discussed. The greater the energy transmitted to the tissues from the injury, the more likely wound healing will become a problem. If the damage is too severe, the tissues die immediately. Invariably there is a gradient of injury from dead, to irreparably damaged, to injured, to healthy tissues. Edema, hypoxia, and infection, if the wound is open, with impairment of host infection and healing responses, lead to post-traumatic problem wounds. In the severe crush injury where bone is involved, osteomyelitis and non-healing of the fracture are often the consequences. Gustilo generated an easy to use open fracture/crush injury classification system that predicts which fractures types will lead to fracture healing complications that include refractory osteomyelitis, non-union, and amputation (Chapter 12).[26]

Host Responsiveness Considerations

A deficiency of the Gustilo classification is that it does not consider the host status in the prediction process. Cierney and Mader get credit for including a host status evaluation in their osteomyelitis classification system. It provides a guide to management and consists of three categories: healthy, compromised (systemic or local), or not relevant

Like the **Goal-Aspiration Score** (Chapter 1), the **Host-Function Score** (Table 2-4) is determined by adding the grades of five assessments each on a 2 (best) to 0 (worst) scale using objective criteria for each grade.

The **Host-Function Score** provides fundamental information that should be included in the initial evaluation of any patient with a wound. It provides guidance as to when collaboration with specialists is indicated, for example, in the decompensated host.

Furthermore, quantifying the patient's level of function provides objectivity to decision making regarding costly and time consuming measures to manage a wound in contrast to a major amputation (or living with a chronic stable wound).

(that is, no treatment is indicated and/or the cure could be worse than the disease).[27] While their contribution was noteworthy for raising the level of awareness to the importance of the host status for healing of wounds with particular reference to osteomyelitis, it does not consider a variety of assessments nor does it quantify the degree the host factors impair healing abilities. Consequently, we generated the **Host-Function Score** based on a 0 to 10 scale (with 10 being optimal) that is both quick to generate and easily quantifies whether the host is healthy, impaired or decompensated (Table 2-4). This score has particular applications in conjunction with the **Goal-Aspiration Score** (Chapter 1) in making decisions whether to employ special considerations to salvage a threatened limb or proceed directly to a lower limb amputation (Chapter 11).

TABLE 2-4. THE HOST-FUNCTION SCORE

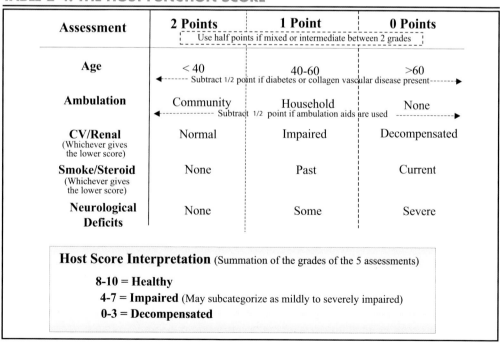

Assessment	2 Points	1 Point	0 Points
	Use half points if mixed or intermediate between 2 grades		
Age	< 40	40-60	>60
	◄------- Subtract 1/2 point if diabetes or collagen vascular disease present -------►		
Ambulation	Community	Household	None
	◄------------- Subtract 1/2 point if ambulation aids are used ---------------►		
CV/Renal (Whichever gives the lower score)	Normal	Impaired	Decompensated
Smoke/Steroid (Whichever gives the lower score)	None	Past	Current
Neurological Deficits	None	Some	Severe

Host Score Interpretation (Summation of the grades of the 5 assessments)

    8-10 = Healthy
    4-7 = Impaired (May subcategorize as mildly to severely impaired)
    0-3 = Decompensated

Deformities from Malunited Fractures

Malunited fractures with resultant deformities can be a cause of problem wounds, especially when the injuries occur in the feet and ankles. Deformities, as previously discussed, amplify stresses to the overlying soft tissues. These can evolve to pressure sores, septic foot wounds, and/or osteomyelitis with weight bearing. The absence of protective sensation may delay the patient's recognition of the problem, but as previously discussed, the neuropathy itself is not the cause of the wound. In the early stages, the superficial ulcer stage of the post-traumatic wound, healing is expected with protective footwear coupled with off-loading techniques. However, once unprotected weight bearing is resumed, the wounds are likely to occur. If wounds do not heal with off-loading, it is likely due to the deformity being too great, the bursa being too large, the bursa being infected, underlying bone infection, or combinations of these. Surgical interventions must then be considered to correct the deformity and/or realign the foot and ankle.

Neuropathy in Post-Traumatic Wounds

Neurological residuals of trauma can also contribute to or be a cause of non-healing wounds for the following reasons: First, loss of protective sensation coupled with a deformity predisposes the site to the development of neurotrophic ulcers as described earlier. Second, if the neuropathy involves motor nerve function, contractures can develop and be a predisposition to the development of wounds. Without correction of the muscle imbalances and resultant deformities, wounds will recur or persist unless the deformities are mild enough to be managed with physical therapy, medications, protective footwear, and/or orthotics. Third, autonomic nerve injury leads to alterations in perfusion. Acutely, this may lead to non-healing of the wounds associated with the trauma. Later, wound healing becomes complicated due to formation of cicatrix in the wound base as a consequence of the hypoxic environment. Alterations in blood flow associated

Clinical Correlation:

A 46-year-old truck driver sustained a crush injury to the dorsum of his right foot when he accidentally dropped a 50-pound jack on it. Several non-displaced fractures of the metatarsals resulted as well as a 5 X 7 cm² slough over the dorsum of the forefoot. The fractures healed, but the forefoot slough wound persisted in spite of optimal wound management.

A year later the patient was referred for hyperbaric oxygen (HBO) treatments. Chronic refractory osteomyelitis of the metatarsals was ruled out with an Indium scan. After two weeks of preparatory hyperbaric oxygen treatments, the wound was debrided and skin grafted. In surgically preparing the graft bed, a 5-mm thick mass of plate-like cicatrix, essentially impervious to blood vessel penetration, was debrided. A split thickness skin graft was placed on the underlying vascular bed.

The skin graft, with some marginal slough, healed completely over a six-month period. The foot itself showed signs of complex regional pain syndrome (reflex sympathetic dystrophy) with coolness, rubor, soft tissue atrophy, and dryness of the skin. This was associated with moderate pain. With pain management and complete wound healing, the patient returned to work two years after the injury.

Comments:

This case exemplifies many of the points made previously with injury, cicatrix formation in hypoxic tissue, the cicatrix becoming a barrier to healing, prolonged healing of the skin graft, and the neurological consequences of the complex regional pain syndrome.

with the complex regional pain syndrome (previously termed reflex sympathetic dystrophy) may be the reason the wounds fail to heal with interventions that normally would be effective.

NEUROPATHY AND WOUNDS

The Role of Neuropathy

Many texts and articles state that neuropathy is the cause of foot wounds.[28-31] We feel strongly that neuropathy has to be put into its appropriate perspective, namely as a contributor to and a reason for failure to notice wounds. From extensive experiences in the management of problem wounds, it is obvious that the majority of patients with neuropathies will heal their wounds and avoid new injuries if sufficiently motivated and compliant (see the **Goal-Aspiration Score**, Chapter 1). There are three types of neuropathies: 1) **Sensory**, 2) **Motor**, and 3) **Autonomic** (Figure 2-13). Most patients with neuropathy present with a combination of these three types, although typically one type is most apparent. Sensory neuropathies alter sensation. They may contribute to heightened awareness of pain termed allodynia (pain perception with light touch) or hyperpathia (exaggerated responses to painful sensations). Conversely, failure to appreciate normal sensation can range along a spectrum from hypesthesia (impaired perception of sensation) to anesthetic (complete loss of sensation). A "quick and easy" 0 (no perception of pain) to 2 (normal sensation) assessment system for pain perception in patients with wounds and wound precursors (Table 2-5) obviates the need for time-consuming and highly subjective Semmes-Weinstein monofilament testing.[32] It provides the essential information for determining the amount of anesthesia needed to perform surgical procedures.

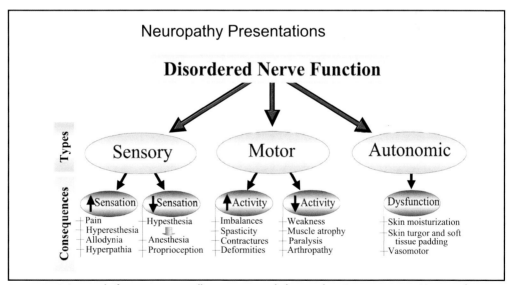

Figure 2-13. Nerve dysfunction—especially as occurs in diabetics—has 3 presentations. Motor and sensory problems can manifest themselves as too much or too little function. Usually combinations of the types of dysfunction occur such as anesthesia, loss of proprioception, deformities, and abnormal vasomotor control in the Charcot arthropathy. Often the consequences represent a continuum of responses, as especially noted with decreased sensation and increased motor activity.

Motor neuropathies are of central or peripheral types. Central motor neuropathies cause balance and weakness problems. Causes include brain injuries from cerebral vascular accident, hypoxic encephalopathy, trauma, infection, neurodegenerative diseases, metabolic disorders (such as diabetes), and demyelinating conditions. Peripheral motor neuropathies lead to imbalances between opposing motor groups such as flexor and extensor muscles. Initially, the manifestations may be those of non-fixed deformities of joints. With persistence they lead to contractures, that is, fixed deformities such as hip and knee flexion contractures, fixed ankle equinus, and clawing of the toes. The role of deformities in the evolution of non-healing wounds was mentioned previously and cannot be over emphasized. Autonomic neuropathies deal with vasomotor regulation and other autonomic nervous system functions. Again, consequences of these problems, such as inability to increase blood flow for wound healing and dryness of the skin make a patient more subject to developing wounds and difficulties with their healing. By far the most frequent presentations of neuropathy are mixed types with motor, sensory and autonomic components.

TABLE 2-5. SIMPLIFICATION OF SENSORY EXAMINATION

1. The "Gold Standard"

- Semmes-Weinstein 5.07 (computed on a logarithmic scale) monofilament test

- "Protective sensation" if the patient feels pressure (equivalent to a 10 gram force) from the end of the monofilament (as the filament begins to bend)

- Laborious, time-consuming, inaccurate; rarely, if ever changes management decisions

2. Pain Evaluation from a Wound Care Perspective ("Quick & Easy")

Grading (Use half points if mixed or intermediate between 2 grades)	"See, Touch, and Go" (No Wound)	Wound "Manipulation" (Wound Present)	Anesthesia Required for Surgeries
2 Points	• No deformities • Sensation: Feet = hands	Normal pain perception	Full
1 Point	• Palpable discomfort of deformities, calluses, etc. • Sensation: Feet = about 50% of hand feeling	Discomfort; able to do procedure(s) with minimal anesthesia	Surface or local with patient awake
0 Points	• No palpable discomfort of deformities, calluses • Anesthetic feet	Able to do procedure(s) without anesthesia	None

RISK FACTORS FOR DEVELOPING WOUNDS

Risk Factors

Five elements, two of which have already been discussed in detail in this chapter, are invariably associated with wounds and can rightly be labeled risk factors or precursors to wound occurrences. These five elements are: 1) **Deformity**, 2) **Dysvascularity**, 3) **Malnutrition**, 4) **Moisture retention**, and 5) **Uncontrolled forces (compressive, shear or tensile)** (Table 2-6). They are listed in alphabetical order to emphasize that no element is more important than another and that in most wound problems the cause of the wound is multifactorial, involving two more of these elements.

TABLE 2-6. FINDINGS THAT CONTRIBUTE TO THE INCIDENCE OF WOUNDS

Findings	Pathophysiology	Vulnerable Sites	Comments
Deformity (Usually associated with neurological deficit)	Callus and/or ulcers develop over bony prominences. Neurological deficits lead to deformities and/or lack of awareness of problem	Presacral, ischial, hip, ankle malleoli, heels, metatarsal head and bunion sites	Usually multiple findings interact to cause a wound
Uncontrolled Forces (Pressure, shear or tension)	Mechanical stresses can generate forces that exceed the skin's tolerance to remain intact and/or exceed the capillary perfusion pressure of approximately 30 mmHg. Same sites as above for deformity.		With 3 or more conditions, the likelihood of a wound greatly increases
Ischemia	Ischemic tissues are subject to injury from minimal trauma, have poor healing abilities and proneness to infection	Sites furthest from the core and/or end-arterial perfusion	
Malnutrition	Systemic considerations of the ischemia patho-physiology above	Poorly perfused bony prominence subjected to repetitive forces	See Table 4-3 for a simplified, easy to use scoring system using these findings
Moisture Retention	Attenuates skin; provides an environment for bacterial proliferation	Perineum; under calluses and around wounds; areas of venous insufficiency	

Shear is characterized by sliding forces. Ordinarily the tough skin on the bottoms of the feet can well tolerate enormous compression stresses and lesser shear stresses, as occur with normal walking. In contrast, abnormal and/or repetitive shear stresses rapidly lead to breakdown of the skin. Shear forces can be very difficult to control in patients with abnormal gaits, partial foot amputations, muscle imbalances, obesity, deformities or combinations of these. Consequently, surgical interventions for these types of wounds, when they occur in the foot, frequently are unsuccessful. Dysvascularity and deformity coupled with malnutrition make the bedridden patient with these problems particularly susceptible to pressure sore development over the portions of their body that transmit the brunt of their body weight to the underlying support surfaces. Moisture retention is the fifth precursor of multi-factorial wound occurrence. It leads to maceration, which diminishes the skin's ability to withstand compressive and shear stresses without injury, as well as provides an environment for multiplication of bacteria. Pressure sores are one of the most significant problems that confront debilitated and infirmed patients and will be discussed further (Chapter 4).

Other Factors that Contribute to Wound Problems

Several other conditions are associated with wound healing challenges, including: 1) **Burns**, 2) **Coagulopathies**, 3) **Elephantiasis**, 4) **Erythralgia**, 5) **Failed surgeries**, 6) **Immunosuppression**, 7) **Medications (especially steroids)**, 8) **Purpura fulminans**, 9) **Pyoderma gangrenosum**, 10) **Radiation injury**, 11) **Venous stasis ulcers**, and 12) **Combinations of these** (Chapter 12). When compared to ischemia/hypoxia, uncontrolled infection, and deformities, these conditions account for only a very small percentage of wound challenges. Regardless of the etiology of the wound challenges, there are general principles for management as will be fully developed in succeeding portions of this text (Chapters 6-12).

CONCLUSIONS

Whereas there are scores of names and terms to describe wounds, recognition of the etiology is a fundamental step in their treatment. This chapter has simplified the process by describing the three most likely etiologies of challenging wounds, namely ischemia/hypoxia, uncontrolled infection, and underlying deformities. Consequently, "a wound by any other name" is still a wound with usually identifiable causes. If the choice lies between naming the wound and identifying its cause, the latter is a far more important consideration. In succeeding chapters, wound descriptions and classifications will be introduced, but the information presented in this chapter and the preceding chapter introduces some of the tools for patient and wound evaluations (**Host-Function Score**, **Goal-Aspiration Score** and "Quick & Easy" Neurological Assessment) as well as providing the fundamentals for understanding the evaluation, management, and prevention of wound challenges.

QUESTIONS

1. How do wound etiologies, descriptions and classifications differ?

2. Why is it desirable to know the etiology of the wound?

3. What are the oxygen requirements for wound healing?

4. What measures does the body initiate to deal with deformities?

5. What are some of the merits of the **Host-Function Score**; what are some of its deficiencies?

6. What advantages does the "Quick & Easy" neurological assessment have over Semmes-Weinstein monofilament testing in patients with wounds and/or wound precursors?

7. What role does the interface have in uncontrolled infection?

8. Why do shear stresses present such a challenge to skin integrity?

9. What are the types and consequences of neuropathies with respect to wound challenges?

10. How can a sensory neuropathy be both a boon and a bane in a patient with a wound challenge?

REFERENCES

1. Guyton AC, Hall JE. Textbook of Medical Physiology, 9th ed. Philadelphia, Pa: WB Saunders Co; 1996:171-172, 1065-1067

2. Babior BM. The respiratory burst of phagocytes. J Clin Invest. 1984;73:599-601

3. Laurnen EL, Kelly PJ. Blood flow, oxygen consumption, carbon-dioxide production, and blood-calcium and pH changes in tibial fractures in dogs. J Bone Joint Surg Am. 1969 Mar;51(2):298-308

4. Leung KS, Sher AL, Lam TW, et al. Energy metabolism in fracture healing. J Bone Joint Surg (Br) 1989;71-B:657-60

5. Hunt TK, Zederfeldt B, Goldstick TK. Oxygen and healing. Am J Surg. 1969; 118:521-525

6. Hunt TK, Pai MP. Effect of varying ambient oxygen tension on wound metabolism and collagen synthesis. Surg Gynecol Obstet. 1972, 135:257-260

7. LaVan FB. and Hunt TK. Oxygen and wound healing. Clin Plast Surg. 1990 Jul;17(3):463-72

8. Peacock EE, Van Winkle W. Wound Repair, 3rd ed. Philadelphia, Pa: WB Saunders Co; 1984:1-104

9. Sevitt, S. Healing of fractures in man. In: Owen R, Goodfellow J, Bullough P (eds.) Scientific Foundations of Orthopaedics and Traumatology. Philadelphia, Saunders 1980:258-273

10. Ueno C, Hunt TK, Hopf, HW. Using physiology to improve surgical wound outcomes. Plast Reconstr Surg, Volume 117(7S) Supplement, June 2006:59S-71S

11. Gottrup F. Oxygen in Wound Healing and Infection. World J. Surg. 2004;28:312-315

12. Reenstra WR, Buras JA, Svoboda KS. Hyperbaric oxygen increases human dermal fibroblast proliferation, growth factor receptor number and in vitro wound closure, Undersea and Hyperbaric Medicine, 1998; #164 25(Suppl):53

13. Eming SA, Brachvogel B, Odorisio T, Koch M. Regulation of angiogenesis: Wound healing as a model. Prog Histochem Cytochem. 2007;42(3):115-70

14. Hunt TK, Van Winkle W Jr. Wound healing: Disorders of repair, in Dunphy JE (ed): Fundamentals of wound management in surgery. South Plainfield: Chirurgecom, 1976:37

15. Peacock EE, Van Winkle W. Wound Repair, 3rd ed. Philadelphia, PA: WB Saunders Co; 1984:102-140

16. Snyder, RJ. Controversies regarding vascular disease in the patient with diabetes: A review of the literature. Ostomy Wound Management, 2007;53(11):40-48

17. Strandness DE. Arteriosclerosis in diabetics. J Vascular Invest. 1995;1(1):50-54

18. Hansen RO, Lundback K. The basement membrane morphology in diabetes mellitus. In: Ellenberg M, Frikin H, eds. Diabetes Mellitus: Theory and Practice. New York: McGraw-Hill; 1970:178-209

19. Dahl-Jørgensen K. Diabetic microangiopathy. Acta Paediatr Suppl. 1998 Oct;425:31-4

20. Guyton AC, Hall JE. O2 Diffusion. In: Textbook of Medical Physiology, 10th ed. Philadelphia, PA: WB Saunders; 2000:454,465

21. Peirce EC II. Pathophysiology, apparatus, and methods, including the special techniques of hypothermia and hyperbaric oxygen. Extracorporeal circulation for open-heart surgery. Springfield, IL: Charles C. Thomas, 1969: 84-88

22. Nimni ME. Polypeptide growth factors: targeted delivery systems, Biomaterials, 1997; 18:1201-1225

23. Newman LG, Waller J, et al. Unsuspected osteomyelitis in diabetic foot ulcers: Diagnosis and monitoring by leukocyte scanning with indium in 111 oxyquinoline. J Am Med Assoc. 1991; 266(9):1246-1250

24. Lipman BT, Collier BD, et al. Detection of osteomyelitis in the neuropathic foot; nuclear medicine, MRI and conventional radiography. Clin Nucl Med. 1998;23:77-82

25. Newman LG, Waller J, Palestro CJ. Unsuspected osteomyelitis in diabetic foot ulcers. JAMA 1991; 266:1246-1251

26. Gustilo R.B., Mendosa R.M., Williams D.N. Problems in the management of type III twenty open fractures. A new classification for type III fractures. J Trauma 24:742-746, 1984

27. Cierny G 3rd, Mader JT, Penninck JJ. A clinical staging system for adult osteomyelitis. Clin Orthop. 2003;414:7–24

28. Boulton A, Kirsner RS, Vileikyte L. Neuropathic Diabetic Foot Ulcers. N Engl J Med. 2004;351:48-55

29. Rathur HM, Boulton AJ. The diabetic foot. Clin Dermatol. 2007 Jan-Feb;25(1):109-20

30. Rathur HM, Boulton AJ. Pathogenesis of foot ulcers and the need for offloading. Horm Metab Res. 2005 Apr;37 Suppl 1:61-8

31. Laing P. Diabetic foot ulcers. Am J Surg. 1994 Jan;167(1A):31S-36S

32. Strauss MB, Miller SS. Addressing foot skin and toenail concerns in diabetes. J Musculoskel Med. 2007;24:312-319

PART **II**

EVALUATION OF WOUNDS

CHAPTER	TITLE	PAGE
3	CLASSIFICATION SYSTEMS FOR THE DIABETIC FOOT WOUND	57
4	CLASSIFICATION SYSTEMS FOR PRESSURE ULCERS/INDOLENT WOUNDS	85
5	THE WOUND SCORE - A SOLUTION FOR THE WOUND CLASSIFICATION DILEMMA	109

INTRODUCTION TO PART II

Evaluation is the first step in dealing with a wound. Information from the evaluation provides the starting point for wound management. An important goal of the evaluation is the establishment of the severity of the wound. From this, logical decisions for management ensue. Many expressions and parameters are used to describe wounds. Perhaps the simplest approach is observation of the wound and determining whether it is a healthy wound, a problem wound, or a futile wound. For the experienced observer, this may be adequate, but it is highly subjective. It does not lend itself to evaluation of outcomes, and if research reports are generated, they are highly subject to bias. For example, with respect to the bias consideration, any wound that fails to heal by the clinician's management might be labeled a futile type, or the failure was because of the patient's non-compliance. Conversely, other observers might say that any wound that heals was fundamentally a healthy wound at the time of its presentation to the clinician and its eventual healing is not a reflection of its initial severity.

A wound grading system results when a group of descriptions or observations of the wound characteristics are combined. In the next two chapters we evaluate over a dozen grading systems for wounds and pressure ulcers from five perspectives, namely objectivity, adaptability, guide for management, validity, and reliability (Part II, Table 1). The wound scoring systems separate themselves into two clearly defined divisions, those designed to evaluate diabetic foot wounds (Chapter 3), and those designed to evaluate pressure ulcers (Chapter 4). A collective examination of the grading systems show that nearly 30 different descriptive terms or evaluation criteria have been used by authors to generate their wound grading systems. Obviously some of the criteria used for wound grading are more important than others, and any scoring system that considers all the possible wound descriptions would be so unwieldy that it would be impractical for clinical applications.

We feel that a grading system should be simple to use and multifaceted. It should provide an all-encompassing and universally applicable approach for determination of the wound severity. The severity becomes intuitively obvious from the score, and the score provides a guideline for wound management. To meet these goals we generated the **Wound Score**, a new paradigm for wound evaluation and formulation of guidelines for management (Chapter 5). While the **Wound Score** is derived from direct observation of the wound, the importance of laboratory and imaging information should not be discounted. Studies such as 1) wound cultures and sensitivities, 2) plain x-rays, 3) nuclear medicine scans, 4) magnetic resonance imaging, 5) Doppler/Duplex evaluations, 6) trans-cutaneous oxygen measurements, and 7) angiography complement the information provided by the **Wound Score** and justify specific interventions for potentially remediable problems. The five assessments used to evaluate wound grading systems (Part II, Table 1) are then applied to the **Wound Score** to show its effectiveness as a comprehensive, yet simple to use system to evaluate and manage wounds.

PART II, TABLE 1. CRITERIA TO EVALUATE WOUND GRADING SYSTEMS

Criteria	Questions to be Answered	Example	Grading
Objectivity	How easy is it to accurately grade each assessment the author uses for grading a wound?	Appearance (color) of the wound base	**2 Points** **Good** Supporting Information
Adaptability	Can the system be used for a variety of wound types and locations?	Malperforans ulcer to necrotizing infection; upper extremity to feet & anything in between	
Guide to Wound Management	Is it applicable for 1) evaluation, 2) treatment, 3) measuring progress, and 4) grading outcomes?	Scores useable for a variety of applications	**1 Point** **Fair** Supporting Information
Validity	How effectively does the grade or score predict the outcome (i.e. criteria-related validity)?	Proffering expectations of healing at the time of the initial evaluation	**0 Points** **Poor** No Supporting Information
Reliability	How consistent are scores made by different examiners (i.e. inter-judge reliability)?	Similar scores from examiners with varieties of experiences	

Interpretations: Wound Evaluation Systems (Summation of the grades of the 5 criteria)

8-10 Points = Useful scoring system

4-7 Points = Scoring system has limited utility

0-3 Points = Probably not useful for evaluation & management of wounds

CHAPTER

3

CLASSIFICATION SYSTEMS FOR THE DIABETIC FOOT WOUND

CHAPTER THREE OVERVIEW

INTRODUCTION 59

WAGNER 59

FORREST AND GAMBORG-NILSEN 66

KNIGHTON 67

PECORARO AND REINBER 69

BRODSKY 70

LAVERY, ARMSTRONG, AND HARKLESS 72

JEFFCOATE AND MACFARLANE 74

FOSTER AND EDMONDS 76

YOUNES, ET AL. 77

CONCLUSIONS 79

QUESTIONS 81

REFERENCES 82

"What you see is not always what you have."

INTRODUCTION

The history of wound evaluation systems is relatively contemporary. In 1976, Meggitt proposed a classification for diabetic foot ulcers.[1] This was the earliest reference to a wound classification system that was discovered in an extensive literature search. Subsequently, over a dozen other classification systems have been reported. The wound classification systems separate themselves into two clearly defined groups: 1) those designed primarily for diabetic foot wounds, and 2) those generated for pressure ulcers. In almost all situations the groups do not overlap in the type of wound they propose to classify; that is, application of a diabetic foot wound classification to a pressure ulcer and vice versa. Aside from the authors' original articles, and with the exception of the Wagner and the four-depth pressure ulcer classifications, there is a dearth of information about the utilization by subsequent wound caregivers of the other classification systems. This chapter focuses on the diabetic foot wound classifications, the first group of wound classifications. The succeeding chapter (Chapter 4) focuses on the second group. We devised a system to evaluate wound grading systems using five criteria that are tabulated in the Introduction to Part II of this text (Part II, Table 1). The five criteria include 1) **objectivity**, 2) **adaptability**, 3) **guide to wound management**, 4) **validity**, and 5) **reliability**. Each wound classification, when feasible, will be reviewed using these criteria.

WAGNER

Historical Perspectives – In 1981, Wagner reported on "A Classification and Treatment Program for Diabetic, Neuropathic and Dysvascular Foot Problems".[2,3] His scoring system was derived from a classification that Meggitt generated five years before the Wagner publication.[1] At that time, Wagner reported that about 80 percent of amputations in patients from first world countries were due to peripheral vascular disease, and of these 80 percent were diabetics. He observed that, with few exceptions, the surgical treatment had been above-knee amputations. With improved sophistication in diagnostic and treatment interventions, above-knee amputations were no longer the predominant level of amputation for this group of patients. He felt that occlusion of major blood vessels was not the cause of most diabetic foot wounds, but rather they were due to microangiopathy manifested as basement membrane thickening. This caused diffusion defects of nutrition and oxygen – our assertion). This made the limb more susceptible to trauma and infection. Neuropathy frequently contributed to the problems by delaying recognition of, or disregard for, early lesions due to absence of pain.

Starting Point – Wagner based his guidelines for management on blood flow to the ankle level. This resulted in two permutations: 1) treatment when vascularity is sufficient, and 2) treatment when vascularity is insufficient. He used Doppler blood pressure measurements to ascertain perfusion to the ankle level. By using a ratio of the systolic pressure readings of the ankle to the brachial artery, a number was generated, named the ischemic index. Wagner stated with respect to diabetic foot wounds that "if the ischemic index is over 0.45, virtually 100% healing results".[2,3] He included eight guide-

Subsequently, the terminology for the ischemic index evolved to ABI or ankle-brachial index.

lines for management when vascularity is sufficient and ten "specific treatment modalities" for using his flow charts in order to "provide the answer to almost any question that should arise within each grade [of six]".[2, 3]

Wagner Grades – Wagner classified foot wounds into six grades (using Roman numerals) based solely on clinical observations that ranged from "potential breakdown" to "total foot destruction." The Wagner Grades with the defining characteristics of each grade are as follows (Figure 3-1):

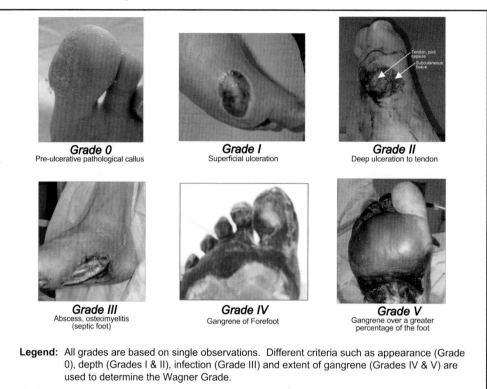

Legend: All grades are based on single observations. Different criteria such as appearance (Grade 0), depth (Grades I & II), infection (Grade III) and extent of gangrene (Grades IV & V) are used to determine the Wagner Grade.

Figure 3-1. Wagner Diabetic Foot Wound Grades.

- *Grade 0:* Intact skin, but a **possible pre-ulcerative condition** such as deformity, hyperkeratotic (callus) formation, and/or neuropathy.
- *Grade I:* **Superficial ulcer** in the skin
- *Grade II:* **Deeper ulcer** that has continuity to tendon, bone, ligament, or joint
- *Grade III:* Deeper lesion with **abscess formation and/or osteomyelitis** (Wagner's algorithm for this grade includes management for systemic sepsis)
- *Grade IV:* **Gangrene** of some portion of the **forefoot**
- *Grade V:* **Gangrene** over the **greater percentage of the foot**

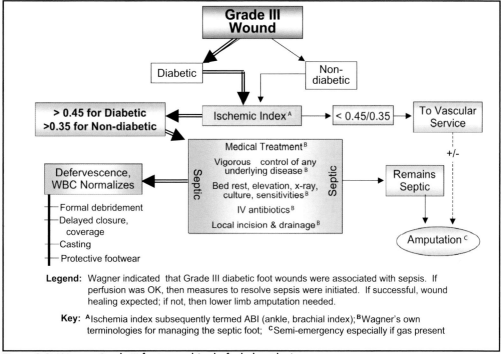

Figure 3-2. Wagner Grade III foot wound (redrafted algorithm).

Wagner supplements each grade by an elaborate algorithm that can have outcomes that range from foot salvage, even for Grade V wounds, to major lower limb amputation, even for Grade 0 pre-ulcerative conditions. As an example, the Grade III wound (deep abscess, osteomyelitis) has three possible end-points including referral to the vascular service, medical and surgical management of the septic foot with wound healing, and lower limb amputation (Figure 3-2).

Evaluation of the Wagner Grading System – When this system is evaluated by the five criteria presented in the introduction to Part II (Part II, Table 1), it does not stand up well to scrutiny. Even so, the importance of the Wagner grading system cannot be discounted. It is the "granddaddy" of all diabetic foot grading systems and is the predominant diabetic foot wound grading system used today. The Wagner Grade III, or greater, diabetic foot wound has now become a criterion for using hyperbaric oxygen therapy as an adjunct to managing these problems.[4] Wagner's algorithms for managing diabetic foot wounds revolutionized the practice of these problems. As he states, his goal was to avoid above knee amputations, a standard of practice at the time, for diabetic foot wounds.[3] He was unquestionably successful because of this goal and deserves the highest accolades for this accomplishment. The following assessments grade the Wagner system from the criteria of objectivity, adaptability, guide to management, validity, and reliability as described in Part II, Table 1. Each assessment is graded from 0 (poor or no supporting information) to 2 (good supporting information).

Objectivity = Fair Supporting Information (1 point) – The grades are highly subject to the observers' impressions with the absence of unambiguous parameters and minimal objective criteria to separate one grade from another. There are no provisions for grading wounds that have components of two or more grades, intermediate between two grades, or are multiple in the foot. Furthermore, the criteria used to establish a Wagner Grade are inconsistent. Grades 0 to II are determined by wound depth, while infection is the criterion used for Grade III. Perfusion as reflected in gangrene and extent of involvement are the criteria used for Grades IV and V. Furthermore, it is assumed that increasing grades reflect worsening situations. This, however, is not so. The Grade III wound associated with sepsis can be much more of a wound healing and limb salvaging challenge than gangrene of the forefoot managed with toe or forefoot amputations (Figure 3-3).

Adaptability = Fair Supporting Information (1/2 point) – The scoring system was designed specifically for diabetic foot wounds, although Wagner's algorithms include a pathway for non-diabetic wounds. The system works well if the diabetic foot wound corresponds to one of the six Wagner grades, but not for wounds in other locations such

> Ironically, lower limb amputations are included as an option in each of Wagner's treatment algorithms for his six grades, and limb salvage is even an option for wounds with a Wagner Grade V. Consequently, objective parameters for determining wound seriousness are not inherent in his 0 to V Grades classification system.

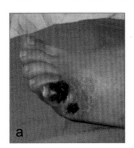 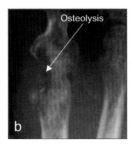 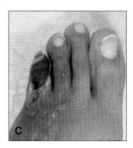

Wagner **III** versus Wagner **IV**

Legend: Photos a and c, based on visual inspection, could both be classified as Wagner Grade IV diabetic foot wounds (forefoot gangrene) with surgical amputation or mummification and auto-amputation of the involved toes being reasonable choices.

Photo b is an x-ray which demonstrates a pyarthrosis with destruction of the metatarsal joint and extensive osteolysis of the metatarsal head, a Wagner Grade III diabetic foot wound. Management in this situation dictates immediate exploration, debridement, toe and partial ray amputation, and decompression of tendon tracts to midfoot and possibly ankle levels.

Obviously, the more serious problem is the Grade III lesion. The x-ray (photo b) was of the metatarsalphalangeal joint of the photo on the left (photo a).

Figure 3-3. Wagner dilemma.

as the ankles, legs or common pressure ulcer sites. Because there are only six options, the system, in terms of grading, should be simple to use if the wound conforms to one of the six grades. However, if the system is used as Wagner intended it to be, that is, with Doppler measurements to determine ischemia (ankle-brachial index) and other information (deformities, leukocyte counts, x-rays, and healing responses), algorithms are to be used for each grade with a combined total of about 50 different treatment decisions. Finally, the Wagner system is not applicable for wounds that start in the feet and ascend proximally such as gas gangrene, necrotizing fasciitis, and tenosynovitis.

If the Wagner system were used for pressure sores, for example in the lower portions of the trunk and the hips, it could be misleading. This is because the "worst possible situations" for these wounds are equated to osteomyelitis, which would be equivalent to a Wagner Grade III, while a superficial slough of skin and subcutaneous tissues covered with a dry thin eschar could be labeled as a Grade IV or V lesion.

Guide to Wound Management = Good Supporting Information (1 ½ points) – Wagner integrates other important wound-related information such as leukocyte counts, cultures, and x-rays to make management decisions in his algorithms. However, all initial decisions are based on the ischemic (ankle-brachial) index derived from Doppler blood pressure measurements

In the 30 years since Wagner first published his system, new evaluation and treatment techniques have been developed, including transcutaneous oxygen measurements, laser Doppler perfusion observations, magnetic resonance angiography, visceral protein

The paradox is that the Doppler information is now rarely, if ever, used as Wagner intended, even thought his six diabetic foot wound grades remain the most widely used diabetic foot wound scoring system.

Doppler blood pressure measurements are notoriously unreliable in diabetics with calcified blood vessel disease. Wagner described four different Doppler flow velocity profiles, which reflect the deterioration in the quality of the Doppler wave as the degree of blockage increases and collateral flow decreases. This not only adds four more management permutations to the approximately 50 that already exist in his algorithm system, but it adds additional subjectivity to the interpretation of Doppler derived information.

Doppler evaluations are notably absent in all succeeding diabetic foot wound evaluations. In a subsequent article, Wagner acknowledged that they were not reliable for assessing perfusion in the diabetic and therefore were not being used.

markers for nutrition assessments, wound dressing agents, bioengineered materials, and the negative pressure wound therapy system which make portions of his evaluation and management technique archaic. Regardless, the Wagner system is fair to good for measuring progress (movement downward on his algorithms), and outcomes (i.e. healed versus amputation), even though it is poor for assessing the initial seriousness of the wound. Finally, Wagner does not utilize other patient related information such as func-

It is noteworthy that Wagner states, "Patient education and prevention are probably the most important aspects of the whole system."[2,3] Also, he mentions that close cooperation is essential between the medical and surgical teams involved in the patient's care. This implies that Wagner appreciates the necessity of using a team approach to manage difficult diabetic foot wounds, but only gives brief testimonial to this by referral to "vascular service," "medical treatment," and "vigorous control of any underlying disease" in his algorithms.

tional potential and patient aspirations (**Host-Function Score** Chapter 2 and **Goal-Aspiration Score** Chapter 1) to make decisions regarding whether to attempt salvage of the wound or proceed directly to a lower limb amputation using the Wagner algorithms.

Validity Measures = Fair Supporting Information (1 Point) – Validity is a term that reflects how well the measuring instrument assesses or evaluates the item to be measured, and can be classified into six types (Table 3-1).[5] In wound healing, we are particularly interested in knowing how well the initial wound grade or score predicts

TABLE 3-1. TYPES OF VALIDITY MEASUREMENTS

Type	Description	Comment, Examples
Concurrent	How well does the score of one test correlate with the score of a non-identical test	Correlations between intelligence and aptitude tests
Construct	Use of related information to define, assess or understand a given observation	Drawing conclusions from test scores
Content	How well does the test or procedure represent what is to be measured	Use of both math & verbal domains to measure intelligence
Criterion-Related	Effectiveness of a test or measurement in predicting outcomes or performance	Predictability of an intelligence test for college grade point average
Face	How well do the items of a classification or test appear to sample what is measured	The weakest validity measurement; development of the Wagner grade
Predictive	Prediction of future performance or outcome	Incorporates elements of construct & criterion-related validity types

Note: Predictive validity is the most important type in terms of proving the usefulness of a wound grading system. As noted, it incorporates elements of criterion-related and construct types of validity. Unfortunately, the Wagner Grading System does not have any validity testing to support its use, and at best, only conforms to face validity, the weakest of all validity types by virtue of its extensive use.

Clinical Correlation:

A healthy 37-year old male sustains a severe open-fracture crush injury to the lower third of his right leg from a motorcycle accident. After initial debridement and stabilization, the patient was told that several additional surgeries including a muscle flap, bone grafting, and intramedullary rodding would be needed if there was to be any chance to salvage the mangled extremity.

The options of lower limb amputation versus attempted salvage were explained to the patient. When he learned that there would be less than a 50 percent chance that the limb could be salvaged and have limited useful function, and it would require more than a year's time for management and convalescence to achieve this expected outcome, he opted for a below knee amputation with an expectation of a quick and almost 100 percent expectation of a good outcome.

Comment:

The above outcome expectations given to the patient were a form of predictive validity. Even though actual statistics were not given to the patient from citations in the literature, the generalizations were sufficient to predict outcomes and aid the patient in making his decision.

Of 153 patients Wagner used for generating the above information, almost 70 percent of the amputations were done at the ankle level or higher. Thirty percent alone were Symes (ankle level) amputations, which today are not considered a good and durable amputation level for diabetic patients, especially those with neuropathy. Of the nine failures reported in his series, one-third were at the Symes level.

Likewise, durability of results was not reported; that is, what happened after healing was completed and functional activities resumed.

outcomes, that is, predictive validity. Does it provide information that we can give to patients so they will know what to expect from our efforts to treat their wounds? The better the predictive validity, the more accurate information that can be given to the patient about what an anticipated outcome will be. This information is useful for explaining treatment options, aiding in the patient's decision making as to what option to choose, and in obtaining informed consents. The Wagner score, by virtue of its widespread use and Wagner's own personal experiences, ranks high in terms of face validity, the weakest of the validity types (Figure 3-4). At most, the elements of the Wagner System are a reasonable attempt to sample what is supposed to be measured. Unfortunately, there are no other validity studies using the Wagner System. The only possible validation information pertaining to Wagner's system was his report that 93 percent of amputations from toes to above knee levels healed when the ischemic index was greater than 0.45.[3]

Reliability Measures = Poor Supporting Information (0 Points) – Reliability is the term used to test how reproducible the observations are. Reliability can be inter-observer (between two or more observers), or intra-observer (repeated measurements by the same person). Reliability implies that if assessments are made by two different people or

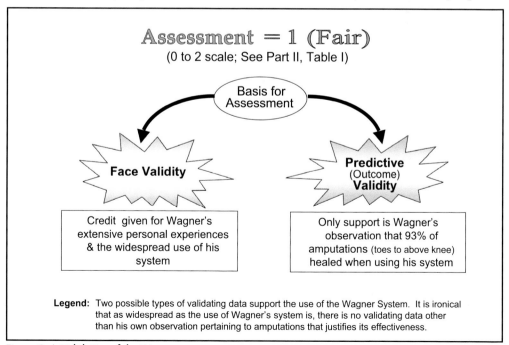

Assessment = 1 (Fair)
(0 to 2 scale; See Part II, Table I)

Basis for Assessment

Face Validity

Predictive (Outcome) Validity

| Credit given for Wagner's extensive personal experiences & the widespread use of his system | Only support is Wagner's observation that 93% of amputations (toes to above knee) healed when using his system |

Legend: Two possible types of validating data support the use of the Wagner System. It is ironical that as widespread as the use of Wagner's system is, there is no validating data other than his own observation pertaining to amputations that justifies its effectiveness.

Figure 3-4. Validation of the Wagner system.

repeated by the same person, the scoring will be the same or nearly the same. The kappa value is a statistical term used to assess the degree of agreement between observers or measurements. If high (0 to 1 scale, with 1 being uniformly identical assessments), the scoring system is said to be reliable. As widespread and long standing as the Wagner grading system is, it is surprising that no inter-observer comparisons of wounds have been reported using this system. Hence, on the reliability criterion, the Wagner system gets a poor (0 point) grade.

Summary of the Wagner Grading System – In an attempt to objectify the appraisal of the Wagner system at this time and other grading systems subsequently, the Criteria to Evaluate Wound Grading systems is a useful tool (Part II, Table 1 and Table 3-7). For the Wagner System using the 0 to 10 point evaluation, the score is a 4 generated from 1 point for objectivity, ½ point for adaptability, 1 ½ points for guide to management, 1 point for validity and 0 points for reliability. Our interpretation of score in the range of 4 to 7 is that it has limited applications as a wound grading system. Presumably for this reason, more than a dozen other grading systems for wounds have evolved. These other scoring systems will now be introduced and evaluated on the same criteria as used above for the Wagner system.

FORREST AND GAMBORG-NILSEN

Characteristics and Basis of the Scoring System – In 1984, Forrest and Gamborg-Nilsen, from Boden, Sweden, published the article "Wound Assessment in Clinical Practice: A Critical Review of Methods and Their Application."[6] The authors gave a review of the subjective and objective methods for wound assessment and presented classification of ulcers based on appearance. This system was specifically designed to determine the need for medical versus surgical treatment strategies. The Forrest System consists of six initial types, which are solely based on the appearance on the wound, and include:

- **Type 1 ulcers:** clean, moist, and granulating
- **Type 2 ulcers:** clean, but have exuberant granulations
- **Type 3 ulcers:** swollen, red, and apparently inflamed, and profuse exudation
- **Type 4 ulcers:** have substantial loss of tissue
- **Type 5 ulcers:** are covered by an adherent film of necrotic material
- **Type 6 ulcers:** are covered by hard black scab

Types 1 and 2 are considered uncontaminated, Types 3 and 4 potentially contaminated, and Types 5 and 6 contaminated. After initial classification, ulcers of Types 2–6 undergo surgical debridement. After this, wounds are re-classified into 3 new types, which determine further management including wet saline compresses for the healthy wounds, dextranomer for wounds intermediate in severity and adhesive zinc oxide tape for the severe wounds. The ultimate goals are for the more severe wounds to improve enough to use wet saline compresses and healing spontaneously or with plastic surgical procedures. In other words, the initial step of classification is differentiation of wounds between those that require surgical management and those that do not require it. The second step is determination of specific treatment strategies after surgical debridement.

Comments – The general description of the wound types in the Forrest and Gamborg-Nilsen classification appears to be relatively understandable and adaptable to wounds in a variety of locations. Each type of wound has its own description. However, some terms, such as "exuberant granulations" and "substantial loss of tissue" are vague and/or ambiguous. The presence of inflammation and necrotic tissue are the main

During the re-classification after surgical debridement, any of the types from 2 to 6 may be classified into one of three subtypes. For example, a Type 3 wound may become sub-type 3, while Type 6 may become sub-type 2, which is less severe than subtype 3. This means that initial wound type does not necessarily reflect severity of the wound, and the initial wound type classification does not give a clear idea about further management.

criteria for determining the wound type. Other important wound descriptors such as wound size, depth, and perfusion status are not included. Interestingly, some of those wound characteristics are discussed in the original article, but the authors did not incorporate them into their system. The classification suggests that the larger the number, the more severe the wound. As the wound type number increases, more complicated management is required. This classification generated a score of 4 ½ out of a possible ten on the criteria we generated for evaluating wound grading systems (Part II, Table 1 and Table 3-7) indicating that it has limited utility as a wound classification system.

Utilization – The Forrest and Gamborg-Nilsen Classification is not widely used. In the available literature, we did not find reports from other authors that utilize this system. One of the possible reasons is that there is little clinical significance (or meaning) of a 6-type subdivision. General management of five types (from 2 to 6) is basically the same—surgical debridement. Results of surgical debridement determine which one of three treatment options will be recommended as the next management step. Another deficiency of the Forrest and Gamborg-Nilsen system is that it does not consider severe ulcers with involvement of deep structures, serious necrotizing soft tissue infections, wet gangrene or combinations of these. The original article does not provide any information about the reliability of this classification. No outcome data is provided. The article concluded that, "experience in wound assessment … is necessary if reliable objective data are to be produced." In other words, the authors conclude that reliability depends on the experience of the evaluator.

KNIGHTON

Characteristics and Basis of the Scoring System – In 1986, Knighton et al. published a classification system specifically developed to analyze wounds for a particular clinical investigation, the outpatient evaluation of autologous platelet-derived wound healing factor.[7] The authors developed a "wound severity index" in order to quantitatively evaluate wounds, follow clinical courses and compare different groups of patients. The system included almost 40 wound descriptors each scored on a different basis divided into three wound characteristics. That is, general wound parameters were scored 0, 2, or 4, anatomic considerations were scored either 0, 2, 5, 7, or 10, while wound measurements were scored with different scales from 0 to 10. The higher the score, the worse the particular descriptor. This generated a total wound score that could range from 0 (best) to 97 (worst). Components of the three wound characteristics included four to seven items as listed below:

- **General Wound Parameters** consisted of periwound erythema, periwound edema, wound purulence, wound fibrin, limb pitting edema, limb brawny edema, and wound granulation (7 components)

- **Anatomic Considerations** included exposed bone, exposed tendon, dorsalis pedis pulse, and posterior tibial pulse (4 components)
- **Wound Measurements** encompassed size, depth, undermining and duration (4 components)

Six diagnostic categories of wounds including decubitus ulcer, diabetes, transplanted diabetic, arterial insufficiency, venous stasis and other comprised the subjects on which he reported his results. Furthermore, an infection score was determined by adding the periwound erythema score, periwound edema score, and wound purulence score to give a range of 14 (worst) to 0 (best).

Comments – Of all the wound classification systems, Knighton's is probably the most comprehensive and deserves high marks for objectivity. However, the lack of consistency in grading the components of the three wound characteristics, the number of descriptors, and the different wound types give this classification so many permutations and combinations that it is unwieldy as a clinical tool for evaluation and management of wounds. Consequently, on a "user-friendliness" scale, it would be among the lowest of all the wound scoring systems. Without a scoring sheet with the wound characteristics and their subcategory descriptors, it would be all but impossible to generate the Knighton wound severity index. Outcomes from his report require scrutiny. Healing times were only given for immediate and delayed applications of PDWHG with the former giving the better results. This classification generated a score of 3 out of a possible 10 on the criteria we generated for evaluating wound grading systems (Part II, Table 1 and Table 3-7), indicating that it probably is not useful as a wound evaluation and grading system. In Knighton's study, wound scores were recorded and tabulated by two

> The professed goal of the Knighton system was to demonstrate the value of his autologous platelet derived wound healing factor (PDWHF). Unfortunately, his data was not convincing since the average initial wound score was 21.6 +/-11.2 (on the 0—best to 97—worst range), suggesting that his wounds were in the most healthy third of the severity index even before starting his autologous PDWHF regimen.

of his clinical and research registered nurse wound-healing specialists. However, the authors did not provide any numbers that would reflect reliability between the two evaluators.

Utilization – Knighton's classification does not appear to be used in clinical practice at this time. Except for Knighton's publications, no other information about the use of his system was found with respect to wound management. There are several possible reasons for this. The system is too complex and time-consuming for every day clinical practice. In addition, the total wound score does not really determine management strategy, nor does it help to predict clinical outcomes. On the positive side, the Knighton's system is applicable to different types of wounds and for wounds in different locations of the body, for which it gets some merits with respect to adaptability. The system might be useful as a research tool because it allows one to follow a wound course and to compare different patients or groups of patients from a variety of descriptors. For example, the edema-evaluation score was used to pair the edema reduction effects of hyperbaric oxygen treatments with transcutaneous oxygen measurements.[8]

At one time, Knighton set up and wholly managed a large group of wound healing centers throughout the United States that utilized his platelet derived wound healing factor coupled with his wound scoring system. None remain in existence at this time.

At best, Knighton deserves credit for raising the awareness of the comprehensive wound healing center concept which is so prevalent in the United States today. At worst, Knighton could be criticized for his entrepreneurial approach to wound management that wrested control away from the clinicians in the hospitals and outpatient facilities that utilized his system.

PECORARO AND REINBER

Characteristics and Basis of the Scoring System – In 1990, Pecoraro and Reinber published their article "Classification of Wounds in Diabetic Amputees."[9] The authors studied three previously described classifications (Wagner, Forrest, and Knighton), conducted an extensive literature search, and developed a new 10-class classification which "encompasses the spectrum from intact skin to deep wounds with extensive necrosis"[9] (Table 3-2). Classes 1, 2, and 3 were further subdivided resulting in 14 choices to classify the wound. According to the authors, the appropriate class was based primarily on structural criteria such as anatomy and morphology and supplemented by secondary historical or physiologic criteria, such as chronicity and infection. The wound class was then recorded on a wound coding sheet that also included 42 site locations, presence or absence of infection, and five levels of edema from none to periwound, to ankle, to mid tibia, to pitting to the knee.

Comments – The authors used different criteria to classify wounds. Classes 1 through 4 are based on depth of the wound, which is not always easy to determine. Classes 5 and 6 are identified by the presence of necrotic film and eschar, respectively, but do not specify the magnitude of wound base involvement with these problems. Class 7 utilizes the term "substantial loss of tissue," a vague term. Class 8 is the only type of wound that is characterized primarily by the seriousness of infection and corresponds closely with Wagner's Grade III septic foot infections. Paradoxically, the authors reported that infection could be present in 8 out of 10 wound classes (Table 3-2). Classes 9 and 10 are defined by the presence of gangrene. Wound perfusion other than the presence or absence of gangrene is not included in the evaluation. This classification generated a score of 2 ½ out of a possible 10 on the criteria we generated for evaluating wound grading systems (Part II, Table 1, and Table 3-7), indicating that it probably is not useful as a wound evaluation and grading system. Its chief virtue is it that it describes and provides a method to precisely locate a variety of wound presentations, that is, it gets fair marks for adaptability. Reliability information is not provided by the authors. The system is not designed to measure the progress of wound healing.

Data published by Pecoraro and Reiber indicated that the Wagner, Knighton, and Forrest systems did not provide precise descriptions for 19 percent to 49 percent of the primary cutaneous lesions encountered in their study of 80 patients.[9] In terms of validity, the authors state that the eventual amputation level was not reliably predicated by the location of the presenting ulceration, with 34 percent of amputations that resulted from non-healing of ulcers of the toes or forefoot, which were performed at the below knee or above knee levels.

TABLE 3-2. SEATTLE WOUND CLASSIFICATION SYSTEM (PECORARO/REIBER)

Class	Description	Comparison Grades	Infection
1	**Intact Skin** 1.1 Superficial or healing minor lesion 1.2 Superficial or healing minor lesion 1.3 Healing minor lesion < 4 weeks duration	Wagner 0	No Yes
2	**Acute Ulcer or Preulcerative Soft Tissue Infection** 2.1 Subcutaneous abscess or cellulitis 2.2 Inflamed, red erythematous ulcer with exudate	Forrest 3	Yes
3	**Partial Thickness Ulcer** 3.1 Partial or early granulations 3.2 Exuberant granulations	Knighton 1 Forrest 1 Forrest 2	Yes
4	**Ulcer Penetrating to Subcutaneous Tissue** (Full Thickness)	Wagner I Knighton 2	Yes
5	**Ulcer Covered by and Adherent Film of Necrotic Material**	Forrest 5	
6	**Ulcer Covered by a Hard Black Eschar**	Forrest 6	Yes
7	**Ulcer with Substantial Loss of Tissue, Penetrating to Tendon, Joint Capsule or Bone**	Wagner II, Knighton 3, Forrest 4	Yes
8	**Ulcer with Deep Tissue Infection**	Wagner III, Knighton 4	Yes
9	**Gangrene Involving Portion of Foot** [Toe(s), forefoot or heel]	Wagner IV, Knighton 5/6	
10	**Entire Forefoot (or Leg) Gangrenous**	Wagner V	Yes

Utilization – The Seattle Wound Classification System is another system not apparently used in clinical practice. However, one additional report utilizing this system was found.[10, 11] Pecoraro and Reiber stated that their system may be useful for clinical investigations, including studies of wound prevalences, validation of treatment protocols and comparison of the results of different clinical trials. With all the permutations and combinations this system has, like the Knighton system, it would take an enormous amount of data to generate conclusions to validate its effectiveness in predicting outcomes. The article suggests that the higher the number of the wound class, the more severe the wound. This is not always true. The failure to differentiate wet from dry gangrene, describe the perfusion status of the involved limb, and specify the wound size are serious deficiencies of this classification system.

> A hard, black eschar covering a wound (Class 6) acts like a biological dressing which would likely be less of a problem to manage and have a better outcome than an ulcer penetrating to subcutaneous tissue (Class 4).
> Likewise, an ulcer with deep tissue infection (Class 8) may have a worse prognosis for healing than gangrene involving a portion of the forefoot (Class 9).

BRODSKY

Characteristics and Basis of the Scoring System – In 1993, Brodsky published a depth-ischemia classification.[12] This system deserves credit for ushering in a number of "matrix" type diabetic foot wound classifications. The matrix classifications pair different domains such as in Brodsky's classification, wound depth (4 grades) with ischemia (4 levels) to generate 16 permutations. Objective criteria are listed for each wound depth and level of ischemia.[13] Brodsky provides specific diagnostic and treatment measures for each depth level and degree of ischemia severity (Table 3-3). Brodsky's system is dynamic in the sense that as the wound depth level improves, the grade decreases and the appropriate management transitions to the new grade.

Comments – Brodsky's classification has many similarities to Wagner's with the main difference being that of using two domains, ischemia and depth, rather than a

TABLE 3-3. BRODSKY'S DEPTH-ISCHEMIA CLASSIFICATION OF DIABETIC FOOT LESIONS

Depth	0	1	2	3
Level	At risk foot, no ulcer	Superficial ulcer	Deep ulcer	Extensive ulceration
Associated findings	Neuropathy, previous wound and/or deformity	Not infected	Open tendon or joint; superficial infection	Exposed bone; deep infection
Management	Education, footwear	Pressure relief; orthotics	Debridement; wound care*	Ray or partial foot amputation*

Ischemia	A	B	C	D
Severity	Perfusion OK	Ischemia without gangrene	Partial gangrene of foot	Complete foot gangrene
Management	None	Vascular evaluation reconstruction as needed	Revascularization; partial foot amputation	Lower limb amputation

*Management moves towards depth levels 1 and 0 as ulcer heals

single criterion to determine the seriousness of the wound. Brodsky provides specific treatments for each of the four items in each domain in contrast to working through rather cumbersome and not always logical algorithms in the Wagner system. However, it is not clear whether management of the depth and ischemia problems is to be done simultaneously, or is to be staged. It would seem logical to address the ischemia problem prior to definitive management of the wound depth problem. The Brodsky numbering (0 best to 3 worst) and ischemia (A best and D worst) grades do not provide intuitive appreciation of the wound's seriousness. Vascular evaluation and possible interventions are given as management choices for three of the four letter classes of ischemia. However, when angioplasty or vascular reconstructions are not feasible, alternatives to augment perfusion and tissue oxygenation are not offered except for some skeptical comments about the usefulness of hyperbaric oxygen.[13] Debridement is given as an option for two

By merely citing numbers and letters, a grade of 0 for depth of the wound could possibly be construed as a worse wound than a grade 3 wound depth. Likewise, without Brodsky's tabulated information, the user or reviewer of the system would likely have little appreciation of the difference, for example, between a 2, B wound and a 0, D wound.

of the four number classes of depth, but confusion could arise as to the urgency of the surgical intervention since severity of infection, especially with respect to the septic foot, is not an inherent component of the classification. Finally, the classification, like Wagner's, is not designed for wounds proximal to the foot. The Brodsky Depth-Ischemia Classification of Diabetic Foot Lesions generated a score of 4 ½ out of a possible ten on the criteria we generated for evaluating wound grading systems (Part II, Table 1 and Table 3-7). This suggests that Brodsky's system has limited utility as a wound classification system.

Utilization – Aside from Brodsky's own presentations and writings, there appears to be little information from others about the utilization of this system. Likewise, we are not aware of any validation or reliability studies using the Brodsky system. With the relative objectiveness of the criteria he provides to establish depth and ischemia, judged to be 1 ½ (on the 0 to 2 scale with 2 being optimal—see Part II, Table 1), his system should be suitable for validation studies to predict outcomes using his initial depth and ischemia grades. The relative specificity of the definitions Brodsky provides for each grade for wound depth and ischemia also makes it adaptable to reliability studies.

LAVERY, ARMSTRONG, AND HARKLESS

Characteristics and Basis of the Scoring System – Lavery, Armstrong, and Harkless generated a matrix wound grading system and published it in 1996 as the University of Texas Health Science Center San Antonio Diabetic Wound Classification[14] designed to predict wound outcomes. Wounds are divided into four depth grades (horizontal scale), from no wound to a wound penetrating to bone or joint and then subdivided into four stages (vertical scale), based on the absence or presence of infection, ischemia, or both (Table 3-4). Like the Brodsky classification, the San Antonio system generates 16 permutations. Since the assessment parameters of infection and ischemia are staged as either absent or present and wound depth is laid out on a continuum of four grades, the generation of a wound score is easy to obtain and fairly objective with this system.

Comments – The San Antonio system has many similarities to the Brodsky system, including 16 permutations and using the depth of the wound and degree of ischemia

TABLE 3-4. LAVERY, ARMSTRONG, AND HARKLESS-UNIVERSITY OF TEXAS SAN ANTONIO DIABETIC WOUND CLASSIFICATION

| | | ← Depth of Wound → | | | |
		0	**I**	**II**	**III**
Infection and/or Ischemia	**Stage A**	Pre- or post-ulcerative lesion completely epithelialized	Superficial wound, not involving tendon, capsule, or bone	Wound penetrating to tendon or capsule	Wound penetrating to bone or joint
	Stage B	Above depth with **infection**	Above depth with **infection**	Above depth with **infection**	Above depth with **infection**
	Stage C	Above depth with **ischemia**	Above depth with **ischemia**	Above depth with **ischemia**	Above depth with **ischemia**
	Stage D	Above depth with **infection and ischemia**	Above depth with **infection and ischemia**	Above depth with **infection and ischemia**	Above depth with **infection and ischemia**

as assessment parameters. Whereas Lavery and the co-authors use grades as the heading for depth and Roman numbers for each succeeding depth, Brodsky uses Arabic numbers with depth as the heading. Regardless, the depth assessments for all practical purposes are identical between the two systems. Like the Brodsky system, the scoring of the San Antonio system is logical, but intuitive understanding that a Grade III, Stage D wound is more serious than a Grade 0, Stage A wound is not inherent in the system. A strong criticism of the Lavery, et al. system is that it fails to consider the severity of infection and the degree of ischemia, and for classification purposes only considers these important parameters as present or absent. This leads to the second major criticism of this system, that it does not provide guidelines for management, where certainly the degree of ischemia and the severity of infection would be fundamental considerations. Other deficits of the San Antonio system include its failure to integrate the classification with other patient-related information (especially severity of infection and degree of ischemia), failure to be used as a tool to evaluate progress, and according to the authors, limited to the foot. The Lavery, et al. San Antonio Classification of Diabetic Foot Lesions generated a score of 5 out of a possible ten on the criteria we generated for evaluating wound grading systems (Part II, Table 1 and Table 3-7). This suggests that this system has limited utility as a wound classification system.

Utilization – Due to the visibility of the authors in podiatric and diabetes organization communities, the Lavery, et al., San Antonio classification has been much publicized.[14-17] Although this classification was criticized for lack of inherent evaluation and management guidelines, other articles by the authors have addressed these important considerations.[15, 18, 19] Unfortunately, their tabulated management format lacks logic as it has eight categories including two subdivisions, is not user-friendly (without the guideline immediately available, the user would be "lost" as to its applications), overuses the hedging adjective "possible" for management in seven of the eight categories, and has no apparent integration with their basic wound classification system. The Lavery, et al. San Antonio system deserves high marks (Graded 2 on the 0 to 2 scale with 2 demonstrating strong supportive information—Part II, Table 1) for the validation information it has generated for predicting outcomes. The authors' reported outcomes deteriorated with increasing stage and grade of the wound and the prevalence of amputation was statistically significant as the wounds increased in depth and stage.[18]

A study by Oyibo and co-workers using the Lavery, San Antonio system showed that increasing stage (presence or absence of infection and/or ischemia), regardless of

The study cited above included a review of 360 medical records. Wounds were tabulated by prevalence of each of the 16 categories and ranged from 0.6 percent for Grades 0 through II wounds with infection and ischemia to 25.8 percent for non-infected, non-ischemic wounds that were superficial and did not involve tendon, capsule, or bone.[18]

The prevalence of amputation ranged from 0 percent in all wounds that were neither ischemic nor infected to 100 percent in wounds that penetrated to tendon or capsule (Grade II) or bone or joint (Grade III) with both infection and ischemia present. Less than 4 percent of patients were in this latter group while almost half the patients were classified in the former group, thus strongly skewing the data collection to the less serious wounds where good outcomes would be anticipated.

grade (depth of wound), was associated with increased risk of amputation and prolonged ulcer healing time.[20, 21] We are unaware of any reliability studies using the San Antonio wound classification system. The organization and logicalness of the classification system should facilitate these types of studies.

JEFFCOATE AND MACFARLANE

Characteristics and Basis of the Scoring System - Jeffcoate and Macfarlane, from Nottingham, England, initially presented their classification of diabetic foot ulcers, "The S(AD) SAD System," in 1993 and later, in 1999, presented the same classification in "The Diabetic Foot".[22, 23]

The authors analyzed previously developed diabetic foot classifications, and felt due to the multiplicity of wounds that some of them were too simple to be practical and others too specific and detailed to be useful. They proposed a new classification that attempted to address these challenges using a matrix format like the two previously discussed for diabetic foot wound classifications (Table 3-5). While Jeffcoate and Macfar-

> The S(AD) SAD letters are an acronym where S = size (AD) = area and depth, S = sepsis, A = arteriopathy and D = denervation.
> The S(AD) terminology reflects the amplification of the authors' original SAD acronym to include size with its subcategories of area plus depth.

lane utilized infection, depth, and perfusion measures similar to the previous two classifications, they add wound size and denervation as two additional descriptive factors. This results in five descriptive factors each graded from 0 (best) to 3 (most severe) generating 20 permutations. The authors felt that a robust classification system is needed for prospective clinical research regarding ulcer management and in a subsequent paper present outcomes using their grading system.[23, 24]

> Sepsis, one of the headings in the S(AD) SAD Systems, has specific connotations including the presence of pathogenic organisms and/or their toxins in the blood and tissues with associated signs and symptoms of malaise, nausea, pain, rubor, swelling, erythema, leukocytosis, dysglcemia, positive blood cultures, or combinations of these.
> The information in the four cells in the sepsis column does not conform to this definition. Furthermore, osteomyelitis, presumably the worst of Macfarlane and Jeffcoate's sepsis conditions, may hardly invoke an inflammatory response in the patient with a chronically draining sinus.

Comments – Macfarlane and Jeffcoate's system is essentially a modification of the Brodsky and San Antonio wound classifications that adds size of wound and neuropathy to the other measurement parameters. However, their selection of descriptors is inconsistent and the criteria they provide for each heading and cell is not always logical.

Similar type inconsistencies and other diagnostic challenges are noted in the descriptions used in the cells under the arteriopathy and denervation columns. For

TABLE 3-5. MACFARLANE AND JEFFCOATE'S CLASSIFICATION OF DIABETIC FOOT ULCERS: THE S(AD) SAD* SYSTEM

Grade	Descriptors				
	Area	**Depth**	**Sepsis**	**Arteriopathy**	**Denervation**
0	Skin intact	Skin intact	No infection	Pedal pulses palpable	Pinprick sensation/VPT** normal
1	< 10 mm²	Skin and subcutaneous tissues	Superficial: slough or exudates	Diminution of both pulses or absence of one	Reduced or absent pin prick sensation, VPT raised
2	10-30 mm²	Tendon, joint, capsule, periosteum	Cellulitis	Absence of both pedal pulses	Neuropathy dominant: palpable pedal pulses
3	>30 mm²	Bone and/or joint spaces	Osteomyeliits	Gangrene	Charcot foot

KEY: * **S(AD) SAD** = Size (area and depth); sepsis, arteriopathy, denervation

** **VPT** = Vibration perception threshold

example, evaluation of perfusion status includes palpation of pulses, which is not always a reliable technique to detect tissue ischemia. Other questions arise about the clinical significance of a 1 square cm (Grade 1) wound versus a 3 square cm (Grade 3) wound. Certainly, massive sloughs such as loss of the plantar flap of a transmetatarsal amputation have clinical significance, but the difference between a 1 and 3 square cm wound is probably negligible. It is arguable whether Charcot foot should be considered the endpoint of the denervation continuum, since other factors such as hyperemia and loss of proprioception may be more important contributors to this problem than loss of sensation. In summary, the Macfarlane and Jeffcoate classification adds two other dimensions to diabetic foot wound analysis, namely size and neuropathy, but it is questionable how this additional information helps define the overall seriousness of the wound or helps as a guide to management. This classification system generated a score of 3 ½ out of a possible ten on the criteria we generated for evaluating wound grading systems (Part II, Table 1 and Table 3-7). This suggests that this system is probably not useful for evaluation and management of wounds.

The classification suggests that gangrene is the endpoint of the arteriopathy continuum and due to ischemia. Gangrene could also be the result of infection, trauma, venous congestion or vasculitis.

Pulses may not be palpable in the edematous, severely deformed, scarified but adequately perfused foot while they may be present even though portions of the foot are gangrenous.

An apparent contradiction is seen in the authors' description of grade 2 arteriopathy pathology as absence of both pedal pulses while palpable pedal pulses are a criteria used for grade 2 denervation pathology.

Utilization – Even though the Macfarlane and Jeffcoate system appears to be user friendly, we did not find any other journal publications that utilized this system in clinical practice. However, the *Diabetic Foot* journal which published this classification contains letters from different specialists that indicate that this system is used in some European countries.[23] The only patient-related clinical parameter that is included in this classification is the presence of neuropathy. Other significant patient-related information such as host function, nutrition assessment or patient motivation factors, as is absent in the other wound matrix formatted classifications previously discussed, are also not integrated into this classification system. A single validity study in 300 patients showed that area, depth and arteriopathy were all independent predictors of outcome.[24] Because of the 25 permutations inherent in the system and the failure of the authors to summate the scores into seriousness categories, meaningful comparisons of wounds could be an unwieldy challenge. The authors do not suggest that their system be used to follow progress over time, although improving grades for most of the five descriptors would be expected as the wound healing progresses. Although no reliablility studies were noted, this system with delineation of specific findings for each grade, like the other two matrix systems, should facilitate this type of study

FOSTER AND EDMONDS

Characteristics and Basis of the Scoring System – In 2000, one year after "The S(AD) SAD System" was published in *The Diabetic Foot*, Foster and Edmonds, from London, England, published their "Simple Staging System" in the same journal. The expressed purpose of their efforts was to develop a system that would help in the diagnosis and management of the diabetic foot.[25] The authors described six stages of the diabetic foot and provided recommendations for management of each stage. Significant events that lead to complications are the basis for the staging system. When viewed in order they describe the natural history of the diabetic foot "on the road to amputation." The stages are as follows:

- **Stage 1:** The diabetic foot **without risk factors** for ulceration
- **Stage 2:** Neuropathy, ischemia deformity, edema and callus, the **well-known risk factors** for ulceration
- **Stage 3: Ulceration** is a pivotal event on the road to amputation and requires urgent and aggressive management
- **Stage 4: Infection** delays healing and can destroy tissue with alarming rapidity
- **Stage 5: Necrosis** is the result of tissue destruction from **infection and ischemia**
- **Stage 6:** When the foot is destroyed, major **amputation** is inevitable; the final stage

The authors give detailed descriptions for each stage. The original article provided recommendations for each stage, including: mechanical control, microbiological control, metabolic control, vascular control, wound control, and educational control.

Comments – Each stage encompasses relatively broad clinical conditions of the diabetic foot and correspondingly lacks specific, objective characteristics that would be helpful to define each stage. This makes the system imprecise. The differences between Stages 1 and 2 are the absence or presence of risk factors. In clinical practice, most of the diabetic patients have risk factors. Diabetes itself is a significant risk factor. Identification of other risk factors may be dependent on the experience of the evaluator and how diligently the risk factors are sought. Consequently, the phrase "diabetic foot without risk factors" is ambiguous. Amputation differentiates Stages 5 and 6, but may be a function of management rather than the natural history of diabetes. Wound severity is not mentioned other than the comment that the higher the stage, the more severe the wound. This system resembles the Wagner system, where for every grade a different criterion was used. In the Wagner system, ulcers or wounds are present in 5 out of 6 stages. Foster and Edmonds' "Simple Staging System" includes ulcers or wounds in 4 out of the 6 stages. The general concensus is that the "Simple Staging System" is oversimplified. This system appears to be more of a description of what could happen to the diabetic foot without appropriate management than a classification system. This classification system generated a score of 3 out of a possible ten on the criteria generated for evaluating wound grading systems (Part II, Table 1 and Table 3-7). This suggests that this system is probably not useful for evaluation and management of wounds.

Utilization – The authors' recommendations for evaluation and management of diabetic foot problems are sound not only for wound management, but also for patient care such as diagnostic procedures, type of local wound care, optimization of metabolic control, and patient education. However, the "Simple Staging System" itself does not include any patient-related information such as mobility status , cardiac function, smoking history, neurological deficits, etc. No information validating or showing the reliability of this system was found. The system presents a number of descriptions rather than a classification. For example, Stage 6 is described as a foot that is "unsalvageable." This term could be used to describe prognosis of the wound, but not the wound itself. Because of the open-endedness of the descriptions, we would predict that the reliability, like that of the Wagner score, would be low. At worst, this grading system is an oversimplified version of a group of wound descriptions. At best, it is a useful diagnostic tool and management guide for diabetic foot infections.

YOUNES, ET AL.

Characteristics and Basis of the Scoring System – In 2002, Younes and his co-authors published a wound scoring system that added a dimension to wound scoring systems that had not been utilized by the previous authors.[26] The dimension was that of using a point system to quantify the severity of the wound (Table 3-6). The authors titled their score the "DEPA" score with "D" representing the depth, "E" the extent, "P" the phase, and "A" the associated etiology for foot ulcers. Four parameters were graded on a 1 (best) to 3 (most severe) scale with the best possible score being three and the worst possible score being 12. Based on the scores, the wounds were classified as low-grade ulcers (DEPA scores =/< 6), moderate grade ulcers (DEPA scores = 7-9), and high-grade ulcers (DEPA score =/>10). Five of the 12 parameter descriptions required additional clarification such as "Necrotizing Infection: infected ulcer with surrounding cellulitis or fasciitis (Table 3-6)." The authors demonstrate how their DEPA score helps them in determining their treatment strategies and predicted outcomes.[27] For example, low-grade ulcers are managed with outpatient care, moderate-grade ulcers with one to two weeks of inpatient hospitalization, and high-grade ulcers with hospital care including surgeries, revascularization, amputations, etc. until the patient is stabilized.

Comments – Younes and his co-authors' general scoring parameters represent a continuum of findings for each DEPA parameter. The first, the depth of the ulcer, is quite logical ranging from skin to soft tissue to bone. However, the other three DEPA parameters have vague components, do not necessarily represent a continuum of find-ings, and contain choices that are not mutually exclusive. Examples of these inconsis-tencies are described in the text box below:

> Infection, given a score of 2 in the extent of bacterial invasion category, could range from a superficial wound exudate, to cellulitis, to an abscess, to floridly infected necrotic tissue with associated systemic sepsis. This overlaps with necrotizing infection which is a 3-score. The authors' criteria for this score are an infected ulcer with surrounding cellutilis or fasciitis.
>
> A timeframe is given for the phase of ulcer category. Each of the parameters (granulating, inflammatory, and/or nonhealing) could fit into the time ranges given by the authors. Granulating and inflammatory terms have overlapping meanings.
>
> Neuropathy, bone deformity, and ischemia of the associated etiology param-eter are also overlapping terms that could be present in any ulcer. Furthermore, the degree of severity and consequences of each of the associated finding could range from inconsequential to limb threatening.

TABLE 3-6. THE DEPTH, EXTENT, PHASE, AND ASSOCIATED ETIOLOGY SCORE FOR FOOT ULCERS

DEPA[1] Criteria	← DEPA[1] Score—General Ulcer Parameters →		
	1-Score	**2-Scores**	**3-Scores**
Depth of the Ulcer	Skin	Soft Tissue	Bone
Extent of Bacterial Invasion	Contamination	Infection	Necrotizing Infection (Infected ulcer with surrounding cellulitis or fasciitis)
Phase of Ulcer	Granulating (Evidence of granulation tissue formation)	Inflammatory (Hyperemic ulcer with no granulation tissue <2 weeks duration)	Nonhealing (Non-granulating ulcer > 2 weeks duration)
Associated Etiology	Neuropathy	Bone Deformity	Ischemia (Clinical signs of acute or chronic arterial insufficiency)

KEY: [1] **DEPA (D=** Depth of Ulcer, **E =** Extent of Bacterial Invasion, **P =** Phase of Ulcer and **A =** Associated Etiology)

DEPA SCORING: 6 Points or less = Low-grade ulcers

7-9 Points = Moderate grade ulcers

10 Points or greater = High grade ulcers

The general ulcer parameters are not intuitive and/or logical enough to be easily remembered; that is, a summary of the information probably needs to be available to generate a score. The authors deserve credit for providing information on how to manage each grade of ulcer (i.e. low, moderate or high-grade) and including the appearance of the wound base (i.e. phase of the ulcer) in their classification.[27] The authors did not state that as the wounds improve, the DEPA scores decrease, thereby making this a static rather than a dynamic classification system. Like the matrix systems, the DEPA scores are not intuitively obvious, with a range of 3 to 12 and, as would not be expected, higher scores are worse than lower scores. The scoring parameters each graded with ordinate numbers from 1 to 3 are not to be proportioned (e.g. giving a score of 1 ½), should a DEPA criterion such as phase of an ulcer need to quantify a wound that is half granulating and half hyperemic.

The DEPA classification system generated a score of 6 ½ out of a possible ten on the criteria generated for evaluating wound grading systems (Part II, Table 1 and Table 3-7). This suggests that this system had utility, although limited, for evaluation and management of wounds. The main concerns with this system are problems with objectivity and logic of the scoring parameters, lack of adaptability to sites other than the foot, and reliability.

Utilization – The grading of wound parameters and classification of wounds by severity has many merits as is reflected by the highest total score of any of the nine wound grading systems analyzed. However, except for the authors' publications, other references to the DEPA score were not found. The authors' own validity study for predicting outcomes gives them high marks (i.e. 1 ½ out of two points) for this criterion (Part II, Table 1 and Table 3-7).[28] Unfortunately, more than half the wounds (49 in 84 patients =58%) were low-grade ulcers, where excellent results would be anticipated regardless of the grading system or standard management practices. Their system predicted outcome of management with a correlation coefficient of 0.78 in the 84 patients studied. Although no reliability studies were provided by the authors, the system, with its relatively objective scoring parameters, would facilitate a reliability study. In summary, this grading system sets a standard for wound classifications by separating wounds into classes of severity based upon relatively objective scoring criteria.

CONCLUSIONS

Wound classification systems should be multifunctional with primary goals to provide objective, reproducible evaluations, and direct appropriate interventions for management. The evaluation of nine different grading systems designed for diabetic foot wounds show that "what you see is not always what you have." That is, the information from one classification system could have quite different interpretations than the information from another system. Different classifications serve different purposes. Some classifications are good for describing the gross characteristics of wounds (e.g., Wagner), some allow prediction of outcome (e.g., Younes), and others facilitate comparisons of wound treatment interventions (e.g., Knighton). Which system is right and which is wrong? The criteria to evaluate wound grading systems (Part II, Table 1 and Table 3-7) is a tool that helps to answer this question. When using these criteria, most

TABLE 3-7. SCORING SUMMARY OF THE WOUND GRADING CLASSIFICATIONS

Grading System	Year	Type	Criteria to Evaluate Wound Grading Systems (Part II, Table 1)					Total
			OBJ	ADAP	MGMT	VAL	REL	
Wagner	1981	Descriptive	1	1/2	1 1/2	1	0	**4**
Forrest	1981	Descriptive	1	2	1 1/2	0	0	**4 1/2**
Knighton	1986	Descriptive	1 1/2	1/2	1/2	1/2	0	**3**
Pecoraro	1990	Descriptive	1/2	1	1/2	1/2	0	**2 1/2**
Brodsky	1993	Matrix	1 1/2	1	1 1/2	1/2	1/2	**5**
Lavery	1996	Matrix	1 1/2	1	0	2	1/2	**5**
Macfarlane	1999	Matrix	1	1	0	1	1/2	**3 1/2**
Foster	2000	Descriptive	1	1/2	1 1/2	0	0	**3**
Younes	2002	Wound Severity	1 1/2	1 1/2	2	1	1/2	**6 1/2**

KEY: **ADAP** = Adaptability, **MGMT** = Management, **OBJ** = Objectivity, **REL** = Reliability, and **VAL** = Validity

of the grading systems discussed are probably not useful for the contemporary evaluation and management of challenging wounds. It is interesting to observe that as time progressed, the scoring systems evolved with almost 100 percent consistency from descriptions of wounds to matrix formatting to classification of wounds by severity based on relatively objective scoring criteria. The number of wound classifications that are currently used indicates that there is still no single-objective, universally accepted classification that quantifies complex information about wounds, guides treatment strategies, predicts outcomes, measures wound progress, and is ideally suited for clinical trials. After discussing the classification systems for wounds of another type, namely pressure sores, in the next chapter, we will introduce a **Wound Score** (Chapter 5) that addresses (and we feel resolves) the deficiencies demonstrated in all of the other wound classifications.

QUESTIONS

1. What are some of the criteria used in the Wagner Grading System?

2. What are the main criteria for determining the wound type in Forrest and Gamborg-Nilsen classification?

3. What are advantages and disadvantages of Knighton's wound system?

4. Why do you think the Seattle Wound Classification System is not widely used in clinical practice?

5. In which way is San Antonio system similar to the Brodsky system?

6. Is Foster and Edmund's "Simple Staging System" oversimplified?

7. Which of the known wound classifications discussed in this chapter would be the best for clinical research purposes?

8. Which of the discussed classifications systems allows physicians to determine the need for amputation vs. limb preservation?

9. Which classification system considers ischemia as an evaluation criterion?

10. Which of the discussed classifications systems provides a tool for monitoring progress?

REFERENCES

1. Meggitt B. Surgical management of the diabetic foot. Br J Hosp Med. 1976;16:227–332

2. Wagner FW. The dysvascular foot: a system of diagnosis and treatment. Foot Ankle 1981; 2: 64–122

3. Wagner FW. Classification and treatment program for diabetic, neuropathic and dysvascular foot problems. Instructional Course Lectures 28. American Academy of Orthopaedic Surgeons;1979

4. Centers for Medicare & Medicaid Services. Coverage of hyperbaric oxygen (HBO) therapy for the treatment of diabetic wounds of the lower extremities. Transmittal AB-02-183. December 27, 2002

5. Smith RG. Validation of Wagner's classification, a literature review, osteotomy wound management, 2003; 49:54-60

6. Forrest RD, Gamborg-Neilsen P. Wound assessment in clinical practice: a critical review of methods and their application. Acta Med Scand. 687:69-74, 1984

7. Knighton DR, Ciresi KF, Fiegel VD, Austin LL, Butler EL. Classification and treatment of chronic nonhealing wounds: successful treatment with autologous platelet- derived wound healing factors (PDWHF). Ann Surg. 204:332-330, 1986

8. Dooley J, Schirmer J, Slade B et al. Use of transcutaneous pressure of oxygen on the evaluation of edematous wounds. Undersea Hyperbaric Medicine 1996;23(3):167-174

9. Pecoraro RE, Reiber GE. Classification of wounds in diabetic amputees. Wounds 1990;2: 65-73

10. Litzelman DK, Marriott DJ, Vinicor F. Independent physiological predictors of foot lesions in patients with NIDDM. Diabetes Care. 1997 Aug;20(8):1273-8

11. Litzelman DK, Marriott DJ, Vinicor F. The role of footwear in the prevention of foot lesions in patients with NIDDM. Conventional wisdom or evidence-based practice? Diabetes Care. 1997 Feb;20(2):156-62

12. Brodsky JW. Outpatient diagnosis and care of the diabetic foot. Instr Couse Lect, 1993; 42:121-139

13. Brodsky, JW. The diabetic foot, in surgery of the foot and ankle, 2007, Ed. MJ Coughlin, RA Mann, CL Saltzman, Mosby, Elsevier, Philadelphia, pp1295-1301

14. Lavery LA, Armstrong DG, Harkless LB. Classification of diabetic foot wounds. J Foot Ankle Surg 1996; 35: 528–31

15. Armstrong DG, Lavery LA, Harkless LB. Treatment-based classification system for assessment and care of diabetic feet. J Am Podiatr Med Assoc. 1996 Jul;86(7):311-6

16. Lavery LA, Armstrong DG, Harkless LB. Classification of diabetic foot wounds. Ostomy Wound Manage. 1997 Mar;43(2):44-8, 50, 52-3

17. Armstrong DG, Lavery LA. Diabetic foot ulcers: prevention, diagnosis and classification. Am Fam Physician. 1998 Mar 15;57(6):1325-32, 1337-8

18. Armstrong DG, Lavery LA, Harkless LB. Validation of a diabetic wound classification system. The contribution of depth, infection, and ischemia to risk of amputation. Diabetes Care. 1998 May;21(5):855-9

19. Lavery LA, Armstrong DG, Vela SA, Quebedeaux TL, Fleischli JG. Practical criteria for screening patients at high risk for diabetic foot ulceration

20. Oyibo SO, Jude EB, Tarawneh I, Nguyen HC, Armstrong DG, Harkless LB, Boulton AJ. The effects of ulcer size and site, patient's age, sex and type and duration of diabetes on the outcome of diabetic foot ulcers. Diabet Med. 2001 Feb;18(2):133-8

21. Oyibo SO, Jude EB, Tarawneh I, Nguyen HC, Harkless LB, Boulton AJ. A comparison of two diabetic foot ulcer classification systems: the Wagner and the University of Texas wound classification systems. Diabetes Care. 2001 Jan;24(1):84-8

22. Jeffcoate WJ, Macfarlane RM, Fletcher EM. The description and classification of diabetic foot lesions. Diabet Med. 1993 Aug-Sep;10(7):676-9

23. Macfarlane RM, Jeffcoate WJ. Classification of diabetic foot ulcers: The S(AD) SAD system. Diabetic Foot 1999; 2: 123–7

24. Treece KA, Macfarlane RM, Pound N, Game FL, Jeffcoate WJ. Validation of a system of foot ulcer classification in diabetes mellitus. Diabet Med. 2004 Sep;21(9):987-91

25. Foster A, Edmonds ME. Simple staging system: a tool for diagnosis and management. Diabetic Foot 2000; 3: 56–62

26. Younes NA, S Alhadidi, AM Albsoul, T AbuSalah. New scoring system for diabetic foot infections, Jordan Med J, 2002; 36:22-28

27. Younes, YA, AM Albsoul, A Hamzeh. Diabetic heel ulcers: a major risk factor for lower extremity amputation, Ostomy Wound Management, 2004, 50(6): 50-60

28. Younes NA, AM Albsoul. The DEPA Scoring System and its correlation with the healing rate of diabetic foot ulcers, J Foot Ankle Surgery, 2004 43(4): 209-213

CHAPTER

CLASSIFICATION SYSTEMS FOR PRESSURE ULCERS/INDOLENT WOUNDS

CHAPTER FOUR OVERVIEW

INTRODUCTION 87

THE SHEA GRADING SYSTEM FOR PRESSURE ULCERATIONS 91

BATES-JENSEN PRESSURE SORE STATUS TOOL (PSST) 93

THE SESSING SCALE FOR PRESSURE ULCER HEALING 95

THE PRESSURE ULCER SCALE FOR HEALING (PUSH) 97

NATIONAL PRESSURE ULCER ADVISORY PANEL (NPUAP)
  STAGING SYSTEM FOR PRESSURE ULCERATIONS 99

WOUND HEALING SCALE 101

THE SUSSMAN WOUND HEALING TOOL (SWHT) 102

MEDICARE CLASSIFICATION OF DECUBITUS ULCERS 104

CONCLUSIONS 104

QUESTIONS 106

REFERENCES 107

"A pressure sore is not always a sore for pressure."

INTRODUCTION

While pressure ulcers have many similarities to diabetic foot wounds, they also have many differences. The differences provide justification for authors and committees to generate pressure classification systems, eight of which will be discussed in this chapter. Many terminologies have been used to describe these conditions (Table 4-1). The common terminology appears to be pressure sores, but other terminology may be more appropriate. Decubitus ulcer is also one of the common descriptive terms.[1] The reality of the situation is that the terms decubitus ulcer and pressure sore in themselves can be

> Decubitus ulcer is defined as a chronic ulcer that appears in pressure areas of skin overlying a bony prominence in debilitated patients confined to bed or otherwise immobilized due to a circulatory defect.[1]
>
> When the phrase pressure ulcer is cross-referenced in this same dictionary citation, the reader is referred to the synonym decubitus ulcer, which suggests decubitus is the preferred terminology.
>
> The term decubitus refers to the position of the patient in bed and can be supine, lateral, semi-lateral, etc. However, not all pressure/decubitus ulcers are associated with lying in bed, as will be explained next.

misleading. Pressure/decubitus ulcers need not be associated with bed rest (that is, lying in the decubitus position), nor from direct pressure itself. First of all, these wounds can occur with wheel chair sitting as is especially seen in spinal cord injured patients. Secondly, many wounds labeled as pressure sores may not be due to pressure over bony prominences (Figure 4-1). Tension (rather than pressure) sores over bony prominences secondary to joint contractures and ulcers from shear stresses are examples. The phrase indolent wound, with the definition as follows, may be a more appropriate, comprehensive, and descriptive term than decubitus ulcer.

> Indolent wound—a difficult to manage, slow to heal and/or non-healing wound associated with inactivity and/or linked to immobility and invariably associated with comorbidities including deformities (usually secondary to neurological deficits), undissipated forces (pressure, shear or tension) over bony prominences, ischemia, malnutrition, and moisture retention.

For these reasons, the phrase "pressure sores/indolent wounds" will be used when appropriate in this chapter.

Scope of the Problem – Pressure ulcers and indolent wounds are an enormous problem in our society. It is understandable why attention to prevention and so many different classification systems exist. These wounds are estimated to affect 1.3 to 3 million new patients each year in the USA alone.[2, 3] With a cost of nearly $40,000 per episode, this could add 40 to 100 billion dollars a year to the health care system.[4] A very proactive

TABLE 4-1. TISSUE DISRUPTION TERMINOLOGIES AND THEIR DESCRIPTIONS [1]

Name	Definitions and Comments (Bolded items have special significance for pressure sores/indolent wounds)
Generic Terms — Erosion	A **wearing away** or a state of being worn away, as by friction or pressure
Sore	A wound, ulcer, or any **open skin lesion**
Ulcer	A lesion through the skin or a mucous membrane resulting from **loss of tissue**, usually with **inflammation.**
Wound	**Trauma** to body tissues, especially that caused by **physical means** and with **interruption of continuity**
Specific Ulcer Terms — Acute Decubitus Ulcer	A severe form of bedsore, of neurotrophic origin occurring in hemipledgia, parapledgia or other **neurologically impaired** patients
Chronic Ulcer	**Long standing** ulcer with **fibrous tissue** in the floor of the ulcer
Decubitus Ulcer	See first text box for this chapter; other synonyms include **bedsore**, decubital **gangrene**, hospital gangrene, **pressure** gangrene, pressure sore, **pressure ulcer**
Indolent Ulcer	A **chronic ulcer** with **hard elevated edges** and few or no granulations and showing no tendency to heal
Trophic Ulcer	Wound from **cutaneous sensory denervation over bony prominence** such as **perforating ulcer** of the foot i.e. malperforans ulcer

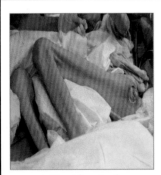
a. Trochanteric Tension Sore

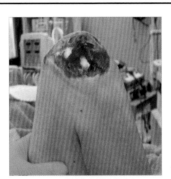
b. Pre-patellar Tension Sore

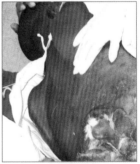
c. Low Back Shear Wound

Legend: These wounds, which might be labeled as pressure sores, have etiologies other than pressure. Wounds in figures a and b are due to tension over bony prominences. The Figure c wound is attributed to sliding forces associated with wheel chair activity.

In almost all indolent wounds, comorbidities such as neurological impairment (stroke, spinal cord injury, degenerative conditions, etc.), peripheral artery disease, and malnutrition contribute to the problem.

Contractures secondary to neurological impairments are particularly pernicious in contributing to indolent wounds and often are impossible to prevent or treat without major surgeries such as contracture releases, lower limb amputations, or complex myocutaneousflaps.

Figure 4-1. Indolent wounds – not decubitus ulcers.

approach is being taken with respect to prevention of pressure ulcers/indolent wounds. When the system "breaks down," there can be legal consequences possibly directed to the family caring for the patient under the guise of elder abuse or ascribed to neglect of the caregivers, if the patient is institutionalized. Evaluation of skin integrity and classification of pressure ulcers/indolent wounds needs to be an essential nursing routine for all "at risk" patients at the time of their admission to a treatment facility and on a regular basis thereafter. Conversely, there are two known risk factors associated with the development of these problems. First, in certain conditions, especially in those patients with multiple comorbidities, the skin may fail as an organ system, just as "end-stage" events occur in other organ systems. The second reason failures occur in maintaining skin

> When "end-stage" events such as severe ischemic strokes in the nervous system, myocardial infarctions with resultant congestive heart failure, and severe malabsorption in the gastrointestinal system develop, interventions do not usually improve the organ systems to their former physiological states. Patients have no choice but to live with the limitations these conditions impose upon them.
>
> When "end-stage" events develop in the skin, should there be a different set of standards than there is for breakdowns in other organ systems? Outcomes of litigation might suggest otherwise. The reality of the situation is that each patient and skin integrity problem has to be dealt with on an individual basis.

integrity is due to the presence of deformities that are so severe that without their corrections, it is almost impossible to prevent wounds from occurring or heal wounds that already exist. Additional information about evaluation and management of the "end-stage" pressure sore/indolent wound is presented in Chapter 12.

Scoring Systems that Measure Risk Factors for Developing Pressure Sores/Indolent Wounds – A number of pressure ulcer risk scales have been developed. These scales are important because they provide predictive value for those at risk for pressure sore/indolent wound development, establish levels of severity and dictate what interventions are needed. In the early 1960's, Norton developed the first risk assessment instrument. It consisted of five subscales including **1) physical condition, 2) mental state, 3) activity, 4) mobility, and 5) incontinence**.

Each subscale was graded on a 1 (worst) to 4 (best) giving a range of scores from 5 (highest risk) to 20 points (lowest risk).[5, 6] Gosnell refined the Norton scale with her own nomenclature including 1) mental status with one to five grades, 2) continence, 3) mobility, 4) activity each with one to four grades, and 5) nutrition with one to three grades. This generated a 5 (lowest risk) to 20 (highest risk) scale.[7] In 1985, Waterlow developed a pressure sore risk scale, which was designed to be used to assess a patient for the risk of developing a pressure sore. It consisted of eight parameters with multiple sub-parameters and eight special risk factors. Grades for each risk factor varied from 0-8 points, with the sum of all variables achieving total score of 0 to >45 points. The author's interpretation was the lower the score the lower the risk factor, with a score of >20 indicating a very high risk for pressure ulcer development.[8] Gosnell also described other information to be recorded such as vital signs, diet, fluid balance, interventions, medications, color, and general skin appearance (with 3 subcategories including moisture, temperature and texture), but did not include these in the actual scoring. It appears that the most widely used instrument for wound risk assessment in the USA is the one developed by Braden.[9-11] In the Braden scale, six criteria that include **1) sensory perception, 2) moisture, 3) activity, 4) mobility, 5) nutrition, and 6) friction and shear** are graded on one (worst possible situation) to three (for friction and shear), or four (for the other 5 criteria) with the higher the number the less concern that the criterion is problematic. This generates a possible scoring range of 6 to 23. The scores are then lumped into risk stratifications as follows: 15-18 points = mild risk, 13-14 points = moderate risk, 10-12 points = high risk, and 9 or less points = very high risk. Unlike the diabetic foot classifications, at least one quality reliability and validity study has been published.[12,13] The Braden Scale generated a predictive efficacy (correct positive and negative predictions combined) of 66.7, the best in the series. However, the Gosnell Scale had the highest sensitivity in predicting pressure sore risk. Inter-rater reliability between the investigators and the research staff was 0.95.

Other Risk Factor Instruments – In 1999 Salzberg, et al. published a scale to predict pressure ulcers during initial hospitalization for acute spinal cord injury.[14] Data was analyzed in 226 patients hospitalized for spinal cord injury with the endpoint criteria being the presence or absence of pressure ulcers during the first 30 days of hospitalization. The authors did univariate analysis of 8 factors including **1) extent of paralysis, 2) level of activity, 3) mobility, 4) urine incontinence, 5) moisture, 6) pulmonary disease, 7) serum creatinine, and 8) albumin**. Various evaluation parameters were used ranging from four for extent of paralysis (paraparesis, quadraparesis, parapledgia and quadripledgia) to yes or no choices for items 4, 5, 7, and 8. Not surprisingly, almost no ulcers occurred in the patients who were in the highest functional levels of the mobility measurements. Autonomic dysreflexia, mental status, tobacco use, diabetes, anemia, or renal disease did not demonstrate statistically significant correlations with pressure ulcer development. The authors reported that their criteria were more accurate in predicting ulcer development than the Braden and other scales they tested. In 2005 Ohura, et al. published an ingenious risk measurement scale for pressure ulcers with demonstration of its usefulness in clinical practice.[15] They considered four parameters: 1) self-sustainability (possible = 0, intermediate = 1.5 and impossible = 3), 2) bony prominence (none = 0, mild = 1.5 and severe = 3), 3) edema (absent = 0, present = 3), and 4) articular contraction (absent = 0, present = 1). This generates scores ranging from 0 (low risk level for ulcer) to 10 (extreme risk for pressure ulcer occurrence). Scores were tabulated into risk level, probability of pressure ulcer, and expected healing period columns (Table 4-2).

A New Tool for Predicting the Occurrence of Pressure Ulcers/Indolent Wounds – With more than 200 risk factors reported for predicting the occurrence of pressure sores, some must be more important than others.[13] In the five systems for ulcer prediction presented in the preceding paragraphs, some parameters are used repeatedly, thus indicating there is some unanimity in what is considered important. However, there is little intuitive logic for scoring except for perhaps the Ohura system. Additionally, without scoring sheets to work from, there is little likelihood that accurate scores for each of the systems could be generated. Finally, without a written summary of the scores ascribed for each risk level, the predictability of pressure ulcer/indolent wound development is not automatically obvious. Consequently, we developed a simple to use, intuitive **Pressure Ulcer/Indolent Wound Prediction Tool** (Table 4-3). By utilizing the 5 most likely factors that contribute to the occurrence of pressure ulcer/indolent wounds and giving each assessment a grade from 0 (worst circumstance) to 2 (best circumstance), a 0 to 10 score is generated with 10 being best and 0 worst. The likelihood of pressure ulcer/indolent wound development becomes obvious from the 0 to 10 score achieved.

We selected the five factors most important for the prediction of pressure ulcers/indolent wound occurrences and the ones most consistently utilized (although with somewhat different terminology) in the systems described above.

These factors (termed assessments to be consistent with other 10 point scores used in this text) include 1) deformity, 2) forces, 3) ischemia, 4) malnutrition, and 5) moisture retention.

Unfortunately, like the Ohura-Hotta system, no validity or reliability scores are available for this system other than our own observations.

The remainder of this chapter analyzes eight published pressure sore/indolent wound scoring systems using the same criteria as used for the diabetic foot wound classifications (Chapter 3). A goal of this analysis is to look for assessments that are uniformly found throughout the current pressure ulcer/indolent wound scoring systems. From this information, it will be seen that the most important assessments have been integrated into our **Wound Score** evaluation tool (Chapter 6).

TABLE 4-2. OBSERVATIONS FROM THE OH (OHURA-HOTTA) SCALE[15]

Total Score	Risk Level	Probability of Pressure Ulcer	Expected Healing Period
0	Very Low	Not applicable	Not applicable
1 to 3	Low	Equal to or <25 %	6 weeks
4 to 6	Intermediate	26-65 %	8 weeks
7 to 10	High	Equal to > 66 %	25 weeks

OH Scoring System: 1) **Self-sustainability** (Possible = 0, intermediate = 1.5 and impossible = 3), 2) **Bony prominence** (None = 0, mild = 1.5 and severe = 3), **Edema** (Absent = 0, present = 3) and **Articular contraction** (Absent = 0, present = 1).

THE SHEA GRADING SYSTEM FOR PRESSURE ULCERATIONS

Basis of the Scoring System – In 1975, Shea published one of the first grading systems for pressure sores.[16] It helped wound care specialists communicate with each other by providing a common language to describe the different appearances of pressure sores. This system has provided a pattern for other classification systems. In fact,

TABLE 4-3. PRESSURE ULCER/INDOLENT WOUND PREDICTION TOOL-STRAUSS

Assessment	2 Points	1 Point	0 Points	Interpretation (Summation of grades from the 5 assessments)
		Use half points if findings intermediate between to grade points		
Deformity (Usually associated with neurological deficit)	None	Minimal-to-moderate (Minimal interference with function)	Severe Severely interferes with function	**8 to 10 Points** Minimal to no risk to generate a PS/IW*
Forces Pressure, shear or tension	None Apparent	Apparent, but no problems have arisen	Present with visible problems	**4 to 7 Points** At risk for generation of a PS/IW*
Ischemia	None (Palpable pulses, skin coloration and capillary refill OK)	Mild to moderate (Doppler pulses, poor skin coloration and capillary refill)	Severe (Necrotic tissue in wound)	
Malnutrition	None	Mild to moderate (Depressed visceral proteins)	Severe (Markedly abnormal visceral proteins)	**0 to 3 Points** Severe risk and/or a PS/IW* already present
Moisture Retention	No Problems	Adequately controlled	Inadequately controlled	

Key: * PS/IW = Pressure sore/indolent wound

all of the pressure ulcer classifications described in this chapter use information from Shea's system to some extent. The Shea system is a five-grade scale that is based on the depth and general appearance of the ulcer (Table 4-4). The system also includes clinical signs and symptoms that may accompany the wound presentation. Shea provides treatment, primarily surgical recommendations, for each of the five grades in his classification.

Comments – Most of Shea's classification criteria are descriptive and not quantifiable. The system primarily targets the depth of the wound, as almost all the other succeeding pressure ulcer classification systems do. The step-wise depth of the wound evaluation makes determination of the wound grade fairly objective. However, in many situations a wound might show components of two or more grades or be in a transition phase between two grades. The author considers the appearance of the wound base and the severity of infection, but does not include other important wound parameters such as size or perfusion. Regardless, the parameters he mentioned are considered either as present or absent with no provision for measuring the degree of involvement such as minimal, moderate, or severe. Shea suggests that the degree of inflammation/infection and the seriousness of the patient's condition are directly related to the depth of the wound. This is not always correct, for superficial wounds may be a source of bacteremia and sepsis while deep wounds may have limited inflammatory signs. The Shea system does not consider systemic conditions such as neurological deficits, diabetes, peripheral artery disease, etc. in the evaluation and management of wounds. The measurement of progress is not a component of this classification system.

Utilization – The system is still widely used in different parts of the world because it is simple, well-known, and provides guidelines for wound management (e.g., local

TABLE 4-4. SHEA GRADING SYSTEM FOR PRESSURE ULCERATIONS[16]

Grade	Findings	Additional Description	Treatment Strategy
I	**Acute inflammatory reaction and/or superficial ulceration**	Involves all soft tissue layers of the skin with erythema of the skin. Moist, irregular, partial thickness ulceration limited to the epidermis. Exposure of underlying dermis may be present	**Local wound care**
II	**Acute inflammatory reaction involving all soft tissue layers**	Full thickness skin ulcer involving the dermis. May extend to but not go into the underlying subcutaneous fat present	**Local wound care**
III	**Ulcer extensively involving the subcutaneous fat**	Undermining of the skin, but limited by the deep fascia. Often necrotic, infected and foul smelling; The patient may be toxic with systemic symptoms	**Surgical debridement**
IV	**Ulcer has penetrated the deep fascia**	Extensive soft tissue spread, osteomyelitis and/or septic and dislocated joints. Patient usually very toxic	**Radical surgical debridement**
Closed	**Large cavity draining through a relatively small sinus**	Typically overlies a bony prominence; With or without muscle and bone involvement	**Surgery with wide excision**

wound care vs. radical surgery). The Shea system has been used to investigate the effectiveness of different therapeutic interventions and in epidemiologic studies.[17, 18] No information was found about validation or reliability studies using the Shea system. The Shea pressure ulcer classification system generated a score of 4 out of a possible ten on the criteria generated for evaluating wound grading systems (Part II, Table 1 and Table 4-4). This suggests that this system has limited utility as a pressure ulcer, indolent wound classification system.

In 1990, a grading scale was generated by Yarkony-Kirk, et al and was compared with the Shea classification. The authors claimed their scale was developed to provide a more complete description of pressure ulcer healing. The Yarkony-Kirk scale has 6 grades: grade 1 is a red area, grade 2 is an ulcer without subcutaneous fat showing, grade 3 shows exposed subcutaneous fat with no muscle observed, grade 4 shows exposed muscle, grade 5 shows exposed bone, and grade 6 indicates joint space involvement. Interrater reliability correlation was a 0.90 for the Yarkony-Kirk scale versus 0.86 for the Shea classification in a study of 72 patients.[19]

BATES-JENSEN PRESSURE SORE STATUS TOOL (PSST)

Basis of the Scoring System – In the early nineties, a group of wound specialists from the University of California, Los Angeles, led by Barbara Bates-Jensen, developed the Pressure Sore Status Tool (PSST). Twenty multidisciplinary experts on wound healing and pressure ulcers assisted in the development of the PSST with the goal of standardizing the assessment and monitoring of pressure ulcers.[20, 21] The PSST consists of fifteen items: two non-scored, and 13 scored (Table 4-5). Each scored item is rated from 1 (best) to 5 (worst). This resulted in a range of scores from 13 to 65 with the higher the score, the more severe the pressure sore. The PSST is dynamic; as the wound improves or worsens, scores change. The ability to quantify progress is one of the stated

TABLE 4-5. BATES-JENSEN PRESSURE SORE STATUS TOOL[20]

Non-Scored Items	Scored Items	Scoring	Interpretations
1. Location 2. Shape	1. Size (length times width) 2. Depth 3. Edges 4. Undermining 5. Necrotic tissue type 6. Necrotic tissue amount 7. Exudate type 8. Exudate amount 9. Skin color surrounding wound 10. Peripheral tissue edema 11. Peripheral tissue induration 12. Granulation tissue 13. Epithelialization	Each scored item* (Column 2) is graded on a 1 to 5 scale 1 = Best (for that item) 2 3 4 5 = Worst Total Score Sum of the 13 scored items	Score Range 13 = Best 65 = Worst (Maximum Score) The higher the score the more severe the findings Scores change as wound improves or worsens

Note: *Objective criteria for grading almost all of the 13 scored items (from 1 to 5) are provided on the scoring sheet used to generate the Pressure Sore Status Tool (PSST)

TABLE 4-6. THE SESSING SCALE PRESSURE ULCER HEALING[26]

Stage	Description	Interpretations
0	Normal skin, but at risk	Scoring (Between 2 successive observations)
1	Skin completely closed; may lack pigmentation or may be reddened	• Minimum score = -6
2	Wound with edges and center filled in; surrounding skin intact and not reddened	• Maximum score = +6 • The higher the score, the better the status of the pressure ulcer
3	Wound bed filling with **pink granulation tissue**; slough present; free of necrotic tissue; **minimal drainage** and odor	
4	**Moderate to minimal granulation tissue**; slough and **minimal necrotic tissue**; **moderate drainage** and odor	
5	Presence of **heavy drainage** and odor, **eschar** and **slough**; surrounding skin reddened or discolored	
6	Breaks in skin around primary ulcer; **purulent drainage**, foul odor, **necrotic tissue** and/or **eschar**; may have septic symptoms	

Scale Score	Interpretation
Negative	Worsening
0	Unchanged
Positive	Improvement

Note: Bold font indicates the 5 parameters (**granulation tissue, infection, drainage, necrosis and eschar**) used in the Sessing Scale to stage wounds

> Giving each of the 13 scored items equal weight might not provide a realistic determination of the seriousness of the wound.
>
> For example, the amount of necrotic tissue in the wound has much more clinical significance than the amount of peripheral edema.
>
> Additionally, skin color, peripheral edema, and induration are terms that have overlapping findings.

goals of the PSST system. A two-page form that is needed to generate a PSST score provides specific descriptions for each of the fifteen parameters. Some parameters, such as size and peripheral tissue induration, are very specific and clearly defined. Other parameters, such as exudate amounts or edge characteristics are less specific, but still adequately described. The PSST does not consider patient related information such as comorbidities.

Comments – The PSST is not as simple to use as the Shea system, but because of criteria provided for each scored item, it is quite objective. With the two-page form, it is possible to generate pressure wound score within a couple of minutes. The details provided to describe the choices for each of the 13 scored items would predict excellent overall accuracy of the observations. The general rule is that the higher the score, the more serious the wound. However, it is difficult to say what the clinical difference between a wound with a score of 35 and one with a score of 45 would be, and how this would relate to management. The 13 scored items address size, depth, and characteristics of the wound base. However, evaluation of perfusion is only indirectly measured by skin color and necrotic tissue. Since the PSST score is a number on an arbitrary range (i.e., 13 to 65) and the authors do not specify wound seriousness categories based on numbers, the PSST score has limited applications as a wound management tool in its present format.

Utilization – The PSST is a well-known system for wound evaluation. Simplicity, objectivity, and ability to quantify the wound process make this tool useful in clinical investigations. It has been used and evaluated in different countries.[22-24] Since the PSST score does not determine specific management strategy, this system does not appear to be widely used in clinical practice. The authors provide detailed information about validity and reliability of the PSST.[20] A nine-member expert panel used objectives and rated relevance of items on a four-point scale. The average content validity rated high with a value of 0.91. The authors reported that an item-by-item inter-rater reliability yielded a correlation coefficient of 0.78, which was above the pre-test agreement criterion of 0.75. Inter-rater reliability was higher (r = 0.89). The methods to evaluate validity and reliability were judged to be appropriate and rigorous.[25] The Bates-Jensen PSST pressure ulcer classification system generated a score of 7 out of a possible ten on the criteria we generated for evaluating wound grading systems (Part II, Table 1 and Table 4-5). This suggests that this system has some utility as a pressure sore/indolent wound classification system and ranks high on objectivity, validity, and reliability criteria.

THE SESSING SCALE FOR PRESSURE ULCER HEALING

Basis of the Scoring System – The Sessing Scale is a seven-stage categorical scale that gives the most attention to the appearance of the wound base with special attention to the five parameters of granulation tissues, infection, drainage, necrosis, and eschar (Table 4-6). Wound care specialists from the University of Southern California Medical

TABLE 4-7. THE PRESSURE ULCER SCALE FOR HEALING (PUSH)[28]

Parameter												Sub-score
1. Surface Area												
Length X width in cm^2	0	<0.3	0.3-0.6	0.7-1.0	1.1-2.0	2.1-3.0	3.1-4.0	4.1-8.0	8.1-12.0	12.1-24.0	>24.0	
Points	0	1	2	3	4	5	6	7	8	9	10	_____

2. Exudate				
Amount	None	Light	Moderate	Heavy
Points	0	1	2	3

Sub-score: _____

3. Tissue Type					
Characteristics	Closed	Epithelial	Granulation	Slough	Necrotic
Points	0	1	2	3	4

Sub-score: _____

Total Score (Summation of the 3 sub-scores; 0 = best to 17 = worst) ☐

Note: 1. The largest pressure ulcer is evaluated. This may be measured at the time of admission and at the time of discharge from an institution

2. Parameters (elements) weighted to produce sub-scores; sub-scores summed

3. PUSH (Pressure Ulcer Scale for Healing) = Summation of the 3 parameter sub-scores

Center and the Sepulveda Veterans Agency Medical Center Los Angeles, California developed the Sessing Scale after interviews with caregivers having expertise in wound management and nurse researchers. It was designed to be a simple, easy-to-use, observational instrument for the assessment of day-to-day progression of pressure ulcers.[26] Each stage has somewhat imprecise descriptions of wound base/peri-wound appearances. Scoring is determined by the observer deciding what stage corresponds best to the appearance of the wound base and the surrounding tissues. Consequently, clinical experience appears to be a fundamental consideration for accurate staging of the wound. As a stage changes with management, the new stage number is subtracted from the original previous stage number to either give a positive number reflecting improvement or a negative number representing worsening. If there is no interval change, then the number is zero.

A moderate-to-strong correlation (r=0.65, p<0.0001) was observed between changes in the Sessing Scale and changes in average wound diameter.[26]

In addition, the authors of the Sessing Scale did a detailed analysis of the content validity of their system. Five experienced clinical nurse specialists in wound care from three institutions evaluated conceptual framework, content, and hierarchy for each wound.[25] Comparison with the Shea Scale was used to evaluate concurrent criterion validity.

The validity of the Sessing Scale to measure wound progression was verified by high correlations with healing measured by changes in the Shea Scale or ulcer diameter (Ferrel BA, et al., 1995). A strong relationship (r=0.90, p<0.0001) was found between changes observed by the two scales.[26]

Comments – The Sessing Scale itself is not complex, but as mentioned above, it requires experience to make accurate assessments. The parameter terms themselves lead to ambiguity; for example, is reddened skin a sign of infection? Does a small, shallow wound without necrotic tissue, but with moderate drainage deserve a higher stage number than a large wound with slough and minimal drainage? How are slough, eschar, and necrosis differentiated? What if different portions of the wound have components of two or more stages? How valid is change of one stage, if one evaluator did the initial inspection while the follow-up was done by a second person? While the Sessing Scale is strong on evaluation of the wound base, other important criteria such as perfusion, size, and depth are all but disregarded. In fact, the authors concluded that the Sessing Scale is an important domain of wound healing that is independent of ulcer size or depth.[27] Unfortunately, objective terms to describe the size, significance, and/or extent of each of the five evaluation parameters are not consistently used. While minimal, moderate, and heavy are used to describe drainage as criteria for differentiating stages, similar terms are not used to describe slough and eschar. Foul odor is more a function of the wound flora than the extent or characteristics of the drainage, but is only mentioned in the worst of the seven stages.

Utilization – The Sessing Scale is relatively well-known, but does not appear to be used to any extent in clinical practice. We did not find studies that utilized this system. While the Sessing Scale has merits for evaluating wound progress, it does not consider patient-related information such as comorbidities or provide guidelines for wound management. It is important to realize that the Sessing Scale and the Shea Scale systems both use descriptions to evaluate wound pathology, and their stages and wound grading characteristics have similarities. The authors performed a pilot study to assess reliability. Ten pressure ulcers were evaluated. Intra-rater reliability was found to be good with a weighted kappa value of 0.90. In longitudinal study (n=50), the weighted kappa value was 0.84. Inter-rater reliability also was found to be adequate with a weighted kappa of 0.80.[25] The Sessing pressure ulcer classification system generated a score of 4 ½ out of a possible ten on the criteria we generated for evaluating wound grading systems (Part II, Table 1 and Table 4-9). This suggests that this system has limited utility as a pressure ulcer/indolent wound classification system even though it rated high on validity and reliability criteria.

THE PRESSURE ULCER SCALE FOR HEALING (PUSH)

Basis of the Scoring System – The Pressure Ulcer Scale for Healing (PUSH) was developed by the PUSH Task Force and sponsored by the National Pressure Ulcer Advisory Panel (NPUAP).[28, 29] The goal of this scale is to monitor the status of the ulcer over time and the response to interventions in clinical practice. A group of wound care specialists from different medical centers developed this scoring system after evaluating 37 subjects with pressure ulcers after conducting a review of the literature and obtaining expert opinions. It is noteworthy that some of the task force members also designed other pressure ulcers classification systems such as the Sessing Scale and The Sussman Wound Healing Tool (SWHT).[26, 30] The task force employed three parameters to measure wound healing 1) ulcer surface area, 2) the character of exudate, and 3) surface appearance of the ulcer. A principal component analysis was conducted to determine the relative importance of each of the three parameters.[28] For example, the ulcer surface area was sub-scored from 0 to 10 while the amounts of exudates and tissue types were scored from 0 to 3 and 0 to 4 respectively. This provided a range of scores from 0 (best) to 17 (worst).

TABLE 4-8. THE SUSSMAN WOUND HEALING TOOL[39]

Categorical Items (Each Graded as Present = 1 or Absent =0)	
Not Good for Healing	**Good for Healing**
1. Hemorrhage	6. Adherence at wound edge
2. Maceration	7. Granulation tissue (Decreased depth)
3. Undermining	8. Appearance of contraction (Decreased size)
4. Erythema	9. Sustained contraction
5. Necrosis	10. Epithelialization

Variables of Depth and Undermining (With individual specifications)	
11. General Depth > 0.2 cm.	16. Undermining @ 12:00 > 0.2 cm
12. Depth @ 12:00 > 0.2 cm	17. Undermining @ 3:00 > 0.2 cm
13. Depth @ 3:00 > 0.2 cm.	18. Undermining @ 6:00 > 0.2 cm.
14. Depth @ 6:00 > 0.2 cm.	19. Undermining @ 9:00 > 0.2 cm.
15. Depth @ 9:00 > 0.2 cm.	

Location and Wound Healing Phase (Abbreviations used with L = Left and R= Right)

20. Location: **UB** = Upper body, **C**= Coccyx , **T** = Trochanter, **I** =Ischial, **H** = Heel, **F** = Foot

21. Wound healing phase: **I** = Inflammation, **P** = Proliferation, **E** = Epithelialization, **R** = Remodeling

Note: A recording sheet with 21 rows is utilized. Items 1 through 19 are recorded as present = + and absent = 0 and the total +'s for "Not good" and "Good" items added up. Items 20 and 21 are recorded as abbreviations. Columns are used for periodic re-evaluations.

Comments – The main value of the PUSH score is that it quantifies healing or deterioration of a pressure sore/indolent wound. With only three parameters to measure, the total score is easy to obtain.[31] The heavy emphasis on wound size and the 11 sub-groupings makes this portion of the evaluation precise, but somewhat tedious. It necessitates the use of a table to convert the surface area calculation to the sub-score point. Also, assignment of points for wound size appears quite arbitrary; that is, do wound sizes ranging from 0 to 4 square cm require six different point categories, while those ranging 8 to > 24 square cm require only three? Important wound characteristics such as depth, perfusion, seriousness of the infection and appearance of the tissue surrounding the wound are not considered. The exudate criteria are quite subjective and the tissue type parameter requires experience by the evaluator for accurate assessment. This parameter does not take into account wounds with several tissue types. The PUSH classification does not provide guidelines for wound management or take into consideration host comorbidities that affect wound healing.

Utilization – The PUSH Tool was designed mainly for clinical purposes. According to Pompeo, the PUSH Tool is not used widely in clinical practice despite its simplicity and ability to evaluate wound progress.[32] In 2001, the authors concluded that the PUSH tool is not a research tool for measuring healing, but studies[32] are reported that it quantifies pressure healing over time.[33-35]

Content validity was established by literature review and expert opinion. In the original article the authors do not provide details of this process and do not disclose its statistical data, but conclude that the PUSH Tool meets requirements of validity.[28] An article published in 2001 by the same group of authors also concludes that the PUSH Tool is a valid measure of pressure ulcer healing, but this paper also does not provide specific statistical data to characterize validity.[33] Concurrent criterion validity was not addressed in either article.

The authors of the PUSH Tool do not address reliability. The PUSH pressure ulcer classification system generated a score of 5 ½ out of a possible ten on the criteria we generated for evaluating wound grading systems (Part II, Table 1 and Table 4-7). This suggests that this system has limited utility as a pressure sore/indolent wound classification system, even though it rated high on objectivity and validity criteria.

NATIONAL PRESSURE ULCER ADVISORY PANEL (NPUAP) STAGING SYSTEM FOR PRESSURE ULCERATIONS

Basis of the Scoring System – In 1989, the Shea Scale was modified by the National Pressure Advisory Panel (NPUAP) consensus conference to a four-level staging system — NPUAP Staging System for Pressure Ulcerations. This staging system has been adopted by the Agency for Health Care Policy and Research (AHCPR, now the Agency for Health Care Research and Quality, AHRQ) Pressure Ulcer Guideline Panels and is published in both sets of the AHCPR Pressure Ulcer Clinical Practice Guidelines.[36] In February 2007, The National Pressure Ulcer Advisory Panel redefined the definition of a pressure ulcer and the stages of pressure ulcers, including the original 4 stages and added 2 stages on deep tissue injury and unstageable pressure ulcers.[37] This is a descriptive, pathology-based scale with the following four elements:

- **Stage I - Non-blanching erythema** of intact skin of a localized area usually over a bony prominence. Darkly pigmented skin may not have visible blanching; its color may differ from the surrounding area.
  Further description: The area may be painful, firm, soft, warmer, or cooler as compared to adjacent tissue. Stage I may be difficult to detect in individuals with dark skin tones. May indicate "at risk" persons (a heralding sign of risk)
- **Stage II - Partial thickness loss of dermis** presenting as a shallow open ulcer with a red pink wound bed, without slough. May also present as an intact or open/ruptured serum-filled blister.
  Further description: Presents as a shiny or dry shallow ulcer without slough or bruising. This stage should not be used to describe skin tears, tape burns, perineal dermatitis, maceration, or excoriation.
- **Stage III - Full thickness tissue loss**. Subcutaneous fat may be visible but bone, tendon, or muscle are not exposed. Slough may be present but does not obscure the depth of tissue loss. May include undermining and tunneling.
  Further description: The depth of a Stage III pressure ulcer varies by anatomical location. The bridge of the nose, ear, occiput, and malleolus do not have subcutaneous tissue and Stage III ulcers can be shallow. In contrast, areas of significant adiposity can develop extremely deep Stage III pressure ulcers. Bone/tendon is not visible or directly palpable.
- **Stage IV - Full thickness tissue loss with exposed bone, tendon or muscle**. Slough or eschar may be present on some parts of the wound bed. Often include undermining and tunneling.
  Further description: The depth of a Stage IV pressure ulcer varies by anatomical location. The bridge of the nose, ear, occiput, and malleolus do not have subcutaneous tissue and these ulcers can be shallow. Stage IV ulcers can extend into muscle and/or supporting structures (e.g., fascia, tendon, or joint capsule)

making osteomyelitis possible. Exposed bone/tendon is visible or directly palpable.

- **Unstageable: Full thickness tissue loss in which the base of the ulcer is covered by slough (yellow, tan, gray, green or brown) and/or eschar (tan, brown or black) in the wound bed.**

  Further description: Until enough slough and/or eschar is removed to expose the base of the wound, the true depth, and therefore stage, cannot be determined. Stable (dry, adherent, intact without erythema or fluctuance) eschar on the heels serves as "the body's natural (biological) cover" and should not be removed.

- **Suspected Deep Tissue Injury** - Purple or maroon localized area of discolored intact skin or blood-filled blister due to damage of underlying soft tissue from pressure and/or shear. The area may be preceded by tissue that is painful, firm, mushy, boggy, warmer or cooler as compared to adjacent tissue.

  Further description: Deep tissue injury may be difficult to detect in individuals with dark skin tones. Evolution may include a thin blister over a dark wound bed. The wound may further evolve and become covered by thin eschar. Evolution may be rapid, exposing additional layers of tissue even with optimal treatment.

Comments – This staging system measures wound depth with secondary considerations for tissue pathology. Depth is not always easy to establish by visual inspection, especially in wounds with sinus tracts or recesses. This detracts from the scoring system's effectiveness, since management decisions require more information than merely the depth of the wound (Figure 4-2). Other important wound considerations such as size,

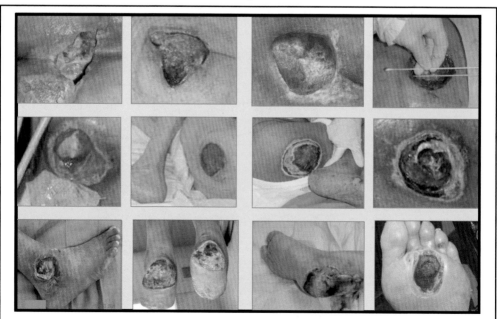

Legend: NPUAP (National Pressure Ulcer Advisory Panel) Stage IV pressure ulcer presentations. About all that can be said is they are all "bad." Without information as to size, bioburden, perfusion and patient comorbidities, appropriate management becomes problematic.

Figure 4-2. A variety of presentations for NPUAP Stage IV pressure sores.

appearance of the wound base, perfusion, and sepsis are not considered. Although specific management interventions are usually obvious for each stage, management recommendations and/or presence of host comorbidities are not incorporated into the NPUAP staging system.

Utilization – The NPUAP system is widely used and is probably the most commonly used system in clinical practice. Because of its simplicity and objectivity, pressure ulcers/indolent wounds are easy to stage without the need for reference materials or scoring tables. The six stages facilitate communications as to pressure sore depth among caregivers. However, without additional information, such as location, bioburden, condition of the surrounding skin, deformities, forces, ischemia, nutrition, and moisture retention, appropriate management requires more than the NPUAP score itself. The system is not designed to quantify wound progress. We found neither validity nor reliability reports in the literature to support the use of NPUAP system. However, because of its widespread and long standing use, like the Wagner grades for diabetic foot infections, it does meet the criteria for face validity. The NPUAP system generated a score of 4 out of a possible ten on the criteria we generated for evaluating wound grading systems (Part II, Table 1 and Table 4-5). This suggests that this system has limited utility as a pressure sore/indolent wound classification system even though it rated high on the objectivity criterion.

WOUND HEALING SCALE

Basis of the Scoring System – The Wound Healing Scale (WHS) was developed in 1997 by Krasner from the University of Maryland School of Nursing, Baltimore, Maryland. It is a descriptive scale for assessing healing in all types of wounds, both acute and chronic.[38] One of the main goals of the WHS was to find a clinical and physiological alternative to reverse staging that describes wound healing. The scale consists of eight alphabetic modifiers as follows:

U = Unstageable; Status/depth cannot be determined
N = Necrotic tissue present
I = Infected
D = Debrided (sharp surgical) during the past 48 hours
G = Granulation; clear wound
C = Contracting
R = Re-epitheliazing
H = Healed

Note: These modifiers are coupled with the original scoring system used to grade the wound.
For Example: Stage IV (NPUAP) that is granulating is designated Stage IV-G; a Stage IV ulcer that is necrotic is designated stage Stage IV-N.
Improvement/Worsening: Movement downward (improvement) or upward (worsening) on the list of the 8 alphabetic modifiers.

A scale score is determined by adding one (or perhaps more) of the alphabetic modifiers to a stage, grade, or score from another wound grading system. As the wound improves (or worsens), the alphabetic WHS modifiers are changed to reflect the progress.[38] In summary, the WHS was designed to assess wound healing, but it is not intended to quantify this process.

Comments – The original article does not include definitions of the eight alphabetic modifiers or the degree of involvement (for example minimal, moderate, or extensive) of each. This suggests the modifiers are self-explanatory in themselves, and for scoring purposes only need to be considered as present or absent. It is unclear if two or more WHS alphabetic modifiers are observed in a wound, all are to be included in the scoring, or separate scores need to be used for each modifier. The eight alphabetic modifiers mainly address the presence of signs of healing; they do not address wound characteristics such as size, depth, vascular status, and degree of infection. The WHS does not include any significant patient-related information. Even though the alphabetic modifier concept of the WHS is easy to understand, a list of the modifiers is needed both by the evaluator and the clinician who might utilize the information to grade and understand the significance of the scale score. Finally, no time frames are recommended for serial evaluations. Consequently, does the WHS provide any more useful evaluation and management information than is provided by merely observing the wound clinically?

Utilization – Clinical applications of the WHS appear to be limited, although the WHS is discussed in different articles.[25] We did not find articles where this scale was used for clinical or research purposes. This would seem an ideal application for evaluating different management interventions. One possible explanation is that this is not an independent classification system, but rather is designed to complement grades and scores from other pressure ulcer scoring systems. In the original article, the author does not present validity or reliability information, although she states that evaluation of these criteria are planned.[38] To date, we are unaware of any such studies. The WHS system generated a score of 2 ½ out of a possible ten on the criteria we generated for evaluating wound grading systems (Part II, Table 1 and Table 4-5). This suggests that this system has limited utility as a pressure sore/indolent wound classification system.

THE SUSSMAN WOUND HEALING TOOL (SWHT)

Basis of the Scoring System – The Sussman Wound Healing Tool (SWHT) was developed by Sussman and Swanson as a physical therapy diagnostic tool to monitor and track wound healing.[39] Based on available publications it appears that this scale is still in development and as of the year 2004, it had not been finalized although a workable version is published in a wound text.[30, 39] The foundation for the SWHT is the acute wound-healing model with the goal of reflecting the changes in tissue status and size over time as a wound progresses. Scores are based on presence or absence of ten categorical items divided into two groups, "not good for wound healing" and "good for wound healing," and four additional variables (Table 4-9).

Comments – The Sussman Wound Healing Tool is labor intensive and despite the comment of the authors that the SWHT is a simple and easy-to-follow system, this is probably one of the most complicated systems available for evaluation of pressure ulcers.[39] There is arbitrariness and repetition in the selection of variables. For example, item 3 is undermining and then repeated in various locations in items 16-19. Adherence at wound edge is a reflection of the absence of undermining. General depth is repeated with depths at specific locations. Why is >0.2 cm the criteria for depth and undermining? Perfusion, bioburden, and size are not considered in the scoring, whereas wound contraction is two permutations (appearance of contraction and sustained contraction).

In addition, the SWHT does not include significant patient-related information or provide guidelines for management.

TABLE 4-9. SCORING SUMMARY OF THE PRESSURE SORE GRADING CLASSIFICATIONS

Grading System	Year	Feature	Criteria to Evaluate Wound Grading Systems (Table II-1)					Total
			OBJ	ADAP	MGMT	VAL	REL	
Shea	1975	Descriptive	1	1	1	1/2	1/2	4
B-Jensen	1992	Scoring	2	1	0	2	2	7
Sessing	1995	Staging	0	1/2	0	2	2	4 1/2
PUSH	1997	Seriousness	2	1 1/2	0	2	0	5 1/2
NPUAP	1989	Staging	1 1/2	1	0	1	1/2	4
Krasner	1997	Descriptive	1 1/2	1	0	0	0	2 1/2
Sussman	1998	Progression	1 1/2	1	0	0	1/2	3
Medicare	2003	Descriptive	1 1/2	1 1/2	0	0	0	3

KEY: ADAP = Adaptability, **MGMT** = Management, **OBJ** = Objectivity, **REL** = Reliability and **VAL** = Validity

Two of the four variables in the SWHT, depth and tunneling/undermining, have five and four subcategories respectively giving a total of 21 wound attributes. Each category item is graded as "present = 1" or "absent = 0" and the total "good" and "not good" items are each summated.

The five depth choices are based on wound depths greater than 0.2 cm in general, and at four different clock positions (i.e. 12:00, 3:00, 6:00 and 9:00). The four undermining/tunneling choices are based on >0.2 cm lengths at the four clock positions noted above.

Location is denoted by abbreviations such as C for coccyx and H for heel. Wound healing phases are arranged in a hierarchy from inflammation to remodeling

Utilization – We did not find information, other than that of the authors, about utilization of this system. The authors stated that "SWHT will be refined and each SWHT variable measured, weighted, and ranked to produce a quantitative tool."[39] To our knowledge, the SWHT has not been finalized and has yet to achieve the goals just stated. In the original article, the authors provide definitions of terms such as validity, reliability, sensitivity to change, and clinical practicality, but do not provide any information on how they were used with their tool.[30] A concern is raised about the content validity of the SWHT since it was based on an acute wound-healing model, but is designed for evaluation of chronic wounds, an entirely different process. The SWWHT system generated a score of 3 out of a possible ten on the criteria we generated for evaluating wound grading systems (Part II, Table 1 and Table 4-5). This suggests that this system has limited utility as a pressure sore/indolent wound classification system.

MEDICARE CLASSIFICATION OF DECUBITUS ULCERS

Basis of the Scoring System – In the October 2008 printing of the ICD-9-CM Official Guidelines for Coding and Reporting document produced by CMS, six stages of pressure ulcer depth are described. The classification is as follows—Stage I (707.21): pre-ulcer skin changes limited to persistent focal erythema, Stage II (707.22): pressure ulcer with abrasion, blister, partial thickness skin loss involving epidermis and/or dermis, Stage III (707.23): pressure ulcer with full thickness skin loss involving damage or necrosis of subcutaneous tissue, and Stage IV (707.24): pressure ulcer with necrosis of soft tissues through to underlying muscle, tendon or bone. Two additional pressure ulcer depth stages are listed, including: 707.20 (unspecified stage) and 707.25 (unstageable). For reimbursment purposes, these codes must be paired to a specific site of pressure ulcer code (707.00-707.09), representing various anatomical sites such as elbow, hip, buttock, heel, unspecified site, other site, etc.[40]

Comments – Although this staging system appears to be neglected in the wound healing and wound classification literature, it is important because so many of the patients with pressure ulcers/indolent wounds have Medicare insurance. The stages, although based on depth, are arbitrary and do not necessarily conform to the anatomical and pathological realities of pressure ulcers/indolent wounds. For example, this staging system does not differentiate between a presacral wound that has necrotic bone in its base versus one that merely tracts to the underlying periosteum. Comorbidities are only indirectly taken into consideration through Diagnostic Related Groups and outliers that likely are present in patients with pressure sores/indolent wounds. Reimbursements for surgical interventions are proportional to the ulcer stage.

> It would be inappropriate to over-classify such a wound as Stage 6 without the presence of bone necrosis. Conversely, under-classifying the wound as Stage 3 (fat layer exposed) does not adequately reflect the seriousness of the problem.

Utilization – Because of the economic implications, the Medicare classification of stages of decubitus ulcers is probably the most frequently used of any pressure sore/indolent wound classifications system. Except for the Medicare Guidelines,[40] we know of no other reports using this system. Consequently, validity and reliability information is non-existent. The Medicare staging of decubitus ulcers generated a score of 3 out of a possible ten on the criteria we generated for evaluating wound grading systems (Part II, Table 1 and Table 4-5). This suggests that this system has limited utility as a pressure sore/indolent wound classification system.

CONCLUSIONS

Summary – Many different pressure sore/indolent wound evaluation systems were discussed in this chapter. Different systems were developed for different purposes. The Shea Grading System for pressure ulcerations was one of the first systems. It was developed to improve communication between wound care specialists and assist with management. It served as a basis for development of other systems. The Pressure Sore Status Tool was developed to standardize the assessment and monitoring of pressure ulcers. The Sessing Scale for Pressure Ulcer Healing was designed to be a simple, observational instrument for the clinical assessment of day-to-day progression of pressure ulcers. The Pressure Ulcer Scale for Healing and the National Pressure Ulcer Advisory Panel

(NPUAP) Staging System for Pressure Ulcerations were designed to monitor the status of the ulcer over time and the response to interventions in clinical practice. The Wound Healing Scale complements the NPUAP Staging System for Pressure Ulcerations and was developed as an alternative to reverse staging. The Sussman Wound Healing Tool was developed mainly to predict and monitor wound healing. The Medicare system is obviously utilized for economic reasons.

Critiques and Plaudits – Each classification system has its own merits and deficiencies (Table 4-5). As a group, the systems are strong on objective evaluation and documentation criteria, but weak on management. This probably reflects that most of the systems were developed and refined by the nurses in contrast to the diabetic foot classifications which were developed largely by physicians and directed towards management. It is a compliment to the nursing field, and in contrast to the diabetic foot wound component, that so many of the pressure sore/indolent wound classification systems have validating and reliable data to support them.

Prospectives – None of the pressure ulcer systems that were discussed in this chapter facilitate simple evaluation of a wound to determine seriousness, predict outcomes, quantify wound progress, and assist with the management. None take into account that pressure ulcers may be an inappropriate term since indolent wounds can arise from other causes such as tension and shear forces, deformities, ischemia and moisture retention. Consequently, "a pressure sore is not always a sore from pressure." Except for the NPUAP four-stage depth evaluation system, none of the scores are intuitively obvious. That is, the scores and their significance can be understood without supporting information from the classification system being immediately available. Finally, there is a great dichotomy between the diabetic foot wound classifications and the pressure ulcer/indolent wound classifications. The challenge of the next chapter (Chapter 5) is to resolve all these conflicts with a **Wound Score** that is simple to use, objective, intuitively reflects the seriousness of the wound, utilizable for a wound in a location of the body, provides a guide for management and makes it easy to objectively quantify progress.

QUESTIONS

1. What findings are predictive of the development of pressure ulcers/indolent wounds?

2. What is the advantage to using the term indolent wound versus pressure sore or decubitus ulcer?

3. What factors are considered in grading pressure ulcers/indolent wounds?

4. What makes the Pressure Sore Status Tool useful for clinical studies?

5. Which of the grading systems are supported by good reliability and validity studies?

6. What is the main value of the PUSH tool?

7. Why is the NPUAP system the most commonly used pressure ulcer scoring system?

8. Why are many of these scoring systems not regularly used in clinical practice?

9. What is the significance of the Medicare Classification of Pressure Ulcer Stages?

REFERENCES

1. Lippincott Williams & Wilkins. PDR Medical Dictionary, Baltimore, 2006; 3rd Ed; pp 1790, 2061

2. Lyder CH. Pressure ulcer prevention and management. JAMA. 2003 Jan 8;289(2):223-6

3. Allman RM. Pressure ulcers among the elderly. N Engl J Med. 1989 Mar 30;320(13):850-3

4. Reger SI, Ranganathan VK, Sahgal V. Support surface interface pressure, microenvironment, and the prevalence of pressure ulcers: an analysis of the literature. Ostomy Wound Manage. 2007 Oct;53(10):50-8

5. Bates-Jensen BM. Pressure Ulcers: Pathophsiology and Prevention, in Wound Care 2nd Edition, 2001; Aspen Publications, Gaithersburg, MD. Chapter 15, pp 325-560

6. Norton D. Calculating the risk: reflections on the Norton Scale. Decubitus 1989; 2(3)24-31

7. Gosnell DJ. Pressure sore risk assessment: a critique. I and II, Decubitus 1989; 2(3):32-39, 40-43

8. Waterlow J. Pressure sores: A risk assessment card. Nurs Times. 1985 (Nov 27); 81 (48): 49-55

9. Braden BJ, Bergstrom N. A conceptual schema for the study of etiology of pressure sores. Rehabil Nurs. 1987;12(1):8-12

10. Bergstrom N, Demuth PJ, Braden BJ. A clinical trial of the Braden Scale for predicting pressure sore risk. Nurs Clin North Am. 1987;22:417-428

11. Braden B, Bergstrom N. Clinical utility of the Braden Scale for predicting pressure sore risk. Decubitus 1989;2(3):40-43

12. Pancorbo-Hidalgo PL, Barcia-Fernandez FP, Lopez-Medina FP, Alvarez-Nieto C. Risk assessment scales for pressure ulcer prevention: a systematic review. J Adv Nurs. 2006;54(1):94-110

13. Bolton L. Valid, reliable pressure ulcer risk assessment, evidence corner. Wounds 2007;19(6):A16-A23

14. Salzberg, CA, Bryne DW, Kabir R, et al. predicting pressure ulcers during initial hospitalization for acute spinal cord injury. Wounds 1999;11(2):Mar-Apr:45-57

15. Ohura T, Hotta Y, Ishii Y, Okamoto Y. A new risk measurement (OH scale) for pressure ulcers and its usefulness for screening and evaluating pressure ulcer patients in clinical practice. Japanese Journal of Pressure Ulcers 2005;7(4):761-772

16. Shea JD. Pressure sores: classification and management. Clin Orthop Relat Res. 1975 Oct;(112):89-100

17. Hondé C, Derks C, Tudor D. Local treatment of pressure sores in the elderly: amino acid copolymer membrane versus hydrocolloid dressing. J Am Geriatr Soc. 1994 Nov;42(11):1180-3

18. Seki M, Takahashi H, Chino N. Treatment of pressure sores accompanied by infection in outpatients with spinal cord injury. Gan To Kagaku Ryoho. 2000 Dec;27 Suppl 3:756-9

19. Yarkony GM, Matthews K, Carlson C, et al. Classification of pressure ulcer. Arch Dermatol. 1990;126(9):1218-1219

20. Bates-Jensen BM, Vredevoe DL, Brecht ML. Validity and reliability of the Pressure Sore Status Tool. Decubitus 1992 Nov;5(6):20-8

21. Bates-Jensen BM, McNees P. Toward an intelligent wound assessment system. Ostomy Wound Manage. 1995 Aug;41(7A Suppl):80S-86S

22. Houghton PE, Kincaid CB, Campbell KE, et al. Photographic assessment of the appearance of chronic pressure and leg ulcers. Ostomy Wound Manage. 2000 Apr;46(4):20-6, 28-30

23. Ohura T, Sanada H, Mino Y. Clinical study using activity-based costing to assess cost-effectiveness of a wound management system utilizing modern dressings in comparison with traditional wound care.[Article in Japanese] Nippon Ronen Igakkai Zasshi. 2004 Jan;41(1):82-91

24. Sanada H, Moriguchi T, Miyachi Y, et al. Reliability and validity of DESIGN, a tool that classifies pressure ulcer severity and monitors healing. J Wound Care. 2004 Jan;13(1):13-8

25. Woodbury MG, Houghton PE, Campbell KE, Keast DH. Pressure ulcer assessment instruments: a critical appraisal. Ostomy Wound Manage. 1999 May;45(5):42-5, 48-50, 53-5

26. Ferrell BA, Artinian BM, Sessing D. The Sessing scale for assessment of pressure ulcer healing. J Am Geriatr Soc. 1995 Jan;43(1):37-40

27. Ferrell BA. The Sessing Scale for measurement of pressure ulcer healing. Adv Wound Care. 1997 Sep;10(5):78-80

28. Thomas DR, Rodeheaver GT, Bartolucci AA, et al. Pressure ulcer scale for healing: derivation and validation of the PUSH tool. The PUSH Task Force. Adv Wound Care. 1997 Sep;10(5):96-101

29. Thomas DR. Issues and dilemmas in the prevention and treatment of pressure ulcers: a review. J Gerontol A Biol Sci Med Sci. 2001 Jun;56(6):M328-40

30. Sussman C, Swanson G. Utility of the Sussman Wound Healing Tool in predicting wound healing outcomes in physical therapy. Adv Wound Care. 1997 Sep;10(5):74-7

31. Berlowitz DR, Ratliff C, Cuddigan J, Rodeheaver GT. National Pressure Ulcer Advisory Panel. The PUSH tool: a survey to determine its perceived usefulness. Adv Skin Wound Care. 2005 Nov-Dec;18(9):480-3

32. Pompeo M. Implementing the PUSH tool in clinical practice: revisions and results. Ostomy Wound Manage. 2003 Aug;49(8):32-6, 38, 40 passim

33. Stotts NA, Rodeheaver GT, Thomas DR, et al. An instrument to measure healing in pressure ulcers: development and validation of the pressure ulcer scale for healing (PUSH). J Gerontol A Biol Sci Med Sci. 2001 Dec;56(12):M795-9

34. Bolton L, McNees P, van Rijswijk L, et al. Wound Outcomes Study Group. Wound-healing outcomes using standardized assessment and care in clinical practice. J Wound Ostomy Continence Nurs. 2004 Mar-Apr;31(2):65-71

35. Gardner SE, Frantz RA, Bergquist S, Shin CD. A prospective study of the pressure ulcer scale for healing (PUSH). J Gerontol A Biol Sci Med Sci. 2005 Jan;60(1):93-7

36. Clinical Practice Guideline, Pressure Ulcers in Adults: Prediction and Prevention (AHCPR Publication No. 92-0047), Rockville, MD: Agency for Health Care Policy and Research, Public Health Service, U.S. Department of Health and Human Services, May 1992

37. National Pressure Ulcer Advisory Panel. Updated staging system. www.npuap.org/pr2.htm. (Accessed December 30, 2007)

38. Krasner D. Wound Healing Scale, version 1.0: a proposal. Adv Wound Care. 1997 Sep;10(5):82-5

39. Sussman C, Bates-Jensen BM. Tools to measure wound healing. In: Wound care: A collaborative practical manual for PTs and RNs. C. Sussman & BM Bates-Jensen. Aspen Pub. 1998

40. International Classification of Diseases, 9th revision Clinical Modification (ICD-9-CM). Chapter 12. October 1, 2008

CHAPTER

THE WOUND SCORE – A SOLUTION FOR THE WOUND CLASSIFICATION DILEMMA

CHAPTER FIVE OVERVIEW

INTRODUCTION 111

GENESIS OF THE WOUND SCORE 112

WOUND SEVERITIES AND MANAGEMENT GUIDELINES 115

THE FIVE COMPONENTS OF THE WOUND SCORE 117

COMPARATIVE ANALYSIS OF THE WOUND SCORE. 122

CONCLUSIONS 125

QUESTIONS 126

REFERENCES 127

"Simplicity is splendid, comprehensiveness is crucial."

INTRODUCTION

Generic problems – All wound management must start with an evaluation. Scoring systems are designed to serve this purpose. Of the multitude of diabetic foot wound and pressure ulcer/indolent wound scoring systems analyzed in the preceding two chapters, none are optimal for evaluation of the wound and as a precursor for the strategic management of problem wounds. This is because of six generic problems:

1. In general, they fail to integrate with other aspects of patient care, utilize information from diagnostic procedures, consider the functional status of the patient (see **Host-Function Score,** Table 2-4), or appreciate the patient's aspirations (see **Goal-Aspiration Score**, Table 1-3).
2. They generally do not consider risk factors known to be predictive of wound development and impediments to healing (Tables 2-6, 4-3).
3. Over fifty findings were used among the previous wound classification systems to evaluate wounds (Table 5.1, Figure 5-1). Obviously, all findings are not of equal value in classifying wounds and providing guidelines for management.
4. The scoring systems do not have generalized applications. They were designed primarily for diabetic foot wounds or pressure sores, with neither working well for the other.
5. Few of the evaluation systems generate numerical scores that are intuitively apparent and facilitate quantifying the wounds by seriousness categories. Some scores are ranked from best to worst, others vice versa; some with high numbers

TABLE 5-1. ALPHABETICAL WOUND DESCRIPTORS FROM "A" TO "V"

Descriptor	Examples	Descriptor	Examples
Anatomy	Structures, location, tissue type	Infection	Bioburden, colonization, cellulitis, contamination, fasciitis, sepsis
Appearance of wound base	Color, drainage, exudate, eschar, filmy, fibrinous, granulation tissue, membranous, slough	Neuropathy	Autonomic, sensory, motor, combinations
Appearance of wound edges	Demarcation, heaped-up, marginal epithelialization	Nutrition	Cachectic, malnourished, morbidly obese, overweight
Characteristics of adjacent skin	Color, ecchymosis, edema, induration, infection, maceration, verrucose	Odor	Foul, none, pungent, putrefactive, sweet, urea-like
		Perfusion	Capillary refill, color, Doppler's, pulses, temperature
Contraction of wound margins	Absent, continuing, initial	Progression	Healed, improving, no change, deterioration
Deformity	Charcot arthropathy, contracture, structural	Risk of skin breakdown	Atrophy, attenuation, hide-bound, hyperkeratotic, hyperpigmented
Depth	Skin, subcutaneous, muscle & tendon, bone, & joint, measurements	Shape of wound	Irregular, longitudinal, oblong, round serpiginous
		Size	Areas—length vs width, small, medium, large; grid patterns
Exudate/Drainage	Amount, color, odor, rate of production, viscosity	Viability	Avascular, healthy, ischemic, necrotic, necrotizing
Granulation tissue	Absent, atrophic, exuberant, hypertrophic		

Note: The descriptors highlighted in yellow are considered the most important of the 19 listed and are the five assessments used for generating the **Wound Score**. The challenge is to provide objective criteria to assess the seriousness of each that is consistent, logical, and easy-to-use as we do with the **Wound Score**

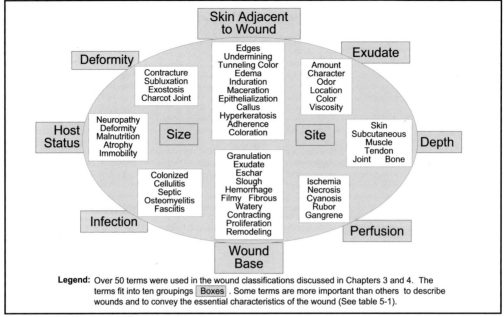

Legend: Over 50 terms were used in the wound classifications discussed in Chapters 3 and 4. The terms fit into ten groupings Boxes . Some terms are more important than others to describe wounds and to convey the essential characteristics of the wound (See table 5-1).

Figure 5-1. Groupings of terms to describe wounds.

being best, while others with low numbers being best; and all with different scoring systems with values that can range from -6 to 97 points and any range in between.

6. Few of the scoring systems are dynamic, or designed to change to reflect improvement or worsening of the wound.

The **Wound Score**, which will be subsequently discussed in this chapter, was designed as a tool that addresses these six generic problems and incorporates the functional status of the patient, and includes management strategies and prevention measures. All this information is integrated into a **Master Algorithm** from which the rest of this text evolves (Figure 5-2).

GENESIS OF THE WOUND SCORE

Goals of a Wound Score – The **Wound Score** remedies the six criticisms just articulated. Several goals provide direction as to how to achieve this. First, a wound score

It is interesting to note that the 50-plus descriptive terms listed in Figure 5-1 fit into ten fairly well defined categories. Of the ten categories, we selected five that were felt to be most useful for describing a wound.

To simplify scoring we used the Apgar scoring system (for assessment of newborn vitality) as a model.[1]

The Apgar scoring system consists of five assessments (each graded as 2 = best to 0 = worst). This generates a 0 to 10 score with ten being optional.

The score is rapidly obtained, objective, and dynamic (i.e. as the newborn improves, the score increases). The significance of a 0 to 10 score is logical without the need for measurement scales to interpret results.

These desirable features of the Apgar scoring approach were incorporated into the Wound Score.

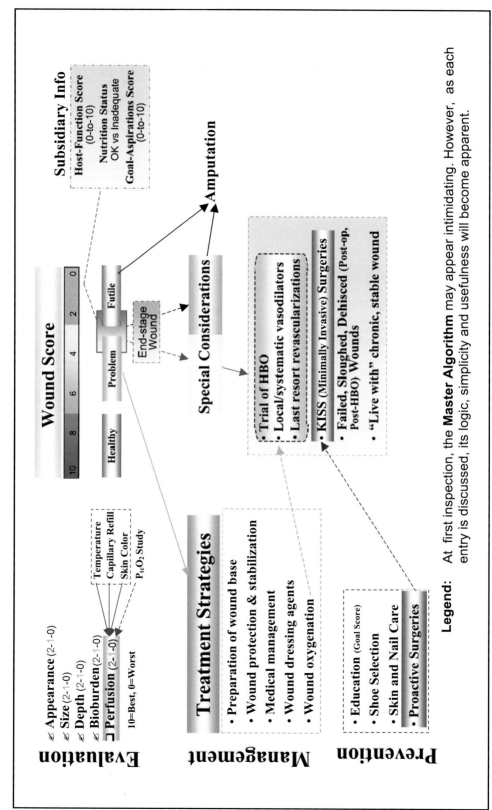

Figure 5-2. The Master Algorithm: Wound evaluation, management, and prevention.

TABLE 5-2. THE WOUND SCORE – A NEW PARADIGM FOR EVALUATION OF WOUNDS

Assessment	2 Points	1 Point	0 Points
	Use half points if mixed or intermediate between 2 grades		
Appearance (Of the wound base)	Red	White/Yellow	Black
Size (Include undermining)	< Thumb	Thumb-to-Fist	> Fist
Depth (Depth of probe)	Skin/SC Tissue	Muscle/Tendon	Bone/Joint
Infection (Bioburden)	Colonization	Cellulitis/ Maceration	Sepsis (↑WBC, bacteremia, fever, ↓malaise, dysglycemia)
Perfusion*	Palpable Pulses (Warm, pink, normal capillary refill)	Doppler (Cool, dusky-pale, sluggish capillary refill)	No Pulses (Cold, purplish-cyanotic, capillary refill > 5 seconds)

Note: *Use secondary techniques (in parentheses) such as skin temperature, skin color, and/or capillary refill to assess perfusion when edema, wounds, or scar tissue interfere with assessment of pulses

Key: SC = Subcutaneous, **WBC** = White blood cell

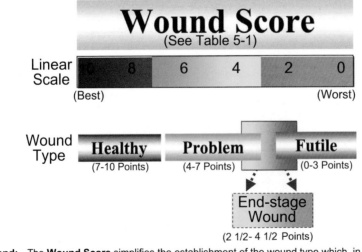

Legend: The **Wound Score** simplifies the establishment of the wound type which, in turn, makes it easy to appreciate the seriousness of the wound and what management is required.

Because the linear scale represents a continuum of responses, it is necessary to consider the end-stage wound, a transitional type between problem and futile. The end-stage wound requires subsidiary information whether to recommend salvage attempts or proceed to major amputation and/or comfort care measures.

Figure 5-3. Using the Wound Score to determine the seriousness of a wound.

should incorporate the most important information of the 50-plus terms used in other scoring systems (Table 5-1, Figure 5-1). Second, objective, unambiguous criteria should be used to grade each assessment from ideal to the worst possible situation. Third, a wound score generated by adding up the individual scores of each finding should utilize a familiar numerical scale so that the seriousness of the wound is obvious and easily categorized from the score. Fourth, a wound score should be simple to use and quick to derive. Fifth, a wound score needs to be dynamic; that is, serial wound scores obtained over the course of time should quantify improvement, no change, or deterioration of the wound. Finally, a wound score should integrate with the other components of management of wounds such as host factors and prevention aspects as it does in the **Master Algorithm** (Figure 5-2).

   Methodology of the Wound Score – From the more than 50 terms placed in ten groupings utilized by other scoring systems, the **Wound Score** uses the five assessments considered to be the most important for describing wounds and making decisions about their management (Table 5.1, Figure 5-1). We modified and fine-tuned the **Wound Score** (and the algorithm derived from it) over a ten-year period to its present form (Table 5-2).[2-7, 15] Each of the five assessments is graded using the most objective parameters possible on a 2 to 0 non-continuous scale. However, when observations are intermediate between two findings or are mixed, that is, components of two finding are present, it is appropriate to use half points to indicate the transition. A score of 2 represents the best possible situation, whereas a score of 0 indicates the worst possible status. When the 0 to 2 grades of the five assessments are summated, a **Wound Score** of 0 to 10 results. With this system, it is clear that a score of 10 is "perfect" and a score of zero is the worst possible situation (Figure 5-3).

> The generation of an objective, easy-to-use, dynamic, wound evaluation system that integrates with patient factors and wound management is one of the two primary reasons for writing *MasterMinding Wounds*.

WOUND SEVERITIES AND MANAGEMENT GUIDELINES

   Healthy and Problem Wounds – Three levels of wound severity: "healthy," "problem," and "futile" become apparent when a **Wound Score** is generated (Table 5-3). The level of wound severity dictates the type of management that is needed to achieve optimal outcomes. "Healthy" wounds generate wound scores of 7 to 10 points. With this type of wound, almost any management that does not damage the healing tissues will have successful outcomes. "Problem" wounds generate scores in the 4 to 7 range. To achieve the best outcomes with this level of wound severity, a strategic approach to management (Part III) is needed. This includes the following five interventions (in alphabetical order): 1) optimal medical management, 2) preparation of the wound base, 3) protection and stabilization of the wound, 4) selection of wound dressings/coverings, and 5) wound oxygenation. For the "problem" wound, each intervention (strategy)

> The optimal management of the five wound management tactics by caregivers most expert for dealing with each epitomizes the philosophical approach we have taken in writing *MasterMinding Wounds* and is the second primary reason for generating this text.

TABLE 5-3. THE WOUND SCORE AS A TOOL TO DETERMINE THE SEVERITY OF A WOUND AND ITS INDICATED MANAGEMENT

Wound Score (Severity)	Likelihood of Healing	Indicated Management
8- 10 Points ("Healthy" Type)	100 %	Basic wound care with hygiene measures, moisturizing agents and covering devices
4-7 Points ("Problem" Type)	80 %	Strategic Management (Part III)*
6-7 Points	> 80 %	Outpatient
4-5 Points	~ 80 %	Inpatient with subsequent outpatient care as **Wound Score** improves
0-3 Points ("Futile" Type)	0 %	Usually lower limb amputation required or a decision to initiate comfort care measures only**

Note: *Strategic Management includes: 1) Optimization of medical management, 2) Protection and stabilization of the wound, 3) Preparation of the wound base, 4) Selection of wound dressings/agents, and wound oxygenation.

Occasionally perfusion can be improved in futile wounds by angioplasty or revascularization. If successful, the **Wound Score would improve and the wound would no longer be classified as a futile type.

Key: ~ = About

should be directed by the caregiver(s) most expert in managing the particular intervention. This precept is the essence of the multidisciplinary approach to management of the "problem" wound.

Futile Wounds – Wound scores in the 0 to 3 range delineate the "futile" wound. "Futile" wounds fail to heal, and in almost all situations major limb amputations are required, or if in other locations, a decision to provide comfort care measures only. A possible exception to this management recommendation is if the limb is successfully revascularized. However, successful revascularization would undoubtedly be reflected by a higher wound score, especially on the perfusion assessment. Consequently, the wound would likely transition from a "futile" wound to the "problem" type. Because the **Wound Score** reflects a continuum of observations, it is possible to generate a number that borders between "problem" and "futile" wounds, that is 2 ½ to 4 ½, which identifies an "end-stage" wound (Part IV). The "end-stage" wound is so named because it is serious enough that lower limb amputation or initiation of comfort care measures only are reasonable recommendations and have been given by one or more caregivers familiar with wound problems. Subsidiary information from the **Host-Function Score** (Table 2-4) and **Goal-Aspiration Score** (Table 1-3), plus establishment and management of the patient's nutritional status, helps to make the management recommendation (i.e. salvage versus amputation) objective.

The "end-stage" wound has special significance because subsidiary information such as host status, nutrition, and patient aspirations are required before a recommendation can be made to salvage the wound or proceed to a lower limb amputation--or comfort care measures only if the wound is in a different location.

THE FIVE COMPONENTS OF THE WOUND SCORE

Appearance of Wound Base – The appearance of the wound base provides information that reflects much about the status of the wound. Objective scoring is accomplished with an almost instantaneous observation (Figure 5-4). A wound with a red base indicates adequate vascularity. It is given two points on the 0 to 2 scale. If the wound base has an exudative or a fibrinous covering that is white or yellow in color, the grade for the appearance finding is 1. An exudate indicates significant bacterial growth in or on the wound base. A fibrinous membrane indicates that the wound base is ischemic but is able to generate a covering, albeit less than desirable compared to that of the vascular-based wound. A wound with a black, necrotic base indicates wound dysvascularity and is ascribed a grade of 0. When the wound base coloration is intermediate between two grades or has mixed findings, that is, partially red based and partially white based, half points are used. Not only does the scoring of this finding merely require a glance at the wound, it is as objective as discriminating red, white-yellow, and black colors. As the wound base evolves to a red, granulating appearance, the **Wound Score** improves. This provides an objective measure of progress and justifies continuing management of the wound.

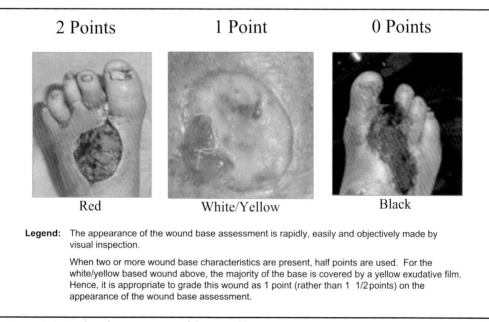

2 Points	1 Point	0 Points
Red	White/Yellow	Black

Legend: The appearance of the wound base assessment is rapidly, easily and objectively made by visual inspection.

When two or more wound base characteristics are present, half points are used. For the white/yellow based wound above, the majority of the base is covered by a yellow exudative film. Hence, it is appropriate to grade this wound as 1 point (rather than 1 1/2 points) on the appearance of the wound base assessment.

Figure 5-4. Grading the appearance of the wound base.

Wound Size – The size of a wound is important, both for predicting how long it will take to heal and how prone it is to developing secondary problems such as infection, sloughs, and cicatrix formation. Although the healing of a closed surgical incision tends to be independent of its length, the larger the size of an open wound, the longer it will take to heal and the more likely complications delaying healing may arise. Wound size changes and with time predicts healing potential.[8] Wound size is also an important consideration in regard to the resources, supplies, and personnel needed to manage the wound. Size can be quantified by length and width measurements, using grids, outlining on cellophane, or with photography that uses measurement scales. For the

Surface areas of wounds that are irregularly shaped may be difficult to measure by the above techniques. Our system considers only three sizes for the purposes of the size assessment and can be easily interpolated from the information we give below.

There are obvious advantages to using this quick, three-reference permutation for wound size, including: 1) The measurement parameters (the patient's thumb and fist) are readily available, 2) Grading is relative to the patient's own thumb print and fist size, 3) It avoids contamination of measuring items such as rulers, grids, cellophane, tape measures, and photography equipment with measurement guides and 4) As with the appearance finding, the wound size grade takes no longer to determine than a glance at the wound.

purposes of the **Wound Score**, size is graded by using the simple references of the patient's thumb print surface area and the size of the fist (Figure 5.5). A wound the size of the patient's thumb print or smaller is considered a small wound and is graded 2 points. If between the size of the thumb and fist, it is a medium sized wound and is graded 1 point. If larger than the fist, it is a large wound and is graded 0 points. If undermining, recesses, tunneling and/or cavitation are present, the wound size is determined by the largest extent of the wound. If findings are borderline between two sizes, half points are used. If a wound is being managed over a long duration, as is the situation with many problem wounds, the surface area and/or wound volume should be used to supplement the size findings and precisely quantify size changes. Nonetheless, for the size assessment of the wound to help generate the wound score and do periodic recalculations of the **Wound Score**, this simple size determination is sufficient, quick to obtain, and accurate enough for scoring purposes.

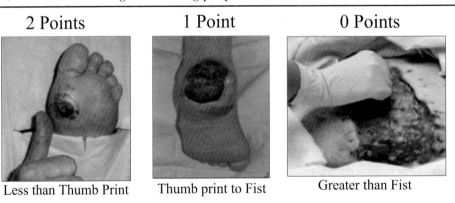

2 Points	1 Point	0 Points
Less than Thumb Print	Thumb print to Fist	Greater than Fist

Legend: The size of the wound base assessment is rapidly, easily and objectively made by comparing the size of the wound with the patient's thumb print and fist.

When wounds are intermediate in size and/or irregular, half points may be used.

For initial and periodic calculations of the **Wound Score**, this size measurement is sufficient and easy to estimate. When following the healing of problem wounds on a frequent basis, surface area and volume measurements may be used to supplement our simple size assessment.

Figure 5-5. Grading the size of the wound base.

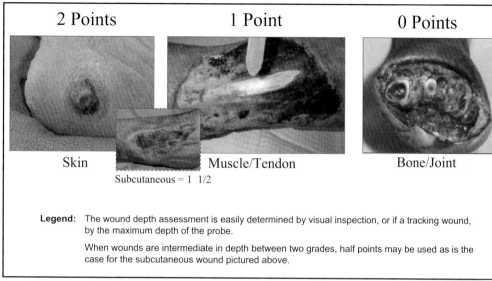

2 Points
1 Point
0 Points

Skin

Subcutaneous = 1 1/2

Muscle/Tendon

Bone/Joint

Legend: The wound depth assessment is easily determined by visual inspection, or if a tracking wound, by the maximum depth of the probe.

When wounds are intermediate in depth between two grades, half points may be used as is the case for the subcutaneous wound pictured above.

Figure 5-6. Grading the wound depth.

Wound Depth – Wound depth is another important cardinal characteristic of a wound. The widely used NPUAP (National Pressure Ulcer Advisory Panel; Chapter 4) pressure sore grading system is based on wound depth. This concept has been modified to reflect the anatomical planes of the wound and integrate with the other findings of the **Wound Score** (Figure 5-6). Pre-wounds, superficial blisters, and healed wounds with the epithelium intact are given a grade of 2 for the wound depth assessment. Wounds that extend to and/or include the subcutaneous tissues are scored 1 ½. If muscle or tendon is visible in the wound base, the score is 1 point, while wounds to the bone or joint level are given a score of 0. When the wound is of the tracking variety, the wound depth grade is determined by the maximum depth or tissue plane a probe reaches. A sterile cotton-tipped applicator can be used for this purpose. As in the appearance and

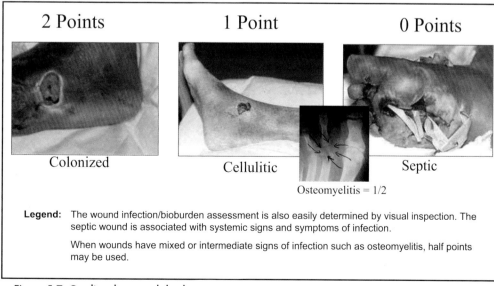

2 Points
1 Point
0 Points

Colonized

Cellulitic

Osteomyelitis = 1/2

Septic

Legend: The wound infection/bioburden assessment is also easily determined by visual inspection. The septic wound is associated with systemic signs and symptoms of infection.

When wounds have mixed or intermediate signs of infection such as osteomyelitis, half points may be used.

Figure 5-7. Grading the wound depth.

size findings, the wound depth grade can usually be determined by direct vision. Only in the tracking and tunneling wounds is a probe needed and, if used, only adds a few seconds to the wound evaluation.

Infection/Bioburden – The determination of the extent of infection in the wound is the fourth assessment used for generating the **Wound Score** (Figure 5-7). If the wound is healthy and without overt signs of infection, a grade of 2 is assigned even though it may be colonized with bacteria. If the wound margins are cellulitic, macerated, or both, the infection assessment is graded 1. If the patient is septic because of the wound, the

> The term bioburden to describe the infection load has become popular. The bioburden is often given as the reason wounds are not showing signs of healing. Many new wound care products have become available that are designed specifically to address this problem. Biofilm is another condition that interferes with control of the bioburden.
>
> Biofilm is a complex structure consisting of colonies of bacteria and usually other microorganisms such as yeast and fungi, which secrete a mucilaginous protective coating in which they are encased. They are typically resistant to conventional methods of infection control.

> Osteitis (infection of only the outer cortex of bone—usually in direct continuity with the wound) and osteomyelitis deserve an intermediate grade of ½ point when not associated with systemic sepsis.
>
> Osteitis is determined by the depth of the wound assessment.
>
> Plain x-rays, possibly supplemented with nuclear medicine studies (triple phase bone scan plus tagged white blood cell scan), almost always can confirm or rule out the diagnosis of osteomyelitis.

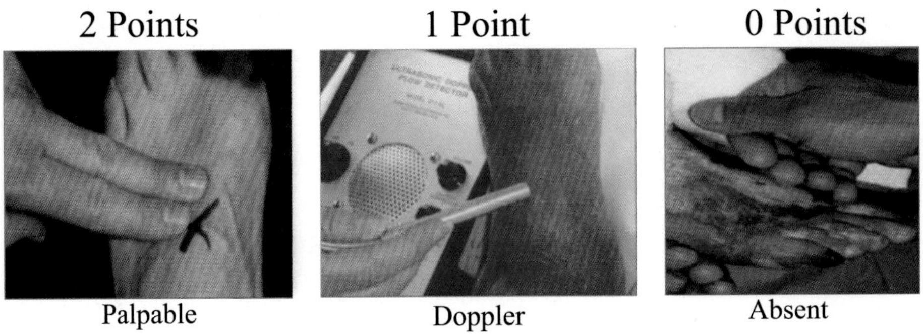

2 Points	1 Point	0 Points
Palpable	Doppler	Absent

Legend: The wound perfusion assessment requires the most clinical skills of all the 5 assessments used to generate a **Wound Score,** and is the only one where physical examination is needed in addition to visual inspection.

Secondary (and tertiary) methods to assess perfusion (Table 5-2) are a reliable adjunct to palpation of pulses.

When perfusion findings are mixed or intermediate between 2 grades, half points may be used.

Figure 5-8. Grading perfusion.

score is 0. The septic state is associated with any one or more of the following findings including fever, leukocytosis, malaise, unstable blood sugars (dysglycemia), and positive blood cultures. Sepsis and cellulitis are among the fastest responders to management interventions. As these conditions resolve, the grades for the infection/bioburden criteria increase. This verifies improvement and demonstrates the dynamic aspect of the **Wound Score**. Other information, such as the amount and character of exudates, wound odor, peri-wound edema, the presence of mixed synergistic organisms, anaerobes, and multiple drug resistant organisms provide additional information about wound infection and should be documented when present. However, the three infection load grades discussed above encompass the necessary information for determining the **Wound Score** and initiating strategic management of the wound problem.

Perfusion – Evaluation of blood flow (and oxygen availability) to the wound is the fifth assessment for completing the determination of the **Wound Score** (Figure 5-8). The importance of perfusion cannot be overemphasized. Problem wounds will not heal unless they have an adequate blood supply. As mentioned in Chapter 2, for healing and infection control, blood supply and metabolic requirements may need to increase twenty fold or more. If these requirements are not met, the wound may not heal and will become labeled as a chronic, non-healing wound. Perfusion is the most difficult to grade of the five assessments that generate the **Wound Score**. If a palpable pulse is present immediately proximal to the wound, a score of 2 points is given. If pulses are not palpable due to wounds, edema, cicatrix, cellulitis, or scarring, secondary methods such as skin temperature, color and capillary refill to the tissues distal to the wound can be used to assess perfusion (Table 5-4). If biphasic or triphasic pulses are detectable by Doppler probes, the perfusion grade is 1. If this equipment is not available, secondary findings for this score include cool temperature of the skin, dusky or pale skin, and/or

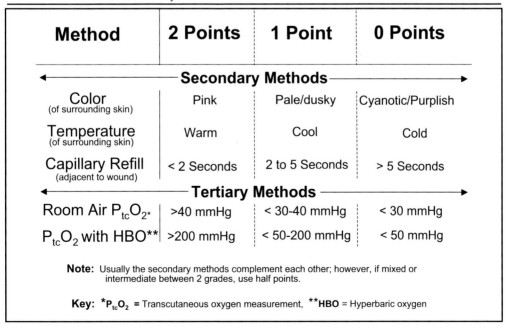

TABLE 5-4. SECONDARY AND TERTIARY METHODS TO ASSESS PERFUSION
(Used when pulses are obscured and/or Doppler equipment not available)

Method	2 Points	1 Point	0 Points
Secondary Methods			
Color (of surrounding skin)	Pink	Pale/dusky	Cyanotic/Purplish
Temperature (of surrounding skin)	Warm	Cool	Cold
Capillary Refill (adjacent to wound)	< 2 Seconds	2 to 5 Seconds	> 5 Seconds
Tertiary Methods			
Room Air $P_{tc}O_{2*}$	>40 mmHg	< 30-40 mmHg	< 30 mmHg
$P_{tc}O_2$ with HBO**	>200 mmHg	< 50-200 mmHg	< 50 mmHg

Note: Usually the secondary methods complement each other; however, if mixed or intermediate between 2 grades, use half points.

Key: *$P_{tc}O_2$ = Transcutaneous oxygen measurement, **HBO = Hyperbaric oxygen sluggish capillary refill (>2 and <5 seconds). Findings that give a perfusion score of 0 include absence of pulses or monophasic Doppler signals, coldness of the skin, absent capillary refill, and/or cyanotic or purplish skin color. Naturally, if no perfusion is detectable proximal to the wound, the likelihood of healing is nil unless revascularization can successfully be done.

Ankle-Brachial Index – Although the use of Doppler-determined ankle-brachial indices (ABI) was once popular, this technique is no longer considered reliable. Ankle-brachial indices are obtained by measuring systolic blood pressures at the arm and ankle levels and generating a ratio. Ratios greater than 0.6 predict healing.[9] The lack of reliability of ABI is attributed to spurious readings that are obtained from transmitted pulsations through calcified blood vessels. Calcified blood vessels, the arteriogram effect on plain x-rays, are a characteristic finding in many diabetics with foot wounds. Juxta-wound transcutaneous oxygen and carbon dioxide measurements provide an indirect assessment of perfusion by measuring tensions of these gases around the wound. Measurements of transcutaneous oxygen tensions in room air and under hyperbaric oxygen conditions provide a tertiary method of assessing perfusions and are highly predictive of wound healing (Table 5-4).[10] Although the clinical assessment of perfusion can be done rapidly, additional time, equipment, and training are required to use the Doppler device as well as obtain transcutaneous oxygen measurements.

COMPARATIVE ANALYSIS OF THE WOUND SCORE

Goals Re: Objectivity – The **Wound Score** resolves the concerns exhibited by the diabetic foot wound and pressure sore/indolent wound scoring systems. The question is, how well does the **Wound Score** stand up to the same scrutiny that was used to evaluate the other scoring systems (Chapters 3 and 4)? By using the same criteria (Part II, Table 1, 3-7, and Table 4-9) that were used before for the other grading systems, the question will be answered. In terms of objectivity, the **Wound Score** earns high marks; that is, 2 on the 0 to 2 assessment grade for evaluating wound scoring systems. This is justified by the use of unambiguous, easy to distinguish criteria, to grade each assessment on the 0 (worst situation) to 2 (best or normal findings) scale. Grades from four of the five assessments including appearance of the wound base, size, depth, and infection/bioburden are easily determined by almost instantaneous visual observations. Palpation, the only other "tool" required, is used for determining the perfusion grade. The end result is that a highly reliable **Wound Score** is obtained almost instantly even by evaluators not experienced with the system. The mnemonic ASDIP where A = appearance of the wound base, S = Size, D = Depth, I = Infection and P = Perfusion (Figure 5-9) makes it easy to recall the five assessments to generate the **Wound Score**. Finally, the 0 (worst) to 10 (best) score from summation of the five assessments provides information regarding the seriousness of the wound. The **Wound Score**, however, meets the objectivity goals, secondary and tertiary goals such as user friendliness, expediency, and documentation are also met.

Goals Re: Adaptability – The **Wound Score** is adaptable for virtually any type of wound including diabetic foot wounds, pressure ulcers/indolent wounds, necrotizing soft tissue infections, refractory osteomyelitis, trauma, venous stasis ulcers, wounds associated with collagen vascular diseases, and almost any other wound type in any location of the body. This is a distinction that the **Wound Score** bridges between the diabetic foot wound and the pressure ulcer/indolent wound grading systems. Even though there are 15 whole number choices (not taking into account the use of half numbers), in actuality

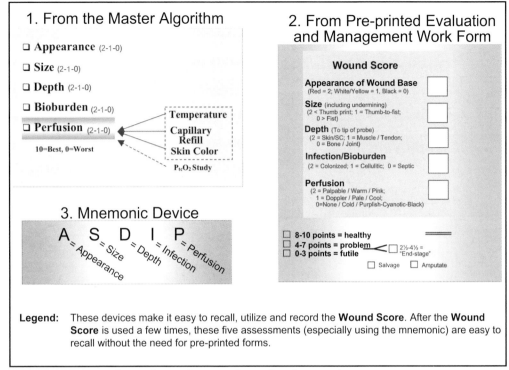

Figure 5-9. Devices for recalling, utilizing, and recording the Wound Score.

there are only three permutations: "healthy," "problem," and "futile" wounds (Table 5-3). These three permutations guide management, directly integrating with the **Master Algorithm** (Figure 5-2). This differentiates the **Wound Score** from all other grading systems (except for Younes' DEPA score, Chapter 3), which are either descriptors of wound characteristics or use matrix formats. For these reasons, the **Wound Score** is graded 2 (on the 0 to 2 scale) on the adaptability assessment.

Goals Re: Guide to Wound Management – The **Wound Score** is multifunctional and designed to incorporate patient related information and laboratory data to make the best possible decisions for evaluation and management of the wound. When decisions need to be made between salvage and amputation of a wound transitional between "problem" and "futile," that is, "end-stage" on the **Master Algorithm**, it integrates with patient related information such as the **Host-Function Score**, nutrition status, and the **Goal-Aspiration Score** to provide objectivity to the decision. For pressure ulcers on the trunk and buttock regions, this ancillary information helps guide decision-making between performing contracture releases, complex flap surgery or providing only comfort care measures for the patient. The five treatment strategies (Part III) for the "problem" wound utilize laboratory and imaging studies to optimize management. Juxta-wound transcutaneous oxygen measurements integrate well with the perfusion assessment and can quantify the benefits of angioplasty and revascularization (Table 5-4).[10]

Wound Management Evaluation of Outcomes – Documentation of progress is another desirable feature of the **Wound Score** and one that is not a feature of most other wound evaluation systems. Improvement in the wound is reflected in increasing **Wound Scores**. This provides a quantitative measure of progress and assists with management.

TABLE 5-5. USE OF THE 0 TO 2 POINT ASSESSMENT SYSTEM TO DOCU-MENT PROGRESS OR DETERIORATION OF THE WOUND

Observation	Grade (Points)	Management (With references to other parts of this text)
Healed	2	Initiate wound prevention measures (Part V)
Improving	1 ½	Continue present management. If wound transitions from "problem" to "healthy", use less complicated dressings
No change	1	Re-evaluate management and initiate Strategic Management (Part III)
Worsening	½	Reassess options & if revascularization/ angioplasty not feasible, consider lower limb amputation or comfort care only (Part IV)
Major amputation or death	0	

For example, if the **Wound Score** improves from "problem" (4 to 7 points) to "healthy" (8 to 10 points), interventions can be reduced from labor intensive, costly dressing changes and debridements to once-a-day or less moist dressing changes. Conversely, if the **Wound Scores** do not improve or worsen, reassessment and change of management are required. For documentation purposes of progress or deterioration, the now familiar 0 to 2 assessment system is highly adaptable (Table 5-5) and coupled with changes in the **Wound Score** meets the criteria for responsiveness as an outcome measuring tool.[11] Other wound outcome-tracking techniques have been proposed, but lack the user-friendliness, simplicity, and objectivity of the **Wound Score** outcome evaluation tool.[12-14] When the **Wound Score** is evaluated as a guide to wound management, it has no equals among the other wound grading systems and desires a 2 on the 0 to 2 assessment scale for this criterion.

 Goals Re: Validity – Outcome studies were conducted on over one hundred of our patients retrospectively and another one hundred patients prospectively. In the retrospective study of "healthy" and "futile" wounds, the accuracy approached 100 percent for healing and failure, respectively. With the "healthy" and "problem" wound groups at the time of the initial assessment, favorable outcomes occurred in approximately 90 percent of the patients.[15] A prospective study of 83 patients with "problem" and "futile" wounds at the time of the initial assessment generated a positive predictive value for healing of 0.80[16] Before it is fair to say that there is good or strong supportive information to validate the **Wound Score**, studies at other institutions need to be done. Consequently, for this wound evaluation assessment, the grade is 1.

 Goals Re: Reliability – Because of the objectivity of the findings used to score each criterion and the ease with which each can be obtained, the reliability of the **Wound Score** should be predictably high. **Wound Score** tallying done by an orderly, a hyperbaric specialist nurse, and a physician were within a half point of each other in over 90 percent of the evaluations. The most discrepancies, as expected, occurred with grading the perfusion parameter. When attendees at a conference were invited to grade a variety of wounds from photographs and some supportive information such as hemograms and

TABLE 5-6. "BEST SCORE" COMPARISONS OF THREE GRADING SYSTEMS

Grading System	Year	Target Wound	Criteria to Evaluate Wound Grading Systems (Part II, Table 1)					Total	Table
			OBJ	ADAP	MGMT	VAL	REL		
Younes (DEPA Score)	2002	Diabetic Foot	1 ½	1 ½	2	1	½	**6 ½**	3-6
B-Jensen (PSST Score)	1992	Pressure Sore	2	1	0	2	2	**7**	4-5
Strauss (Wound Score)	1999	Any Wound Any Site	2	2	2	1	1	**8**	5-2

KEY: **ADAP** = Adaptability, **DEPA** = Depth, extent, phase of ulcer and associated etiology, **MGMT** = Management, **OBJ** = Objectivity, **PSST** = Pressure Sore Status Tool, **REL** = Reliability and **VAL** = Validity

perfusion assessment, the accuracy was in the 75 percent range. Before the **Wound Score** deserves more than one point for the reliability assessment, more studies are required. Consequently, the **Wound Score** at this time generates an overall score of 8 on the criteria to evaluate wound grading systems (Part II, Table 1) and exceeds the best scores for the diabetic foot wound and pressure ulcer/indolent wound classification systems (Table 5-6).

CONCLUSIONS

Merits of the Wound Score – The **Wound Score** is a new paradigm for wound evaluation. It provides objectivity for wound management. Although the **Wound Score** utilizes information that other diabetic foot wound and pressure ulcer/indolent ulcer scoring systems have used, the selection of the most important assessments, its objectivity, and simplicity, make it unique. The **Wound Score** is easy to master and scores are quick to obtain. The 0 to 10 point scale simplifies interpretations and provides numerical information to quantify the seriousness of the wound; that is, it is easy to appreciate and integrate with patient factors, laboratory data and management in the **Master Algorithm** approach. Another feature of the **Wound Score** is that it facilitates wound studies by making it easy to evaluate progress. Since the seriousness of the wound is quantified, comparison of wounds and management techniques with similar wound scores becomes possible. This enhances the prospects of generating valid studies to determine the effectiveness of treatment interventions. Indeed, "simplicity is splendid and comprehensiveness crucial," and the **Wound Score** illustrates this maxim in all respects.

QUESTIONS

1. What are some of the reasons the **Wound Score** was developed?

2. What are the five assessments used to generate the **Wound Score**?

3. What are the merits and disadvantages of using the thumb print/fist surface area for determining the size assessment of a wound to generate a **Wound Score?**

4. What are the findings used to differentiate the various infection/bioburden grades?

5. How does the **Wound Score** help to predict wound-healing outcomes?

6. What assessments of the **Wound Score** are easiest to obtain?

7. How can the **Wound Score** be used as a research tool?

REFERENCES

1. Apgar V. A proposal for a new method of evaluation of the newborn infant. Anesth Analg. 1953; 32:260–7

2. Strauss, MB. Problem wounds, practical solutions, J Muscle-Skeletal Med, 2000; May:267-283

3. Strauss MB. Diabetic foot and leg wounds. Principles, management and prevention, Primary Care Reports, 2001; 7 (22), 187-197

4. Strauss MB. Hyperbaric Oxygen as an adjunct to surgical management of the problem wound, Hyperbaric Surgery, Perioperative Care, 2002, Eds DJ Bakker, FS Cramer, Best Publ, Flagstaff AZ, Chap 15:383-396

5. Strauss MB. IV Aksenov, Evaluation of diabetic wound classifications and a new wound score, Clinical Orthop Related Res, 2005;439:91-96

6. Strauss MB. Problem Wounds, Practical solutions [revised & upgraded article from 200] , J MusculoskeletalMedicine 2006;23-251-262

7. Strauss, MB. SS Miller, Diabetic foot problems: Keys to effective, aggressive prevention, Consultant, 2007; 47(3):245-252

8. Lavery, LA, SA Barnes, MS Keith, et al. Prediction of healing for postoperative diabetic foot wounds based on early wound area progression. Diabetes Care 2008; 31:26-29

9. Wagner, WF Jr. 1979. A classification and treatment program for diabetic, neuropathic and dysvascular foot problems. [Orthopaedic]. Instructional Course Lectures. 28:143–165

10. Strauss, MB, Bryant BJ, and Hart GB. Transcutaneous oxygen measurements under hyperbaric oxygen conditions as a predictor for healing of problem wounds. Foot &. Ankle Internat. 2002; 23(10):933–937

11. Martin RL, Irrgang JJ, Lalonde KA, Conti S. Current concepts review: foot and ankle outcome instruments. Foot Ankle Int. 2006 May;27(5):383-90

12. Lazarus GS, Cooper DM, Knighton DR, et al. Definitions and guidelines for assessment of wounds and evaluation of healing. Arch Derm. 1994; 130(4):489-493

13. McCrary BF. A proposed final post-treatment wound outcome-tracking tool. Wounds 2006; 18(5):117-118

14. Matousek S, Deva AK, Mani R. Outcome measurements in wound healing are not inclusive: a way forward. Int J Low Extrem Wounds 2007 Dec;6(4):284-90

15. Strauss, MB, Strauss WG. Wound scoring system streamlines decision-making. BioMechanics 1999; VI(8):37–43

16. Borer KM, Borer Jr RC, Strauss MB. Prospective evaluation of a clinical wound score to identify lower extremity wounds for comprehensive wound management. Undersea Hyperbaric Med. 2000; 27(Suppl):34

<u>NOTES</u>

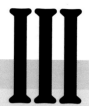

PART

THE STRATEGIC MANAGEMENT OF PROBLEM WOUNDS

CHAPTER	TITLE	PAGE
6	MEDICAL MANAGEMENT STRATEGIES	133
7	PREPARATION OF THE WOUND BASE	165
8	PROTECTION AND STABILIZATION OF THE WOUND	193
9	SELECTION OF WOUND DRESSING AGENTS	219
10	WOUND OXYGENATION AND HYPERBARIC OXYGEN THERAPY	253

INTRODUCTION TO PART III

The "problem" wound is a wound that presents healing challenges and corresponds to a 4 to 7 point score on the **Wound Score** evaluation. To meet these healing challenges and achieve the best possible outcomes, a multidisciplinary management approach is strongly recommended. The multidisciplinary approach includes five strategies: 1) **medical management interventions, 2) preparation of the wound base, 3) protection and stabilization of the wound, 4) selection of wound dressings/coverings, and 5) wound oxygenation.** They are listed in alphabetical order to emphasize that all must be given consideration in managing the "problem" wound and no single strategy is more important than another. However, some strategies may be more challenging to manage than other medical management interventions for the patient with serious comorbidities, such as difficult to manage diabetes mellitus with "end-stage" renal disease, or wound oxygenation in patients with advanced peripheral artery disease.

Management of the "problem" wound is an integral component of the **Master Algorithm** (Figure 5-2 and Part III, Figure 1). Each strategy with its goals, implementation, and challenges is included as a separate chapter in this part (Part III) of the text. Each strategy should be managed by the caregivers most expert in that aspect of the patient's wound management. This is the essence of the multidisciplinary approach to the management of the "problem" wound. Even though there is enough information to generate a textbook for each of the five problem wound management strategies, the information is condensed to chapter length discussions with the goals of emphasizing the essential information needed to manage each strategy and to appreciate the caregivers' skills to make appropriate decisions in their own areas of expertise. As an example, there are several thousand proprietary wound dressing/covering agents. To generate a list of every product, its costs, merits, disadvantages, special application tricks, etc. would be a daunting task. However, by listing generic products that have similar mechanisms (Chapter 9), wound care dressing/covering specialists can select the product which they believe will be most beneficial for their patients and with which they are most comfortable using.

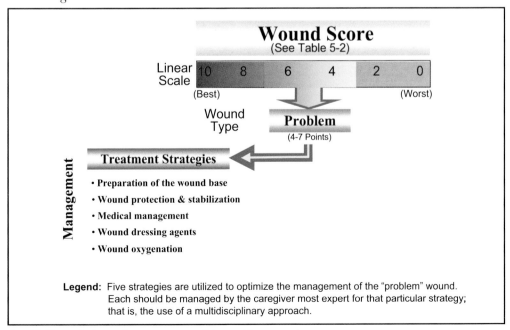

Part III, Figure 1. Strategic management of the problem wound.

NOTES

CHAPTER

MEDICAL MANAGEMENT STRATEGIES

CHAPTER SIX OVERVIEW

INTRODUCTION 135
CARDIOVASCULAR 136
ENDOCRINE 139
HEMATOLOGICAL 143
INFECTIOUS DISEASE AND OSTEOMYELITIS. 146
NEUROLOGICAL 150
NUTRITION. 152
PSYCHIATRIC 157
PULMONARY AND CRITICAL CARE 158
RENAL 158
RHEUMATOLOGICAL 159
CONCLUSIONS 160
QUESTIONS 161
REFERENCES 162

"Care for the wound is only part of the story. Success depends on how you manage the rest of the patient's problems."

INTRODUCTION

Medical problems are important considerations in the pathogenesis and refractoriness of healing "problem" wounds. The wound itself may merely represent the "tip of the iceberg" of multi-organ and multi-system disturbances. Early identification and appropriate management of these problems requires an integrative approach. Some of the problems are acute and require immediate therapeutic interventions; others are chronic and necessitate long-term management. In addition to the primary care physician's role, collaboration with specialists is often needed to manage these medical problems, especially when they are in their decompensated or "end-stages." **The Host-Function Score** (Chapter 2) is an abbreviated assessment tool that provides information as to the functional potential of the patient. It contributes to making appropriate decisions regarding salvage or amputation of "end-stage" wounds, as will be discussed in Part IV. However, the **Host-Function Score** is not a substitute for the evaluation and management of medical comorbidities that can interfere with wound healing for any wound type from "healthy" to "futile." This chapter discusses many of the medical problems and management strategies that need to be considered in every patient with "problem" wounds. It is not our intention that the information in this chapter be used as a guide to comprehensive medical management or a substitute for the information found in medical texts. Throughout this chapter we use the terminology "normal," "impaired," and "decompensated" to designate the severity of the comorbid condition and as a guide to when consultants are needed. These terms are not intended to be a substitute for the standard classification systems utilized in the medical literature. It is

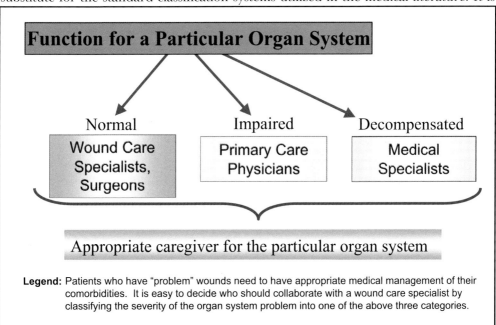

Legend: Patients who have "problem" wounds need to have appropriate medical management of their comorbidities. It is easy to decide who should collaborate with a wound care specialist by classifying the severity of the organ system problem into one of the above three categories.

Figure 6-1. Hierarchy of caregiver involvement for medical management of comorbities in patients with "problem wounds."

our intention that the information provides guidelines for wound care providers as to when consultation with primary care physicians or specialists is required to provide optimal management of their patients with "problem" wounds.

Significance of Comorbidities - Are some of the medical problems (listed alphabetically) in the chapter topics above more important than others with respect to the healing of "problem" wounds? The severity of each medical problem can be placed on a continuum from "normal" to "impaired" to "decompensated" (Figure 6-1). It is obvious that some medical problems are more significant than others because of the frequency in which they are found as comorbidities in patients with "problem" wounds. This is especially true for cardiovascular, endocrine, infectious disease, renal, and nutritional problems, where elements of these problems are frequently present in patients with "problem" wounds. However, any one of the above-mentioned comorbidities can be serious enough to be the reason the strategic approach to problem wound management fails. Failures in management of "problem" wounds may include death, major limb amputation, or persistence of a pressure ulcer/indolent wound.

Hierarchy of Comorbidities - Objective criteria are available, and will be presented in subsequent headings, to distinguish which level of severity ("normal," "impaired," or "decompensated") each medical problem should be assigned. In essence, the medical problems listed in the chapter topics above encompass a review of organ systems, an essential component of the database needed to appropriately manage every patient. Hence, for optimal management of the patient with the "problem" wound, it is necessary to establish if any of the ten organ systems discussed are "impaired" or "decompensated" (Figure 6-1). If the system or status is "normal," collaboration with other physicians is not necessary. If a problem is present, but not a serious impediment to wound healing, the medical condition is considered an "impairment." The medical care at this level is appropriately managed by the patient's primary care physician. If the medical problem is "decompensated" or "end-stage," the patient could die from the problem or be seriously incapacitated by it. Typically, a specialist is required for this level of care and collaborative management is essential.

CARDIOVASCULAR

Evaluation - Cardiovascular problems are among the most frequent of all medical conditions and undoubtedly account for substantial morbidity and mortality. Much can be done to diagnose and manage cardiovascular problems. The history and physical examination are the starting point for recognizing cardiovascular, as well as other medical conditions. Information from this portion of the patient's database provides the justification for ordering other diagnostic studies and/or obtaining specialist consultation. Several items in particular need to be considered when one evaluates the cardiovascular status of the patient with a "problem" wound. These include cardiac history, especially with respect to myocardial infarction, congestive heart failure, peripheral vascular disease, rhythm abnormalities, cardiac medications, necessity for anticoagulation, or combinations of these. Additional useful information is gained from a determination of cardiovascular risk factors and the lipid profile. Every patient with a "problem" wound and a comorbid cardiovascular condition requires multiple laboratory tests, including a hemogram, basic metabolic profile, lipid profile, chest x-ray, and electrocardiogram. Additional studies such as an echocardiogram, cardiac stress tests, and cardiac catheterization may be necessary before the patient can be cleared for surgical interventions for the "problem" wound. These latter studies are usually done after

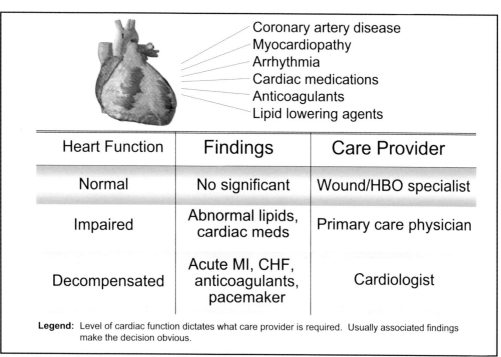

Coronary artery disease
Myocardiopathy
Arrhythmia
Cardiac medications
Anticoagulants
Lipid lowering agents

Heart Function	Findings	Care Provider
Normal	No significant	Wound/HBO specialist
Impaired	Abnormal lipids, cardiac meds	Primary care physician
Decompensated	Acute MI, CHF, anticoagulants, pacemaker	Cardiologist

Legend: Level of cardiac function dictates what care provider is required. Usually associated findings make the decision obvious.

Figure 6-2. Cardiac function and care providers.

consultation and upon the recommendation of the cardiologist and/or critical care specialist.

Functional Status of the Cardiovascular System - This database makes it easy to determine where the patient's cardiovascular status lies on the seriousness continuum (Figure 6-2). Criteria for establishing "normal" function include absence of cardiac symptoms, normal exercise tolerance, and no requirement for cardiac medications. Patients with essentially normal heart function but who require heart medications, lipid lowering medications, anticoagulation, or combinations of these to maintain this level of function and/or prevent cardiovascular complications are considered to have "impaired" cardiac function. Patients in heart failure, having an abnormally low injection fraction, or convalescing from an acute myocardial infarction are classified as "decompensated" with respect to heart function. Peripheral vascular disease is another problem related to the cardiovascular system that can interfere with wound healing. This subject will be discussed further in the hypoxic wound chapter (Chapter 11).

Management - Management of cardiac problems is obviously one of the highest priorities in the patient's hierarchy of care. With the sophistication of medical care that is now available, all but the most serious heart problems can be effectively managed with medical and surgical interventions. Cardiac management in the patient with "decompensated" heart function and a concomitant "problem" wound should be directed at achieving two goals. First is the improvement of cardiac output to optimize perfusion to the wound site. The second goal is to reduce edema, which so often accompanies right-side heart failure. Edema interferes with healing by increasing the diffusion distance of oxygen from the capillary through tissue fluids to the wound site (Chapter 2). Oxygen is very diffusion limited as compared to carbon dioxide, which has twenty times more diffusion capacity through tissue fluids. Hence, edema reduction is an important contributor to improved oxygenation. In the hypoxic "problem" wound, edema reduction may make the difference between healing and non-healing. Patients with "problem" wounds who have implanted pacemakers may require hyperbaric oxygen treatments (Chapter 10) as an adjunct to management of their "problem" wounds. Presence of a pacemaker is not a contraindication to hyperbaric oxygen therapy.[1] Nearly all modern pacemakers are designed and tested to withstand the treatment pressures used for hyperbaric oxygen therapy. If a question arises about this matter, the pacemaker manufacturer should be contacted for their recommendations.

Wound Care and Surgical Considerations - For the patient who requires medications for "impaired," but not "decompensated," cardiac function, it is imperative that these medications are continued during wound management. In the zeal to manage the wound, especially if limb threatening, these medications may initially be overlooked,

> This dictum of discontinuation of anticoagulation before surgery may be modified if the patient has severe peripheral artery disease and surgery is being performed distal to the ankle level. In these situations, bleeding is usually so sparse that control is easily achieved with items immediately available in the operating room such as tourniquet, electrocautery, suture ligatures, vascular clips, and local hemostatic agents (i.e. Gelfoam and thrombin).
>
> If the patient has had recent coronary artery stent placement, or has another condition requiring continuous anticoagulation, and surgery is urgent such as the need for a below knee amputation, then collaboration between the surgeon, cardiologist, and anesthesiologist should be done pre-operatively. The risks and benefits of surgery need to be adequately explained to the patient. Blood and fresh frozen plasma need to be available before performing the surgery when it is necessary to maintain anticoagulation.

especially if the patient is unaccompanied and unable to communicate because of other comorbidities. If the patient is on anticoagulants, they need to be stopped prior to any major surgery because of concerns of uncontrolled bleeding during surgery and the post-operative period. If anticoagulation is critical, longer acting anticoagulants such as Warfarin (Coumadin®) and/or anti-platelet agents such as Clopidogrel (Plavix®) should be stopped at least three to four days prior to surgery while anticoagulation is main-

> Heparin and low molecular weight heparins, because of their short duration of action, can be stopped four to six hours prior to surgery, or have their effects neutralized with protamine sulfate during surgery.
>
> With these alternatives, surgery can be performed without concerns of excessive bleeding from the effects of these anticoagulants while minimizing the threats of thromboses from prolonged discontinuation of them.

tained with intravenous or subcutaneous heparin. Because of their short action, they can be stopped a few hours before surgery and then resumed immediately after surgery. A day or two post-op, oral anticoagulants are typically restarted and heparin or the fractionated heparins discontinued after the oral anticoagulants reach therapeutic levels.

ENDOCRINE

Diabetes - Diabetes mellitus is a very frequent comorbidity in patients with "problem" wounds. About 15 percent of patients with diabetes mellitus develop "problem" wounds.[2] It is our observation that over 50 percent of patients being treated at wound healing centers have diabetes, while approximately 80 percent of patients admitted to hospitals for management of "problem" wounds have diabetes as one of their comorbidities. Complications of diabetes such as gangrene, critical limb ischemia, uncontrolled infection, unmanageable deformities, and neuropathy pain make this diagnosis the most frequent cause of lower-limb amputations.[3] Diabetes is associated with 25-90 percent of all lower limb amputations. With our strategic management approach, approximately 80 percent of patients with diabetes who present with "problem" wounds (**Wound Scores** in the 4 to 7 range) heal their wounds and avoid amputations.[4, 5] Without it, amputation rates as high as 50 percent are reported in diabetic patients with "problem" wounds.[6] Other endocrine problems such as hypo- and hyperthyroidism, parathyroid disorders, and adrenal gland dysfunction occasionally occur as comorbidities in patients with problem wounds.

Diabetic Predispositions for Wounds - Elevated blood glucose associated with diabetes mellitus causes well-known pathophysiological effects that predispose patients to wound formation and impair wound healing (Figure 6-3). These include: 1) Angiopathy with microvascular and macrovascular complications,[7, 8] 2) Peripheral neuropathy,[9] 3) Glycosylation,[10] and 4) Impaired phagocytic function of neutrophils.[11, 12] Neutrophil functions that are impaired in hyperglycemia include phagocytosis, bactericidal activity, chemotaxis, and adherence.[13] In one study, post-operative infections after coronary artery bypass surgery decreased by 90 percent (10% down to 1%) when blood sugars were kept below 200 mg/dL beginning before anesthesia and continuing for 12 hours after surgery.[14] Additional studies have shown that tight glucose control lowers the risk of wound infection and reduces mortality in diabetic patients after open heart operations.[15-18]

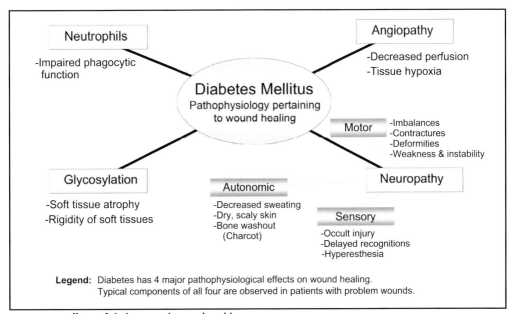

Figure 6-3. Effects of diabetes and wound problems.

Mechanisms Contributing to Diabetic Complications - The mechanisms by which chronic hyperglycemia contribute to diabetic complications are not fully explained.[19] Glycosylation of tissues from hyperglycemia is one possible explanation. It may decrease flexibility and resistance of tissues to tensile, compression, and shear stresses. Fat pad atrophy under bony prominences is another finding in diabetic patients that predisposes to wound formation. Whether this is a consequence of neuropathy, hyperglycemia, ischemia, or combinations of these is not fully known. Another hypothesis is that peri-nerve edema contributes to diabetic neuropathy, because surgical decompression of peripheral nerves has been reported to improve symptoms.[20] The prospective Diabetes Control and Complications Trial (DCCT) and the UK Prospective Diabetes Study (UKPDS) provided strong evidence that strict glycemic control delays the onset of microvascular complications (primary prevention) and slows the rate of progression of already present complications (secondary intervention) in insulin-dependent diabetes.[21,22] These studies confirmed that diligent monitoring and rigorous control of blood sugars effectively delay the onset and slow the progression of diabetic retinopathy, nephropathy, and neuropathy in patients with insulin dependent diabetes mellitus.

Diabetes Effects on Healing of Problem Wounds - The effects of diabetes on healing of "problem" wounds is a complex subject. In some patients, the obvious problem is that of impaired perfusion from the accelerated atherosclerotic process. In some patients, too much blood flow is the problem as is frequently associated with the Charcot arthropathy (Chapter 12). In other patients, the wound problem arises secondary to neuropathy, with two probable mechanisms. On the motor side, a sequence of events starts with muscle imbalances leading to contractures and deformities and then evolving to mechanical problems and subsequent wound development over the deformities. Second, loss of sensation often delays recognition and management of actual or impending wound problems. The history and examination are the starting point for recognizing these problems. There are multiple laboratory tests to monitor diabetic patients. One measure in particular which is of value to the wound care specialist is the hemoglobin A1c (HbA1c) blood test. This test reflects the level of glycemic control over the preceding three months. In both insulin-dependent and non insulin-independent diabetes, the goal is to keep HbA1c below 6.5-7.0%. Normal values are six percent or less. The risks of complications from diabetes decrease proportionately as the HbA1c level approaches normal values.

Management of Type 1 Diabetes - Medical management of patients with diabetes should be done in conjunction with the primary care physician and/or endocrinologist. Much can be done to manage diabetes and optimize the healing responses for "problem" wounds with respect to this disorder. Although the management goals are similar, there are differences between Type I and Type II diabetes (Table 6-1). In Type I diabetes the onset is typically earlier in life than Type II, and there is eventual total absence of insulin production by the beta cells of the pancreas. End organ involvement, such as retinopathy, nephropathy, angiopathy, and neuropathy is frequently observed. Type I diabetes appears to be independent of the components of the metabolic syndrome, which include: 1) Abdominal obesity, 2) Atherogenic dyslipidemia, 3) Elevated blood pressure, 4) Insulin resistance or glucose intolerance, 5) Proinflammatory state, and 6) Prothrombotic state. Treatment of Type I diabetes includes administration of insulin with dosing and timing based on blood glucose levels. For optimal management, three to four blood glucose checks per day are needed. In general, Type I diabetes patients should be managed with at least two injections of mixtures of short/rapid-acting and

TABLE 6-1. COMPARISONS AND CONTRASTS OF TYPE I AND TYPE II DIABETES

Item	Type I Diabetes	Type II Diabetes
Incidence	In the USA, Canada, and Europe, over 80 percent of diabetic patients are Type 2, 5 to 10 Percent are Type 1, and the remainder due to other causes	
Onset	Usually early in life	U sually late in life
Association with the metabolic syndrome	Infrequently	Frequently
Pathophysiology	Destruction of the pancreatic beta cells, leading to absolute insulin deficiency	Variable degrees of insulin deficiency and resistance
End organ involvement	Angiopathy, retinopathy, neuropathy, nephropathy, and myopathy	
Wound problems	Usually a later event in life	May be the presenting finding
Lower limb amputations	Relatively low	Rates approach 50 % in some reviews
Management	Insulin replacement therapy, diet	Oral hypoglycemic agents primarily; insulin secondarily

TABLE 6-2. MAIN CHARACTERISTICS OF ORAL HYPOGLYCEMIC AGENTS

Oral hypoglycemic agents	Main mechanism of action	Side effects	Possible combinations with
Sulfonylureas (2ⁿᵈ generation) - Glyburide - Micronized glyburide - Glipizide - Glipizide-GITS - Glimepride	Increase pancreatic insulin secretion	Weight gain Hypoglycemia	- Biguanide - Glucosidase inhibitor - Thiazolidinedione - Insulin
Meglitinides (non-sulfonylurea secretagogues) - Repaglinide - Nateglinide	Increase pancreatic insulin secretion	Weight gain Hypoglycemia	- Biguanide
Biguanides - Metformin - Metformin extended release	Decrease hepatic glucose production	Nausea Diarrhea Abdominal pain Lactic acidosis	- Meglitinide - Biguanide - ǎ-glucosidase inhibitor - Insulin
ǎ-glucosidase inhibitors - Acarabose - Miglitol	Decrease intestinal carbohydrate absorption	Gas Abdominal pain Diarrhea	- Sulfonylurea - Biguanide
Thiazolidinediones - Rosiglitazone - Pioglitazone	Increase peripheral glucose disposal	Edema Weight gain	- Sulfonylurea - Biguanide - Insulin

long/intermediate-acting insulin. Better control is always achieved with "intensive" regimes, which include 3–4 injections a day. Also, long-acting insulin (up to 24-hour duration of action) such as Lantus® (insulin glargine [rDNA origin] injection) is now available. Lantus® is usually administered once a day. The insulin pump/glucose monitor provides optimal management of blood sugars with its continuous monitoring and infusion of insulin based on blood glucose levels.

Management of Type 2 Diabetes - As stated in the previous paragraph, medical management of patients with diabetes should be done in conjunction with the primary care physician or endocrinologist. Treatment of Type II diabetes requires a step-wise approach. The first step entails lifestyle modification, diet management, and exercise. If those measures are insufficient, the second step is monotherapy with an oral hypoglycemic agent. Oral hypoglycemic agents have a variety of mechanisms of action, including increasing the pancreatic secretion of insulin, decreasing the hepatic production of glucose, reducing the intestinal absorption of carbohydrates, and augmenting the peripheral utilization of glucose (Table 6-2). Initially, a sulfonylurea agent or a biguanide is often recommended to either increase pancreatic insulin secretion or decrease hepatic glucose production, respectively. The third step is using a combination of two oral agents. The fourth step is the use of insulin and one or more oral agents. The final step in the hierarchy is the use of insulin alone as is described above for the Type I diabetic.

Management of Diabetic Complications - Management of the complications of diabetes, not withstanding the "problem" wound, is challenging and frequently requires collaboration with other specialists, such as endocrinologists, nephrologists, cardiologists, neurologists, ophthalmologists, gastroenterologists, vascular surgeons, etc. Treatment of diabetic nephropathy includes blood pressure control, protein restriction, and administration of angiotensin-converting enzyme inhibitors,[23] angiotensin-receptor blockers,[24] and calcium channel blockers.[25, 26] While renal protective effects of angiotensin-converting enzyme inhibitors and angiotensin-receptor blockers in the treatment of diabetic nephropathy are well established, the therapeutic efficacy of calcium channel blockers still remains controversial. Treatment of diabetic neuropathy is difficult and mainly directed towards tight glucose control and pain management. Available treatments for the peripheral and autonomic neurological complications of diabetes are only partially effective and provide modest improvement at best.[27, 28] Gastrointestinal problems, including gastroparesis and mal-absorption syndromes, may require special diets, foot supplements, feeding tubes/percutaneous enteral gastrostomy tubes, or hyperalimentation in order to meet the patient's metabolic needs.

Preparation of the Diabetic Patient for Surgery - For the patient with impaired glucose metabolism, but not "decompensated" diabetes, management by the primary care physician is usually sufficient. This group of patients typically has stable blood sugars with medical management and does not have major "end-stage" organ involvement from diabetic complications. Surgeries for management of their "problem" wounds generally are no more risky than surgeries in patients with normal glucose metabolism. Pre-operative management includes: 1) Maintaining the patient NPO (nothing per os) six to eight hours prior to surgery, 2) Holding their scheduled insulin doses on the day of surgery, 3) Monitoring blood sugars with finger stick glucose testing while NPO and using regular insulin subcutaneously as needed to keep blood sugars in an optimal range, and 4) Slow (50 to 100 cc/hr) infusion of intravenous fluids with glucose solutions while awaiting surgery. A repeat blood glucose measurement is done immediately upon arriving at the post-anesthesia care unit (recovery room), and then institution of insulin or supplementation of glucose is done according to the glucose levels. For surgeries longer than two hours, intra-operative blood glucose monitoring is recommended.

The complexity of diabetes management is exemplified by the diabetic patient with malnutrition (hypoalbuminemia) and renal insufficiency. Obviously, for management of the "problem" wound, optimal protein substrates are essential. However, the augmentation of protein intake and the elimination of their waste products by the kidneys may exceed these organs' capacity to handle the increased load and lead to renal insufficiency or failure.

Management requires a "balancing act" between protein intake and the kidney's ability to handle the challenge. In these situations, input from the clinical nutritionist is essential to select diets that optimize protein intake without placing the impaired kidneys at increased risk of deterioration or failure.

Preparation of the Brittle Diabetic for Surgery - "Decompensated" diabetes is established by the history of repetitive hypoglycemia, hyperglycemia, and/or ketoacidosis episodes. The term "brittle" diabetic is used for this group of patients. Typically, diabetic patients with this severity of involvement are under the care of an endocrinologist-diabetes specialist. Another criterion that may be used for defining "decompensated" diabetes is the use of an insulin pump. Again, the endocrinologist is the specialist who typically manages this aspect of diabetes care. When surgeries for "problem" wounds are performed on the diabetic patient, the peri-operative management described for the patient with impaired glucose metabolism should be followed. In addition, every effort should be made to schedule the surgery as early in the morning as possible in order to reduce the time the patient is NPO and to re-establish the patient's normal eating and insulin management routines as soon as possible.

HEMATOLOGICAL

Scope of Hematological Problems - Hematological problems are frequently present in patients with "problem" wounds. Usually they are secondary to other disease processes. Anemia is often observed in patients with "problem" wounds who have other comorbidities, such as diabetes, collagen vascular diseases, neoplasms, chronic infections, renal insufficiency or failure, malnutrition, and sickle cell disease. Leukocyte functions are also affected by comorbid conditions. Diabetes interferes with leukocyte functions such as adherence, chemotaxis, and phagocytosis. Hypoxia compounds these problems by interfering with leukocyte oxidative killing and migration. Coagulopathies are another group of hematological disorders that are associated with wound problems. Blood clotting deficiencies that lead to hematomas, ecchymoses, or both from minimal trauma may result in wound problems. These problems may arise from tissue necrosis, sloughs, compartment syndromes, and infections associated with the injury site. At the other extreme, hypercoagulable states can be the etiology of wound problems (Table 6-3). These problems can affect arterial, venous or both sides of the vascular system.[29] The most florid examples of wound-associated coagulopathies occur with disseminated intravascular coagulation and purpura fulminans (Chapter 12). As the result of these coagulopathies, the wounds are often so severe that major limb amputations are required.

Hierarchy of Management - In general anemias, leukocytosis and thrombocytopenia are easy to recognize and are appropriately managed by the primary care physician in collaboration with the specialist managing the "problem" wound. Hematologist-oncologists are needed to optimize management when the hematological

TABLE 6-3. DISEASE STATES AND RISK FACTORS PREDISPOSING PATIENTS TO THROMBOEMBOLISM

Abnormality	Affected Vascular Beds		
	VENOUS	VENOUS AND ARTERIAL	ARTERIAL
Defects in coagulation factors	Resistance to activated protein C (factor V Leiden) Deficiency of protein C Deficiency of protein S Deficiency of antithrombin III Mutation of prothrombin		
Defects in clot lysis	Deficiency of plasminogen Deficiency of tissue plaminogen activator	Dysfibrinogenemia* Deficiency of plasminogen-activator inhibitor type I*	
Metabolic defects		Homocysteinemia	
Platelet defects		Herparin-induced thrombo-cytopenia and thrombosis Myeloproliferative disorders Paroxysmal nocturnal hemo-globinuria* Polycythemia vera (with thrombocytosis)	
Stasis	Immobilization Surgery Congestive heart failure		
Hyperviscosity	Cancer (Trousseau's Syndrome)	Polycythemia vera Waldenstöm's macroglobu-linemia Sickle cell anemia Acute Leukemia	
Defects in vessel walls	Use of oral contraceptives	Trauma Vasculitis	Atherosclerosis Turbulence
Other	Estrogen therapy Pregnancy or puerperium Nephrotic syndrome	Antiphospolipid syndrome Foreign bodies Cyclooxygenase-2 inhibitors†	Hypertension Diabetes Smoking Atrial fibrillation Hyperlipidemia Chronic inflammation Systemic Lipus erythe-matosus‡

*In this disorder, the venous involvement far exceeds the arterial involvement.
†Specific inhibitors of cyclooxygenase-2 reduce systemic production of the anithrombotic prostaglandin prostacyclin. A recent series described four patients with secondary antiphospholipid syndrome in whom acute thrombosis developed in conjunction with a cyclooxygenase-2 inhibitor
‡A prothrombotic effect of systemic lupus erythematosus, separate from antiphospholipid antibodies, has been suggested but not definitely established

From Levine JS, Branch DW, Rauch J. The antiphospholipid syndrome. N Engl J Med 2002 Mar 7l346(10):752-63.

problem is "decompensated," as in the situation of difficult-to-manage anemias, blood dyscrasias, immunocompromised states, obscure coagulopathies, and neoplasms.

Hematological Considerations for Surgery - Patients who require surgery for their

> Anemias associated with sickle cell disease and chronic kidney diseases are especially challenging to manage. Usually, these problems are managed by hematologist-oncologists or when kidney problems are the primary etiology, by nephrologists.
>
> These diseases frequently require serial administrations of erythropoiesis stimulating products (Erythropoietin (Epogen®; Procrit®) and Darbepoetin (Aranesp™)), which are genetically engineered agents that increase the production of red blood cells.
>
> In many hospitals, ordering the erythropoiesis stimulation agents is under the auspices of the hematologist-oncologist, nephrologist, or critical care specialist.

"problem" wounds and have associated hematological abnormalities must have these problems addressed appropriately. If moderately anemic, hematocrits in the 30 +/- 3 percent range, or profoundly anemic, hematocrits less than 25 percent, blood should be available during surgery to be transfused as indicated. Considerations for blood transfusion include the duration of the anemia, the extent of the surgery, the stability of the patient's vital signs, and presence of other comorbidities, particularly cardiovascular problems such as coronary artery disease. Patients with "end-stage" renal disease and hematocrits in the 22 to 27 percent range typically are accommodated to this level of

> What is the ideal hematocrit for optimizing perfusion, yet providing adequate delivery of oxygen to tissues? The viscosity of blood increases proportionately to increases in the hematocrit. Conversely, as blood viscosity increases, blood flow decreases through relatively poorly perfused regions, as is so often associated with "problem" wounds. Sludging, atherosclerosis, vasoconstriction, and thrombosis contribute to low flow states.
>
> The more fluid the blood is, that is the less viscous, the better the perfusion through regions of low flow. It has been reported in a multi-variate analysis that patients with preoperative hematocrits of > 36 percent have a higher risk of failed amputations.[30, 31] This supports the recommendation to defer blood transfusions (PRBC's) preoperatively if hematocrits are >25 percent in patients with stable vital signs.
>
> This is a circumstance for which hyperbaric oxygen (Chapter 10) is ideally suited. Hyperbaric oxygen adds oxygen to the plasma so oxygen delivery is increased without increasing the viscosity of blood.

anemia and usually do not require transfusions for their "problem" wound surgeries. Minimally invasive surgeries (Chapter 11) such as percutaneous tenotomies, lesser toe amputations, percutaneous drilling and controlled osteoclasis for realignment of metatarsal heads are not usually associated with significant blood loss. Hence, the decision for transfusion needs to be based on the stability of the vital signs and comorbidities.

The other major hematological consideration for "problem" wounds with respect

Not infrequently, patients with infected, limb-threatening wounds such as necrotizing fasciitis and major wounds secondary to severe lower extremity contractures have marked drops in their hematocrits after surgery, even though their blood loss was negligible from the surgery.

This apparent paradox is attributed to a contracted fluid volume from their underlying condition, which is managed with crystalloid infusions by the anesthesiologists during surgery, thus causing a dilution effect.

In such situations, the decision to transfuse needs to be based on the patient's vital signs rather than the level of anemia. If the vital signs are stable, iron and mulitvitamin supplements are started. If profoundly anemic and there is associated kidney disease and/or ongoing infection, Erythropoietin or similar products (used to stimulate red blood cell production) may be given in the presence of these conditions. If hypotensive and tachycardic, then packed red blood cell transfusion is indicated.

to surgeries is the use of anticoagulation. Not infrequently, patients with "problem" wounds are on anticoagulants. Reasons include atrial fibrillation, history of venous thrombosis, recent revascularization and/or angioplasty procedures, deep vein thrombosis prophylaxis, and hypercoagulable states. If the surgeries are minimally invasive, as described above, anticoagulation does not need to be stopped. If anticoagulation needs to be discontinued because of concerns about excessive intra- and post-operative bleeding, discontinuation and resumption of anticoagulation can be done to minimize risks of thrombosis using heparins (see cardiovascular section above).

Occasionally, intra- and post-operative bleeding is a problem even though the patient is not anticoagulated. Hemostasis with electrocautery is often ineffective regardless of the intensity setting of the electrical current in diabetic and atherosclerotic patients, especially those with "end-stage" renal disease and/or on immunosuppressors.

Possible explanations for this observation include the ineffectiveness of electrocautery for the cauterization of calcified vessels and the presence of occult coagulopathies associated with the disease processes.

When bleeding is at other than the capillary level, ligatures are usually effective to achieve hemostasis. When bleeding is at the microcirculation level, that is an apparent "capillary ooze," closing with drains, flap approximation, and compression dressings usually effectively manages this problem. Sometimes bleeding continues for three to four days postoperatively, but invariably stops by this time with the above measures.

INFECTIOUS DISEASE AND OSTEOMYELITIS

Continuum of Infection Using the Wound Score - Infection is present to some extent in every "problem" wound. It may merely be colonization of the wound base, which is considered a normal finding and graded 2 points on the infection/bioburden assessment of the **Wound Score** (Table 5-2). The next level in the continuum is the cellulitic/macerated wound. It is characterized by exudate production in the wound base, erythema around the wound margins, infected, moist skin edges adjacent to the

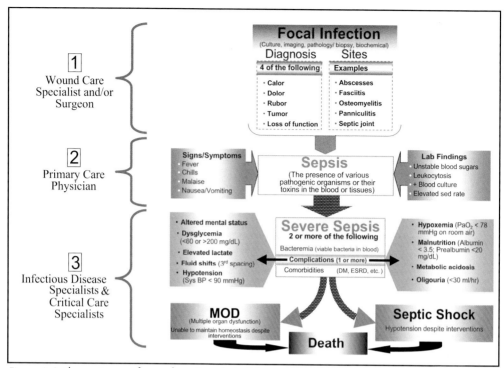

Figure 6-4. The continuum of wound sepsis and physician management.

TABLE 6-4. ANTIMICROBIAL THERAPY FOR "PROBLEM" WOUNDS BASED ON VIRULENCE OF THE INFECTION

Mild* (OSSA, Streptococci and sensitive gram negative bacilli)	Moderate (Mixed aerobic and anaerobic infections)	Severe (O/MRSA, VRE, ESBR and other multiple drug resistant organisms)
Dicloxacillin Oxacillin (Prostaphlin)	Ampicillin/Sulbactam (Unasyn)	Vancomycin
Amoxicillin/clavulanate (Augmentin)	Piperacillin/Tazobactam (Zosyn) Levofloxacin (Levaquin) and Cefazoline (Ancef)	Linezolid (Zyvox) Quinupristin/dalfopristin (Synercid)
Cefadroxil (Duricef) Cephalexin (Keflex)	Clindamycin	Daptomycin (Cubicin)
Levofloxacin (Levaquin) or Ciprofloxacin Ampicillin	Cefepime (Maxipime) or Ceftazidime (Fortaz) and Clindamycin or Metronidazole (Flagyl)	Tigecycline (Tygacil)
Metronidazole (Flagyl) Penicillin Doxycycline or Trimethoprim and Sulfamethoxazole (Bactrim) + Rifampin (O/MRSA suppression)	Ancef or Methicillin and Imipenem or Ertapenem Clindamycin and Gentamycin Cephalexin (Keflex), Metronidazole (Flagyl) and Levafloxacin (Levaquin)	Above with Tobramycin, Amikacin (Amikin), Cefepime (Maxipime), or Ceftazidime (Fortaz) or Pipercillin/Tazobactam (Zosyn)

KEY: *Mild = Absence of systemic signs of infection; oral antibiotics usually sufficient, **ESBL** = Extended spectrum beta-lactamase resistance, **O/MRSA** = Oxacillin/methicillin resistant Staphlococcus aureus, **OSSA** = Oxacillin sensitive Staphlococcus aureus, **VRE** = Vancomycin resistant enterococcus

wound, or combinations of these (graded 1 point on the infection assessment of the **Wound Score**). Wet gangrene and progressive necrotizing soft-tissue infections reflect the extreme end of the wound infection continuum. In these situations, the patient is invariably septic, with findings of fevers, chills, malaise, leukocytosis, unstable blood sugars, positive blood cultures, or combinations of these in association with the wound (graded 0 points on the infection assessment of the **Wound Score**). Each level of infection is associated with specific diagnostic criteria and the physician who should be primarily responsible for its management (Figure 6-4). When the infections are mild or moderate and the infection assessment grade of the **Wound Score** is 1 or 2 points, management by the primary care physician and/or the surgical specialist is usually sufficient. Collaboration with an infectious disease specialist is advisable in the "decompensated" situations, such as patients with multiple drug-resistant organisms, sepsis (graded 0 points on the infection assessment of the **Wound Score**), renal and/or hepatic insufficiency, immunological compromises, or combinations of these. In these situations, not only is control of the infection at the wound site imperative, but prevention of potential serious infection complications (i.e. subacute bacterial endocarditis, septic embolization, etc.) is essential. In many institutions, prescribing the newer more expensive antibiotics for the serious group of infections is limited to the infectious disease specialist in order to ensure the highest possible quality control, cost benefits, and prevention of the emergence of drug resistant organisms.

Refractory Osteomyelitis - Refractory osteomyelitis is commonly found in "problem" wounds of the foot and ankle. Whenever a seemingly benign appearing wound fails to heal with antibiotics in the absence of an underlying bony deformity, osteomyelitis should be the presumed diagnosis. In addition to persistence of the wound, other clinical features help to confirm the presence of chronic osteomyelitis. These include induration around the wound margins, lichenification/mammilation of the adjacent skin, an elevated erythrocyte sedimentation rate and C-reactive protein, and/or a fibrinous membrane and/or biofilm over the wound base. If the wound base tracks to

When perfusion is poor, osteopenia and osteolysis may not be observed in infected bone. This is due to inactivity of the osteoclast, the bone cell responsible for resorption of dead and infected bone. Osteoclastic activity is arrested in the hypoxic environment. This is because it is the most oxygen dependent of the bone cells, with 100 times the metabolic activity of the osteocyte, the bone cell embedded in ossified tissue.

It is easy to appreciate why the metabolic and oxygen demands of the osteoclast are so high. The osteoclast is a macrophage (multinucleated giant cell) that has migrated to bone. When in contact with bone, enzymes such as acid and alkaline phosphatases are induced, which dissolve the diseased bone and allow its mineral contents to be carried away by perfusion. Like the neutrophil, its metabolic demands are high in order to function. Without perfusion, the bone's mineral contents will not be removed.

Hyperbaric oxygen (Chapter 10), used in the presence of suspected osteomyelitis, has helped to confirm this diagnosis. In dysvascular, hypoxic wounds that have failed to demonstrate x-ray evidence of osteomyelitis after a course of antibiotics, bone resorption has been observed after ten-to-fourteen hyperbaric oxygen treatments (Figure 5-7).

bone, there is at least a 75 percent likelihood that the bone is infected.[32, 33] Imaging studies are also helpful. Plain x-rays confirm the diagnosis of osteomyelitis when there is radioleucency of the bone over the ulcer and/or there is a disruption in the cortical margin of the bone. "Soft signs" suggesting osteomyelitis on plain x-rays include soft tissue swelling over the suspected bone infection site, soft tissue ulceration to the cortical margin of the bone and osteopenia. An aspiration needle biopsy of bone for culture and sensitivities is the "Gold Standard" for confirming the presence of osteomyelitis. However, swabs of the wound base, sinus tract, and bone biopsy cultures are usually similar as long as the wound base or sinus tract is cleansed of its exudate and necrotic debris (usually secondarily infected) has been removed.[34, 35] In the operating room, initial debridement of the infected granulation tissue should be done before submitting a bone sample for cultures and sensitivities. Both aerobic and anaerobic cultures should be obtained. Upon recommendation of the infectious disease consultant, specimens may be sent for fungi and acid-fast bacilli. If the suspected site is not obvious on physical examination, the biopsy should be done under radiological (fluoroscopic) control. From the results, antibiotics should be selected according to the organisms' sensitivities in collaboration with the infection disease specialist.

Imaging Studies for Refractory Osteomyelitis - Nuclear medicine studies are the next level in the hierarchy for confirming the presence or absence of refractory osteomyelitis. A bone (Technectium) scan reflects bone remodeling and inflammation, hence it is not specific for osteomyelitis. An Indium scan using autologous-labeled neutrophils is more specific for bone infection. By superimposing congruous images and looking for concordant activity from the two scans, osteomyelitis can be differentiated from bone remodeling and adjacent soft tissue infections. Usually, by the time nuclear medicine scans are ordered, the diagnosis of osteomyelitis can be confirmed by clinical and plain x-ray findings. The great value of the nuclear medicine scans is to confirm the diagnosis and demonstrate the extent of the bone infection. This helps in decision making for surgery; that is, defining the extent of the (infected) bone that needs to be debrided. In general, magnetic resonance imaging (MRI) for osteomyelitis in "problem" wounds is not recommended. Although extremely sensitive in detecting bone edema, it is unable to differentiate between infection and remodeling. Too often, the MRI reports are returned stating that osteomyelitis is suspected and should be confirmed by clinical correlation and nuclear medicine scans. Decisions based on MRI findings alone could result in unnecessarily extensive debridements and/or amputations.

Virulence - Another infectious disease consideration in dealing with "problem" wounds is the virulence of the organism. Virulence is a measure of the severity of the disease the organism is capable of causing. Some organisms cause minimal disease while others, like those causing gas gangrene, are highly virulent. The picture becomes confusing, however, when other factors are co-existent, such as comorbidities in the host or the presence of implants, bone grafts, and bone cement. In these situations, organisms with minimal virulence can be very pernicious, as observed in patients who are immunocompromised, have peripheral vascular disease, "end-stage" renal disease, and/or collagen vascular diseases. In addition, organisms that generate a biofilm are notoriously difficult to eradicate because the biofilm acts as a barrier to antibiotic and leukocyte penetration. Concern about the seriousness of the infection is thus judged by these considerations as well as the type and complexity of the antibiotic required (routes of administration, requirements for monitoring, and the expense) rather than the virulence of the organism itself. Consequently, infections can be considered as mild, moderate, or severe based on what antibiotics are required to manage them (Table 6-4). In all situations where organism virulence or perniciousness of the infection is a concern, the infectious disease consultant should manage the antibiotic selections, the monitoring of side effects from antibiotics, and the duration of antibiotic treatment.

Immunological Competence - The immunological competence of the patient must always be considered when managing "problem" wounds. Cardiovascular, diabetic, and hematological factors that affect host responsiveness were discussed previously. Patients with "problem" wounds may be on immunosuppressors for various medical conditions. Infections that otherwise would be considered as innocent become very serious matters. In such situations, aggressive antibiotic treatment and appropriate surgical interventions must be initiated as soon as the infection is recognized with input from the infectious disease consultant. The same recommendations are made for patients with human immunodeficiency virus (HIV) and acquired immunological deficiency syndrome (AIDS). A variety of antiviral and immunological-complementing medications are now available. When managing a "problem" wound, these medications need to be optimized to improve the patient's lymphocyte count and ensure the best chances of healing.

Recurrent Oxacillin-resistant Staphlococcus aureus Infections - Occasionally, diabetic patients with osteomyelitis caused by Oxacillin-resistant Staphlococcus aureus (ORSA) fail to respond to the strategic management of their "problem" wound. Despite

> The abbreviations ORSA (Oxacillin resistant Staphlococcus aureus) and MRSA (Methicillin resistant Staphloccus aureus) can be use interchangeably. The reason ORSA is the preferred terminology is because the sensitivity testing is actually done with Oxacillin rather than Methicillin. However, MRSA is the more common terminology.
>
> Likewise, OSSA (Oxacillin sensitive Staphlococcus aureus) and MSSA (Methicillin sensitive Staphlococcus aureus) are also interchangeable terms.

extended courses of organism-sensitive antibiotics, surgical debridements, hyperbaric oxygen therapy, and wound care, the infection recurs after the course of antibiotics is completed. These patients act as if they have a genetic deficiency in their immune systems for dealing with ORSA, and even with optimal management the infected bone and adjacent soft tissues never become sterilized. Once a course of antibiotics is completed, the infection recurs weeks to months later even though the wound site appears healed and infection free while the patient was on antibiotics. Because of the recurrences after optimal management, amputations one joint level above the recurrence site, that is, at the lower limb level, may be required to control the infection.

NEUROLOGICAL

Neurological Problems and Wounds - Neurological conditions contribute to wound healing problems. Much has already been said about neuropathy, but a few points need to be reiterated. First, neuropathy is an important contributor to "problem" wounds, but it is not the reason for non-healing. Countless numbers of patients with profound neuropathies and concomitant wounds heal their wounds and with prevention measures (Part V) avoid developing new wounds. Second, neuropathies as they pertain to wounds are manifested in three ways: sensory, motor, and autonomic (Figure 2-13). Each presentation is associated with specific problems and each requires specific interventions in order to avoid the development of wounds. Third, neuropathies that contribute to the development of "problem" wounds are not unique to diabetics. Severe joint contractures, which predispose to heel, hip, ischial, and presacral pressure ulcers, are a complication of strokes, multiple sclerosis, and Parkinsonism (Chapter 12). A multitude of other neurological problems such as Charcot-Marie-Tooth disease, leprosy, cerebral palsy, encephalopathies of various etiologies, reflex sympathetic dystrophy/complex regional pain syndrome, and spinal cord injuries predispose the patient to developing joint contractures and deformities. All are precursors to the development of "problem" wounds in vulnerable areas. Finally, the neurological status of the patient is one of the five assessments of the **Host-Function Score** (Table 2-4). If the neurological status of the patient is normal, a grade of 2 points (on a 0 to 2 scale) is assigned. A grade of 1 point is given to neurological conditions that cause minor to moderate sensory losses, muscle weaknesses/imbalances, or deformities. When these problems are severe, the neurological assessment component of the **Host-Function Score** is 0 points.

The sensory examination of a patient with a wound or wound predisposition such as a deformity can be done expediently with a "Quick & Easy" sensory evaluation (Table 2-5).

Neurological Problems: A Boon or a Bane? - While neurological deficits are undesirable, they have two consequences that facilitate wound care management and wound

Frequently, the patients with diabetic neuropathy, spinal cord injuries, and complex regional pain syndromes have disabling symptoms due to hypersensitivity from their nerve injuries. Often the wound site is anesthetized and allows debridements of the wound site to be performed without discomfort to the patient.

The neuropathic pain in these patients needs to be managed aggressively in a step-wise fashion. Initially, pain is managed with non-narcotic analgesics. If not effective, then the following agents may tried:

- Tricyclic antidepressants, such as amitriptyline, imipramine, and desipramine (Norpramin, Pertofrane)
- Other types of antidepressants, such as duloxetine (Cymbalta), venlafaxine, bupropion (Wellbutrin), paroxetine (Paxil), and citalopram (Celexa)
- Anticonvulsants, such as pregabalin (Lyrica), gabapentin (Gabarone, Neurontin), carbamazepine, and lamotrigine (Lamictal)
- Opioids and opioid-like drugs, such as controlled-release oxycodone, an opioid; and tramadol (Ultram), an opioid that also acts as an antidepressant

Agents may be applied to the skin, such as capsaicin cream and lidocaine patches (Lidoderm, Lidopain).

Finally, if these measures are not successful, local injection of lidocaine of the nerve immediately proximal to the symptom site should be tried. If there is temporary complete relief of pain, then justification for surgical transection of the nerve should be considered.

healing (Figure 6-5). First, impaired sensation in the area of a wound facilitates wound care. It allows for painless or nearly painless debridements and dressing changes.

Second, increased blood flow is associated with Charcot arthropathy which invariably has neurological components. Typically in this condition, wounds heal once deformities are corrected and the foot is stabilized. Consequently, neurological deficits must be recognized and addressed in all patients with "problem" wounds or the propensities for developing wounds (Part V). Knowledgeable, motivated patients with neuropathies usually can avoid wound problems once complications from the neuropathy, such as deformities, are appropriately managed. Primary interventions appropriately done by the

> Neuropathy is not a confounding factor with respect to healing of the "problem" wound. Deformity, ischemia/hypoxia, and uncontrolled infection are the three primary reasons wounds fail to heal (Chapter 2).
> Neuropathy is a risk factor for developing a "problem" wound.

wound care specialist include education in foot, skin and toenail care, appropriate activity level, and selection of proper footwear. When muscle imbalances, spasticity, and contracted joints are present, the primary care physician can initiate physical therapy, splinting, muscle relaxants, and pressure ulcer preventative measures. When deformities are severe, the surgical specialist is required to do tenotomies, release contractures, correct deformities, and/or realign the foot and ankle. When these fail, amputations by the surgeon may be the end-point.

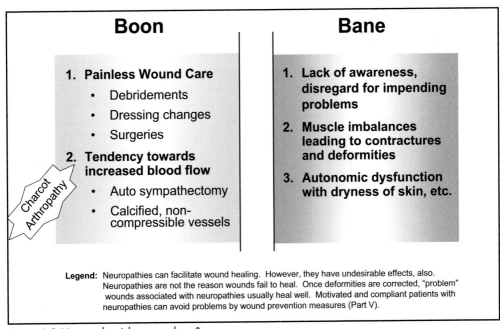

Boon	**Bane**
1. **Painless Wound Care** • Debridements • Dressing changes • Surgeries 2. **Tendency towards increased blood flow** • Auto sympathectomy • Calcified, non-compressible vessels	1. **Lack of awareness, disregard for impending problems** 2. **Muscle imbalances leading to contractures and deformities** 3. **Autonomic dysfunction with dryness of skin, etc.**

Charcot Arthropathy

Legend: Neuropathies can facilitate wound healing. However, they have undesirable effects, also. Neuropathies are not the reason wounds fail to heal. Once deformities are corrected, "problem" wounds associated with neuropathies usually heal well. Motivated and compliant patients with neuropathies can avoid problems by wound prevention measures (Part V).

Figure 6-5. Neuropathy: A boon or a bane?

NUTRITION

Causes of Malnutrition in the Patient with a Wound - The patient's nutrition status always needs to be assessed in the management of "problem" wounds. Malnutrition is often a contributing factor to wounds that are not responding as expected, and/or new wounds, especially pressure ulcers, that develop while the patient is being managed for a "problem" wound at a different site.[36] Malnutrition contributes to decreased or compromised immunocompetence and increased susceptibility to infection. Although much attention has been given to cancer and burn patients with regard to maintaining adequate nutrition, this critical consideration is sometimes ignored in the patient with the "problem" wound.

Chronically infected "problem" wounds are frequently associated with malnutrition, even though the wound may be small in size. There are several reasons for this: First, sepsis, which may be associated with "problem" wounds, is an appetite suppressant and can be a reason for inadequate nutrient intake. Second, co-existing conditions such as gastroparesis and malabsorption syndromes, as are frequently observed in diabetic patients, may interfere with food absorption in the gastrointestinal tract. Third, other co-existing conditions such as chronic renal insufficiency may be a cause of accelerated protein losses from the body. Fourth, neurological conditions such as stroke can cause dysphagia and severely limit or even disrupt the swallowing of food. Fifth, age-related changes in the body may be associated with poor dentition, inadequate salivation, weakness of jaw muscles for chewing, or combinations of these and may be the reason the patient selects or is fed a non-nutritious diet. Sixth, because of ignorance about nutrition, lack of money, or combinations of these, less expensive, less-nutritious foods are selected. Finally, psychiatric problems such as depression are observed in patients with "problem" wounds and can interfere with appetite. Usually the causes of malnutrition are multifactorial in the patient with a "problem" wound.

Special Features of Nutrition Problems - Nutrition problems have three special features. First, they are among the easiest to diagnose of all the medical problems in patients with serious wounds. This is because the patient's nutrition status can be readily assessed with anthropometric measurements (body mass index), biochemical tests, clinical evaluation and review of dietary history. Serum albumin is a biochemical indicator of visceral protein stores. Prealbumin provides analogous information. The advantage of monitoring prealbumin is that it responds much more quickly to interventions than albumin does. Whereas prealbumin levels will show changes in two to three days after implementing nutrition interventions, it may take three to four weeks for these effects to be reflected in the albumin levels (half-life 21 days). Second, weight and/or body mass

> The biochemical responses must be considered in the context of the patient's inflammatory response as monitored by the C-reactive protein.[37] Spuriously low prealbumin and albumin values occur in conjunction with the acute inflammatory response.

index are poor indicators of a patient's nutrition status. This paradox is often observed in the obese patient with a "problem" wound whose nutrition status, in terms of protein stores, is critically low. In addition, the caloric costs of the metabolic stress, such as wound healing, must be added to the basal energy expenditure (BEE) when determining caloric requirements for patients. For wounds and infections, the BEE must be multiplied by factors of 1.1 to 1.8 (depending on various factors such as trauma, stress, extent of wound, etc.) to determine total energy expenditures (TEE).[38] Third, unlike many of the other medical problems found in patients with "problem" wounds, nutrition problems can always be managed and corrected. That is, nutrition need never be an "end-stage," non-remedial problem in a patient where the decision has been made to treat the wound (Part IV).

Clinical Correlation:

A 79-year-old female with a persistent wound over the anterior aspect of her left leg following trauma to the area about 18 months before was referred for a wound care evaluation. Two previous skin grafts to the area had failed. The wound base was clean and viable, but devoid of granulation tissue.

Cultures grew skin flora and pulses were palpable in her feet. Aside from mild coronary artery disease and moderate obesity, the patient was healthy.

Hyperbaric oxygen treatments were started for the reason of failed skin grafts, and nutritional parameters were obtained. Initial albumin and prealbumin levels were about 50 percent of normal. The clinical nutrition consultant initiated a calorie reduction program with protein supplements.

After ten days the wound base began to develop granulation tissue. The prealbumin level had normalized although the albumin level was still low. On the 14th day after the above measures were started, a third split thickness skin graft was done with 100 percent take and excellent durability over the five years the patient returned for yearly follow-up evaluations.

Comment:

The patient's obesity masked her protein depletion state. It was no coincidence that the appearance of healthy granulation tissue coincided with normalization of the prealbumin level. The failure for the albumin to normalize at that point in time reflected its 21-day half-life. This observation has been observed repeatedly in patients whose wounds were not developing granulation tissue. Hyperbaric oxygen complements this process through its angiogenesis enhancement mechanism (Chapter 10).

The patient was followed semiannually to ensure she continued skin hygiene and lubrication for her legs and used venous stasis prevention support hose.

Nutrition Problems and Oral Supplementation - There are four levels of nutrition problems each with its own special interventions (Figure 6-6). For those patients who are able to eat and drink adequately, the first level of intervention is the addition of oral supplements. Generally, the oral supplements are milkshake-like drinks that have added vitamins, minerals, and protein (Table 6-5). Multivitamins and other nutrients may also be used for their specific effects (Table 6-6). The role of Vitamin C for wound healing is well recognized. Specific deficiencies such as iron deficiencies in anemic patients and zinc and magnesium deficiencies in diabetic patients can be confirmed with laboratory tests and can be managed appropriately. Patients on steroids should be supplemented with Vitamin A. Generally, supplementing mega-doses of vitamins and minerals is not recommended if overall nutrition intake is adequate, nor will it speed up wound healing.

For patients with persistently poor appetite, Megestrol acetate (Megace®) oral suspension, a synthetic derivative of the naturally occurring steroid hormone progesterone, can enhance appetite and is often given in conjunction with the oral supplements. Dronabinol (Marinol®), a marijuana derivative, and periactin (Cyproheptadine), an antihistamine-antipuritic agent, have also been used for appetite stimulation. Oxandrolone (Oxandrin®), a steroid, is sometimes prescribed to increase lean body mass. In overweight patients, the goal is to provide adequate protein intake to support wound healing and visceral protein repletion while reducing the overall calorie intake to achieve gradual weight reduction.

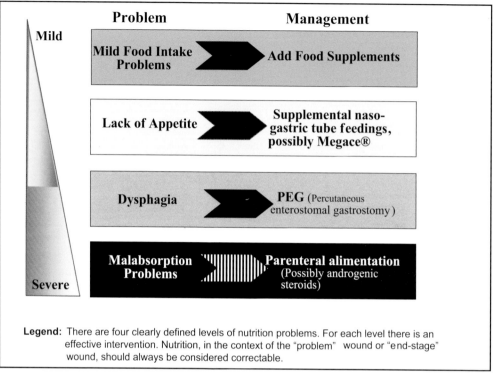

Legend: There are four clearly defined levels of nutrition problems. For each level there is an effective intervention. Nutrition, in the context of the "problem" wound or "end-stage" wound, should always be considered correctable.

Figure 6-6. The hierarchy of nutrition problems and their managment.

TABLE 6-5. CALORIE AND PROTEIN CONTENTS FOR 8 FLUID OUNCE DIET SUPPLEMENTS

Name	Kilocalories	Protein (Grams)	Purpose/Disease Type
Ensure Plus, Boost Plus	355-360	13-14	General
TwoCal HN	480	~20	General
Resource or Enlive (Clear Liquid)	250-300	9-10	General
Glucerna Shake	~230	10	Diabetes mellitus
Suplena	475	7	Renal insufficiency/ pre-dialysis
Nepro	475	~17	End-stage renal disease/dialysis

Comment: There are many comparable diet supplements. Those listed above are ones with which the authors are most familiar.

TABLE 6-6. VITAMIN, MINERAL, AND OTHER NUTRIENT SUPPLEMENTS FOR WOUND HEALING

Name	Effects	RDA (Recommended Dietary Allowance)	Supplementation for Wound Healing
Vitamin A	Healthiness of skin, and resistance to infection counteract the effects of gluticocorticosteroids	1000 mcg	3000 mcg
B Complex	Metabolism, skin and nervous system function, red blood cell formation	1-2 mg (3 mcg for B12)	Double RDA
Vitamin C	Wound healing, counteract undesirable effects from smoking	60-90mg (Add 35 mg/day for smokers)	Up to 1000mg BID
Vitamin D	Bone formation	5-10 mcg	Not recommended
Vitamin E	Protection from oxygen radicals may inhibit angiogenesis	8-10 mg	400 (~150 mg) international units twice daily
Vitamin K	Blood clotting	70-140 mcg	Not recommended
Zinc	Insulin metabolism	8-11 mg	40 mg
Arginine	May benefit immune function, nitrogen retention and wound healing; avoid in septic patients	NK	NK
Glutamine	Fuel source for rapidly diving cells	NK	0.57 grams per kilogram daily
HMB (B-hydroxy B-methylbutrate)	May increase collagen deposition, inhibit muscle breakdown	NK	NK

KEY: mcg = micrograms, **mg** = milligrams; **NK:** not known; **Yellow highlight** = particular importance for wound healing

Micronutrient requirements must be modified for patients with chronic liver and/or kidney disease as well as whether the patient is taking the agents by mouth or by parenteral routes.[39, 40]

In these situations, the recommendations from the dietician are essential and further establish the dietician as an integral member of the multidisciplinary wound care team. The clinical pharmacist is another essential wound team member who usually collaborates on dosing with the dietician and formulates the parenteral nutrition solutions.

Other Routes of Nutrition Administration - The second level of intervention is to supplement the patient's voluntary oral intake of food with nasogastric or nasojejunal feedings through a feeding tube. An effective technique is to allow the patient to eat and drink during the day and then use the feeding tube to provide additional nutrition during the night while sleeping. The dietician is the wound team member that manages these stages of the patient's nutrition problems. The third level of intervention is that of nutrition through a PEG (percutaneous enterostomal gastrotomy) tube. This intervention is needed when dysphagia is severe enough that adequate oral nutrition becomes impossible, complications arise from continuing the use of feeding tubes and/or the patient is at risk of aspirating food when swallowing, as frequently occurs with patients with residual neurological deficits from stroke. The gastroenterologist's input is needed for making the final decision about insertion of a PEG. The final level of nutrition intervention is parenteral feeding. In the presence of malabsorption syndromes or a nonfunctional GI tract in general, this may be the only way adequate nutrition can be achieved. Usually, the decision for using parenteral nutrition is a collaborative one with the primary care physician, the clinical dietitian, the pharmacist, the gastroenterologist, and the surgeon managing the wound care. When this hierarchy of interventions is used, virtually any malnutrition problem can be managed.

Summing-up Nutrition - As just described, the recognition and management of nutrition problems can be objective with much science to support the decision-making. The appropriate nutrition therapy care plan to promote adequate protein stores is fundamental to wound healing. Close associations have been observed between wound improvement and visceral protein levels. As the prealbumin begins to increase, the appearance of the wound base is frequently observed to change from a chronic non-healing appearance to one that is forming healthy granulation tissue. As the wound improves and the inflammatory response decreases (as reflected by a decrease in the CRP level), there is often a concomitant improvement in the prealbumin level.

The majority of nutrition challenges in patients with "problem" wounds occur in four forms: First is the morbidly obese patient that requires adequate protein intake, but a diet low enough in calories to result in weight reduction. Second is the patient with renal insufficiency who must follow a reduced protein diet in order to not cause deterioration in the function of their kidneys. Third, in those patients with hepatic encephalopathy where ammonia levels are elevated and the use of Lactulose does not adequately control this problem, protein restrictions are necessary. Fourth is the patient whose oral intake is inadequate, is unable to swallow or absorb food. These problems become remedial with assistance of the clinical dietitian and the hierarchy of nutrition interventions that are available (Figure 6-6).

PSYCHIATRIC

Mild and Serious Psychiatric Conditions that Contribute to "Problem" Wound Challenges - Although psychiatric problems may seem far removed from the obvious causes of non-healing wounds, they may contribute to wound healing problems both directly and indirectly. Unfortunately, they tend to be disregarded due to focusing attention to the wound. With reference to wounds, psychiatric problems in their milder forms may be manifested as denial that the wound is so serious; anxieties to the point of refusal of treatment interventions, especially hyperbaric oxygen therapy; non-compliance with care, and unrealistic expectations, such as refusing amputation surgery in hopes that a gangrenous foot will come back to life. In their more serious forms, patients may use their wounds for manipulative purposes, that is to control the activities of their care-givers or actually generate wounds (Munchausen's syndrome) to gain sympathy or avoid responsibilities. Life and limb threatening wounds are also seen in patients with antisocial personality disorder and or substance abuse problems that develop at infected street drug injection sites. Finally, the patient may be oblivious to the wound due to severe depression, schizophrenia, or dementia. These may cause indirect problems such as malnutrition and direct problems such as inability to follow directions or self-destructive behavior that further harms the tissues in the "problem" wound.

Hierarchy in the Management of Psychiatric Problems Associated with Wounds - Milder psychiatric problems are appropriately managed by the wound care specialist, typically with discussions of management options and anticipated outcomes and the prescribing of anti-anxiety agents and sedatives. This is usually done in conjunction with support from the primary care physician, especially when the medications are required on an ongoing basis. Dementia to the point of being oblivious to the wound problem, the requirement for major psychoactive medications to control behavior, the use of wounds to manipulate others, or wounds that are self-induced are all factors that qualify the psychiatric problems as "decompensated" from the patient's mental status perspective. For these problems, as well as drug addiction/detoxification, collaboration and follow-up care with a psychiatrist is needed.

PULMONARY AND CRITICAL CARE

Pulmonary Issues in Wound Healing - Pulmonary problems are rarely a concern in wound healing. However, if they are serious enough to cause hypoxemia, they could adversely affect wound healing. In addition, medications, such as steroids and immuno-suppressors that are needed to manage the pulmonary condition can interfere with wound healing. Usually pulmonary problems are associated with other serious medical problems such as cardiovascular, endocrine, infectious disease, and rheumatological, and frequently require management by the pulmonary and critical care medicine specialist. This is observed in patients with life and limb threatening necrotizing soft tissue infections. In patients who have "problem" wounds with pulmonary conditions such as pneumonia, chronic obstructive pulmonary disease, asthma, and bronchitis and with normal or only mildly abnormal pulmonary function tests, it is appropriate for the primary care physician to manage these conditions. Significantly abnormal pulmonary function studies, critically low tissue oxygen saturations and/or requirement for assisted ventilation define "decompensated" lung function and the indication for collaboration with the pulmonary medicine specialist. Consequently, as in the medical conditions previously described, there is a hierarchy of seriousness of pulmonary conditions and rather well defined levels of care for each in patients with "problem" wounds.

Patients who retain carbon dioxide should also be considered in the "decompensated" pulmonary function group.

This latter problem has important ramifications if the patient is receiving hyperbaric oxygen therapy (HBO). Since these patients have lost the carbon dioxide respiratory drive, respiration is initiated by low blood oxygen tensions.

With HBO, blood oxygen levels will be increased so much that the hypoxemia drive to breathe is no longer present. If the patient falls asleep during the HBO treatment, breathing may cease and the patient will not adequately ventilate.

This problem does not pose an absolute contraindication for hyperbaric oxygen therapy, but rather it requires diligence on the part of staff to keep the patient awake and remind the patient to breathe during the HBO exposure.

RENAL

Renal Disease Challenges for Wound Healing - Chronic kidney disease in conjunction with diabetes is associated with high percentages of failures in the management of "problem" wounds. Several explanations are offered, including: 1) Azotemia and protein losses interfere with the wound healing environment, 2) The angiopathy that led to the kidney problem also affects the vasculature in the wound healing area, 3) Immunosuppression for preservation of kidney allografts interfere with healing and infection control and 4) Arterial-venous fistulas for dialysis when proximal to the wound "steal" blood from the wound-healing area. Due to protein loss, the lower limit of normal for prealbumin in the azotemic patient is about 20 percent higher than for the non-azotemic patient. Approximately thirty percent of patients with chronic kidney disease (renal insufficiency or "end-stage" renal disease) have advanced peripheral artery disease.[41, 42] In most of these patients the vascular disease is so severe that they are not candidates for revascularization or angioplasty or previous revascularizations have not resolved the perfusion problems.

Classification of the seriousness of renal disease using the previous format is probably more objective than for any of the other medical problems discussed. If the patient has renal insufficiency, as manifested by elevated blood urea nitrogen and creatinine levels and decreased urinary creatinine clearance, the label of "impaired" renal function is appropriate. If the patient requires dialysis, then renal function is "decompensated" and a nephrologist is needed for management. Occasionally, acute renal failure occurs in patients with "problem" wounds, typically associated with severe sepsis and/or trauma. In patients who were previously healthy, renal function usually improves as the patient's other problems resolve. Patients who have had renal transplants present additional wound healing challenges primarily due to the requirement for immunosuppressors to prevent rejection of the allografted organ. Because of the need to protect the transplanted organ all medication use, dietary management and vitamin and mineral supplementation requires collaboration with the patient's nephrologist.

RHEUMATOLOGICAL
Wound Healing Challenges from Rheumatological Conditions - Rheumatological problems, like pulmonary conditions, are infrequently associated with serious wounds. Yet, when wounds are present in patients with underlying rheumatological problems, they can be very difficult to manage. The rheumatological conditions that are associated with the most challenging wound problems are the collagen vascular and autoimmune diseases such as rheumatoid arthritis, psoriasis, lupus, scleroderma, dermatomyositis, and mixed connective tissue disorder. This is because vasculitis at the microcirculation level is often a component of these diseases. The other serious problem is abnormal collagen formation and metabolism, which directly interferes with wound healing. A not-unusual finding is the presence of palpable pulses, yet the wound is non-healing distal to the pulse because of the microangiopathy and collagen metabolism problems. A further complicating feature is that steroids, disease-modifying anti-rheumatic drugs (DMARDs), and antimetabolites may be required to control the rheumatological problem. All these medications interfere with wound healing and control of infection. Collagen vascular diseases frequently affect the kidneys and further complicate wound healing from this perspective. Any patient with a collagen vascular disease should be considered as an "impaired" host with respect to wound healing and requires collaboration, at the minimum, with the patient's primary care physician with respect to management of the wound. Criteria for labeling the rheumatological condition as "decompensated" include the disease is serious enough to require steroids, DMARDs or antimetabolites, multi-organ involvement is present, and/or there are marked joint deformities. At this level of seriousness, collaboration for wound management should be done with the rheumatologist. Patients with concomitant infected total-joint arthroplasties and associated collagen vascular diseases are among the most difficult to salvage of all infected joint arthroplasties and require management jointly by orthopaedic surgeons, infectious disease specialists, and rheumatologists.

CONCLUSIONS

Medical Strategies - There is little question that the care for the medical problems in patients with serious wounds is an essential strategy for the management of "problem" wounds. Consequently, the maxim "Care for the wound is only part of the story; success depends on how you manage the rest of the patient's problems" could not be more important for expressing the essence of this chapter. The use of the simple classification of the medical condition as "normal," "impaired" or "decompensated" provides an immediate tool as to the seriousness of the problem, how much it will interfere with wound healing, and the level of expertise needed to manage it (Figure 6-7). If the patient is classified as "normal," the wound specialist usually does not need to request help from consultants. If "impaired," management can usually be done at the primary care physician level. If serious enough to be classified as "decompensated," the medical specialist is usually required to manage the problem. Some of the medical problems are remedial, such as nutrition, certain hematological conditions, and infectious diseases. Others may remain stable, such as neurological conditions, "end-stage" renal disease, cardiac disease, and psychiatric problems. Peripheral artery, rheumatological, and pulmonary problems may continue to worsen as time progresses and present increasingly severe challenges for wound healing. The main dilemma with respect to the medical management strategy is that while the patient is hospitalized, complete control and collaboration from multi-disciplines is easy to accomplish, but compliance and follow-up is often times difficult to achieve on an outpatient basis. In summary, the goals of the medical management strategy for "problem" wounds are to optimize management of medical comorbidities, to provide medical clearances for surgery, and to prevent future complications.

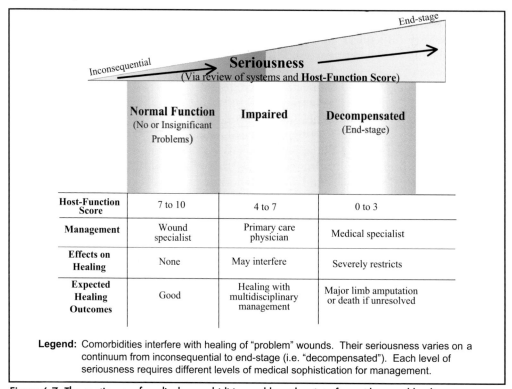

	Normal Function (No or Insignificant Problems)	Impaired	Decompensated (End-stage)
Host-Function Score	7 to 10	4 to 7	0 to 3
Management	Wound specialist	Primary care physician	Medical specialist
Effects on Healing	None	May interfere	Severely restricts
Expected Healing Outcomes	Good	Healing with multidisciplinary management	Major limb amputation or death if unresolved

Legend: Comorbidities interfere with healing of "problem" wounds. Their seriousness varies on a continuum from inconsequential to end-stage (i.e. "decompensated"). Each level of seriousness requires different levels of medical sophistication for management.

Figure 6-7. The continuum of medical comorbidities and how they interfere with wound healing.

QUESTIONS

1. How do the classification tools "normal," "impaired," and "decompensated" help to decide the level of care needed for comorbid conditions?

2. How is the designation "impaired" differentiated from "decompensated" when assessing the cardiac status of a patient with a "problem" wound?

3. How does hyperglycemia contribute to diabetic complications?

4. When should a hematologist be consulted as part of the wound healing team?

5. When should an infectious disease specialist be consulted as part of the wound healing team?

6. How do neurological conditions contribute to the development of wounds and interfere with wound healing?

7. What are the four levels of intervention for managing nutrition deficits?

8. How can psychiatric problems interfere with wound healing?

9. What possible mechanisms contribute to poor wound healing responses in patients with "end-stage" renal disease?

10. Which medical comorbidities are likely to be remedial? Which are likely to remain stable and unchanged? And which are likely to deteriorate during the course of managing the "problem" wound?

REFERENCES

1. Moon RE, Hart BB. Operational use and patient monitoring in a multiplace hyperbaric chamber. Respir Care Clin N Am. 1999 Mar;5(1):21-49

2. Reiber GE, Lipsky BA, Gibbons GW. The burden of diabetic foot ulcers. Am J Surg. 1998 Aug;176(2A Suppl):5S-10S

3. Global Lower Extremity Amputation Study Group. Epidemiology of lower extremity amputation in centres in Europe, North America and East Asia. The Global Lower Extremity Amputation Study Group. Br J Surg. 2000 Mar;87(3):328-37

4. Strauss, MB, Strauss WG. Wound scoring system streamlines decision-making. BioMechanics 1999 VI(8):37–43

5. Borer KM, Borer Jr RC, Strauss MB. Prospective evaluation of a clinical wound score to identify lower extremity wounds for comprehensive wound management. Undersea Hyperbaric Med 2000 27(Suppl):34

6. Strauss MB. Hyperbaric oxygen as an intervention for managing wound hypoxia; its role and usefulness on diabetic foot wounds. Foot Ankle Internal. 2005; 26(1):15-18

7. Reichard P, Nilsson BY, Rosenqvist U. The effect of long-term intensified insulin treatment on the development of microvascular complications of diabetes mellitus. N Engl J Med. 1993 Jul 29;329(5):304–9

8. Clark, CM Jr, DA Lee. Prevention and treatment of the complications of diabetes mellitus. N Engl J Med. May 1995 4;332(18):1210–17

9. Dyck P, Thomas PK, eds. 1999. Diabetic neuropathy. 560 pp. Philadelphia: W.B. Saunders

10. Buckingham BA, Uitto J, Sandborg C, et al. scleroderma-like changes in insulin-dependent diabetes mellitus: clinical and biochemical studies. Diabetes Care. 1984 Mar-Apr;7(2):163-9

11. Mazade MA, Edwards MS. Impairment of type III group B Streptococcus-stimulated superoxide production and opsonophagocytosis by neutrophils in diabetes. Mol Genet Metab. 2001 Jul;73(3):259–67

12. Perner A, Nielsen SE, Rask-Madsen J. High glucose impairs superoxide production from isolated blood neutrophils. Intensive Care Med. 2003 Apr;29(4):642–5. Epub 2003 Jan 28

13. Wall SJ, Sampson MJ, Levell N, Murphy G. Elevated matrix metalloproteinase-2 and -3 production from human diabetic dermal fibroblasts. Br J Dermatol. 2003 Jul;149(1):13-6

14. Lazar HL, Chipkin SR, Fitzgerald CA, et al. Tight glycemic control in diabetic coronary artery bypass graft patients improves perioperative outcomes and decreases recurrent ischemic events. Circulation 2004 Mar 30;109(12):1497-502. Epub 2004 Mar 8

15. Zerr KJ, Furnary AP, Grunkemeier GL, Bookin S, Kanhere V, Starr A. Glucose control lowers the risk of wound infection in diabetics after open heart operations. Ann Thorac Surg. 1997 Feb;63(2):356-61

16. Guvener M, Pasaoglu I, Demircin M, Oc M. Perioperative hyperglycemia is a strong correlate of postoperative infection in type II diabetic patients after coronary artery bypass grafting. Endocr J. 2002 Oct;49(5):531-7

17. Furnary AP, Gao G, Grunkemeier GL, Wu Y, Zerr KJ, Bookin SO, Floten HS, Starr A. Continuous insulin infusion reduces mortality in patients with diabetes undergoing coronary artery bypass grafting. J Thorac Cardiovasc Surg. 2003 May;125(5):1007-21

18. Li JY, Sun S, Wu SJ. Continuous insulin infusion improves postoperative glucose control in patients with diabetes mellitus undergoing coronary artery bypass surgery. Tex Heart Inst J. 2006;33(4):445-51

19. Nathan DM. Long-term complications of diabetes mellitus. N Engl J Med. 1993 Jun 10;328(23):1676–85

20. Dellon AL. Treatment of symptomatic diabetic neuropathy by surgical decompression of multiple peripheral nerves. Plast Reconstr Surg. 1992 Apr;89(4):689-97

21. The Diabetes Control and Complications Trial Research Group: The effect of intensive treatment of diabetes on the development and progression of long-term complications in insulin-dependent diabetes mellitus. N Engl J Med. 329:977–986, 1993

22. UK Prospective Diabetes Study (UKPDS) Group. Intensive blood-glucose control with sulphony-lureas or insulin compared with conventional treatment and risk of complications in patients with type 2 diabetes (UKPDS 33) 1998 Lancet; 352:837

23. Lewis EJ, Hunsicker LG, Clarke WR, Berl T, Pohl MA, Lewis JB, Ritz E, Atkins RC, Rohde R, Raz I. Collaborative Study Group. Renoprotective effect of the angiotensin-receptor antagonist irbesartan in patients with nephropathy due to type 2 diabetes. N Engl J Med. 2001 Sep 20;345(12):851-60

24. Brenner BM, Cooper ME, de Zeeuw D, Keane WF, Mitch WE, Parving HH, Remuzzi G, Snapinn SM, Zhang Z, Shahinfar S; RENAAL Study Investigators. Effects of losartan on renal and cardiovascular outcomes in patients with type 2 diabetes and nephropathy. N Engl J Med. 2001 Sep 20;345(12):861-9

25. Gashti CN, Bakris GL. The role of calcium antagonists in chronic kidney disease. Curr Opin Nephrol Hypertens. 2004 Mar;13(2):155-61

26. Moriyama T, Oka K, Ueda H, Imai E. Nilvadipine attenuates mesangial expansion and glomerular hypertrophy in diabetic db/db mice, a model for type 2 diabetes. Clin Exp Nephrol. 2004 Sep;8(3):230-6

27. Nathan DM. Prevention of long-term complications of non-insulin-dependent diabetes mellitus. Clin Invest Med. 1995. Aug;18(4):332–39

28. Nathan DM. The pathophysiology of diabetic complications: how much does the glucose hypothesis explain? Ann Intern Med. 1996. Jan 1;124(1 Pt 2):86–89

29. Levine JS, Branch DW, Rauch J. The antiphospholipid syndrome. N Engl J Med. 2002 Mar 7;346(10):752-63

30. Eneroth M, Persson BM. Risk factors for failed healing in amputation for vascular disease. A prospective, consecutive study of 177 cases. Acta Orthop Scand. 1993 Jun;64(3):369-72

31. Hansen ES, Wethelund JO, Skajaa K. Hemoglobin and hematocrit as risk factors in below-the-knee amputation for incipient gangrene. Arch Orthop Trauma Surg. 1988;107(2):92-5

32. Newman LG, Waller J, Palestro CJ, Schwartz M, Klein MJ, Hermann G, Harrington E, Harrington M, Roman SH, Stagnaro-Green A. Unsuspected osteomyelitis in diabetic foot ulcers. Diagnosis and monitoring by leukocyte scanning with indium in 111 oxyquinoline. JAMA. 1991 Sep 4;266(9):1246-51

33. Newman LG, Waller J, Palestro CJ, Hermann G, Klein MJ, Schwartz M, Harrington E, Harrington M, Roman SH, Stagnaro-Green A. Leukocyte scanning with 111In is superior to magnetic resonance imaging in diagnosis of clinically unsuspected osteomyelitis in diabetic foot ulcers. Diabetes Care. 1992 Nov;15(11):1527-30

34. Mousa HA. Evaluation of sinus-track cultures in chronic bone infection. J Bone Joint Surg Br. 1997 Jul;79(4):567-9

35. Patzakis MJ, Wilkins J, Kumar J, et al. Comparison of the results of bacterial cultures from multiple sites in chronic osteomyelitis of long bones. A prospective study. J Bone Joint Surg Am. 1994 May;76(5):664-6

36. Ord H. Nutritional support for patients with infected wounds. Br J Nurs. 2007 Nov 22-Dec 12;16(21):1346-8, 1350-2

37. Demling, R.H., DeSanti, L. (2000). The stress response to injury and infection: Role of nutritional support. Wounds: A Compendium of Clinical Research and Practice, 12(1), 3-14

38. Clinical Nutrition. A Resource Book for Delivering Enteral and Parenteral Nutrition for Adults. University of Washington. Academic Medical Centers, Harborview Medical Center, University of Washington Medical Center, Seattle, Washington, 1997. http://healthlinks.washington.edu/nutrition/ Accessed on January 7, 2008

39. Ross V. Micronutrient recommendations for wound healing. Support Line 2002; 24:3–9

40. Thompson C, Fuhrman MP. Nutrients and wound healing: still searching for the magic bullet. Nutr Clin Pract. 2005 Jun;20(3):331-47

41. Kohlhagen J, Kelly J. Prevalence of vascular risk factors and vascular disease in predialysis chronic renal failure. Nephrology (Carlton). 2003 Dec;8(6):274-9

42. Leskinen Y, Salenius JP, Lehtimaki T, Huhtala H, Saha H. The prevalence of peripheral arterial disease and medial arterial calcification in patients with chronic renal failure: requirements for diagnostics. Am J Kidney Dis. 2002 Sep;40(3):472-9

CHAPTER

7 PREPARATION OF THE WOUND BASE

CHAPTER SEVEN OVERVIEW

INTRODUCTION 167
WOUND BASE DESCRIPTIONS 169
MANAGEMENT OF THE WOUND BASE. 174
HEALING STAGES OF THE "PROBLEM" WOUND. 178
MANAGEMENT OF SPECIAL WOUND BASE PROBLEMS 184
CONCLUSIONS 189
QUESTIONS 191
REFERENCES 192

> ## *"A wound without a healthy base*
> ## *is like a tree without roots."*

INTRODUCTION

Appropriate preparation of the wound base is essential for managing the "problem" wound. In contrast to the previous chapter that dealt with medical aspects of the "problem" wound, the management of the wound base needs to be considered from a surgical perspective. The base must be made clean enough and sufficiently free of unhealthy tissue so that other treatment strategies can become as effective as possible. In addition, preparation of the wound base needs to be done so that coverage or closure of the wound becomes feasible after taking into consideration the healing potential of the wound site. Wounds that are not healing or are problematic for healing may be given labels such as indolent, limb threatening, refractory, or use etiologies such as burns, post-traumatic, toxic, vasculitic, etc. We prefer the use of the terms "problem," "end-stage," and "futile" wound since they can be quantified by the **Wound Score** with each having special management interventions (Figure 5-3). "Problem wounds" fail to heal for three primary reasons: 1) deformities, 2) uncontrolled infection, and 3) ischemia/hypoxia (Chapter 2). Invariably, elements of the three reasons given above explain why they are wound healing challenges (Table 7-1). As stated before, neuropathy is not a reason a "problem" wound fails to heal. It may contribute to the development of a deformity secondary to muscle imbalances or delay diagnosis because of loss of pain awareness. This chapter describes the management required to optimize the appearance and quality of the wound base. Although this aspect of the strategic management of the "problem" wound usually employs surgical procedures, other techniques to achieve these two goals will be discussed.

Why Wounds Persist – "Problem" wounds persist for many reasons. Underlying bony deformities are a primary reason. Wounds arising because of these deformities, especially in the feet, are termed malperforans ulcers. In other locations they are called pressure ulcers (over the site of involvement, e.g. trochanter, ankle, ischium, or presacral), or indolent ulcers. Management of the deformity is often all that needs to be done to initiate healing of these types of problem wounds. Many times, especially in the feet and toes, this can be done with minimally invasive surgeries (Chapter 16). Chronically infected wounds are invariably due to underlying osteomyelitis (usually avascular) or other poorly vascularized tissue such as bursae and cicatrix (dense scar tissue). When "problem" wounds arise secondary to acute infections such as necrotizing fasciitis, ischemia/hypoxia is an important contributor to the problem. In either acute or chronically infected wounds, surgical interventions are an integral part of the wound base management strategy. As discussed before, ischemia may be due to central causes such as cardiac impairment, large vessel disease, small vessel disease (angiopathy), venous insufficiency, or combinations of these. Although wound base management would seem to be best managed by the surgical disciplines of the wound team (general surgeons, plastic surgeons, orthopaedic surgeons, and podiatrists), other members of the wound team can perform many surgically related activities to prepare the wound base.

TABLE 7-1. PRIMARY & SECONDARY REASONS WOUNDS DO NOT HEAL OR BECOME HEALING PROBLEMS

Problem	Reason	Considerations, Comments
Deformity	Primary	Frequently due to muscle imbalances secondary to neuropathy, trauma (malunited fractures), or hereditary conditions
Uncontrolled Infection	Primary	Usually due to avascularity of bone (osteomyelitis), bursa or cicatrix, or foreign material in the wound complicated by ischemia/hypoxia at the infection site
Ischemia/ Hypoxia	Primary	Inadequate circulation (impaired heart function), edema, inadequate perfusion (peripheral vascular disease), and/or microangiopathy (thickened basement membrane)
Burn	**Secondary** (All have 1 or more of the primary reasons wounds do not heal)	Irreversible thermal damage to the skin; **ischemia** due to blood vessel damage, stasis, and edema
Post-op		**Ischemia** from tissue injury; **infection**
Post-traumatic		Same as for post-op; **ischemia** and **infection**
Pressure Sore		Underlying **deformities** (bony prominences) and/or contractures (muscles imbalances) secondary to neurological deficits
Shear		Repetitive trauma usually over bony prominences (**deformities**), compromised skin (**ischemia**), or abnormal motion secondary to neurological impairment
Toxic		Secondary to toxin or foreign material introduction (snake bite, spider bite, extravasation of drugs, or high-pressure injection injuries) causing tissue damage and **ischemia**
Vasculitic		Associated with collagen vascular diseases; non-healing due to **ischemia** (microangiopathy and/or sympathetic vasomotor over-activity); **infection** secondary to immunosuppression (steroids, antimetabolites, non-steroidal anti-inflammatory agents)
Venous stasis		Venous insufficiency leading to edema (a **deformity** in some respects) and **ischemia** (from increased diffusion distance of oxygen through the edema fluid and nearly avascular cicatrix formation under the ulcer base)

Note: Diabetes mellitus (as in "diabetic foot wounds") and peripheral neuropathy are not reasons "problem" wounds fail to heal and, consequently, are not included in the above table.

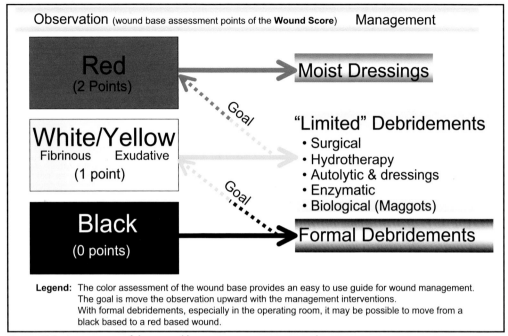

Observation (wound base assessment points of the **Wound Score**)   Management

Red
(2 Points)

→ Moist Dressings

White/Yellow
Fibrinous   Exudative
(1 point)

"Limited" Debridements
• Surgical
• Hydrotherapy
• Autolytic & dressings
• Enzymatic
• Biological (Maggots)

Goal

Black
(0 points)

Goal

→ Formal Debridements

Legend: The color assessment of the wound base provides an easy to use guide for wound management. The goal is move the observation upward with the management interventions. With formal debridements, especially in the operating room, it may be possible to move from a black based to a red based wound.

Figure 7-1. Appearance of the wound base as a management guide.

WOUND BASE DESCRIPTIONS

Describing the Wound Base – The wound base appearance assessment of the **Wound Score** provides an easy, objective, and efficient method for evaluating the wound base and initiating appropriate management of this component. It merely requires discriminating between the colors red, white (or yellow), and black (Figure 7-1). This simplified classification system provides the basis for interventions to manage the wound base (described in the next section of this chapter). Also, it contributes to the dynamic aspect of the **Wound Score**. The goal for management of the wound base is for it to evolve to a red, healthy, granulating appearance that becomes ready for coverage or closure. As the color of the wound base improves, the grade rises, contributing to an improved **Wound Score**. This explains how the **Wound Score** is dynamic; that is, improvements (or deterioration) in each of the five components is reflected in a change in the **Wound Score**.

> The additional wound information (Table 7-2) should be included in the wound description of the initial medical record notes, and amended in subsequent notes as the wound and surrounding skin characteristics change.
>
> The description of the wound in the chart notes should be so lucid that the reader of the note will be able to "visualize" what the wound looks like even without photographs.
>
> The **Wound Score** is a scoring system to quantify the seriousness of the wound and help make management decisions (**Master Algorithm**, Figure 5-2). The wound base assessment provides a simplified method to establish a grade point for the many characteristics (Tables 5-1 & 7-2 and Figure 5-1) that can be used to describe a wound.

TABLE 7-2. ADDITIONAL INFORMATION TO SUPPLEMENT THE DESCRIPTION OF A WOUND

I. Type of Wound Base

1. Healthy, granulating tissue
2. Hypovascular ("anemic" appearing granulation tissue)
3. Vascular, non-granulating (e.g. exposed muscle after fasciotomy)
4. Gelatinous membrane, biofilm
5. Fibrinous membrane (thick or thin)
6. Transudate, ichor (thin watery discharge)
7. Exudate, ischoroid discharge (purulent discharge; scant, moderate, large)
8. Thin eschar (viable tissue underneath)
9. Thick eschar (full thickness slough)
10. Necrotic soft tisssue (wet gangrene)
11. Advancing necrosis (progressive necrotizing soft tissue infection)

II. Shape of Wound Margins

1. Round
2. Oval, ovoid
3. Oblong
4. Triangular
5. Dumbbell (two larger portions connected by a narrow isthmus)
6. Serpiginous (snake-like, multiple smooth curves)
7. Crescent (semi-lunar, falcate, hemispherical, sickle shaped)
8. Saw toothed (jagged, irregular)
9. Bi-lobed, pear or gourd shaped
10. Narrow, slit-like
11. Dehisced (post-op separation along suture line—superficial or full thickness)

III. Characteristics of Surrounding Skin

1. Normal, smooth, flat
2. Verrucose (wart-like), papillomatous (bumpy)
3. Rutted (narrow furrows), grooved, (single or wide furrows)
4. Corrugated (cardboard-like), wrinkled (especially after edema reduction)
5. Filamentous (filament projections)
6. Edematous; pitting vs brawny, diffuse vs localized
7. Induration; firm edema with associated erythema warmth and tenderness
8. Varicosities, telangiectases
9. Wound margins: 1) Thin crust, 2) Callus/hyperkeratosis (firm & dry or moist & soft), 3) Epithelialized
10. Necrotic soft tisssue (wet gangrene)
11. Advancing necrosis (progressive necrotizing soft tissue infection)

IV. Color of Surrounding Skin

1. Normal, (pink, rosy)
2. Dusky (dark, dark-shade)
3. Cyanotic (bluish, dark blue)
4. Black
5. Pale
6. Piebald (two colored)
7. Variegated (multicolored)
8. Bronzed, hyperpigmented
9. Erythematous (cellulitic, hyperemic)

V. Geometry (contours) of Wound Base

1. Flat at the level of the skin surface
2. Cavitary (depth of cavity)
3. Recessed (extent and clock location)
4. Tracking (depth and clock location)
5. Tunneling (from where to where)
6. Fistula (track between 2 cavities)

Additional Wound Base Information – The wound site should always be accurately localized using anatomical terms such as segment (e.g. toes, foot, ankle, leg, etc.), position (e.g. dorsal, plantar, posterior, medial, middle, lateral), and portion of the segment (e.g. proximal, middle or distal thirds). Additional information can be added to the red, white/yellow, black description of the wound base to further its depiction (Table 5-1, Figure 5-1 and Table 7-2). This information includes the type of wound base, the shape of the wound margins, the characteristics of the surrounding skin, the color of the surrounding skin and the topography (contours) of the wound base. This information is useful for documentation purposes and for describing an individual wound, but

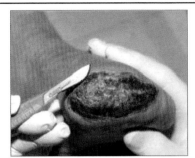
Thin Serous Crust

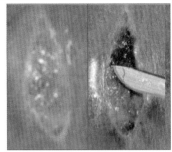
Thin Filmy Exudate

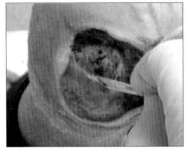
Fibrinous Membrane/ Biofilm

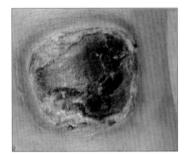
Thin Firm Eschar

Legend: Additional information is useful for describing the wound base and documenting progress

Figure 7-2. Vascular-based wounds with different appearances.

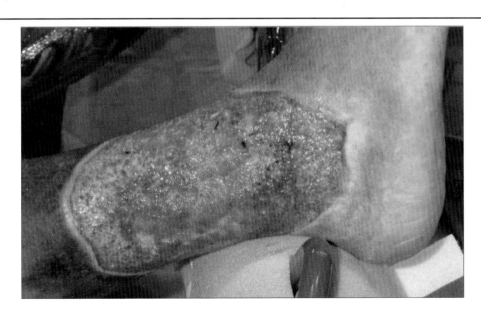

Legend: The wound base is ready for skin grafting. Note the epithelialization (white rim) that is occurring around the wound margins. **Wound Score** = 6 1/2 points **Appearance of wound base** = 2, **Size** = 0, **Depth** = 1 points, **Infection/Bioburden** = 1 1/2 points and **Perfusion** = 2 points

Figure 7-3. Vascular-based wounds covered with healthy granulation tissue.

should be considered as an adjunct to the **Wound Score** grading assessment and for guiding management of the wound base.

Red Based Wound – A red-based wound is indicative of a good vascular supply (Figure 5-4). However, not all wounds with vascular, viable bases are ready for coverage or closure (Figure 7-2). The formation of healthy-appearing granulation tissue in the wound base is the sign that the wound is ready for coverage or closure (Figure 7-3). This finding is highly predictive that skin grafting or secondary surgical closures will be successful. The healthy granulating wound base is characterized by a homogenous, red, velvety-like appearance somewhat resembling finely ground, uncooked hamburger meat. Although healthy granulating wounds are colonized by bacteria, no exudates are present and the portions of the dressings that contact the wound base have a faint reddish pink stain on them. Another characteristic observed in healthy granulating tissues is that dressing changes are no longer painful. Finally, epithelial in-growth begins to appear around the wound margins of the healthy granulating wound.

"Frustrated" Granulation Tissue – At times "frustrated" forms of granulation tissue develop in wound bases. This type of granulation tissue is often found over fibrinous membranes or ischemic underlying tissues. It is pale in color and does not have the beefy red appearance of healthy granulation tissue. Many times it will also be covered with a thin exudate (ichoroid discharge). These findings are often found in the bases of chronic, non-healing wounds. A pale, anemic appearing wound base is often associated with malnutrition. With appropriate wound base management (next section), these wounds can usually develop healthy enough bases that healing will occur either by epithelialization at the margins or with surgical techniques. Initiation of an inflammatory response with increased blood flow, angiogenesis, and development of healthy granulation tissue is a fundamental objective of the preparation of the wound base strategy.

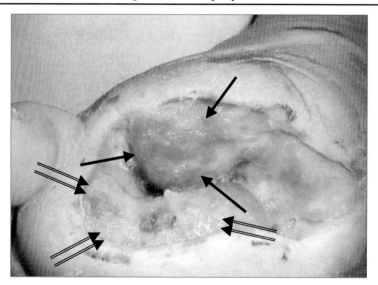

Legend: The wound base appears ischemic. Areas of vascularized wound base are present (single arrows), but are not covered with healthy granulation tissue. Other areas are covered with a fibrinous membrane. **Wound Score** = 5 points (**Appearance of wound base** = 1 point, **Size** = 1 1/2 points, **Depth** = 1/2 point (due to tract), **Infection/Bioburden** = 1 point and **Perfusion** = 1 point).

Figure 7-4. Ischemic-based wound.

White or Yellow Based Wound – The white or yellow based wound represents the intermediate type (Grade 1 on the 0 to 2 scale) of wound base (Figure 5-4). These findings indicate that the wound is not ready for coverage or closure and more needs to be done to improve the wound base. If the wound base assumes this appearance after debridement, it may only be a matter of time before it evolves into a healthy-based wound. This is especially true if initially the base was a Grade 0, that is, had a black, necrotic base (Figure 5-4). Yellow coloration in the base of a wound is typically from an exudate, a biofilm, and is usually indicative of infection flourishing in the wound base. The underlying causes of persistent exudates, a biofilm in wound bases, are wound ischemia/hypoxia, necrotic material in the wound base, bacteria that are not sensitive to the antibiotics the patient is receiving, or combinations of these. The white base of a wound may be either due to an exudate, a biofilm, or from interruption of healing due to the causes described above. Persistent or recurrent formation of fibrin (scabs), fibrin crusts (dried scabs), fibrinous membranes, and cicatrix formation suggest that the wound base is too hypoxic to form healthy granulation tissue.

Black Based Wound – When the base of wound is black, it is obvious that the tissue covering the wound base is necrotic. If it is thin, such as crust or thin eschar, it is usually indicative of healthy underlying tissue, especially if the surrounding skin is okay. The eschar can be used as a biological dressing. However, if it is thick, soft, and/or fluctuant, it indicates that dead tissue, suppuration, or both are under the wound base (Figure 7-5). This requires surgical debridement to viable tissues. Many times the demarcation is not clear; that is, there is a transition from necrotic to compromised—viable, but unhealthy—to healthy tissue. By debriding to compromised but viable tissue and leaving the wound open with appropriate dressing selections (Chapter 9) and application of the other components of strategic management, tissues are more likely to be conserved and

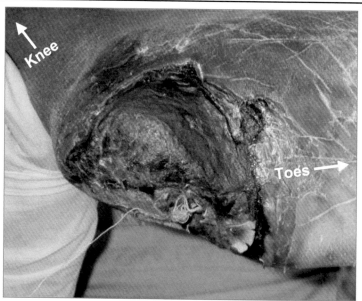

Legend: The soft eschar covering the wound base indicates full thickness necrosis to the underlying calcaneus. Although no exudate is evident, the eschar margins were moist and had a very foul smell. **Wound Score** = 4 points (**Appearance of wound base** = 0 points, **Size** = 1 point, **Depth** = 1 point, **Infection/Bioburden** = 1/2 point and **Perfusion** = 1 1/2 points).

Figure 7-5. Soft eschar over an infected, necrotic heel wound.

amputations avoided. The debridement usually results in immediate conversion of the wound from the 0 (black base) grade point to the 1 (white or yellow base) grade point or even the 2 (red base) grade point with respect to the wound base appearance assessment. This is another example of the dynamic aspects of the **Wound Score** and demonstrates how interventions modify the score and quantify improvement.

MANAGEMENT OF THE WOUND BASE

Debridement, Surgical Debridement – Debridement is the term used for the removal of devitalized tissue from a wound. This may involve all layers of tissue from skin, to subcutaneous, fascia, muscle, tendon, joint, or bone. From the perspective of problem wound management, debridement need not be limited to the removal of devitalized tissue. It may involve removal of deforming bony elements and other tissues that could interfere with closure, or present mechanical problems that would lead to wounds in the future. Fortunately, the majority of wound debridements require the removal of only the most superficial portions of the wound base. There are five techniques to achieve this goal. Surgical debridement is the first and most common debridement technique. Scalpel, scissors, and forceps are the instruments used for soft tissue debridements. For bony tissue, curettes and ronguers are usually required (Table 7-4). Outpatient surgical debridements are usually speedy and effective. The goal is to remove the unhealthy superficial tissue covering the wound base, but not necessarily establish healthy surgical margins. This allows the wound to establish its own line of demarcation and conserve as much tissue as possible. Serial debridements at weekly or biweekly inter-

TABLE 7-3. FREQUENTLY USED SURGICAL PROCEDURES TO MANAGE WOUND BASES (AND TOENAILS)

Procedure (CPT® Code[1])	Reimbursement[2]	Venues[3] for Procedures	Global Days[4]
Debridement, skin, partial thickness (11040)	$47.91	IC, IO, OW	None
Debridement, skin , full thickness (11041)	$55.91	"	None
Debridement including sub-cutaneous tissues (11042)	$75.78	"	None
Debridement including muscles (11043)	$275.40/ $237.85	IC, IO, OW/ OR	10
Debridement, including bone (11044)	$376.64/$328.04	"	10
Debridement of dystrophic toe nails (11721)	$44.84	IC, IO, OW	>5 nails; 60 days
Percutaneous tenotomy of toe, single tendon (28010)	$237.79/$221.45	IC, IO, OW/ OR	90
Amputation, toe, interphalangeal joint (28820)	$533.09/$360.34	"	90
I&D below fascia; foot, single location (28002)	$507.32 /$394.64	"	10 (foot); varies w/ site
Debridement of underlying bone of foot (28005)	$633.32	OR	10 (foot); varies w/ site
Drilling and osteoclasis of lesser metatarsal (28308)	$388.99	"	90
Achilles tendon lengthening (27606)	$301.74	"	90
Intramedullary ankle rodding (27848)	$850.21	"	90

(This table is generated for illustrative purposes. Refer to the cited documents for comprehensive billing information.)

NOTE: [1]CPT = *Current Procedural Terminology* from the American Medical Association (AMA) - 2009

[2] Reimbursement amounts are from the 2009 *Center for Medicare & Medicaid Services* (CMS) website, physician fee schedule look-up for Los Angeles, California (www.cms.hhs.gov/PFSLookup/) (The allowable amount will vary according to region.)

[3] **IC** = In-clinic, **IO** = In-office, **OW** = On-ward, **OR** = Operating room

[4] Global days include one preoperative day, the day of surgery, & non-reimbursable follow-up days of care. If other procedures are done (e.g., debridements), it is appropriate to bill accordingly. Global days for surgical procedures are specified in the *Federal Register*.

vals are usually sufficient to meet this goal. In contrast, the goal for debridement in the operating room is the establishment of viable surgical margins. This may require the removal of bony elements, partial amputations, and large quantities of questionably viable soft tissues. In this sense, the surgeon establishes the line of demarcation.

Other Debridement Techniques – After surgical debridement, enzymatic debridement is probably the most commonly used technique for necrotic material in the wound base. This requires application of enzymatic debriding agents with papain/urea or collagenase derivatives and is especially useful for the wound base with a fibrous covering[1] Hydrotherapy is the third technique for wound debridement. Whirlpool or pulsatile lavage softens and removes debris and loosely attached tissues. Care has to be exercised

> After November 2008, the manufactures of the papain enzymatic debriding agents were instructed by the Food and Drug Administration (FDA) to stop the production of topical papain products.
> This decision was based on 37 serious adverse events using topical papain since 1969; some of which were allergic hypersensitivity reactions.

to avoid cross contamination of other patients or infection of health care personnel when using this technique.[2-4] Hydrotherapy followed by sharp surgical debridement is an effective method to remove pedunculated and fibrillated material in the wound base. The fourth debridement technique is autolytic. In this technique, substances generated by the wound itself such as proteases, collagenases, matrix proteins, etc., act as auto debriding agents. With dressing changes, the debris is removed. Biological debridement using maggots is a fifth debridement technique.[5-6] It is effective for removing devitalized tissue while not damaging the viable margins. New maggot application techniques such as biobags that confine the maggots to localized areas makes this less repulsive than allowing the maggots to crawl uncontrolled over the wound. In most situations with problem wounds, a combination of the first four therapies are utilized. While in the hospital with necrotic based wounds, daily sharp debridements are recommended after hydrotherapy followed by enzymatic or autolytic wound dressing techniques. With outpatients, sharp surgical debridements are done periodically with use of enzymatic debriding agents, negative pressure wound therapy or combinations of these between visits.

Red Wound Base – The appearance assessment of the **Wound Score** serves as a guideline for the debridement and dressing selection interventions that are indicated for managing the wound base. If the wound base is red (wound base assessment grade = 2) and granulation tissue is forming, vascularity is adequate (Figure 7-3). The wound is expected to heal by epithelialization at the margins or after skin grafting or closure of flaps. The management maxim is to keep the wound as close to the normal environment of the body tissues as possible. This defines the principle of "moist healing." Appropriate wound dressing selections (Chapter 9) achieve this goal effectively.

Wound hygiene is important. Dressings need to be changed frequently enough so bacteria do not colonize the dressings. The wound base needs to be cleansed of debris on a regular basis with physiological solutions. Gauze moistened with normal saline is an excellent choice for cleansing and gentle debridement of superficial debris from the wound base. Often crusts form over the new epithelium growing at the margins of the wound. These should be debrided at weekly or bi-weekly intervals with a scalpel to prevent the build-up of debris and bacteria growth under the crust. Also, removal of a

TABLE 7-4. DOCUMENTING DEBRIDEMENTS FROM LEAST COMPLICATED TO MOST COMPLICATED CONSIDERING SOPHISTICATION OF INSTRUMENTS USED, SIZE (FROM WOUND SCORE) AND DEPTH (FROM WOUND SCORE)

Factor \ Points	2	1 1/2	1	1/2	0
Instrument(s) (complexity)	Scalpel	Scalpel + forceps	Scissors	Curette	Ronguer
Size[1]	Small	*	Medium	*	Large
Depth[2]	Partial skin (PT) Full thickness (FT) skin	Subcutaneous	Muscle and/or tendon	(Bursa and /or deep ciatrix)	Bone and/or Joint
Relative Reimbursement[3]	Baseline (PT) = 1 FT Skin =1.2	1.6	5.0	---	6.9

NOTE: Each in-office, in-clinic or on-ward procedure should be documented by indicating the following: 1) Instrument(s) used, 2) size, and 3) depth. Points can be ascribed for each factor for expediency; for billing purposes, the depth of the debridement must be specified.

*Use half points when intermediate between two size grades

[1] Same grading system as used for size assessment for the **Wound Score**

[2] Same grading system as used for the depth assessment of the **Wound Score**; Medicare ICMS bases reimbursements on depth of wound only

[3] Relative reimbursements are ratios determined by assigning partial skin thickness (PT) as the baseline (equals 1) and then using the increments in reimbursements to show the relative increases in payments, e.g. bone debridement is reimbursed 6.9 times that of a partial skin debridement. Bone debridement would require use of curettes or ronguers.

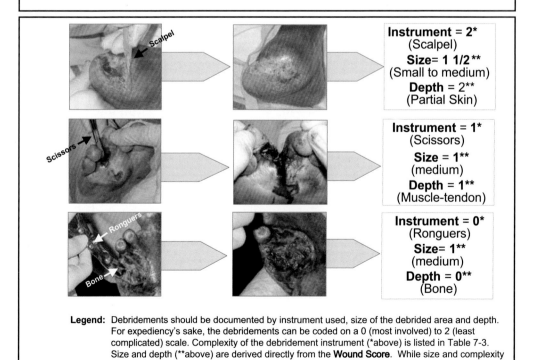

Instrument = 2*
(Scalpel)
Size= 1 1/2**
(Small to medium)
Depth = 2**
(Partial Skin)

Instrument = 1*
(Scissors)
Size = 1**
(medium)
Depth = 1**
(Muscle-tendon)

Instrument = 0*
(Ronguers)
Size= 1**
(medium)
Depth = 0**
(Bone)

Legend: Debridements should be documented by instrument used, size of the debrided area and depth. For expediency's sake, the debridements can be coded on a 0 (most involved) to 2 (least complicated) scale. Complexity of the debridement instrument (*above) is listed in Table 7-3. Size and depth (**above) are derived directly from the **Wound Score**. While size and complexity of the instruments used are important, reimbursements are based on depth of debridement .

Figure 7-6. Debridements and their documentation.

rigid crust, especially if thick, will allow wound contracture to proceed. Wound contracture reduces the surface area of the wound and further contributes to healing.

Mechanical Problems – Mechanical problems such as deformities, open joints, exposed ("proud") bone, and joint contractures need to be corrected by surgical means to achieve successful healing and prevent recurrences. Necrotic tissue, including portions of or entire toes, must be removed also. These principles are essential for managing the other (white/yellow = 1 and black = 0) grades of the wound base also. Surgical techniques to manage the mechanical problems include ostectomies, osteotomies, joint resections, and/or tenotomies (Table 7-3).[7] Although these procedures require surgical skills, most can be done in an office or clinic setting, thereby obviating the time and costs of using an operating room. All procedures should be suitably documented with complexity of the instrument(s) used for the debridement, the size of the wound, and the depth of the wound (Table 7-3, Figure 7-6). For reimbursement purposes, the Center for Medicare/Medicaid Services (CMS, formerly known as Medicare) only considers the depth of the debridement. In the diabetic with profound sensory neuropathies, these procedures can be done with minimal or no local anesthesia.

White and/or Yellow Based Wound – If the wound base is white or yellow (wound base assessment grade = 1 point), debridements are required. In contrast to the black based wound (grade = 0 points), where the goals of surgery are the removal of obviously necrotic tissue and the establishment of viable margins, immediate establishment of a vascular based wound is not required for the white/yellow based wound. Serial debridements to debulk the exudative and fibrinous material on the wound base are very effective and conserve the maximal amount of underlying tissue (Figure 7-2). Characteristically, angiogenesis occurs under the wound base, so removal of the exudative or fibrinous material accelerates the formation of a healthy, granulating wound. Hydrotherapy such as pulsatile lavage or whirlpool, typically done by physical therapists, is helpful in cleaning the wound base, the surrounding skin and softening (hydrating) the debris in the base of the wound. This latter effect facilitates superficial debridements. Since it takes a couple of weeks for angiogenesis to occur in hypoxic based wounds, the superficial debridements of the necrotic material on the surface of the wound complement the healing processes taking place underneath. The goal is to achieve a healthy, vascular based wound (grade = 2 points).

Black Based Wound – Management of the black based/necrotic wound base (wound assessment grade = 0) was described above. Usually, management of the necrotic based wound, especially if the gangrene is of the wet type, needs to be done in the operating room. In septic, necrotic based wounds, infection often tracks along tendon sheaths and fascial planes so exploration and decompression of these structures may be required in addition to the debridement of dead tissue. Amputations may be required; often they need to be creative. Unconventional procedures (such as longitudinally oriented flaps for forefoot and toe wounds, compound midfoot-fore foot amputations, dorsal flaps to cover midfoot wounds, complete medial and lateral ray removals, subtotal calcanectomies, split thickness skin grafting directly onto cancellous bone, and middle ray resections with narrowing of the forefoot) are surgical options that achieve healing in the problem wound with necrotic elements and preserve the function of the foot (Chapters 11 and 16). Patients with black, necrotic based wounds are at risk of lower-limb amputations. This is especially true in the presence of risk factors for lower-limb amputation including prior amputation, concurrent foot wound, peripheral artery disease, neuropathy and deformity (Chapter 13). A **Wound Score** in the 0 to 3 range defines the futile-type wound and correlates highly with the need for a lower-limb amputation. In fact, black based wounds with a grade of zero points for perfusion are sufficient findings to justify a major amputation. Only if perfusion can be improved with revascularization and/or angioplasty will lower limb amputation possibly be avoided. Another strong justification for a lower limb amputation is intractable, uncontrollable rest pain, regardless of the characteristic of the wound itself.

HEALING STAGES OF THE "PROBLEM" WOUND

Staging the Healing of Problem Wounds – Unlike the three clearly defined stages of healing in the uncomplicated wound that occurs over well-defined time periods (Chapter 2, Figure 2-4), the "problem" wound heals by a continuum of responses over variable time periods (Figure 7-7). The continuum of responses separate into three clearly defined stages: latency, angiogenesis, and coverage-closure (Figure 7-8). "Problem" wounds can additionally be separated into three subtypes: 1) non-healing, 2) necrotizing soft tissue infection, or 3) indolent (Figure 7-9). Each "problem" wound type requires different interventions for management of the wound base. In the indolent type, the patient has such severe comorbidities that wound management is only a secondary consideration or cannot be optimally done because of the seriousness of the other problems. Although healing of the "problem" wound, regardless of the subtype, is a continuous process, there are predominant findings for each stage (latency angiogenesis, or coverage - closure). When the majority of the wound base conforms to one of the stages, it is appropriate to describe it based on the majority finding. If the wound is in transition almost equally between two stages, this can be so indicated.

Latency Stage – The latency stage is the initial stage of healing of the "problem" wound (Figures 7-7 and 7-8). The latency stage represents the time from the initiation of strategic management until angiogenesis becomes evident. It may vary in duration

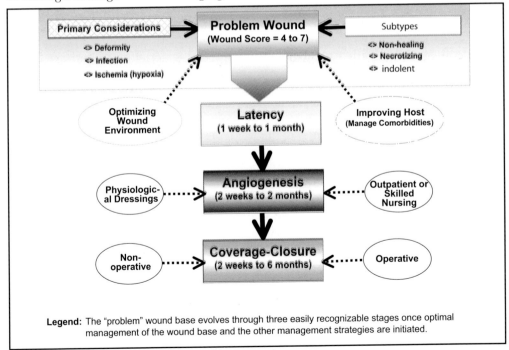

Figure 7-7. Stages in the healing of the "problem" wound.

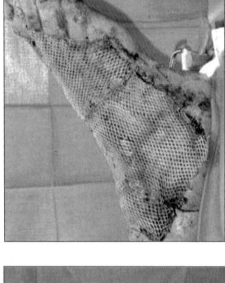

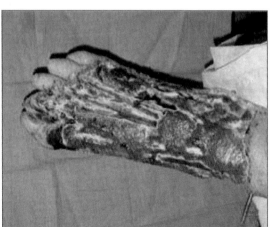

Coverage/ Closure
(**Wound Score** = 9 points)

Angiogenesis
(**Wound Score** = 6 points)

Latency
(**Wound Score** = 4 points)

Early Angiogenesis

Legend: This post-traumatic slough wound evolved through the three well-defined stages. The latency period, the time from initiating the five management strategies to the angiogenesis stage, required about four weeks. Even though the healing process was continuous, elements of early angiogenesis were evident in the latency stage and necrotic tissue was still present in the angiogenesis stage. Note how the **Wound Score** quantifies progress; the only assessment that did not change was perfusion which remained 1 (Doppler pulses) throughout.

Figure 7-8. Stages in the healing of the problem wound.

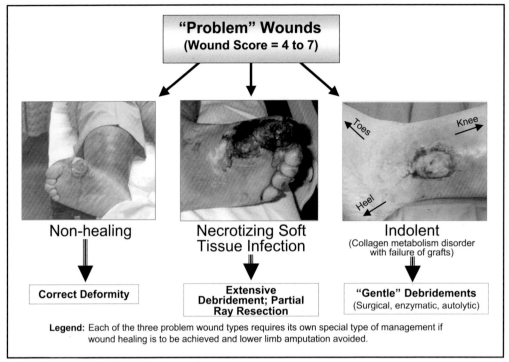

Figure 7-9. Subtypes of "problem" wounds.

from as short as a few days up to a month or more. The term latency suggests, in this context, that the wound is "at rest"; that is, from a clinical perspective, few changes are apparent in the appearance of the wound base. However, during this time, changes are taking place within the wound and around its environment so that the wound can progress from non-healing to healing. It is essential that the management of the wound base be integrated with the other wound management strategies during this stage. During the initial portions of this stage, hospitalization is usually required in order to integrate evaluation and management most efficiently. The goals during this stage are two-fold: First, the host status must be optimized so that the internal environment of the wound becomes as healthy as possible. This includes attention to the medical management strategy discussed in the preceding chapter. Second, the wound environment must be made as optimal as possible. This is achieved by the measures described in this chapter and succeeding chapters on wound protection and dressing selections. Different approaches must be utilized for managing the latency stage for each of the three clinical types of "problem" wounds (Figure 7-9).

Non-healing Wound Subtype – For the non-healing wound, measures must be introduced to initiate the responses needed for healing (Figure 7-9). Because of infection, hypoxia, and mechanical problems, (the problems most frequently observed), and to a lesser extent, deficient substrates (including growth factors) and matix metalloproteinase inhibitors in the wound, the chronic problem wound responds as if it is in a state of suspended animation. It does not improve; conversely, it does not worsen. In order to change the status quo, the above problems must be recognized and measures to correct them introduced. This can be as simple as removing a deformity or the other measures described for managing the wound base in this chapter, or as complex as trying to ascertain whether or not growth factor deficiencies or wound inhibitors are the cause of the non-healing. The majority, observed to be over 90 percent in our experiences, of chronic non-healing wounds fail to heal because of the reasons mentioned previously of deformities, osteomyelitis, hypoxia, or combinations of these. Once these problems are addressed, an inflammatory response develops and the wound, previously described as non-healing, can proceed through the other two stages of healing.

Necrotizing Soft Tissue Wound Subtype – For the second situation, the progressively advancing, necrotizing soft tissue infection, management is directed at controlling the infection and establishing viable tissue margins with debridements (Figure 7-9). Invariably, host compromising factors, including malnutrition, dehydrations) peripheral artery disease, diabetes, drug injection sites (especially with the use of street drugs) and combinations of these are associated with the progressively advancing, necrotizing soft tissue infection. Management of these problems is fundamental to successful outcomes. Multiple organisms, including aerobes and anaerobes, are often cultured from the wound. This is the reason the problem is sometimes labeled a combined synergistic infection.[8] Appropriate antibiotics are required. The other fundamental to managing the progressively advancing, necrotizing soft tissue infection is surgery. Once sepsis is controlled, viable margins are established (usually requiring multiple debridements), and the other strategies for managing the "problem" wound are initiated, the wound generates an inflammatory response, evolves through the latency period and proceeds through the other two stages of wound healing.

Indolent Wound Subtypes in Patients with Critical Comorbidities – The indolent wound in the patient with comorbidities that have important consequences with respect to wound healing represents the third type of non-healing "problem" wound (Figure 7-9). The management of the comorbidities requires as much emphasis in these situations as managing the wound itself. Problems such as nutritional deficits, hemopoietic conditions, renal insufficiency, heart disease, hypoxemia, immunological problems, collagen vascular disease, endocrine-metabolic disorders, obesity, and peripheral vascular disease must be addressed. Smoking may also be a contributing cause of non-healing in indolent wounds as well as other "problem" wounds. In some patients such as those with Buerger disease (thromboangiitis obliterans), major lower limb amputations, often bilateral, may be the consequences.[9, 10] Even though comorbidities are likely to be present in other "problem" wound types, the indolent nature of these latter types of wounds is as much due to the comorbidities as the conditions that directly interfere with wound healing such as deformities, uncontrolled infection, ischemia/ hypoxia or combinations of these. Every endeavor must be made to mitigate the comorbidities in order to optimize wound healing. Of the three "problem" wound subtypes, this is the least frequently observed.

Angiogenesis Stage – Angiogenesis defines the second stage of healing of the "problem" wound (Figures 7-7 and 7-8). Unlike the latency stage, the angiogenesis stage is similar for the three clinical "problem" wound types (non-healing, necrotizing soft tissue infection, and comorbidities). By the time the angiogenesis phase begins, sepsis has been resolved, edema controlled, and nutrition improved. The precursors of angiogenesis occur during the latency stage, when fibroblasts are mobilized, multiply, and begin to lay down a matrix for new blood vessels to grow into. As mentioned before, fibroblast function and angiogenesis are oxygen dependent. Without oxygen tensions of approximately 30 mmHg in the tissue fluids adjacent to the wound site, healing will not occur.[11-13] If oxygen tensions are below this level, work-up and interventions to resolve the ischemia/hypoxia problem are required (Chapters 10 and 11). In the optimal situation, the angiogenesis stage evolves within a couple of weeks, but in the hypoxic wound, it may take months to occur.

Wound Management in the Angiogenesis Stage – Management of the wound changes from the latency to the angiogenesis phase. The goal of wound management in the latency phase is to keep it as free of debris and bioburden as possible. For the angiogenesis phase, wound management is directed to keeping the wound base as physiological as possible. With proper dressing selections (Chapter 9), wound care can be reduced to as infrequently as one dressing change every two to three days, without interfering with the progression of wound healing. Consequently, during this stage of healing, the patient can be transferred from the hospital to a lower level of care such as the skilled nursing facility or home. Rechecks by those directing the wound management need to be done only once every week or two. If the wounds are not under loading areas of the foot, such as the metatarsal heads and the heel, full weight bearing on the lower extremity is permissible. When the wound base becomes covered with healthy granulation tissue, coverage-closure options must be considered. This is discussed in the following section.

> Once wounds evolve to the angiogenesis stage, they rarely deteriorate. Usually, antibiotics and oxygen perfusion supplementing measures are no longer required.
> However, attention to management of the wound base, comorbidities and nutrition must be maintained to keep the wound evolving toward the coverage-closure stage.

Coverage-closure Stage – Once the wound has a healthy, granulating base, decisions for coverage-closure need to be made (Figures 7-7 and 7-8). Wound coverage implies that the wound closes by epithelialization from around its margins or by skin grafting. Closure suggests that the soft tissues around the wound are of sufficient amount and good enough quality that they can be mobilized and approximated in a delayed closure fashion. In between is the choice to allow the wound to heal-in by secondary intention. Many times the best choice is obvious. At other times, decisions need to be made as to which choice for coverage-closure is the best for the particular wound. The choice has to be consonant with the patient's desires. Factors that need to be considered are perfusion to the wound and surrounding areas, size of the wound, location of the wound, and mobility of the patient. Usually patients with superficial, small-to-medium sized wounds prefer to maintain their level of activity, avoid hospitalization for wound closure-coverage, and allow the wound to cover by epithelialization from the margins. Epithelialization in these wounds proceeds from the periphery of the wound inward in a centripetal fashion. Maximum epithelial in-growth from the margins of the wound is about one millimeter a week. Many times it is slower because of comorbid factors.[14]

Metabolic Requirements for Wound Coverage-closure Choices – A second factor to consider when making a decision about the coverage-closure choice is the metabolic and oxygen requirements of the particular technique. Previously, it was stated that metabolic demands and oxygen requirements may need to increase 20-fold or more in order for healing to occur (Chapter 2). This estimate is probably valid for some closure techniques, whereas other choices may not have such high demands. Regardless, there is a hierarchy of oxygen and metabolic requirements for the choices of wound coverage and closure (Table 7-5). The wound with the lowest requirements is the one covered by a thin, dry crust. Epithelialization occurs under the margins of the crust. This is nature's own Band Aid®; it is the optimal situation for wound healing. By the time the crust separates, the wound base is usually fully epithelialized. The next level in the hierarchy is the healthy granulated-based wound where epithelialization is proceeding around the margins. Other wound coverage-closure techniques, in their order of increasing metabolic and oxygen demands include: 1) split thickness skin grafting, 2) simple skin approximation with sutures, staples or tape strips where the skin edges are easily brought together, 3) mobilization of flaps where retention sutures or multi-plane closure may be needed, such as in transmetatarsal amputations, 4) rotation or microvascular free flaps where the flaps bring their own blood supply to the wound base, and 5) healing by secondary intention of large cavitary wounds.

Special Techniques for Cavitary Wounds – Special techniques may need to be employed for achieving closure of the cavitary wound that is not healing. It is the most challenging of the wound healing closure-coverage hierarchy. Before these techniques are utilized, the three primary reasons wounds fail to heal, namely, deformity, uncontrolled infection, and ischemia/hypoxia must be addressed. If healing is still not occurring after these have been managed, special techniques should be used to reduce the size of cavitary wounds. If the margins are pliable and mobile, simple sutures to partially approximate the wound, but not close it completely, are effective. This avoids sequestering sepsis in the wound base while substantially reducing the volume of the wound. Partial wound approximation, although little appreciated, is very effective in rapidly reducing the volume of a cavitary wound without compromising the other care that

TABLE 7-5. HIERARCHY (BY INCREASING METABOLIC AND O_2 DEMANDS) OF WOUND COVERAGE-CLOSURE TECHNIQUES

Rank	Wound Description	Technique (For Closure-Coverage)	Activity Restriction	Comments
1	Thin crust	Epithelialization of wound margins	None[1]	Least metabolic and O_2 demands for healing[2]
2	Healthy, superficial wound, small	Same as above	None[1]	Requires dressing changes
3	Healthy superficial wound, large	Split thickness skin graft	3 weeks	Improved "takes" by meshing & adjunctive HBO
4	Simple flaps (Skin & SC tissue only)	Skin closure	3 weeks	Closure with sutures, staples or Steri-strips®
5	Full thickness flaps	Mobilization of flaps, layer closure	4 weeks	Examples, TMA, & lower limb amputations
6	Cavernous, especially with exposed bone at the base	Muscle rotation or microvascular free flap	6 weeks	Technically demanding; flaps have their own extrinsic blood supply
7	Cavitary wound	Healing by secondary intention	Weeks to months	Most demands for healing; techniques can reduce wound size[2]

Notes: [1]None; that is, community ambulation and traveling is permitted; avoid water immersion
[2]Other techniques include 1) Negative pressure wound therapy, 2) Casting or wraps, or 3) Partial wound approximations with sutures to reduce wound size
Abbreviations: HBO = Hyperbaric oxygen, **O_2** = Oxygen, **SC** = Subcutaneous, **TMA** = Transmetatarsal amputation

needs to be given to the wound. Placement of two or three sutures across the wound and reducing the size of open area immediately reduces the volume of a wound by a third or more. When the patient returns a week later, the sutures are typically loose. This is due to the viscoelasticity (stress relaxation) of the tissues. At this time, or after a week or two later, a second set of sutures can be placed to further reduce the volume in a serial closure fashion. A second technique is to use well-fitting casts and/or wraps to narrow the size of the wound (Chapter 8). Negative pressure wound therapy (NPWT) is a third intervention for dealing with difficult to manage "problem" cavitary wounds (Chapter 9). NPWT has appreciably advanced the management of the indolent presacral and hip pressure sore, as well as difficult to heal wounds in other locations, more than any other technique that has become available within the last ten years.

MANAGEMENT OF SPECIAL WOUND BASE PROBLEMS

Distal Toe Tuft Wounds – These wounds are usually found in the insensate foot with proximal interphalangeal joint flexion contractures. Pressure plus shear forces on

In-office Surgical Procedures – Many toe and foot procedures can be done safely and appropriately in an office, or non-operating room setting. As in all surgical procedures, informed consents, after discussion of treatment options and expected outcomes, need to be obtained from the patient. Prepping and draping of the operative site should be appropriate for the procedure along with the use of sterile instruments. If anesthesia is needed, local infiltration, metatarsal blocks or foot blocks can be used. In most patients with wounds of this type, the sensory neuropathy is so profound that minimal, if any, anesthesia is needed (Table 2-5). The body part removed must be disposed of properly—preferably by the pathology department of a hospital.

Partial Toe Amputations – For partial toe amputations, fish mouth incisions are effective. The end of the incision should be as far distal to the joint as possible; essentially to the end of healthy appearing skin. The dorsal and plantar flaps are raised to the distal interphalangeal joint level and the joint capsule incised along with the flexor and extensor tendons. When this is completed, the toe distal to the incised joint capsule can be removed from the field. With a ronguer, the bulbous head of the phalanx and articular cartilage is debrided to a round, smooth surface. The fish mouth flaps can then be approximated with sutures, staples, or adhesive skin closures; redundant skin is trimmed as needed.

Auto-amputations of Toes – If the toe becomes a dry, firm eschar with sharp demarcation between healthy and unhealthy tissues–that is, mummifies–it can go onto auto-amputation. Successful auto amputation conserves the greatest amount of tissue possible since bone shortening proximal to the line of demarcation and mobilization of flaps is unnecessary. Just as a dry thin crust is "nature's own Band Aid®," auto-amputation is "nature's consummate surgeon."

the tip of the toe, with standing and walking, leads to a blister that progresses to ulceration. Although the wounds may be small, tracking to the distal phalanx is very suggestive that osteomyelitis is present. Fusiform enlargement of the toe is a reliable confirmatory sign that osteomyelitis is present.[15] Because of the injury, swelling, and distal vessel disease, there is a high likelihood that the tuft is avascular (osteonecrosis). At this stage, management requires partial toe amputation at the interphalangeal joint level or complete toe amputation at the metatarsal-phalangeal joint level. Except for the great toe, these procedures can be done in-office or in the clinic. If the wound is at the superficial blister or pre-ulcer stage, padded inserts in the shoes may be helpful in healing the wound and preventing recurrences. Correction of the toe contracture with a percutaneous flexor tenotomy will correct the deformity and prevent recurrences.

Wounds over the Apices of Interphalangeal Joints – These wounds are invariably associated with muscle imbalances secondary to motor neuropathies. The imbalances cause joint contractures, leading to clawed and hammer toe deformities. Pre-ulcers and ulcers occur when the apices of the deformities rub against the toe boxes of improperly fitting footwear. Consequently, the first step in management is prescribing shoes with large toe boxes. The second step is correction of the flexion contracture with the tenotomy described above. If the joint is infected, that is a pyarthrosis is present, infection is rarely controlled with antibiotics alone. Interphalangeal joint resection is the third step and should be done in the operating room setting. This will shorten the toe by about 20 percent of its length. If the interphalangeal joint resection is not feasible due to dysvascularity or fails, toe amputation is the next alternative.

> Toe Flexor Tenotomy - For toe flexor tenotomies, the patient is asked to actively flex the toe as forcefully as possible while counter pressure in the upward direction is placed on the toe tip to make the flexor tendon as taut as possible. A transverse 3 mm incision using a #11 (spear point-like) scalpel blade is made just proximal to the plantar metatarsalphalanageal joint crease. The tip of the blade is penetrated to the bone level.
>
> The scalpel tip is swept transversely across the tendon using the skin incision as a pivot point, thereby not enlarging the incision. The release of the tendon is confirmed by both an audible "twang" and a palpable release of tension, similar to cutting a bowstring. After this, the toe no longer postures in the flexion attitude. To further straighten the toe, the interphalangeal joints are manipulated into the hyperextension position. Bleeding, which is usually minimal, is controlled with direct compression over the incision for a few minutes.
>
> A small gauze dressing is placed over the operative site and the patient is allowed to leave the office as it was entered (i.e. full weight bearing if the patient is ambulatory.) Because of the non-sterile office setting, the patient is prescribed oral antibiotics for a couple of days and instructed to return for follow-up one week later. Usually tenotomies for one toe only are done during an office visit. If additional tenotomies are required, they can be done in a serial fashion at weekly intervals.

Ulcerations along the Medial Side of the Great Toe – These wounds are invariably associated with underlying hypertrophy of the medial condylar eminences of the interphalangeal joint or bony spurs at this level. Removal of the offending bone deformities would seem to be an easy solution, but unfortunately in the patient with impaired circulation to the foot there is only a fifty percent likelihood of successful healing. Once the ulcer is excised and the deformity removed, it is difficult to mobilize and approximate the skin flap tissues along the medial aspect of the toe. The other alternative, a partial amputation of the hallux at the interphalangeal joint level, will usually heal primarily even in the patient with comorbidities that can affect wound healing.

Malperforans Ulcers under Metatarsal Heads – This is the "classic" example of a wound forming because of an underlying deformity. The deformity arises from the depressed metatarsal head that occurs as a consequence of the clawed toe deformity. The clawed toe causes dorsal subluxation of the metatarsalphalangeal joint, resulting in depression of the metatarsal head. The depressed metatarsal head becomes a point of pressure concentration with weight bearing. Callus formation under the depressed metatarsal head is a precursor to ulcer formation. Callus debridement and protective footwear is the first intervention for management of this problem (Chapter 15). Total contact casting is often used for the management of the superficial ulcer stage. Although the ulcer may heal, total contact casting does not correct the underlying deformity, and recurrences are to be expected when using this technique. Correction of the clawed toe deformity can be done as in-office procedure by doing a flexor tenotomy as described above to correct the flexion contracture coupled with an extensor tenotomy to correct hyperextension at the metatarsalphalangeal joint level. When the ulceration persists after correction of the clawed toe or in the absence of a clawed toe, a minimally invasive metatarsal neck osteotomy (especially indicated in the patient with impaired wound healing and infection control conditions) will correct the depressed position of the metatarsal head and thereby alleviate the pressure concentration forces (Chapter 16).

Closed Space Foot Infections and Ascending Tenosynovitis – These two problems are usually found in conjunction with each other. The patient presents with a septic foot usually secondary to one of the wounds described in the above paragraphs. Systemic signs of sepsis, such as unstable blood sugars, leukocytosis, fever, malaise, and/or positive blood cultures are usual accompanying findings. If a small and seemingly innocuous wound seals over, an abscess forms, leading to a closed space infection. As the suppuration expands, sepsis dissects proximally along the tendon sheaths. If not expediently decompressed (surgical incision and drainage, exploration and debridement), the problem can progress to a necrotizing soft tissue infection. Once decompressed, wound base management is implemented as previously described. These problems most frequently develop in patients with comorbidities such as diabetes, peripheral

Toe Extensor Tenotomy—Toe extensor tenotomies can be done in a fashion analogous to the flexor tenotomy described previously. Informed consents and operative site preparations are done as described before.

The patient is asked to dorsiflex the toes as forcefully as possible. Counter pressure is placed on the distal portion of the toe in the plantarward direction. A transverse 3 mm incision is made on the dorsum of the foot at about the metatarsal neck level. The tenotomy is completed by sweeping the tip of the #11 scalpel blade transversely across the taut tendon as done for the flexor tenotomy. Post-tenotomy management is the same as for the flexor tendon.

The percutaneous extensor tenotomy may be difficult to execute in the edematous foot or in the foot with hidebound, scarified skin and subcutaneous tissues on its dorsum. If this is observed, the tenotomy should be done in the operating room with a longitudinal incision and release of the tendon under direct vision.

neuropathy, malnutrition and peripheral artery disease. Cultures tend to be of the mixed aerobic and anaerobic variety. Consequently, multidisciplinary management for optimizing management of the comorbidities and antibiotic choices is essential to avoid lower-limb amputations and preserve a functional extremity.

Bunions and Bunionettes – Wounds from these problems arise because of their associated deformities. The bunion is a protuberance of hypertrophied bone and bursa along the medial aspect of the first metatarsal head usually in conjunction with a hallux valgus deformity of the big toe metatarsalphalangeal joint. The bunionette is the little toe counterpart of the bunion. Ulcers develop because of trauma and attenuation of the skin over the apex of the deformity. Although these problems are commonly associated with the neuropathic foot, there is undoubtedly a large genetic component to their etiology. Management of wounds from these problems starts with protective footwear to relieve contact pressures over the apex of the deformity. When wounds are present, surgery becomes necessary. Although 50 or more procedures have been described for managing bunions, in the patient with peripheral artery disease and other host compromising conditions, surgery for this problem should be as minimally invasive as possible. In this group of patients, surgical options range from excision of the ulcer, ostectomy, and realignment of the hallux to partial first ray amputation.

Wounds Associated with Midfoot Hyperpronation and Dropout – Charcot arthropathy (Chapter 12) and posterior tibial tendon insufficiency are the major causes of these difficult to manage foot deformities. Superficial wounds can usually be managed with off-loading and appropriate footwear. When bursa and bone become infected, debridement and ostectomy are required. When the wounds are large and associated with uncontrollable deformities, two options arise. The first is complex foot and ankle reconstruction which takes a year or more convalescence and has a 75 percent likelihood of a good outcome (Chapter 16). The second is lower limb amputation. With respect to lower limb amputation, two major options are available: a Symes amputation at the ankle level, or a below knee amputation. For the dysvascular patient with peripheral neuropathy and other comorbidities, we strongly recommend the latter. At one time, the Symes amputation was strongly recommended when lower limb amputation was necessary because of unresolved foot wounds. For the reasons listed in the text box, it is now rarely done in favor of the below-knee amputation, especially in the dysvascular, neuropathic patient.

Hind Foot Wounds – Wounds in the region of the heel are particularly difficult to manage. Off-loading may almost be impossible, especially for the weak and/or obese patient. Usually there is a shear (twisting, torque) component to the etiology of plantar heel ulcerations. Even if ambulation is limited to a wheelchair, it is almost impossible to prevent loading and shear stresses during transfers. Heel pressure sores in the bedridden patient tend to occur on the backs (posterior aspects) of the heels due to inadequate off-loading. They are invariably associated with peripheral arterial disease, lower extremity contractures and malnutrition. With off-loading, many hind foot wounds heal with the five wound healing strategies (Part III). If bone infection is present, it is usually superficial; that is, an osteitis with only involvement of the outside cortex of the bone. Excision of the ulcer, partial calcanectomy and mobilization of flaps for closure is an alternative to lower limb amputation. Successful outcomes from this surgery are a function of the severity of the wound (**Wound Score** - Table 5-2), the health of the patient (**Host-Function Score** - Table 2-4), and patient aspirations (**Goal-Aspirations Score** - Table 1-3).

Concerns Re: the Symes Amputation—Although the Symes amputation can be very functional in the properly selected patient, it is not recommended as an amputation choice for the patient with a problem wound of the foot. Reasons for this are as follows:

1) The vascularity of the ankle-level surgical site is not likely to be much better than that of the site of the problem wound in the foot. Consequently, healing of the surgical site may be difficult. New wound development is likely to occur if weight bearing is done to any extent on the stump end. The small surface area of the Symes stump end concentrates forces during loading onto a surface that is probably less than one fourth the loading areas of the foot.

2) Because of the likelihood of weakness and balance difficulties in the patient population with problem wounds associated with peripheral arterial disease, useful ambulation without a prosthesis (such as for walking to the bathroom from the bedroom at night) probably is not feasible due to five centimeters (two inches) of limb shortening from the Symes amputation.

3) For the obese patient, fitting and donning of the Symes prosthesis is more challenging than for the below knee prosthesis, which requires little more than "stepping" into the prosthesis from the sitting position.

4) Even though the Symes prostheses is designed to be patellar tendon bearing, loading does occur at the end of the stump. The protective soft tissue mantle, muscle, and subcutaneous tissue and resultant surface area in contact with the prosthesis is many-fold greater at the below knee leg amputation level than at the Symes, distal tibial level. Consequently, the breakdown of skin over the end of the Symes is much more likely to occur with the Symes amputation than with a below knee amputation.

5) For the non-ambulator, sitting balanced in a chair is not likely to be enhanced by the longer length of the Symes as compared to the below-knee (transtibial) amputation.

6) Although energy demands and cadence are better in the Symes ambulator as compared to the below-knee amputation ambulator, the ambulation requirements of the patient who had a "problem" wound (because of other comorbidities) will probably be limited to household or limited community activities (Chapter 2).

7) New technologies for the artificial foot and ankle components of the below knee prosthesis have significant functional advantages. Because of the length of the Symes prosthesis, most are not adaptable for this artificial limb.

Ankle Wounds – Ankle wounds often have similar causes and generate similar management problems as the hind foot wound. Frequently, they are associated with minor trauma such as a bump or a scratch. Because of limited ability to mobilize the soft tissues over the bony prominences of the medial and lateral malleoli, wound coverage-closures are challenging. Debulking bone is a limited option, since removal of a malleolus will result in ankle instability and likely lead to further problems. A possible solution is the minimally invasive but technically demanding surgery of intramedullary ankle fusion in conjunction with resection of the malleoli (Chapters 12 and 16).

Leg Ulcers – Most commonly, these are due to chronic venous insufficiency. In their simplest forms, they can usually be managed with appropriate dressing materials (Chapter 9), possible debridements, and compression wraps. When these techniques are unsuccessful, components of arterial insufficiency and/or underlying cicatrix, which causes a barrier to angiogenesis, are present. In these situations, methods to augment wound oxygenation (Chapters 10 & 12) and surgery to remove the cicatrix barrier, usually in conjunction with skin grafting, result in successful coverage.

Hip, Ischial, and Presacral Pressure Sores – Invariably, the causes of these indolent problem wounds are multifactorial. Problems include malnutrition, bony deformities, loss of protective sensation, moisture control, and joint contractures. Joint contractures are particularly pernicious in the bed-ridden patient. They lead to uncontrolled forces (compression, shear and/or tension) over bony prominences. Severe contractures of the hips and knees resulting in fixed lower-extremity posturing in the knee-chest position make turning and off-loading the patient's vulnerable sites for developing pressure sores almost impossible. Although above-knee amputations have been proposed for the end-stage contracture, a better technique is percutaneous hip and limited open flexion contracture releases around the knee (Chapter 16). Negative pressure wound therapy has simplified the management of these wounds and is remarkably effective as long as untreated osteomyelitis is not present in the wound base. In the bedridden patient, it is difficult to justify flaps and grafts to cover large indolent presacral and hip pressure sores in contrast to the spinal cord injured patient where flap closure is frequently indicated. When sepsis occurs in the hip joint, resection arthroplasty (Girtlestone procedure) or hip disarticulation are alternatives to living with a chronically infected wound.

CONCLUSIONS

Preparation of the wound base is such a fundamental concept that this strategy is hardly ever overlooked in management of the "problem" wound. However, two paradoxes become evident when considering the preparation of the wound base strategy. First, the wound care specialist must not neglect to address the three fundamental reasons wounds can be labeled (or quantified using the **Wound Score**) as problems, namely deformities, uncontrolled infection and ischemia/hypoxia. The second paradox is that preparation of the wound base encompasses an extensive spectrum of interventions. The spectrum ranges from simple debridements in the outpatient setting to lower limb amputations at every level from partial toe resections to hip disarticulations. Although an amputation might not be considered a preparation technique, in reality it may be the ultimate solution for management of the "problem" wound base. Obviously, for amputations other than at toe levels, a surgeon experienced in amputation techniques becomes an integral member of the wound team.

Three goals are evident for preparation of the wound base. The first is to make the base as healthy as possible. This goal is visually evident as well as documented by using the wound base grading assessment of the **Wound Score**. This goal is realized when the wound base transitions from black to white/yellow to red and then onto coverage-closure (Figure 7-1). The second goal is to conserve tissue to maintain function and facilitate coverage-closure. The third goal is to expedite healing by making the wound base as healthy as possible. These goals are implemented by debridements which range from simple scraping of the wound base to lower limb amputations at all levels and by coverage-closure techniques (Table 7-5). Dilemmas for managing the wound base resolve around doing too little, as may occur in the outpatient setting because of pain considerations and/or inadequate equipment versus doing too much to establish healthy surgical margins in the expensive, time consuming operating room setting. If the choice is available, the former approach is preferred since this conserves the most tissue by allowing the wound to establish its own lines of demarcation plus avoiding expenses of hospitalization and operating room services.

A wound without a healthy base will remain a problem. In many respects it is "like a tree without roots." The wound will remain unchanged and eventually deteriorate (analogous to the branches and leaves of a tree devoid of its roots, which will not grow and flourish). Like the tree cut from its roots, the "problem" wound will not "bear the fruits" of wound healing without a healthy base. All nourishment and healing (growing/improving to the point of coverage-closure) must come via the wound base just as is necessary for the tree via its roots. Just as the gardener must ensure that the roots of the tree remain moist, well nourished, properly covered and healthy, the wound specialist must make sure that the management of the wound base is optimal especially in the "problem" wound where wound healing challenges are anticipated.

QUESTIONS

1. What are the three primary reasons "problem" wounds fail to heal?

2. How is color recognition in the wound base assessment of the **Wound Score** used to give a point grade?

3. What are the healing stages of the "problem" wound?

4. What are the three sub-types of "problem" wounds?

5. What are some of the coverage-closure options for managing the "problem" wound?

6. What is the pathophysiology of a malperforans ulcer under a metatarsal head?

7. How does the anatomy of the hindfoot and ankle regions predispose these areas to wound development and complicate their management?

8. What are the benefits and disadvantages of the Symes (ankle level) amputation?

9. What special techniques can be used for managing the cavitary wound?

REFERENCES

1. Alvarez OM, Fernandez-Obregon A, Rogers RS, Bergamo, L, Masso J, Black M. Chemical debridement of pressure ulcers: a prospective, randomized comparative trial of collagenase and papain/urea formulations. Wounds, 2000;12(2):15–25

2. Stanwood W, Pinzur MS. Risk of contamination of the wound in a hydrotherapeutic tank. Foot Ankle Int. 1998 Mar;19(3):173-6

3. Simor AE, Lee M, Vearncombe M, Jones-Paul L, Barry C, Gomez M, Fish JS, Cartotto RC, Palmer R, Louie M. An outbreak due to multiresistant acinetobacter baumannii in a burn unit: risk factors for acquisition and management. Infect Control Hosp Epidemiol. 2002 May;23(5):261-7

4. Maragakis LL, Cosgrove SE, Song X, Kim D, Rosenbaum P, Ciesla N, Srinivasan A, Ross T, Carroll K, Perl TM. An outbreak of multidrug-resistant acinetobacter baumannii associated with pulsatile lavage wound treatment. JAMA. 2004 Dec 22;292(24):3006-11

5. Graner JL. S.K. Livingston and the maggot therapy of wounds. Mil Med. 1997 Apr;162(4):296-300.

6. Steenvoorde P, Jacobi CE, Van Doorn L, Oskam J. Maggot debridement therapy of infected ulcers: patient and wound factors influencing outcome - a study on 101 patients with 117 wounds. Ann R Coll Surg Engl. 2007 Sep;89(6):596-602

7. Strauss MB. Surgical treatment of problem foot wounds in patients with diabetes. Clin Orthop Relat Res. 2005 Oct;439:91-6

8. Grainger RW, MacKenzie DA, MaLachlin AD. Progressive bacterial synergistic gangrene: chronic undermining ulcer of meleney. Can J Surg. 1967 Oct;10(4):439-44

9. Cooper LT, Tse TS, Mikhail MA, McBane RD, Stanson AW, Ballman KV. Long-term survival and amputation risk in thromboangiitis obliterans (Buerger's disease). J Am Coll Cardiol. 2004 Dec 21;44(12):2410-1

10. Ohta T, Ishioashi H, Hosaka M, Sugimoto I. Clinical and social consequences of Buerger disease. J Vasc Surg. 2004 Jan;39(1):176-80

11. Niinikoski J. Effect of oxygen supply on wound healing and formation of experimental granulation tissue. Acta Physiol Scand Suppl. 1969;334:1-72

12. Gordillo GM, Sen CK. Revisiting the essential role of oxygen in wound healing. Am J Surg. 2003 Sep;186(3):259-63

13. Hunt TK, Ellison EC, Sen CK. Oxygen: at the foundation of wound healing--introduction. World J Surg. 2004 Mar;28(3):291-3

14. Donahue, K and Flanaga, V. Healing rate as a prognostic indicator of complete healing: a reappraisal. Wounds 2003 Mar;(3):71-76

15. Rajbhandari SM, Sutton M, Davies C, et al. 'Sausage toe': a reliable sign of underlying osteomyelitis. Diabet Med. 2000 Jan;17(1):74-7

CHAPTER

8

PROTECTION AND
STABILIZATION OF THE WOUND

CHAPTER EIGHT OVERVIEW

INTRODUCTION 195
THE SOFT COMPRESSION DRESSING. 196
SPLINTS 200
CASTS 203
ORTHOSES. 209
SURGICAL STABILIZATION 210
COMPLICATIONS FROM PROTECTION AND
    IMMOBILIZATION DEVICES. 212
CONCLUSIONS 215
QUESTIONS 216
REFERENCES 217

> *"Every living thing needs rest and protection—*
> *the problem wound is no exception."*

INTRODUCTION

Of the five wound strategies, protection and stabilization of the wound is the one most likely to be overlooked at worst, or to be given insufficient attention at best. Although some attention may be given to this strategy by wound care providers, often it is not ideal for the particular wound problem. There are several reasons for this. First, so much emphasis is placed on the other strategies, especially the selection of wound dressing agents, that stabilization and protection of the wound is mistakenly thought to be inherent in wound dressing management. Second, those who are most expert in making stabilization and protection decisions and interventions for the problem wound, such as orthopedic and podiatric surgeons, are frequently not part of the multidisciplinary wound team. Many times, their services are only requested when failures occur with wound management and surgery is needed. Third, there is the misconception that protection and/or stabilization devices interfere with wound care. Fourth, applications of stabilizing and protection devices for the wound may be intimidating to the caregivers, generating concerns that they will lead to complications such as pressure sores and pin tract infections. This chapter puts the wound protection and stabilization strategy into its proper perspective and presents the techniques to meet this goal in a hierarchy from the least complicated, most fundamental devices to the most complicated, most challenging ones.

Desirable Features of a Restful Environment – Why is a restful environment conducive to healing the "problem" wound (Figure 8.1)? Motion is detrimental to healing. It interferes with fibroblast bridging and angiogenesis across the wound gap. If the new blood vessels at the wound margins are repeatedly sheared off by motion, healing of the wound will be frustrated. This is analogous to performing construction work on a new building each day, and then having the day's progress destroyed by a demolition crew each evening. Motion across a wound contributes to edema of the hyperemic tissues due to capillary leakage. The restful environment at the microcirculation level is more likely to encourage flow and avoidance of transudation and bleeding than is an environment where motion may kink, compress, and/or shear off vessels. Edema in the wound base is harmful. If confined, it can interfere with capillary perfusion by compressing the capillary bed and thwarting blood flow at the level where all exchange of oxygen, nutrients, and waste products take place. Another harmful effect of edema is that it increases the diffusion distance of oxygen, which is about 1/20th as diffusible through tissue fluids as the waste product carbon dioxide is.[1] This effect interferes with oxygen availability to fibroblasts and leukocytes in the wound healing environment. Finally, free blood and edema fluid in the wound provide ideal media for bacteria growth and multiplication.

Considerations – Of the five management strategies for the "problem" wound, the protection and stabilization of the wound strategy is the one requiring the most creativity by the caregiver as well as the one fraught with the most hazards. Because of the multiple varieties of wounds, their locations, and their severities, ingenuity is often required to determine the most effective protective and immobilization device for the wound. These

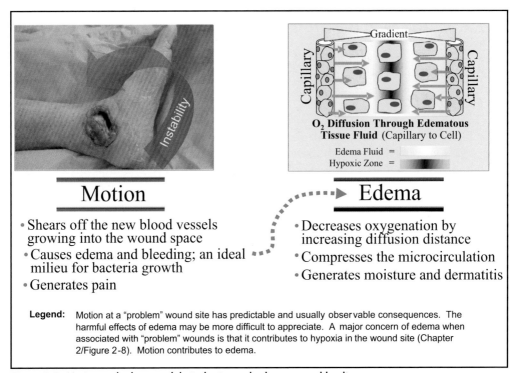

Figure 8-1. Motion and edema and their detrimental role on wound healing.

can range from soft compression dressings to surgical stabilization (Figure 8-2). Intermediate measures include splints, orthoses, and casts. Any time an immobilization, protective device is applied, the caregiver must be cognizant of the potential complications it can cause. These include new pressure sores, interference with circulation, delay in the recognition of a necrotizing infection, contribution to deformities such as ankle contractures, and pain. Consequently, any time a protection and/or immobilization device is utilized, the patient and his/her caregivers must be instructed about the potential complications of the device and seek immediate advice if any questions arise about the development of possible complications. Consequently, the wound protection and stabilization strategy is the strategy that is most likely to be inadequately managed, the least well-defined, the strategy requiring the most creativity, and the one most likely to cause complications (Figure 8-3).

THE SOFT COMPRESSION DRESSING

First Considerations – The wound dressing is the first consideration in stabilizing and protecting the wound. Often, it is not appreciated for these reasons. The wound dressing needs to be differentiated from the almost countless number of agents that are used to cover the wound base (Chapter 9). The wound dressing overlies the dressing agent, which actually comes in contact with the wound. A variety of choices are available for covering and wrapping a wound (Table 8.1). Usually gauze is used to cover the wound dressing agent, although other items such as sponges or non-adherent coverings may be used as the first layer. It is important that the first layer of the soft dressing comes in contact with the entire extent of the wound. This helps stabilize the flaps and minimizes motion of the wound. The wound environment should be made as restful as

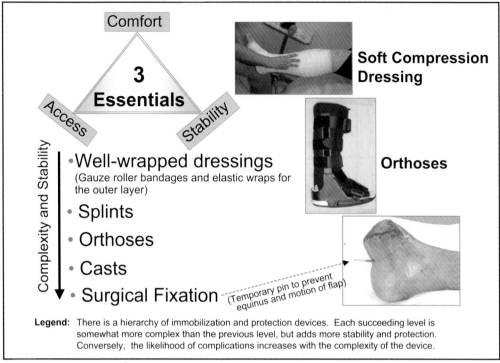

Figure 8-2. Requirements for and complexity of protection and immobilization devices.

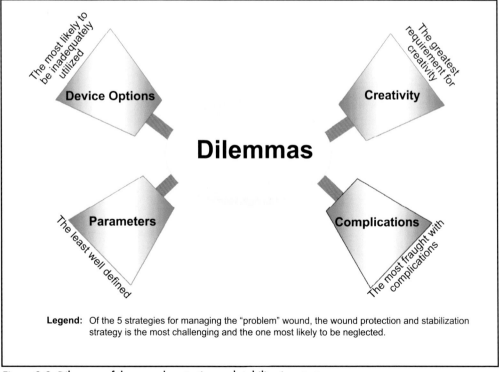

Figure 8-3. Dilemmas of the wound protection and stabilization strategy.

TABLE 8-1. CHOICES FOR DRESSING MATERIALS TO COVER WOUNDS

Role/Function	Examples	Comments
1. Direct contact with wound base or incision	-Gauze sponge -Ribbon gauze -Non-adherent coverings -Rubberized sponge materials*	Gauze dressings in contact with the open portion of a wound are usually moisturized with saline or other agents (Chapter 9) Dressing materials may be impregnated with lubricants (petrolatum, anti-microbial agents, silicones, etc.) to achieve special effects
2. Padding and/or additional absorption	Dry gauze, abdominal pads, fluffs, cotton wadding, lambs wool, sheep skin, cast roll	
3. Compression & stability (i.e. to keep the underlying dressings in place and minimize motion at the wound site)	-Non-stretch roller bandage -Stretch roller bandage -Elastic wrap -Non-stretch, rubberized wrap -Bias-cut stockinet -Tubular stockinet	May have a tourniquet effect if applied too tightly and/or swelling occurs after the dressing is applied
	-Surgical netting	Very useful for holding dressings in place over irregular surfaces

Note: *Rubberized or polyvinyl foam materials are commonly used in conjunction with negative pressure wound therapy. They may be coated with antimicrobial agents for additional bioburden control

possible, a first consideration in wound protection and stabilization, as discussed above. Dry padding is then placed over the portion of the dressing that actually comes in contact with the wound. A variety of choices are available including additional gauze, abdominal (ABD) pads, fluffs, cotton wadding, sponge materials, and cast padding. The outer portion of the dressing usually is the deciding factor for what padding is to be used. For example, if a cast, then cast padding would be used.

The Circular Wrap – If the wound is in an extremity, the circular wrap becomes the next layer of covering (Figure 8-4). The circular wrap serves several functions. It holds the gauze dressings in place, provides compression over the layers of gauze, and helps to stabilize the wound. Finally, the circular wrap is held in place with an elastic bandage, bias cut stockinet or surgical netting, which is a fish net-like elastic netting that conforms to almost any shape. Surgical netting is very effective in stabilizing dressings over sites that are difficult to wrap, such as the abdomen, a hip disarticulation site, the head, and the neck. The stabilizing effects of the well-padded dressing are affirmed by the effectiveness and common usage of the Bunnell hand dressing and the Jones dressing for knee injuries.[2,3] Often, a plaster or fiberglass splint is incorporated into the soft dressing to increase stability. The immobilization and gentle compression effects of the well-applied soft dressing are effective in relieving pain and providing comfort for the patient. Finally, these types of dressing for the extremities complement other wound care measures such as elevation and mobilization. For example, pillows placed under well-padded dressings facilitate elevation of the extremity and prevent pressure concentrations and shear over vulnerable sites such as the heel and the malleolar prominences of the ankle. When the patient is ready to be mobilized, a sling supports the upper extremity dressing while crutches, walkerette, or wheelchair allow partial or non-weight bearing ambulation with the light weight lower extremity dressing.

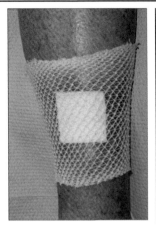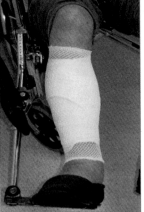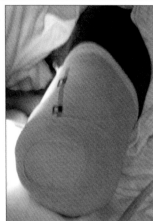

Legend: The gauze dressing over the wound is held in place without using tape. Uniform compression is achieved with the circular gauze wrap. Surgical netting holds the dressing in place. This facilitates removal of the dressing for wound inspections and dressing changes. Additional compression can be achieved by wrapping elastic bandages over the circular wrap.

Figure 8-4. Surgical netting and circular wraps to cover wounds.

Ease of Application and Removal – Other requirements for dressings include ease of application, ease of removal, and stability. The roller bandage choices are particularly useful for holding dressings in place. They are easy to apply because they simply need to be rolled on. Several short strips of tape or surgical netting suffice to keep the dressing from unwrapping. Dressings where the outer wraps are elastic bandages or surgical netting usually stay in place even in the most active patients. Use of encircling bandages such as roller gauze and elastic wraps eliminate the need to place tape on the skin to hold the dressing in place. Not infrequently, skin is avulsed when removing the tape, especially in those patients with atrophic, thin, friable skin. Repetitive application of tape to the same site can lead to contact dermatitis from the adhesives in the tape. The final requirement for the ideal protective and stabilizing dressing is that it is as easy to remove as to apply. Scissors, a source of contamination, become unnecessary when only a couple of pieces of tape or surgical netting are used to hold the wrappings in place. After this, the roller portion of the dressing is unrolled and the gauze coverings removed. If cast padding or cotton wadding is used under the roller bandage, it is easy to tear the padding, one layer at time, avoid the need for scissors, and provide access to wound without removing the entire bulky dressing and/or immobilization device. After the wound site dressing is inspected, cleansed, and redressed, the padding can be closed (analogous to closing a book) over the wound site and then held in place with the same wrapping materials, if clean, that were used for the original dressing. These techniques save resources while facilitating wound hygiene and regularly scheduled application of the wound base dressing agent.

Use of scissors to cut through the dressing is not advised. The small scissors found in dressing sets quickly dull after the first few cuts through gauze materials. Usually only one or two layers can be cut at a time, which makes the dressing removal tedious. As the disposable scissors dull, it becomes increasingly time consuming and frustrating to "chew" through the dressing. If bandage scissors are used, they can be a source of contamination and need to be sterilized between patients. This can present logistical challenges in active wound care clinics or hospital wound care wards. Use of the techniques described above eliminates these problems, while meeting all the goals of the optimal soft, protective, and stabilizing dressing.

SPLINTS

Protection and Immobilization with Splints – Splints represent the next step in the hierarchy of protection and immobilization devices (Figure 8-5). They are rigid devices that stabilize and immobilize joints, which make them a useful tactic for this wound strategy. Typically they are planar; that is, they cover the posterior or anterior surface of an extremity part rather than being circumferential, as a cast is. Splints are user friendly by virtue of their ease of application and removal and are safer for immediate post-operative or post-traumatic applications, because swelling in a splint is unlikely to interfere with circulation, as a cast might. There are two types: individually fabricated and prefabricated. Individually fabricated splints, as the name implies, are generated for the needs of the patient. They are made to conform to the anatomy of the patient and the needs of the wound. Modern fiberglass splint materials come in fixed lengths and widths, and they merely need to be removed from the hermetically sealed package, soaked in water, squeezed until no longer dripping wet, molded to the site of application, and held in place with bias-cut stockinet or an elastic wrap. The fiberglass hardens, becoming rigid in approximately five minutes. Plaster can be used in the same fashion but is not as durable. If it gets wet after hardening, it loses its rigidity. Often, the fabri-

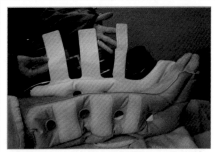

Inflatable Waffle Air Cushion Boot

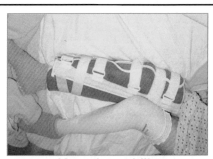

Knee Immobilizer

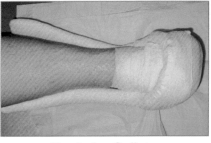

Posterior Splint

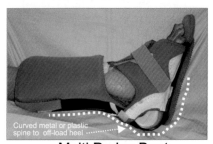

Multi Podus Boot

Legend: These examples of immobilization and protection devices all have common features. The features include protection and immobilization of the wound site, stabilization of the joints adjacent to the wound, easy access for wound management, prevention of contractures and comfort.

Figure 8-5. Immobilization and protection devices.

cated splint is incorporated into the post-op dressing, being applied in the operating room at the conclusion of the surgery. In most situations, splints are used as temporary immobilizing devices. Once the operative or wound site is ready for a non-bulky dressing, more rigid immobilizing devices such as orthoses and casts are used.

Joint immobilization – Immobilization of joints prevents motion at the wound site. This can be especially important for the immediate post-op management of split thickness skin grafts and for wounds over muscle-tendon units. Another goal of the prefabricated splint is to prevent deformities such as equinus contractures of the ankle and flexion contractures of the knees. Prefabricated splints serve many of the same purposes, but are not as versatile. They may not accommodate the bulky post-op dressing or a major deformity. Typically, prefabricated splints for the lower extremities are posterior shells made of plastics and held in place with Velcro® straps. Usually, they are padded with foam like material to prevent pressure sores. The primary purposes are the same as for the fabricated splints. Since they are made out of more durable materials, weight bearing usually will not interfere with their effectiveness. There is a continuum of protective footwear devices that transition into orthoses (Chapter 15). The following are some splints that have applications for wound healing.

Fiberglass (or plaster) splint – This is the standard by which splints are judged. It can be molded to accommodate almost any deformity of the foot and ankle. Padding such as cotton, foam, fleece-like material, or ABD pads can be placed between the splint and the patient's skin to avoid pressure concentrations. The splint is held securely in place with an elastic wrap or bias-cut stockinet. Pressure sores can arise from creases in the splint or inadequate padding over bony prominences such as the posterior aspect of the heel and the malleoli of the ankle. The junction of the splint between the leg and the foot, that is the ankle region, tends to fail, which leads to ineffective immobilization of this joint and equinus deformities.

Knee immobilizers – These devices are multi-functional. They help to maintain the knee in extension, facilitate elevation of the lower extremity with the aid of pillows under the calf, and prevent hip adduction contractures when pillows are placed between the knees. Their ease of adjustment and application with Velcro® sided panels and fasteners allow them to conform to almost any sized extremity. In patients with deformities and/or compromised skin integrity, pressure sores can develop at points of stress concentration. These occurrences may be avoided by bending the malleable metal stays that are incorporated into the splint and placing additional padding such as ABD pads under the proximal and distal ends of the knee immobilizer.

Multipodus Boot – This is a front entry, boot-type device lined with artificial fleece-like material and that uses Velcro® straps to hold the flaps together. The heel area is open. Pressure is relieved over the posterior aspect of the heel by a metal stay bent outward in the heel area. In effect, this suspends the heel in air. Outriggers from the rigid foot plate can be adjusted to control rotation of the lower extremity. This device effectively off-loads the heel. It is easy to apply and remove for dressing changes, skin hygiene, and inspections for pressure sores. In patients with compromised skin integrity, pressure sores may develop from the straps or from trying to derotate a lower extremity with a rotation deformity. Finally, in those patients with equinus deformities, pressures will be concentrated under the forefoot, subjecting it to ulcer formation, if indeed the splint will be able to accommodate the equinus deformity at all.

Pillow splints – These are the simplest of all splints and the most multifunctional. Their universal availability and ease of application do not negate their effectiveness. They are particularly effective for stabilization of minimally or non-displaced fractures in neurologically impaired extremities. Elastic wraps, tape, or Velcro® straps can be used to hold the pillows in place and add to the stabilizing effects. When placed under the calves, pillows are one of the most effective methods for off-loading the heels to prevent or manage pressure sores in these areas. In conjunction with knee immobilizers and/or splints, they are ideal for elevating the extremity to prevent edema formation. A disadvantage of pillows is that they require frequent checks and adjustments to insure that they remain properly placed, especially in the actively moving patient.

Posterior shells of bivalved casts ∠ This is an inexpensive, effective immobilization device. The site to be immobilized is casted. The cast is bivalved, and the anterior half discarded. The remaining portion is padded and used as a fabricated splint. The lamination and cross weaving of the fiberglass (or plaster), coverage of about half the circumference of the limb, and molding to the exact contours of the leg make this splint strong enough to resist almost any deforming force. Additionally, it can be made strong enough to allow weight bearing ambulation.

Prefabricated plastic shell splints – They are more rigid than fabricated fiberglass and plaster splints, but are much are more expensive. Although different sizes may be available, they are not designed to accommodate deformities. They may come with foam or fleece-like padding, usually removable for cleaning or replacement and with Velcro® straps for easy donning and removal of the device. If permanent splints are indicated, for example in a drop foot deformity, they can be custom adjusted and molded with heat malleable plastics, and are termed AFOs (ankle foot orthoses). Frequent inspections are necessary when these splints are used in insensate feet to avoid ulcers from pressure concentrations and shear stresses.

Inflatable Waffle Air Cushion Boot – This orthosis is a front entry, air-filled boot with an opening over the heel area. The manually inflated waffle construction is designed to avoid pressure concentrations in the skin that comes in contact with the boot. The edges of the boot are held together with Velcro® straps. This is a user-friendly device that is easy to apply and remove. However, it is ineffective if not inflated to the proper pressure. It requires frequent inspections to ensure that it has not rotated or partially slipped off the patient's foot. If the rotation is not correct, heel pressure and shear sores can arise.

Disadvantages of Splints - As versatile as splints are, they do have disadvantages. Many of the disadvantages were discussed with the individual splints described above. A chief concern with splints is the development of pressure sores, especially in those that are fabricated at the time of application. There is a tendency for folds and creases to form where the splint is bent to conform around the posterior aspect of the ankle. Too much molding may excessively load the bony prominences of the heel and make them vulnerable to generating pressure sores. Splints are not effective in correcting deformities; they maintain corrections after deformities have been improved by surgery or injections. Frequently, the use of a splint is ineffective in maintaining the passive correction of an ankle equinus deformity obtained while the patient is under anesthesia. When the patient emerges from anesthesia, the powerful plantar flexors of the ankle can deform the splint or slide the splint distally so it no longer conforms to the contour of the foot and ankle. This is a precursor to pressure sore development. In general, splints, especially the fabricated ones, are not designed for walking. Of course exceptions exist, especially with ankle foot orthosis, and when the posterior half of a cast is used as a splint. Some prefabricated splints such as the multipodus boot have modifications that allow standing, transferring, and walking. If the extremity area is subject to dependent edema, edema may form in the areas not covered by the splint when the patient is out of bed.

Also, if out of bed without the splint and wraps, edema may accumulate to such an extent that the splint cannot be reapplied until the edema is resolved. Finally, compliance especially when the patient is out of the hospital or nursing facility setting is a concern with splint use, because they are so easy to remove. If immobilization is required after hospital discharge, for example after an Achilles tendon lengthening, other immobilization devices such as casts are recommended.

CASTS

Advantages of Using Casts for Immobilization – Casts are immobilization devices applied to meet the individual requirements of the site of application. Consequently, casts can be applied to meet almost any size, shape, deformity, or wound healing need (Table 8-2).[4] Fiberglass and plaster are the two materials used to construct casts. Fiberglass has many advantages, including strength, lightness, durability, and ability to maintain its structural integrity even if it gets wet.[5] Plaster has the advantages of being more moldable, such as for club foot casting, and is less expensive, being about one quarter the cost of fiberglass. Casts in general, and fiberglass casts in particular, have many indications for immobilizing and protecting the "problem" wound, such as 1) affording access to wounds through windows or recesses in the cast without losing its strength, 2) tolerating wetness such as from wound extravasation or accidental immersion without disintegrating, 3) maintaining correction of deformities while effectively immobilizing the site, 4) allowing weight bearing without breaking, and 5) minimizing the need for frequent cast changes and edema control because of their uniform, circumferential compression effects.

Cast Complications – Complications can arise when using casting for "problem" wounds. These include: 1) Maceration and cellulitis of the skin margins adjacent to the wound. This problem occurs in exudative wounds and in wounds in patients with edematous extremities. The moisture wets the adjacent cast padding materials.

TABLE 8-2. CAST MODIFICATIONS TO FACILITATE WOUND CARE

	Modification	Purpose	Comment
Wound Access	Oblong (ovoid) shaped window	For access to small circular-shaped wounds in the foot	Maximum exposure to the wound with minimal weakening of cast
	Diamond shaped window	Provides access to long, narrow wounds on the leg	Preserves cast strength by minimizing stress risers generated by the window
	Rectangular window	Access to larger wounds as well as the skin adjacent to the wound	Weakens cast; used for exudative wounds requiring thick dressings and exposure of adjacent skin
	Ninety-90 heel cup window	Full access to plantar and/or posterior (pressure sore) heel wounds	Easy to replace and maintain compression over the heel with an elastic wrap or similar bandage
	Medial or lateral forefoot recess	Provides access to forefoot and distal midfoot wounds near end of cast	Requires strong reinforcement of forefoot-plantar portion of the cast to prevent collapse and skin injury
Special Casts	PTB (patella tendon bearing)	Minimizes rotation stresses between the leg & ankle; allows knee flexion as well as weight bearing	Useful especially for ankle wounds & in patients with large, obese legs
	Lower extremity with 35-45° of knee flexion	Prevents weight bearing of lower extremity	May be required for non-compliant patients especially with temporary transcalcaneal-tibial pin to stabilize ankle
	Cylinder cast for lower extremity	Prevents bending of knee for wound closures around the knee especially for non-compliant patients	Tends to slip distally; knee immobilizers are more versatile
Foot Plate	Rocker bottom	Aids in walking; compensates for loss of ankle motion with a cast	Curved bottoms make easier toe-off & heel strike for walking
	Heel build-up	Off-loads forefoot; compensates for residual ankle equinus	May make patient feel off-balanced and/or add increased stresses to hips & back when walking
	Foot plate extension beyond end of toes	Protects toes; eliminates motion at metatarsal-phalangeal joint level with weight bearing	Strong plantar forefoot reinforcement required to prevent softening of cast end & pressure sores over forefoot

The constant contact of the moist padding irritates the skin as well as provides a medium for bacterial growth. 2) The development of pressure sores at sites other than the wound are always a concern when using a cast in the neuropathic extremity. 3) Alterations in fluid retention in the extremities, as often seen in patients with heart failure and/or renal disease, may result in the cast becoming so loose that it pistons upward and downward and generates wounds, or it becomes so tight that it interferes with circulation. 4) The cast, like many other unilateral immobilization devices, may generate wounds on the contralateral extremity from accidental kicking, bumping, or prolonged contact, such as when sleeping with the casted leg lying on the opposite limb.[6]

Special Cast Types – "Problem" wounds often require special cast types and modifications to meet the requirements for wound care. These include the needs for immobilization and protection of the multitude of locations and variety of wounds, and to prevent complications from these devices. The following are special casting techniques that have applications for the problem wound.

Creative Casts – These are casts that have design features that make them special (Table 8-2, Figure 8-6). The simplest is the cast with a window cut into it to provide access to the wound.[7] They are special for several reasons. First, the window has to be on target over the wound. Second, the cast must be strong enough that it will maintain its immobilization and protection properties even with the window. For a large wound or several wounds in different locations, this can be a challenge. Third, the window should be large enough to provide access to the entire wound and a narrow rim of adjacent skin. Finally, the window needs to be intact, complete, and replaced after each dressing change in order to prevent window edema through the opening. An elastic bandage works well for holding the window in place while maintaining compression to

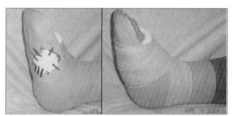
Window with Wrap to Hold in Place

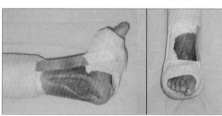
Strut to Provide Access to 2 Wounds

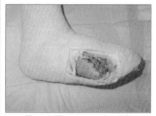
Foot Enclosed with a Window

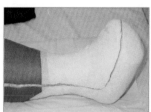
Bivalved Cast with Foot Enclosed

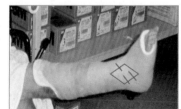
Patellar Tendon Bearing to Prevent Rotation

Legend: Ingenuity is required in order to optimally immobilize wounds, yet allow access for wound care. When windows are made, the cast usually has to be reinforced so it will not break with the stress risers generated by the window.

Figure 8-6. Creative casting.

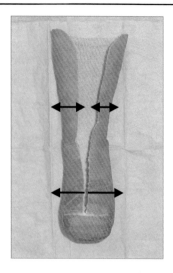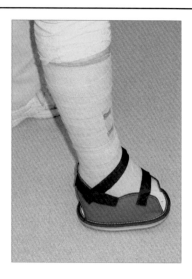

Legend: The edges (arrows) of the univalved elasticized fiberglass cast can be easily pulled apart to remove the flexible fiberglass cast or squeezed together to approximate each other. When the edges are approximated and the cast wrapped with an elastic bandage, a rigid construct results. Removal of the univalved flexible cast provides complete access to the wound for dressing changes and skin hygiene.

Figure 8-7. Flexible fiberglass casting.

prevent edema at the window site. A stirrup or metal strut can be used creatively to maintain the integrity of cast when a large window is required (Figure 8-6) or a plantar wound needs to be off-loaded.[8]

Flexible Fiberglass Cast (FFC) – The FFC is a special variation of the fiberglass cast (Figure 8-7). By using newly engineered fiberglass technology, elastic properties of the fiberglass are retained after it hardens (cures). The result is an immobilization and stabilization device that combines the accessibility of the splint with the strength and durability of the cast. When used for "problem" wounds, the FFC is applied in the same fashion as a cast, and is then univalved anteriorly. The edges of the univalved portion of the elasticized fiberglass are spread so the FFC can be removed. This provides optimal access for wound care and skin hygiene. Once the wound is dressed, the FFC is replaced. Strength sufficient to allow full weight-bearing ambulation with the FFC is achieved by snuggly wrapping it with an elastic bandage. This brings the univalved edges together, restores the cylindrical geometry of the cast, and results in immobilization and strength properties similar to the traditional fiberglass cast.

Serial casts – Serial cast applications are done for several reasons. First, they provide a means of complete inspection of the wound and surrounding tissues. During cast changes, the skin that was under the cast can be cleansed and lubricated. Second, if a non-rigid deformity or joint contracture is present, serial casting can gradually correct the problem. This reduces the chances of pressure sore development by overzealous correction of the deformities with a single casting. Third, serial casting can correct the deformity that caused the wound and thereby eliminate the underlying reason the wound failed to heal.[9] Fourth, if wounds protected by the cast are highly exudative, the cast padding will be wetted, foster the growth of bacteria, become smelly, and cause maceration of the adjacent skin. If cast changes need to be done at more than weekly intervals for the above reasons, techniques other than serial casts should be utilized to protect and immobilize the "problem" wound site.

Total contact casting (TCC) – TCC is a modification of a leg cast that is widely used for superficial wounds in neuropathic feet. The total contact cast is designed to reduce pressure concentrations under wounds to distribute force concentrations, that is, load share uniformly over the entire weight bearing surface of the foot. Although the goals and principles are similar, there are many variations to applying TCC. Typical TCC starts with a two to three layer thickness of cast padding. This is followed by padding the sole of the foot and other bony prominences, such as bunions, malleoli, and the spine of the tibia, with felt. Next, a thin, carefully molded leg cast is applied that totally encloses the toes. Traditionally, plaster is used for this layer because of its better molding properties as compared to fiberglass. Finally, a strong outer layer of fiberglass is added for strength and durability. This layer may be modified with a rocker bottom contour or wedges to provide a plantigrade surface for the bottom of the foot.

Concerns Regarding Total Contact Casting (TCC) – The TCC has both advantages and disadvantages (Table 8-3, Figure 8-8). Healing of superficial wounds in the forefoot is observed in approximately 80% of neuropathic feet if the recommended protocols are followed.[10-12] This requires an initial cast change after one week, then weekly or biweekly thereafter until healing is achieved. Healing of the superficial ulcer with a TCC may take three to six months or more. After healing has occurred with the cast, and shoe wear is resumed, recurrence rates are high, approaching 50% or more.[13] This is because the underlying deformity is not corrected with TCC, nor is the neuropathy changed. However, once healing has occurred in motivated patients (**Goal-Aspiration Score**, Part IV), recurrences do not always occur. One important reason is that once a wound is healed, the blood supply and energy requirements for maintaining the steady state, healed wound are about 1/20 of those required during the actual healing process. Experiences with TCC demonstrate that stabilization and protection

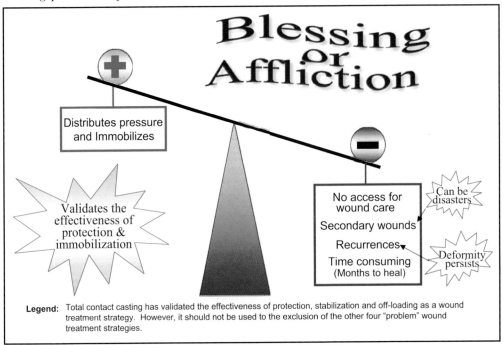

Legend: Total contact casting has validated the effectiveness of protection, stabilization and off-loading as a wound treatment strategy. However, it should not be used to the exclusion of the other four "problem" wound treatment strategies.

Figure 8-8. Total contact casting.

TABLE 8-3. SPECIAL FEATURES (ADVANTAGES) AND DISADVANTAGES OF THE TOTAL CONTACT CASTING

Advantages	Disadvantages
1. Comfortable	1. Time consuming and technically demanding to apply
2. Allows full weight bearing	2. Covers wounds so wound care is only done with cast changes
3. Load shares weight over the entire foot	3. Requires cast changes initially at weekly, then bi-weekly intervals
4. Obviates the need for dressing changes	4. If infection develops under the cast, it may go unrecognized until the next cast change and by then evolve into a serious problem
5. Good results in healing of superficial forefoot wounds	5. Not advised for other than superficial wounds limited to the forefoot and midfoot
	6. Healing of superficial wounds may take three to six months
	7. Because the deformity is not corrected, recurrent wounds at the same location are likely
	8. May lead to wounds at other sites from cast pressure sores
	9. Limits foot hygiene and skin care to the time cast changes are done
	10. Tends to disregard or not utilize other strategic management interventions.

of the wound (the most overlooked, under-utilized of the five treatment strategies) many times by itself results in healing of wounds.[14, 15] With windows in casts, as we advocate, remarkable healing of "problem" wounds is observed. The reality of the situation is that the off-the-shelf removable cast walker boot appears to be as efficient as a TCC in managing diabetic foot ulcers.[16, 17]

Ironies of Total Contact Casting (TCC) – It is ironical that the advocates of TCC almost use this technique to the exclusion of the other four wound strategies (i.e. preparation of the wound base, medical management, selection of wound dressing agents, and wound oxygenation). Total contact casting interferes with wound care by preventing access to wounds at the recommended intervals for dressing changes. Agents with demonstrable effects such as silver-impregnated dressings, bioengineered skin substitutes, negative pressure wound therapy, growth factors, alginates, sponges, and enzymatic debriding agents (Chapter 9) often require wound hygiene and changes more frequently than weekly or biweekly as would be the situation if they were used with TCC. As mentioned before, persistence of a deformity is one of the three primary reasons (in addition to ischemia/hypoxia and unresolved infection) that wounds fail to heal. With surgical interventions (Chapters 6 and 16), wound healing is anticipated in a matter of days in contrast to months with TCC. The indications for TCC are quite limited and include minimally exudative wounds, wounds no deeper than their widths, and wounds with no more than a limited amount of marginal erythema. A final concern about TCC is that it may delay the diagnosis of an aggravated infection such as deep abscess formation or necrotizing fasciitis in the neuropathic patient until the next cast change is due. This is a circumstance that can lead to an unmitigated disaster and culminate in a major lower limb amputation.

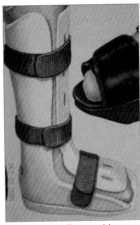

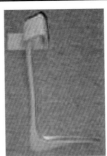

Plastic Ankle Foot
Orthosis (AFO)

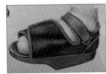

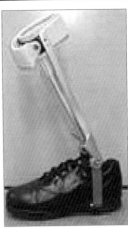

Plastic Removable
Walker Boot

Ortho Wedge Shoe

Klenzak Double
Upright Brace

Legend: Orthoses may be off-the-shelf items such as the wedge shoe and removable boot or customized to counteract the deformity and/or protect the wound such as the AFO and Klenzak brace

Figure 8-9. Examples of orthoses.

Patella Tendon-Bearing (PTB) Cast – The PTB Cast is another special casting technique. It is very useful for controlling rotation and/or adduction-abduction deformities at the foot and ankle level. The deformities are usually due to Charcot arthropathy, ligamentous disruptions, neuropathy, bone deformities or combinations of these. By extending the cast to the knee level with the knee in 45 degrees of flexion and carefully

> When it is not feasible to apply a PTB cast for rotational control purposes due to wounds or fractures around the knee or when external/internal rotation of the hip is an issue, rotation can be controlled with an outrigger device. This is accomplished by using fiberglass to attach a hollow cylinder (for example a spool from a 3 inch roll of fiberglass) to the posterior aspect of cast at the junction of the middle and distal thirds of the cast.
>
> A 12 to 16 inch rod is placed through the spool while the patient is lying in bed. This keeps the forefoot in alignment with the knee. When the patient is sitting, the rod is removed since undesirable rotation is usually controlled with the knee in 90 degrees of flexion.

molding the anterior portion of the cast around the patella, the patella tendon and the flairs of the proximal tibial metaphysis, rotation at the foot-ankle level is controlled as effectively as with a lower extremity (long leg) cast. The portion behind the knee is trimmed to allow knee flexion to 90 degrees. Even with windows for access to wound care, the cast is durable enough to permit weight bearing while controlling rotation with the knee in full extension.

ORTHOSES

Usefulness of Orthoses – Orthoses are protective devices that have multiple functions including protection, stabilization, deformity correction and enhancement of mobility (Figure 8-9). In many respects, orthoses are a more permanent counterpart of the splint. For immobilization and protection purposes, orthoses need to be differentiated from inserts used in footwear to add extra padding, off-load, and compensate for deformities of the foot. For wound protection and immobilization, prefabricated splints such as the knee immobilizer (Figure 8-5), cylinder casting of the lower extremity, and plastic orthoses/splints serve almost identical functions. Orthoses can be either off-the-shelf items or custom designed. Off-the-shelf items come in a variety of sizes and usually are designed so adjustments can be made to accommodate most sizes and shapes of the site to be protected. These are the devices that have the most applications for problem wounds. Custom designed splints, in contrast to orthoses, are usually applied after a wound has healed and are used to compensate for deformities, such as AFOs (ankle foot orthosis) used for drop foot deformities.

Advantages and Disadvantages of Orthoses – Orthoses have many advantages as well as some disadvantages for use with problem wounds. Advantages include 1) ease of application, 2) design features to prevent pressure concentrations, 3) comfort, 4) quick removal and reapplication for wound care and skin cleansing, 5) simplicity for adjusting when edema diminishes or bulky, absorbent dressings are no longer required, 6) ability to be cleaned and sanitized if soiled, 7) durability, and 8) cost benefits. The costs of off-the-shelf orthoses are comparable to those of casts when considerations are given for materials, cast technicians' time, and cast changes. Disadvantages of using orthoses for problem wounds are two-fold. First, when marked deformities, massive girths of legs, and/or partial foot amputations are present, orthoses may not be able to accommodate to these shapes. If used in such circumstances, the orthosis may lead to complications such as new pressure sores and loss of alignment. Second, in the non-compliant patient, the orthosis may not be used as instructed, because it is so easy to apply and remove. Suspicions of non-compliance are confirmed when progress with wound management does not proceed as expected and/or the orthosis looks in brand new condition at follow-up evaluations. Full compliance for orthoses use can be achieved by placing a few wraps of fiberglass or plaster around it or by using non-removable plastic ties that must be cut off to remove the orthosis. The following examples are commonly used orthoses available off-the-shelf or with a minimum of special fabrication.

Ankle foot orthosis (AFO) – Typically, these orthoses are used to control drop foot deformities and are not used for wound healing purposes. They are made of thermal moldable plastics and shaped to accommodate the contours of the patient's leg and foot. They are light-weight, thin, and easily fit into a patient's shoes. Usually, a single Velcro® strap at the proximal edge of the AFO is sufficient to keep this orthosis in place. The leg portion may be lined by a fleece-like material. Extreme caution is required when using an AFO in the patient with a sensory neuropathy because of the formation of pressure sores without the usual warning sign of pain.

Klenzak (double upright) brace – The Klenzak brace is a double upright brace that attaches proximally by a leg cuff and inserts distally into the patient's shoe. Hinges may be applied to allow ankle motion. If hinges at the ankle joint are used, spring action in the hinge assists with foot dorsiflexion. Even though this orthosis has largely been replaced by the AFO, it still serves a useful role in the neuropathic foot. This is because the AFO is unable to control rotation or angular deformities at the ankle or foot level (foot inversion/supination, hyperpronation/foot eversion, varus or valgus deformities of the hindfoot, excessive abduction and/or adduction of the forefoot). The Klenzak brace by virtue of its attachment to the shoe can usually keep the ankle and foot in the neutral and plantigrade position. Sometimes straps are placed to control varus or valgus sagging of the ankle. The stabilizing properties of the Klenzak brace with a custom fitted shoe can facilitate wound healing when underlying deformities are the cause and can prevent new wounds from appearing.

Ortho wedge shoe (OWS) – The OWS is a modification of the post-op shoe (Figure 8-9). The foot plate has a 2½ inch (6.4 cm) build-up under the heel portion. The side portions/flaps of the shoe provide easy access for entry and removal with velcro® straps even if the foot is bandaged. The OWS is designed to off-load the forefoot and midfoot when weight bearing, thereby making it useful for protecting wounds in this area. Walking and balance control may be difficult for the marginal ambulator because of the heel elevation and the reduced surface area to floor contact of the foot plate. In addition, some patients modify the stance phase/weight bearing portion of the gait cycle in the OWS by rolling off the forefoot portion. If this occurs, the OWS no longer off-loads the forefoot.

Post-op shoe – This orthosis is designed to prevent motion through the forefoot and midfoot. It has a shoe portion attached to a rigid foot plate, usually made of wood or plastic. Like the OWS, the post-op shoe is easy to apply and remove with large side flaps and Velcro® straps. It is most commonly used after surgeries with closed operative sites in these areas. Walking with the post-op shoe requires a flat foot gait. The sole may be modified to a rocker bottom shape to allow roll-on and roll-off of the heel strike and toe-off portions of the stance phase of the gait cycle. While it reduces motion at the forefoot and midfoot joints, it does not prevent off-loading, which is a goal of the OWS.

Removable walker boot – This is a cast-like boot with a rigid plastic splint attached to a thick rocker-bottom sole plate. The boot is lined with foam rubber. Adjustable Velcro® straps secure the rigid frame and the foam boot around the patient's leg and foot. Modifications include the addition of adhesive-backed foam pads to improve fitting, hinged ankle joints to aid in walking, removable hexagonal rubber pegs in a sole insert to off-load localized pressure concentrations, and foam fillers for heel defects and equinus contractures. This is a very versatile orthosis that meets almost all the requirements needed to immobilize and protect the problem wound, while providing access to the wound for dressing changes and sufficient stability to allow weight bearing. Other modifications include inflatable liners, gel pads, toe coverings, and adjustable side portions to accommodate and improve stabilization of a variety of deformities. These modifications and features make the removable walker boot essentially as protective as the total contact casting for healing of superficial wounds.[16, 17]

SURGICAL STABILIZATION

The Ultimate Immobilization – Surgical stabilization provides the ultimate in immobilization. When coupled with correction of deformities and wound debridement, healing of wounds otherwise thought to be unsalvageable can result. Further discussion of this is found in the discussion of "end-stage" Charcot arthropathy (Chapter 12). In general, internal fixation devices such as plates and screws are not feasible when wounds penetrate to bone that is graded zero points (on the 0 to 2 scale) of the wound depth component of the **Wound Score**. This is because the hardware acts as a foreign object in the wound and serves as a nidus for infection and a substrate for formation of a biofilm. Another relative contraindication for internal fixation is osteopenia. If severe, fixation with screws will not hold in the soft bone. Loss of fixation leads to recurrent deformity, wound formation, and likelihood of a lower-limb amputation. This succession of complications is especially observed in patients who have advanced neuropathy with loss of pain and proprioception sensation.

Stabilization of Joints with Pinnings – Temporary external fixation is another alternative to maintain correction of deformities and stabilize wounds. This is accomplished by two techniques. The first is the placement of large Steinmann pins across joints (Figures 8-2). This technique is used after contracture releases of the knees and ankles (Achilles tendon lengthenings), deformity corrections after osteotomies and ostectomies, and stabilization of digits after joint resections. Typically, the ends of the pins protrude beyond the skin level. This allows for easy removal without the need to return the patient to the operating room. Pin tract care is essential for preventing infection ascending along the pin tract. Pin tract care is best done by cleansing the pin/skin interface with hydrogen peroxide or normal saline and then wrapping the pin snuggly with dry gauze. The wrap should be tight enough to gently depress the skin around the pin. This prevents pin tract edema, oozing of fluid around the pin, colonization of the fluid by bacteria, invasion of the adjacent skin, and cellulitis (Figure 8-10). When a percutaneous pin is in place, the patient should be strictly non-weight-bearing on the extremity. If there are concerns about patient compliance, a lower extremity (i.e. long leg cast) should be applied with the knee maintained in 45 degrees of flexion. This effectively prevents weight-bearing through the foot. A significant complication of a pin tract infection is inoculation of the pin-bone junction and the development of osteomyelitis. Lower-limb amputations can result from this complication.

Duration of Pin Immobilization – The time that temporary pins remain across joints varies depending on the circumstances. Usually, for joint resections and contracture releases, three weeks is adequate. This is sufficient time to allow the wound flaps to heal, for a soft tissue mantle to develop around the joint, or for the soft tissues to

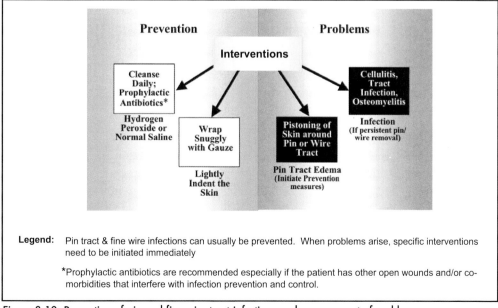

Legend: Pin tract & fine wire infections can usually be prevented. When problems arise, specific interventions need to be initiated immediately

*Prophylactic antibiotics are recommended especially if the patient has other open wounds and/or co-morbidities that interfere with infection prevention and control.

Figure 8-10. Prevention of pin and fine wire tract infections and management of problems.

accommodate to the reduced position after joint contracture releases. In the patient with a history of a "problem" wound, prophylactic antibiotics are continued during the time the percutaneous pin remains in place. When the pin or pins are removed, the corrected positions may be maintained by using casts, splints or orthoses. Ideally, these immobilizing devices are removed two or three times a day, so passive and active joint motions can be done under the supervision of a therapist or a caregiver. If a pin tract infection is noted, the pin needs to be removed immediately, and the corrected position maintained with a cast for a three-week period. When wounds are present, the pins are maintained until the wound has healed enough that adequate wound care can be done through a cast window. This may take three weeks to three months or more. Does temporary pin placement across major joints such as the ankle and knee lead to joint stiffness and/or arthritis? The answer is that for the clinical demands of the patient, temporary pin placements across joints have not lowered their rehabilitation endpoints as would be predicted from their pre-wound, pre-operative level of function.

External Skeletal Fixation – The other temporary fixation immobilization technique is that of external fixation. This technique, although surgically demanding, is a very effective way to immobilize, stabilize, and maintain corrections of deformities in association with "problem" wounds. Typically, pins or fine wires are placed in the leg to be used as anchors for the ring (Ilizarov) external fixation frame. Distally, fine wires are placed across the heel and forefoot and attached to the external frame. This fixation technique provides rigid immobilization, yet allows access for wound care. The goal is to keep the fixator in place for a three-month period. By this time, osteotomies have healed and the soft tissue mantle has matured enough to maintain the correction with casting techniques.[18] If the wound is not completely healed by this time, a window is placed in the cast to provide access for wound care. This approach is especially advocated for the "end-stage" Charcot arthropathy wound (Chapter 12).

COMPLICATIONS FROM PROTECTION AND IMMOBILIZATION DEVICES

Diligence with the Use of Immobilization Devices – Of all the strategic management interventions for "problem" wounds, wound protection and stabilization require the most diligence. This is because devices such as casts and splints are applied to extremities that already have problems, and these problems may increase the chances of inherent complications arising from their use. In the preceding sections, special concerns and complications from protection and stabilization devices were mentioned. Frequently observed problems and/or complications, their predispositions and their prevention are summarized as follows.

Pressure Sores: Pressure sores arise from pressure concentrations under these devices. Frequently, they are associated with slippage of the devices. Peripheral artery disease, atrophic skin, sensory neuropathy, and deformities are precursors to the development of these problems. If casts are applied, they should be well padded. When splints and orthoses are used, they need to be checked frequently for slippage and removed at least twice a day so the skin under the splints can be checked for evidence of pressure concentrations. Any complaint of discomfort in these devices is reason to check the area of complaint, or if it is in a cast, make a window over the site of the complaint. If the precursors described above are present, increased diligence and attention to any complaint with the device wear must be addressed.

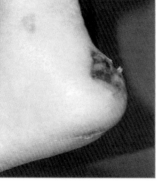

Ulcer from crease in elastic wrap

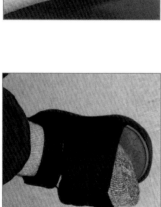

Inadequate wrap

Heel ulceration from posterior splint

Inadequate immobilization for the deformity

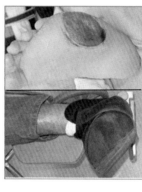

Slippage

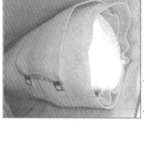

Blister from strap

Legend: Use of protection and immobilization devices are fraught with inappropriate applications and complications. Of the five management strategies for the "problem" wound, this strategy is the one that requires the most vigilance and monitoring.

Figure 8-11. Complications from immobilization and protection devices.

Compliance Issues: Splints and orthoses are subject to removal by the patient. Reasons include the fact that they are a nuisance to wear, they are not comfortable, they are too hard to put on and remove for hygiene purposes, and they slip when the patient is active. Clues as to non-use include the pristine appearance of the device when the patient is checked at follow-up visits, loss of correction of the deformity, lack of improvement of the wound, and the onset of new wounds. The adherence to device wear is one of the measures to judge patient compliance for the **Goal-Aspiration Score** (Table 1-3).

Inappropriate Use: Due to misunderstandings, ignorance, or willful neglect, the removable devices may not be optimally placed. This is frequently observed in knee immobilizers, where the patient reapplies the device as distally as possible and knee extension is no longer maintained. When bilateral orthoses are used, they occasionally are used on the wrong sides. Splints are sometimes reapplied in a rotated position so they no longer provide the desired immobilization as well as lead to pressure sores due to lack of conformability. Most removable devices have a tendency to slip with ordinary usage. This requires awareness by the patient and/or the caregivers and repositioning when necessary. As in compliance issues, inappropriate usage is prevented by education of the patient and family and frequent return visits to insure the devices are being worn appropriately.

Breakage, Wear, and Tear: Patients must be instructed that if the cast breaks or the orthosis no longer appears effective, reevaluation must be immediately obtained. Posterior plaster splints to immobilize the ankle and prevent equinus are notorious for fracturing at the ankle level. This can be prevented by diagonally reinforcing the sides of the splint at the ankle level or using double thickness splints. Pressure sores occur over the dorsal aspect of the distal portion of the forefoot in walking casts when the plantar end of the cast softens and collapses. When the patient walks with the broken cast, the dorsum of the forefoot is pushed upward on the edge of cast and quickly leads to ulceration. For removable walker boots, Velcro® straps lose their ability to securely fasten the boot resulting in slippage with repetitive usage. Likewise, padding loses its effectiveness, that is bottoms out, with prolonged compressive and shear stresses. When these occur, the device must be refurbished or replaced.

Skin Hygiene: Failure to maintain skin hygiene when protection and immobilization devices are used can lead to complications in itself. Typically, patients with neuropathy have dry, scaly skin (Chapter 14). This leads to crusts, moisture accumulation under the crusts, skin maceration and finally ulceration. With cast wear, skin cleansing and lubrication should be an integral part of any cast change. When removable devices are used, the patient and/or caregivers should be instructed in skin hygiene and moisturization techniques (Chapter 14). Their adherence to this is another measure of the compliance assessment of the **Goal-Aspiration Score** (Table 1-3).

Improper Selection of Devices: Not infrequently, the device the physician or other caregiver selects for the immobilization and protection strategy is improper. Examples are as follows: rotational and angulation deformities are not adequately controlled by a leg cast. Post-op shoes are, likewise, inadequate for these purposes. Lower extremity (long leg) or patellar tendon bearing casts may be required. Knee immobilizers can not control pervasive knee flexion contractures. They will lead to pressure sores in the leg from the end of the knee immobilizer. Off-loading with pillows, that is, accepting the contracture, casting, or surgical releases may be alternatives for dealing with this problem. Pressure sores at the apices of markedly clawed toes and at the tips of the toes may not be manageable with protective footwear. Surgical interventions may be required in these situations. Surgery may likewise be required for management of malperforans ulcers that persist after off-loading or recur after total contact casting.

CONCLUSIONS

The fundamental aspect of wound protection and stabilization – Wound protection and stabilization is so fundamental to the principles of wound healing that it is often overlooked or disregarded, perhaps by benign neglect. This latter phrase implies that the patient will assume responsibility for resting and protecting the wound because of the very nature of the wound itself. With the techniques described in this chapter, protection and stabilization can be optimized. For the "problem" and "end-stage" wounds, proper stabilization and protection often will make the difference between healing and failure. There is no question that "every living thing needs rest and protection—the problem wound is no exception." Although wound healing nurses and technicians have expertise in selecting and applying soft dressings, the surgeon with expertise in managing "problem" wounds of the lower extremity needs to manage splints, casts, orthoses, and surgical stabilization. The selection of immobilization and protection devices is a dynamic process. As the wound improves, the optimal immobilization and stabilization devices change. For example, they may proceed from rigid stabilization such as external fixation to casts, then orthoses, and finally to protective footwear.

Three-fold goals of protection and stabilization – In summary, the goals of the wound protection and stabilization strategy are three-fold: first, the establishment of an optimal environment for wound healing through rest, off-loading, and protection; second, provision for easy access for wound care; and third, prevention of deformities. These goals are achieved by proper selection of dressings, splints, casting, orthoses and using temporary stabilization by pinning of joints or with external fixation. As the wound improves, the selection of devices changes from the more complicated, more care-demanding to the least complicated and more user-friendly choices. The four dilemmas of the protection and stabilization strategy, namely adequate management of this strategy, creativity, awareness of parameters or goals to be achieved, and avoidance of complications (Figure 8-3) are mitigated by understanding the pathomechanics of the problem, knowledge of the choices available, attention to detail, and close supervision. As stated before, the surgeon experienced in dealing with these problems is the member of the wound healing team that will most likely make the decisions for management of this strategy. The other team members contribute to the execution of the protection and immobilization choices and the prevention of their complications.

QUESTIONS

1. Why is the wound protection and stabilization strategy the most overlooked of the five strategies used for managing "problem" wounds?

2. What are the main concerns about using protection and immobilization devices for wound management?

3. What are the desirable and undesirable features of the soft compression dressing/stabilization and immobilization device?

4. What are the desirable and undesirable features of splints?

5. Why are casts so useful in the management of "problem" wounds?

6. What are the benefits and hazards of total contact casting?

7. What are the differences between splints and orthoses?

8. When does surgical stabilization need to be considered in patients with "problem" wounds?

9. What are the potential complications of wound protection and immobilization devices?

10. What are the three main goals of the protection and stabilization strategy in "problem" wound management?

REFERENCES

1. Guyton AC, Hall JE. O2 Diffusion. In: Textbook of Medical Physiology, 10th ed. Philadelphia, PA: WB Saunders; 2000:454,465

2. Bunnell S. The early treatment of hand injuries. J Bone Joint Surg Am. 1951 Jul;33-A(3):807-11

3. Jones R. Injuries to Joints. Oxford War Primers, 2nd Ed, p 23, Henry Frowde and Hodder & Stoughton, London,1918

4. Browning D. Using a cast to manage a pressure sore. J Wound Care, 1997; 6:315

5. Caravaggi C, Faglia E, De Giglio R, et al. Effectiveness and safety of a nonremovable fiberglass off-bearing cast versus a therapeutic shoe in the treatment of neuropathic foot ulcers: a randomized study. Diabetes Care. 2000 Dec;23(12):1746-51

6. Halanski M, Noonan KJ. Cast and splint immobilization: Complications. J Am Acad Ortho Surg, 2008; 16(1): 30-40

7. Agas CM, Bui TD, Driver VR, et al. Effect of window casts on healing rates of diabetic foot ulcers. J Wound Care. 2006 Feb;15(2):80-3

8. Tamir E, Daniels TR. Off-loading neuropathic plantar heel ulcers with a metal stirrup brace: case report. Foot Ankle Int. 2007 Mar;28(3):385-7

9. Pohl M, Rückriem S, Strik H, et al. Treatment of pressure ulcers by serial casting in patients with severe spasticity of cerebral origin. Arch Phys Med Rehabil. 2002 Jan;83(1):35-9

10. Guyton GP. Advantages of TCC offset limitations, BioMechanics, 2003; X(4):55-66

11. Myerson M, Papa J, Eaton K, et al. The total-contact cast for management of neuropathic plantar ulceration of the foot. J Bone Joint Surg, 1992; 74-A:261-269

12. Hartsell HD, Fellner C, Saltzman CL. Pneumatic bracing and total contact casting have equivocal effects on plantar -pressure relief, Foot Ankle Itnl 2001, 22(6):502-506

13. Frigg A, Pagenstert G, Schäfer D, et al. Recurrence and prevention of diabetic foot ulcers after total contact casting. Foot Ankle Int. 2007 Jan;28(1):64-9

14. Ha Van G, Siney H, Hartmann-Heurtier A, et al. Nonremovable, windowed, fiberglass cast boot in the treatment of diabetic plantar ulcers: efficacy, safety, and compliance. Diabetes Care 2003 Oct;26(10):2848-52

15. Nabuurs-Franssen MH, Sleegers R, Huijberts MS, et al. Total contact casting of the diabetic foot in daily practice: a prospective follow-up study. Diabetes Care. 2005 Feb;28(2):243-7

16. Pollo FE, Brodsky JW, Crenshaw SJ, et al. Plantar pressures in fiberglass total contact casts vs. a new diabetic walking boot. Foot Ankle Int. 2003 Jan;24(1):45-9

17. Piaggesi A, Macchiarini S, Rizzo L, et al. An off-the-shelf instant contact casting device for the management of diabetic foot ulcers: a randomized prospective trial versus traditional fiberglass cast. Diabetes Care 2007 Mar;30(3):586-90

18. Ilizarov, GA. The tension-stress effect on the genesis and growth of tissues. Part I. The influence of stability of fixation and soft-tissue preservation, Clin Orthop Relat Res. 1989 238:249-281

<u>NOTES</u>

CHAPTER

SELECTION OF WOUND

DRESSING AGENTS

CHAPTER NINE OVERVIEW

INTRODUCTION 221

GOALS FOR THE WOUND DRESSING AGENTS 222

MOISTENED GAUZE DRESSINGS 229

COVERING AGENTS FOR THE HEALTHY-BASED,
   NON-SECRETION PRODUCING WOUNDS 233

DRESSING TACTICS FOR SECRETION PRODUCING WOUNDS 237

GELS, SALVES, OINTMENTS, AND SOLUTIONS WITH ADDITIVES 241

MYTHS, MISCONCEPTIONS, AND FALLACIES ABOUT WOUND
   DRESSING AGENTS 247

CONCLUSIONS 249

QUESTIONS 250

REFERENCES 251

"So many choices, so many opportunities."

INTRODUCTION
Dressing Agent Selection

The selection of the dressing agent that covers the wound base requires knowledge of the available products as well as the characteristics of the wound itself. Preparation of the wound base with debridement and other techniques has been described previously (Chapter 7). The appearance assessment of the **Wound Score** provides easy-to-use, tangible criteria for evaluating the wound base and is useful for making intelligent decisions regarding the selection of dressing agents to cover the wound base. Conversely, the selection of the particular dressing agents is a daunting one. This is because there are so many choices available. There are hundreds of different dressing products for covering wounds. In addition, there are over a half dozen considerations that must be evaluated in the selection of the agent used to cover the wound base (Figure 9-1). These include: 1) comfort, 2) cost-effectiveness, 3) wound location, 4) size, 5) characteristics of the secretions/bioburden, 6) cost benefits, and 7) frequency of dressing changes. Many wound care product manufacturers have a full range of products that are similar to the full range of products of other manufacturers. How does one decide which agent to use when so many choices are available?

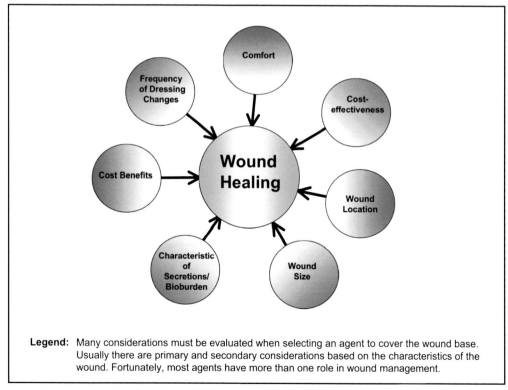

Legend: Many considerations must be evaluated when selecting an agent to cover the wound base. Usually there are primary and secondary considerations based on the characteristics of the wound. Fortunately, most agents have more than one role in wound management.

Figure 9-1. Considerations for selecting the agent to cover the wound base.

Categorization of Dressing Agents

The purpose of this chapter is to present a classification system that categorizes the products by the type of wound base for which they are most applicable. Many of the products have primary and secondary benefits (Table 9-1). Wound dressing agents can be categorized into four types based on their mechanisms (Figure 9-2). Each category of wound dressing agent has its own advantages and disadvantages (Table 9-2). The four categories include: 1) gauze moistened with aqueous solutions, 2) impermeable coverings, 3) products to absorb secretions and 4) agents with special additives. Several of the wound dressing agents in each category have more than one function and many of the newer products are specifically designed to be multi-functional (Table 9-1). From this categorization paired with the assessment of the wound base, the selection of an appropriate agent can readily be made. The dilemma arises in choosing which company's product to use. The decision is usually made based on the experiences of the wound care provider with the agent selected and the options made available by the third party payer/insurance company for the wound care product.

TABLE 9-1. PRIMARY CONSIDERATIONS FOR AND SECONDARY BENEFITS OF WOUND DRESSING AGENTS

Primary Considerations for Selecting the Dressing Agent	Secondary Benefits						
	Bioburden Management	Costs	Reduced Frequency of Dressing Changes	Maintenance of Moist Environment	Odor Control	Pain Management	Psychological Effects
Absorption of Secretions	✓				✓		✓
Bioburden Management	--				✓		✓
Comfort			✓	✓		✓	✓
Costs (materials and nursing)		--	✓				
Debridement Effects	✓				✓		✓
Ease of Dressing Changes		✓	✓		✓	✓	✓
Independence (doing own* dressing changes)		✓					✓
Maintenance of Moist Environment		✓	✓	--		✓	
Occlusiveness (barrier effects)		✓	✓	✓	✓	✓	✓
Size of Wound	✓	✓		✓		✓	

*Own implies patient and/or family member being able to do wound care without visiting nurse or other paid caregivers.

GOALS FOR THE WOUND DRESSING AGENTS

Selection Goals

The goals of the wound dressing agent selection strategy may, at first consideration, be confused with those of the wound protection and stabilization strategy (Chapter 8). Each complements the other, but each has specific objectives. The goals of the wound

TABLE 9-2. ADVANTAGES AND DISADVANTAGES OF THE FOUR CATEGORIES OF DRESSING AGENTS FOR THE WOUND BASE

Category	Advantages	Disadvantages
Moist (aqueous) **gauze dressings**	Inexpensive; applicable to almost all wound sizes, shapes and types	Labor intensive; frequent dressing changes required; maceration of adjacent skin
Coverings for healthy (red) **based wounds***	Infrequent dressing changes; comfort; economical	Fluid accumulations under coverings lead to infections Applicable only for superficial wounds
Products (absorbents) **for secretion producing wounds**	Less labor intensive than moist dressings; often serve multiple purposes	Relatively expensive; often inappropriately used as a substitute for needed surgical interventions
Gels, salves, ointments and solutions with or without additives	Easy-to-use, comfortable; ideal for the final stages of wound healing; often specific effects	Generally for uncomplicated wounds; great variation in prices; some are very expensive

Note: *Corresponds to a grade of 2 points on the wound assessment of the **Wound Score**

Many times combinations of dressing agents from two or more categories are used.

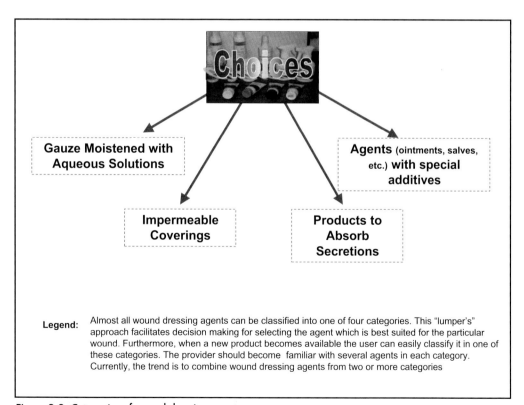

Legend: Almost all wound dressing agents can be classified into one of four categories. This "lumper's" approach facilitates decision making for selecting the agent which is best suited for the particular wound. Furthermore, when a new product becomes available the user can easily classify it in one of these categories. The provider should become familiar with several agents in each category. Currently, the trend is to combine wound dressing agents from two or more categories

Figure 9-2. Categories of wound dressing agents.

dressing agent selection strategy are fourfold and include, first, to achieve and maintain a moist, physiological covering to optimize the wound environment; second, to decrease the bacterial load in the wound, commonly referred to as the bioburden; third, to make the application of the dressing agent as easy and comfortable as possible (i.e. convenience); and fourth, to select the wound-dressing agent that is most cost-effective and cost beneficial. With such an enormous selection of choices for wound dressing agents, these goals should always be considered whenever selecting a specific wound-dressing agent.[1]

Moist Healing

The concept of moist wound healing is fundamental to the management of "problem" wounds.[2, 3, 4] All body tissues within the skin envelope are bathed in tissue fluids. The tissue fluids provide a physiological environment for cell function. It is logical that for wound healing to progress, the wound healing environment needs to be made as close to the normal physiological environment as possible. This means keeping the wound moist with physiological substances. The best physiological substances are crystalloid fluids that have electrolyte concentrations similar to tissue fluids. Other agents, such as gels, help maintain a moist environment by placing a protective coating over the wound base to keep it from drying out. Of all the wound coverings, the thin dry firm eschar provides the most physiological environment to the underlying wound base (Figure 9-3). Even though the outer layer is dry, the eschar maintains a sealed, bacteria-free, moist environment between its under surface and the base of the wound. The thin dry eschar wound base covering requires the least oxygen and metabolic requirements of any of the wound coverage-closure choices (Chapter 7). Less than ideal physiological types of moist wound bases are from edema fluid oozing through the wound base or from exudate secondary to infection. Excessively moist wound bases are commonly found in wounds in dependent portions of the body, especially in edematous lower extremities, and are analogous to fluid leaking out of a hole in the bottom of a barrel. Compounding factors to this problem are venous stasis disease, edema secondary to heart failure, obesity, lymphatic obstruction, and hypoproteinemia. Usually, the leakage is so perfuse that it saturates the dressing as well as macerates the surrounding tissues. In these situations, a first step in successful management of the wound is that of edema control (Chapter 6).

Bioburden

The surfaces of open wounds are usually colonized with bacteria, as are the skin and mucus membranes covering all the other parts of our body.[5, 6, 7] This is a normal finding, which equates to a grade of 2 points (on the 0 to 2 scale) of the infection/bioburden assessment of the **Wound Score**. When bacteria invade and multiply in the wound base, an exudate is produced. Even though the exudate may make the wound base moist, it is not physiological because of the bacteria it contains, as well as the metabolic waste products of the bacteria and the breakdown products of tissues from the bacterial invasion. The bacterial load equates to the bioburden.[8] When bacteria invade and multiply in the surrounding skin, cellulitis occurs. With exuberant exudate or marked leakage of fluid, the skin margins adjacent to the wound macerate. The findings of cellulitis and/or maceration equate to a grade of 1 point on the infection/bioburden assessment of the **Wound Score**. If the bacteria invade and multiply in deeper tissues and they or their products enter the blood stream, sepsis results (grade of 0 points on the infection/bioburden assessment of the **Wound Score**). Many wound dressing agents have bacteriostatic/bacteriocidal effects. Their goal is to reduce the bioburden. There are

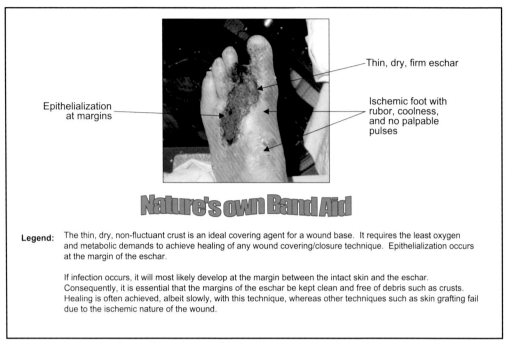

Epithelialization at margins

Thin, dry, firm eschar

Ischemic foot with rubor, coolness, and no palpable pulses

Nature's own Band Aid

Legend: The thin, dry, non-fluctuant crust is an ideal covering agent for a wound base. It requires the least oxygen and metabolic demands to achieve healing of any wound covering/closure technique. Epithelialization occurs at the margin of the eschar.

If infection occurs, it will most likely develop at the margin between the intact skin and the eschar. Consequently, it is essential that the margins of the eschar be kept clean and free of debris such as crusts. Healing is often achieved, albeit slowly, with this technique, whereas other techniques such as skin grafting fail due to the ischemic nature of the wound.

Figure 9-3. A thin, dry, firm eschar - the "ideal" wound covering.

many choices available for products with bacteria killing effects.[9] While these agents may control superficial infections and multiplication of bacteria in the normal wound, they are not effective with deeper infections or when biofilms develop.[10] Other interventions such as systemic antibiotics, wound debridements, and wound oxygenation must be addressed when infection extends deep to the base of the wound and/or extends into the peripheral tissues.

Ease of Wound Dressing Agent Application

Methods to achieve this goal include optimizing the accessibility of the wound, making the dressing change as comfortable as possible for the patient, and making it as convenient as possible for the caregivers. As mentioned in the previous chapter, a dressing should be easy to apply, remain in place without losing its effectiveness, commensurate with the patient's activity, and be easy to remove (Chapter 8). To improve the accessibility of difficult-to-reach wounds, position the patient in the lateral decubitus or prone position if the wound is around the ankle or on the posterior heel, back, buttocks, or hip. Use an assistant or family member to keep the patient on his or her side or to keep the lower extremity in an elevated position. All the wound dressing materials should be staged at the bedside or in the examination room to expedite the process.

Comfort

Comfort with dressing changes must always be a prime consideration. There is a wide range of patients' pain responses to dressing changes, from no discomfort whatsoever to the requirement for dressing changes to be done in the operating room under anesthesia (Table 9-3). For the majority of "problem" wounds in diabetic patients, dressing changes are not painful because of significant sensory neuropathies. In patients with normal sensation, the initial dressing changes after surgery can be excruciatingly painful. Wetting the portion of the dressing in contact with the wound with normal saline or during a hydrotherapy treatment (whirlpool or pulsatile lavage) is helpful when removing dressings where the dressing adheres to the wound base due to crusted blood or fibrinous material. As the wound improves, the dressing changes typically become less painful to the point that when they are nearly painless, the wound is usually ready for coverage-closure. At the opposite extreme is the patient with the hyperesthetic, hyperpathic (exaggerated pain response) wound. These situations are seen in patients with profound ischemia in their lower extremities and those with CRPS/RSD (complex regional pain syndrome/reflex sympathetic dystrophy) who have associated wounds. Pain control for dressing changes is managed by the physician directing the care and administered by the patient or caregiver doing the dressing change.

TABLE 9-3. HIERARCHY OF PAIN RESPONSES AND MANAGEMENT FOR DRESSING CHANGES

Pain Response	Examples	Management	Points*
Insensateóno significant pain with dressing changes	Diabetic patients with profound sensory neuropathies Spinal cord injuries resulting in paraplegia or quadriplegia	No pain management required	0
Minimal discomfort	Moderate sensory neuropathies Superficial wounds Nearly healed wounds	No analgesics with verbal reinforcement and/or mild oral analgesics	½
Moderate discomfort	Minimal sensory neuropathies Post-op dressing changes a week or more after surgery	Intravenous analgesics such as morphine before dressing changes	1
Severe discomfortó with or without unabated pain, even between dressing changes	Normal sensation in post-op patients Patients with drug-seeking behavior Hyperesthetic/hyperpathic wounds; dysvascular patients Patients with CRPS/RSD** Apprehensive pediatric patients	Patient controlled analgesics Continuous epidural analgesia Strong maintenance analgesics supplemented with strong IV analgesics during dressing changes Dressing changes (with or without debridements) in the operating room	1½ -2 (Patients with hyperesthesia, hyperpathia and/or allodynia need to be recognized & so designated)

*0 (no pain) to 2 (normal) **"Quick & Easy"** Pain Assessment (Table 2-5; Chapter 2)

**CRPS = Complex regional pain syndrome; RSD = Reflex sympathetic dystrophy.

Frequency

The frequency of dressing changes is another important consideration in selecting dressing materials. Some dressing materials require changes three or four times a day in order to be effective. For some choices, dressing changes once a day is sufficient. Others only need to be changed every two or three days. Finally, some dressings only require one application, such as impermeable membranes or other coverings used over split thickness skin graft donor sites. However, if the outer protective covering becomes stained or soiled, it should be changed as needed without disturbing the wound dressing agent that is in actual contact with the wound. The decision of which dressing material to use is multifactorial (Figure 9-1). In general, the more secretions (including blood and transudates as well as exudates generated at the wound base) and the greater the bioburden, the more frequently dressing changes need to be done. As the wound improves and generates fewer secretions, the frequency of dressing changes decreases. When this occurs, the wound dressing agents are usually changed to products requiring less frequent applications. This, of course, has many ramifications, including less discomfort for the patient, fewer needs for caregivers to change dressings, decreased quantities of dressing supplies, and the reduced necessity for hospitalization in an acute care facility.

Cost-Effectiveness versus Cost-Benefit

The fourth consideration in the selection of wound dressing agents is their cost-effectiveness and cost-benefit analysis. These are confusing, somewhat overlapping terms (Figure 9-4). Cost-effectiveness implies that the intervention and its outcome are cost-effective in terms of dollars and cents expended, in the short term, for those paying for and those being reimbursed for the care provided; that is, they are getting the most cost-effective use of their money. As an example, the most cost-effective method for dealing with a limb threatening "problem" wound might be an amputation instead of extended hospitalizations and long-term use of expensive wound dressing agents. The patient could be out of the hospital after four or five days. This would be very cost-effective for the hospital and payer. However, subsequent charges and responsibilities will be shifted from the hospital to other facilities, payers, the patient and/or family members. Consequently, the overall cost to the health care system might be much more than for salvaging the limb if the costs of the prosthesis, rehabilitation, loss of independence, and need for assisted living are factored in. Regarding cost-benefit analysis, the perspective is changed to what is most beneficial for the patient in terms of quality of life issues. This implies that cost-benefit analysis refers more to the benefit to the patient and their long-term consequences than does cost-effectiveness, which typically takes a short-term perspective.

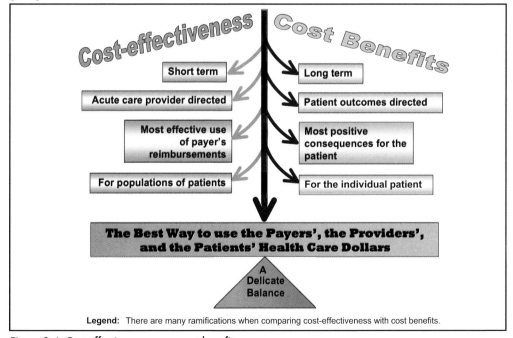

Legend: There are many ramifications when comparing cost-effectiveness with cost benefits.

Figure 9-4. Cost-effectiveness versus cost benefits.

Cost Considerations Regarding Wound Dressing Agents

Cost-effectiveness and cost-benefit need always to be considered when making decisions about managing wounds. The selection of wound dressing agents is no exception. The ideal situation is when the intervention is both cost-effective and cost-beneficial. Subsequently in this chapter, the basis for making cost-effective, cost-beneficial decisions for selecting wound dressing agents will be described. Unfortunately, of the five strategies for managing the "problem" wound, the selection of dressing agents to cover the wound base is the one most influenced by the economic interests of the manufacturers of the products. This is reflected by the industry's heavy investment in the promotion of wound dressing products. The result is that many misconceptions, fallacies, and myths have arisen about the use of wound dressing agents (Table 9-4).

TABLE 9-4. MYTHS, MISCONCEPTIONS, AND FALLACIES REGARDING WOUND DRESSING AGENTS

1. The moist gauze wound dressing is archaic and serves no useful role in the contemporary management of "problem" wounds.

2. The more frequent the dressing changes, the better the chances of wound healing.

3. One dressing agent is ideal for all wounds.

4. Wound size, shape and depth need not be considerations (vs. appearance of the wound base) when making decisions about the selection of wound dressing agents.

5. The use of expensive wound dressing agents is the best assurance that wound management will be successful.

6. When scientific data supporting the benefits of a particular wound dressing agent is reported, it is incontestable.

7. Failures with the use of a particular wound dressing agent can always be attributed to lack of patient compliance and/or failure to follow the manufacturer's instructions.

8. There is only a small range of costs among the different wound dressing agents.

9. If one wound dressing agent is effective, it is not appropriate to change to another even if the wound improves.

10. Wound dressing agents that have two or more functions should be avoided. Likewise, the use of two or more agents on the same wound is counterproductive.

Multiple Functions of Wound Dressing Agents

Wound dressing agents often have two or more functions. Criteria can be established to evaluate effectiveness and help define indications for choosing a particular agent and include adaptability for a variety of wound types, availability, costs, effectiveness, and versatility (Table 9-5). Usually, multiple functions are a desirable feature of the agent, but there can be complications from multi-function wound dressing agents. This is usually attributed to one or more of the ingredients being tissue toxic, an irritant, or allergenic. Although the standard of practice is moving towards using wound dressing agents with multiple functions, there can be disadvantages in addition to the complications described above. These include increased costs, the lack of indications for the secondary effects of the wound dressing agents or the secondary effects interfering with the overall management of the wound. The latter consideration is frequently observed when an antibiotic ointment is used for an exudative wound. The vehicle to carry the antibiotic, usually petrolatum based, may act as an occlusive agent and consequently retain exudative material in the wound. The remainder of this chapter discusses the four categories of wound dressing agents based on their primary mechanisms, considers their other effects and provides answers to myths, misconceptions and fallacies about wound dressing agents (Table 9-4).

TABLE 9-5. STANDARDS FOR EVALUATING WOUND DRESSING AGENTS WITH SPECIFIC REFERENCE TO AQUEOUS (MOISTENED) GAUZE

Criteria	Moistened Gauze Dressings	Comments
Adaptability	It can be applied to any size or shape of wound. It works well for wounds with tunneling, tracking, bridging, or recesses	The more complex the wound, the more expertise required for application of a dressing
Availability	Usually universally available; when not, clean cloths sterilized in boiling water can suffice	Many choices available including: ribbon, mesh, conforming, roller, compression, and absorbent varieties
Costs	In terms of supplies alone, no dressing agent is less expensive	Materials alone are but one item that needs to be factored-in when considering costs of dressings
Effectiveness	Widespread usage with predictable outcomes; i.e. has face validity (Chapter 3)	The moistened gauze dressing should always be considered when deciding which dressing to use for the acute wound
Versatility	Applicable for all wound base findings from healthy, red based (grade = 2 points) to necrotic (grade = 0 points) Dressing changes remove wound debris	The moist gauze dressing is often the only logical option for the initial i.e. acute management of the challenging* wound

*Examples of challenging wounds include large wounds, deep wounds, wounds after surgical debridements and wounds associated with necrotizing soft tissue infections.

MOISTENED GAUZE DRESSINGS

The Moist Gauze Dressing as a Standard and Its Paradoxes

We feel the moist gauze dressing is the standard by which all wound dressing agents should be measured. This dressing agent merely requires moistening gauze with normal saline with or without the addition of other ingredients, and then covering the wound base, if flat, or packing it into the wound, if cavitary. It is the standard because of its adaptability, availability, costs, effectiveness and versatility, especially for the acute wound (Table 9-5).[11] Even so, there are a number of paradoxes associated with the use of the moist gauze dressing. These include:

Bioburden management: Bacteria thrive in the moist dressing. Exudative material in the moist dressing provides an ideal medium for bacteria growth. While additives to the aqueous agent, such as acetic acid, may impede bacteria proliferation, they are not as effective as agents specifically designed to address the bioburden in the exudative wound and their durations of action may be short-lived.[12, 13] The changing of moistened gauze dressings with additives two to four times a day maintains a moist environment for the wound base while reducing the bioburden.

Cost-effectiveness: Although the dressing materials themselves may be the least expensive of any choice, nursing care to perform the dressing change three or four times a day may make the aqueous gauze dressing agent more expensive than other choices.

Evaporative heat loss: The normal body temperature is the ideal temperature for wound healing. Cooling from evaporative heat loss from the moist dressing may lower the temperature of the wound base. This coupled with poor perfusion, as associated with peripheral artery disease, may contribute to cooling of the wound site and slow metabolic reactions. This concern is probably only realized in very large wounds.

Material choices: Although the moist gauze dressing implies that fine mesh gauze is used, there are other options. These include gauze ribbon, coarse mesh, roller (stretch and non-stretch), and thick-absorbent padded gauze. Each has its own special uses. For example, ribbon gauze is useful for small tracking wounds, fine mesh for optimal contact with the wound base, roller gauze for large cavernous wounds, thick-absorbent padding for oozing, and stretch gauze to apply compression.

Skin maceration: Moisture from the dressing may extend onto the adjacent skin and cause maceration. The macerated skin harbors bacteria and is a precursor to cellulitis. In addition, it may interfere with wound contraction and epithelialization at the wound margins, thereby interfering with wound healing.

Wound moisturization: Because of evaporation, the moist dressing may dry out between dressing changes, especially if not done frequently. While this may be desirable for exudative wounds and may facilitate removal of debris when the dried dressing is changed, it is not optimal for the vascularized-based, non-exudative wound. The cells responsible for wound healing and infection control may die in a desiccated environment.

Wound severity: It is paradoxical that the wounds least suited for moist gauze dressings are those that are the healthiest, smallest, most long-standing, and the most superficial. Because of their small size, the moist gauze is likely to dry out before the next dressing change. When the patient is mobilized, the gauze dressing is prone to slip off the superficial wound, especially if on the foot and ankle. Conversely, the moist gauze dressing is ideally suited for the cavitary wound because of its conformability; it can accommodate almost any wound size or shape.

Side effects: Agents such as acetic acid, bleach, hydrogen peroxide, etc. have varying degrees of toxicity to fibroblasts, keratinocytes, and leukocytes.[14, 15, 16] When used in diluted solutions, their value in control of the bioburden appears to outweigh their potential toxicities. As the bioburden is controlled, the wound dressing agents should be changed to more physiological solutions, such as normal saline, then transition to agents that require less frequent applications, such as hydrogels (Figure 9-9).

Techniques to Improve the Effectiveness of Moistened Gauze Dressings

The effectiveness of the moist gauze dressing can be improved by several techniques. To deal with the bioburden, bacteriostatic, and bactericidal agents, as mentioned above, are added to the solution (Table 9-6). These are helpful for the purposes intended, but may have side effects such as cellular toxicity, desiccation and interference with coagulation. Wetting agents, such as surfactants help maintain moisture in the desiccated wound. Maceration of the adjacent skin can be reduced by using drying agents, such as zinc oxide preparations around the margins of the skin adjacent to the wound. Moisture in the dressing and heat in the wound can be maintained with a non-permeable barrier, such as cellophane placed over the gauze layers that come in contact with the wound. This technique is inappropriate for exudative wounds, but useful for healthy wounds free of exudates. When used in this situation, the frequency of the moist dressing change can be reduced. Elastic wraps provide compression over the wound. This improves contact between the dressing material and wound base and helps to control edema in the extremity. With edema reduction, fluid leakage through the wound base decreases.

TABLE 9-6. AGENTS TO MOISTEN THE GAUZE DRESSING
(Listed in approximate order of frequency of selection)

Agent (Generic name)	Composition	Primary Effect	Other Effects	Miscellaneous (Costs*, side effects, comments)
Normal Saline (NS)	0.9% sodium chloride solution	Maintains a moist environment (Humectant)	Softens debris; debridement with dressing changes	Inexpensive; minimal side effects 2 to 3 changes daily to maintain moist environment
Ringer's Irrigation Solution	Similar to NS with potassium and calcium	SAA **	SAA	SAA; electrolyte composition is more similar to serum than NS
Acetic Acid Solution	0.25% acetic acid solution	Antibacterial Humectant	Acidifies; especially for *Pseudomonas sp.* Mild desiccating effects	SAA for NS; Made by adding 30 cc of white (table) vinegar to 1 liter of NS
Bunnell's Solution	(30 cc 50% glycerin, < 1% acetic acid, and < 1% benzalkonium chloride per liter)	Humectant Antibacterial (acetic acid)	Glycerin (an emollient) prevents dressing adherence & maceration Benzalkonium chloride maintains sterility	SAA, but more expensive than NS ($40 per liter); Popularized by Dr. Sterling Bunnell for serious hand infections
Dakin's Solution	Diluted sodium hypochlorite solution Full strength = 0.45%; ¼ strength = 0.125%	Antibacterial Humectant	Dissolves necrotic tissue & clots Deodorizes odors from coliforms & anaerobes	Costs similar to Bunnell's solution Toxic to tissues, ¼ strength recommended; switch to less toxic agents as soon as the wound warrants it
Flagyl® Solution	2 grams of metronidazole in 1 liter NS	Antibacterial Humectant	Less toxic to tissues than Dakin's & Acetic Acid Solutions	Easy to compound; not frequently used, consider using for wounds with anaerobes
Silver Nitrate Solution	0.1% silver nitrate	Antibacterial	Primarily used in burn management	Inexpensive, about $10 a liter; Stains everything black with which it comes in contact
Domeboro's Solution	2% Acetic acid/ Aluminum acetate	Astringent (constricts engorged tissues) Humectant	Antibacterial	Costs similar to Bunnell's solution Frequently used for external auditory canal infections

*Costs are estimates for purchases through a pharmacy. Other considerations include dressing supplies and the caregiver's time needed to change the dressing.

** **SAA** = same as above

The Moist Dressing as a "Work of Art"

The proper application of the moist dressing is as much a "work of art" as it is a routine nursing skill. Clean technique, that is using disposable clean gloves (and gowns if drug resistant organisms are growing in the wound) is required for those managing the dressing change. All dressing supplies should be staged at the patient's bedside before beginning the dressing change. The old dressing should be removed in as painless a fashion as possible and disposed of properly. Disposal of the dressing should be in labeled, biohazard bags for contaminated non-sharp materials. Pain is controlled with a combination of methods, including oral and/or intravenous bolus analgesics, gentle removal of the old dressing, and use of normal saline to wet the adherent portions, if necessary. The dressing is especially a "work of art" when the wounds are deep, irregularly shaped and have recesses or tracts. Wetting of the gauze that is to come in contact with the wound base can be done by pouring the aqueous solution onto it or by soaking it in a small container. In either case, soaking wet gauze should be squeezed to remove excess liquid to the degree that it remains moist. However, the gauze should neither be so wet that fluid drips from the dressing and macerates the adjacent skin margins nor so dry that the wound base desiccates between scheduled dressing changes. The dressing should be applied so that all parts of the moist dressing come in contact with the wound base. If this is not done properly, secretions and exudates can collect in the interstices of the wound and become a source of on-going sepsis and lack of improvement. The moistened dressing should remain in the confines of the wound; that is, it should not moisturize the skin margins surrounding the wound. Experience and motivation are needed to properly pack the moistened gauze into the wound cavity. This insures that all surfaces of the wound base come in contact with the dressing, provides gentle compression, and avoids interfering with wound contraction. The wound should not be tightly packed, except temporarily to achieve hemostasis. When the wound is irregularly shaped, the well-applied moist dressing looks like a "work of art" with its contours perfectly conforming to the shape of the wound and not bulging above the skin surface (Figure 9-5). Finally, creativity is required to apply the remainder of the dressing so it remains in place, applies compression and is easy to remove. This includes dry gauze padding, gauze roller wrapping and an elastic bandage, bias cut stockinet or surgical netting (Chapter 8).

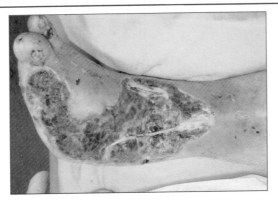

Legend: This irregularly shaped wound was managed with moist dressing changes. Notice the non-desiccated vascular appearance of the wound base and the healthy skin margins that are free of maceration. The patient's family became very adept at doing the dressing changes.

In terms of economies and efficiencies, the moist dressing technique cannot be surpassed especially for acute wounds. Soon thereafter, the wound was ready for skin grafting.

Figure 9-5. The moist dressing change as a "work of art."

Wound Care by the Patient or Other Caregivers

The final component in the art of applying the moist dressing is motivation. Motivation is required to execute the above techniques for applying the dressing. However, this goal need not be limited to the nursing staff. The patient, family members and/or the patient's other caregivers can be instructed in wound dressing techniques. Although they may not be professionals with respect to wound care, when motivated they can learn to perform the dressing changes very effectively. Some of the most resounding successes with managing slowly healing wounds have been achieved by patients and family members who assume responsibility for the dressing changes. Usually the criteria for discharging the patient with a "problem" wound to a lower level of care are three-fold. First, sepsis has been controlled. Second, the wound base is vascular and beginning to generate granulation tissue and third, the dressing changes are no longer painful.

When these goals have been reached, the motivated patient, family or other caregivers can assume the responsibility, if so willing, for the patient's dressing changes or supplement dressing changes between home health care nursing visits.

COVERING AGENTS FOR THE HEALTHY-BASED, NON-SECRETION PRODUCING WOUNDS

Wound Base/Covering Agents

Once a wound develops a vascular base, additional options become available for wound dressing agents. The covering selections described in this section (Table 9-7) work well for healthy appearing, non-exudative, superficial wounds (wound base assessment grade = 1 1/2 points for the **Wound Score**.) "Covering" implies that the dressing is placed over the entire wound and may even extend beyond its margins to include the adjacent skin. The goals for covering agents are that they remain in place for sustained periods of time, keep the wound base moist and prevent contamination. These agents are usually impermeable or semi-permeable. A representative type of wound that uses this group of dressing agents is the donor site for a split thickness skin graft. Other wounds that are appropriate for "covering" selections as described above include superficial pressure ulcers, healing wounds that have progressed to the point where closure-coverage options need to be considered, non-exudative burn wounds, abrasions, venous stasis ulcers with healthy bases, and wounds associated with epidermolysis. The common denominator for these wounds is that they are healthy enough that the covering agent can remain in place over the wound for several days or more without jeopardizing wound healing. These wound dressing agents are also appropriate for covering "healthy" wounds that require casting for protection and/or stabilization of the wound site.

Advantages and Disadvantages of Covering Agents for Healthy-based Wounds

The main advantage of this choice is that it reduces the frequency of dressing changes. This is especially important for those patients whose dressing changes are painful. Another important advantage of the covering selections is that they substantially reduce the nursing care costs associated with dressing changes. Covering selections also help maintain a moist environment over the wound, which is ideal for epithelialization, the final stage of healing. Disadvantages include increased costs of supplies for each dressing change. However, this is only a relative consideration, because decreased frequency of dressing changes and associated health care provider costs can make this dressing agent choice cost-effective. Another problem is that fluid may accumulate under those coverings that are sealed to the skin surrounding the wound. This acts like a bulla, which in turn may be a source of discomfort and infection. Bacteria growing in the fluid can lead to cellulitis, maceration of the surrounding skin and damage to the surrounding epithelium. A final consideration for covering this type of wound is the use of bioengineered skin substitutes and autografts (split and full thickness skin grafts). These interventions are expensive. The bioengineered agents are receiving much attention in the wound healing literature and are heavily promoted by their manufacturers (Table 9-8 and 9-9).[17, 18] The products alone cost hundreds of dollars or more for each application. Some can be applied in the clinic or office setting, while others require the use of an operating room. With large wounds, which require multiple

TABLE 9-7. WOUND COVERING AGENTS FOR WOUNDS WITH HEALTHY, SUPERFICIAL BASES

Agent/ Categories	Examples*	Primary Effects	Other Effect(s)	Miscellaneous (Costs**, Side Effects, Comments)
Semi- permeable Membrane Coverings (Impregnated and non-impregnated)	Adaptic® Parachute silk Scarlet red gauze Telfa® Vaseline® gauze Xeroform™ gauze	Maintain a moist environment Fluids able to ooze through to the next layer	Comfort Antibacterial for the impregnated choices Less frequent need for dressing changes Changes of outer dressing possible without disturbing the covering	Minimally expensive (< $10 per application) Minimal side effects; occasional infections develop under the coverings Removal may be painful due to adhesions Outer coverings changed as needed, some daily, some remain until healed
Non- permeability Membrane Coverings	OpSite® Tegederm™	Maintain a moist environment over the wound (i.e. hermetic seal)	Comfort Occlusive, non-absorptive, membrane-like covering	Minimally expensive; Fluid collections under the membrane can be a source of pain and a site for infection to develop; they may require aspirations Changed as needed (weekly) for wound hygiene
Hydrocolloid Dressings and Foams	Duoderm® Lyoderm®	SAA (same as above) Impervious	Padding over pressure points Resist shear & abrasion stresses Comfort	Minimally-to-moderately expensive ($10-to-$20 per application); Occlusiveness of dressing may retain exudates and macerate tissues; Changed usually one to three times a week
Matrix Metallo- proteinase Inhibitors	Promogran®	Inhibits formation of matrix metal-protein enzyme complexes. These complexes interfere with wound healing	Semi-permeable membrane-like covering	Moderately expensive No methods currently exist to ascertain which wounds are failing to heal due to matrix metalloproteinase inhibitors; Changed weekly
Tissue- engineered Skin Substitutes	See Tables 9-8 & 9-9	Induce epithelialization and collagen formation	Semi-permeable membrane-like covering Growth factors in the agents may induce angiogenesis, epithelialization & healing	Expensive ($100 to $1000 or more per application for small surface areas) Usually stabilized with a second covering such as Xeroform® and protective dressings which are reapplied as needed Reapplications are frequently required Some require application in the operating room in conjunction with debridements
Biological Skin Substitutes (Allografts and xenografts)	Human cadaver skin allograft Porcine skin xenografts	Reduce fluid & protein losses (in the presence of large skin deficits)	Comfort Induce epithelialization	Expensive; operating room applications increase expenses manyfold Usually limited to burns and other conditions where skin losses may be massive Changes done as needed, usually 1-to-2 week intervals
Split Thickness Skin Grafts	Human skin autograft	Definitive wound healig	Comfort Permanence	Very expensive (thousands of dollars) when operating room time, hospitalization and physicians' charges are considered Deferred until wound healthy enough for the skin graft to "take" Donor site management required

* These are examples of coverings with which the authors and their reviewers have had experiences. The list is not designed to be all-inclusive. Consequently, the omission of a covering is not intended to deprecate the value of the product nor suggest it does not have effects equal to or better than those in the above table. The goal of this table is to allow the prescriber to make informed decisions about which products to choose based on categories of products.

** Costs are based on estimates of the charges for the purchase of the initial quantity of the agent. Other considerations that need to be factored into the costs are those of operating room time to apply the agent (when needed), additional supplies (gauze, padding and wraps) and caregiver time needed to manage the dressing.

quantities of the product and the operating room for applications, extra costs are substantially greater than simple moistened gauze dressing changes. As stated before, the great majority of wounds fail to heal or their healing is delayed because of three reasons: persistent deformity, uncontrolled infection (osteomyelitis), and/or wound ischemia/hypoxia (Chapter 2). Bioengineered skin substitutes should be used for their specific indications and not as substitute for the other strategies used for management of "problem" wounds.

TABLE 9-8. MONOLAYER BIOENGINEERED WOUND DRESSING AGENTS

Name (Manufacturer)	Source	Components	Uses	Comments
Alloderm® (Lifecell Inc.)	Cadaver skin	Dermal matrix (acellular)	Burns, soft tissue padding, support	Fills defects; other formulations are Cymetra™, and Repliform™; not rejected; 2-year shelf life
Celladerm™ (Celadon Science, LLC)	Human foreskin	Cultured allogenic keratinocytes	Partial/full thickness wounds	Cells do not divide; > 6 month shelf life, not Food and Drug Administration approved
Dermagraft® (Advanced BioHealing, Inc.)	Human neonatal foreskin	Fibroblasts + polyglactin mesh	Dermal equivalent for deep wounds	Living cells secrete matrix proteins, growth factors and cytokines; mesh absorbed after 3-4 weeks; multiple applications; cryopreserved; about $800.00/application
Epicel® (Genzyme Corporation)	Autologous skin	Cultured keratinocytes	Deep burns	High percentage of permanent takes; one day shelf life; grown with mouse cells, considered a xenotransplant product by FDA
GRAFTJACKET™ (Wright Medical Technology, Inc.)	Human	Acellular dermal framework	Support tissue	Acellular, freeze dried; temporary coverage for wounds, tendon, ligament, and bone; another Alloderm® product
EZ DERM™ (Brennen Medical, LLC)	Porcine	Cross-linked collagen	Partial thickness burns/diabetic ulcers	Temporary covering; potential immune and disease transmission as with any allograft or xenograft; shelf life 18 months
FlexHD™ (Ethicon, Inc.)	Human	Dermal matrix	Scaffold	Acellular, pre-hydrated, no refrigeration; minimal elasticity; supports cellular replication and vascularity
Laserskin® (Fidia Advanced Biopolymers S.r.l.)	Autologous keratinocytes	Hyaluronic acid template	Burns, venous stasis ulcers	Template perforated using laser techniques; incorporates into wounds; pores enhance drainage
NeoForm™ (Mentor Corporation)	Cadaver	Dermal product	Scaffold for tissue expansion/reconstruction	Solvent hydrated, 5 year shelf life, no refrigeration; removal unnecessary before skin grafting
Oasis® (Healthpoint, Ltd.)	Porcine small intestine	Submucosal acellular collagen	Burns; diabetic, venous, pressure & ischemic ulcers	Provides an acellular dermal scaffold for tissue growth; application in clinics; about $400 per 6 x 6 inch square sheet
Permacol™ (Tissue Science Laboratories, Inc.)	Porcine	Dermal collagen and elastin	Soft tissue repair	3-dimensional collagen matrix after DNA removed; cross-linked; meshed for vascular in-growth
PriMatrix™ (TEI Biosciences, Inc.)	Bovine	Fetal dermis tissue	Ulcer bases	Dermal repair scaffold; Acellular; vascularizes quickly; shelf life - 3 years
SurgiMend® (TEI Biosciences, Inc.)	Bovine	Fetal dermis	Soft tissue reconstruction for weak or damaged tissues	Native, non-denatured acellular collagen; biological mesh provides structural support and a scaffold; porosity allows cell and blood vessel penetration
TissueMend® (TEI Biosciences, Inc.)	Bovine	Fetal dermis	Repair, reinforce soft tissues e.g. tendons	For wounds with poor tissue quality; new tissues integrate with matrix; used for rotator cuff repairs
Unite® Biomatrix/ OrthADAPT (Pegasus Biologics, Inc., Synouis® Orthopedic and Wound Care, Inc)	Equine	Pericardium	Wound coverage	De-cellularized; stabilization controlled collagen cross-linking; resists enzymatic degradation; fenestrated; must be kept moist; recently renamed OrthADAPT®

Note: Other names for these types of products include Human Skin Equivalents and Bioengineered Alternative Tissues

This listing is believed to be accurate and as comprehensive as possible at the time it was generated by the authors. Even so, new products, changes in product names, and manufacturers occurred during the process of generating this table.

For more complete descriptions of the products and their costs, information should be obtained from the manufacturers. The internet was found to be a useful starting point for obtaining information to generate this table.

Evaluation Criteria for Wound Covering Agents

When wound covering agent selections for healthy wound bases are evaluated with the five criteria used for the moist dressing agents, namely; adaptability, availability, costs, effectiveness, and versatility (Table 9-5), they compare favorably for properly selected wounds as summarized below:

- **Adaptability -** These dressing selections are adaptable to almost any small or medium-sized wound corresponding to the size assessment grade (1 or 2 points) of the **Wound Score**. They work well with regular as well as irregularly shaped wounds. When the wound size exceeds the dimensions of the selected wound covering agent, it is often better to use a different category of wound dressing agents. Some of the wound covering selections have adhesive around their

TABLE 9-9. BI-LAYERED BIOENGINEERED WOUND DRESSING AGENTS

Name (Manufacturer)	Source	Components	Uses	Comments
Apligraf® (Organogenesis, Inc.)	Human skin	1. Living human keratinocyges 2. Fibroblasts	Living skin equivalent; venous stasis ulcers; diabetic ulcers	Human fibroblasts in a bovine collagen lattice to produce a matrix of proteins; needs to be applied within 15 minutes of opening package; mimics function of dermis.
AWBAT™ (Aubrey, Inc.)	Porcine	1. Type I collagen mobile peptide 2. Silicone-nylon membrane	Superficial burns; donor sites; coverage for meshed autografts	AWBAT = Advanced Wound Bioengineered Alternative Tissue Collagen interacts with host fibrin; precise porosity and occlusiveness to reduce fluid accumulation; several types for different applications
Biobrane® (Mylan Laboratories, Inc.)	Porcine	1. Type I collagen mobile peptide 2. Silicone-nylon membrane	Superficial burns; donor sites; coverage for meshed autografts	Similar to AWBAT; Autoclaved; FDA approval in 1979
GammaGraft® (Promethean LifeSciences, Inc.)	Cadaver	1. Epidermis 2. Dermis	Temporary dressing for 2-6 weeks	Irradiated; 2 year shelf life at room temperature
Integra® Dermal Regeneration Template (Integra LifeSciences Corp)	Bovine	1. Type I collagen cross-linked with GAGs (glycosaminoglycans) 2. Silicone covering	Coverage of poorly vascularized structures including tendon and bone	Silicon covering prevents moisture loss, must be removed for definitive skin coverage; GAGs mask binding sites and prevent inflammation; controlled degradation Requires application in operating room; 2 x2 square inch = $1,400 → 8 x 10 = $4,225
OrCel® (Forticell Bioscience, Inc)	Human skin cells	1. Neonatal Keratinocytes 2. Neonatal dermal fibroblasts	Venous stasis ulcers; diabetic wounds, severe burns, STSG donor site coverage	Bovine collage cross-linked sponge; matrix contains viable cells to secrete growth factors and cytokines; can be cryopreserved Vascularizes quickly to provide a scaffold for new tissues. Gradual/complete resorption in 2 weeks
TransCyte® (Smith & Nephew, Inc)	Neonatal foreskin + porcine collagen	1. Fibroblasts 2. Silicone-covered nylon mesh	Burns, partial thickness wounds	Cryo-preserved; temporary skin substitute; may require multiple applications Silicone must be removed

Note: Please refer to note/comments at the end of Table 9-8

edges to secure them to the surrounding skin. If the wound is larger than the dimensions of the covering selection, the adhesive will lie on the wound base and not attach to the surrounding skin. If coverings without adhesive around their margins are used for larger wounds, then patchwork applications are required. For some of the selections, this can become increasingly expensive for very large wounds.

- **Availability -** The covering selections are generally available at hospitals and wound clinics. They can be obtained for use in private offices, also. Because of the costs of some of these agents, especially the tissue-engineered products, the selections are not inventoried, but rather obtained on an as-needed basis from pharmacies or their manufacturers, or can be delivered to the patient via home health nursing services. The formularies of payers may also dictate which products are available.

- **Costs -** The costs of covering agents vary from inexpensive to quite expensive. However, with single or infrequent applications, they can be cost-effective compared to less expensive agents that require frequent dressing changes by wound care providers.

- **Effectiveness -** For properly selected wounds, that is a "healthy" wound (**Wound Score** of 8-10 points), these wound covering selections are very effective. Wound healing is observed and predictable with a minimum of wound care. In some instances healing is reported, especially with tissue-engineered coverings, when the wound did not improve with other types of dressing agents.

- **Versatility -** Of all the wound dressing agents, the wound covering choices are the least versatile. Basically, they can only be used for healthy, vascular based, non-exudative wounds that do not have underlying deformities that interfere with wound healing or osteomyelitis. These wounds correspond to a wound base assessment grade of 1 1/2 points on the **Wound Score**.

DRESSING TACTICS FOR SECRETION PRODUCING WOUNDS

Concerns Regarding Secretions

Secretion producing wounds are those that generate discharges beyond the normal tissue moisturization of a healthy wound base. The secretions may be exudates (fluids rich in protein and cellular elements, usually infected with bacteria), transudates (watery fluids from tissues or edema), blood, or combinations. Although secretions may appear to be desirable because they keep the wound base moist, they have many undesirable features. When exudative, they often contain bacteria, breakdown products of tissues, waste products of metabolism, enzymes, cytokines, leucocytes, and matrix metalloproteases. All interfere with healing, at the least, and can cause deterioration of the wound, at the worst. Transudates wet the wound. When large, they keep the wound too moist. Dressings quickly become saturated, which leads to maceration and cellulitis of the surrounding skin. Because transudates contain glucose, protein and other components of tissue fluid, they provide an ideal environment for the growth of bacteria. Special interventions, including surgical procedures, may be required to manage secretion-producing wounds (Table 9-10).

TABLE 9-10. INTERVENTIONS FOR MANAGING THE SECRETION PRODUCING WOUND

Categories	Examples*	Primary Effects	Other Effects	Miscellaneous (Costs**, side effects, comments)
Absorbents	Aquacel® PolyMem® (Coated polyurethane material) Kaltostat® (Calcium sodium alginates) Mepilex® (Silicone contact layer)	Absorption of secretions	Convenience, reduced frequency of dressing changes; Comfort; Desiccating effect;	Minimally expensive (< $10 per application); Minimal side effects Heavily secretory wounds may overwhelm the absorbing capacity of the agent Not practical for large wounds; Dressing changes every 1 to 3 days
Absorbents with bioburden control additives	Acticoat™ (Silver coated) Aquacel® Ag (Silver impregnated) Iodosorb™ (Cadexomer dressing with iodine)	SAA (same as above) Control of bacteria growing on the surface of the wound	SAA	About 1 ½ times more expensive than the absorbents alone (above row); Same side effects as above, but contraindicated in those with allergies to the bactericidal ingredients (silver or iodine); Dressing changes every 1 to 3 days
Continuous wound irrigation	Plastic or silicone catheter placed in wound base; irrigation with normal saline	Washout of secretions and debris Maintains moist environment	Reduction of bioburden Comfort (No dressing changes while employed)	Minimally expensive Used for several days after debridement of septic wounds Side effects include maceration of tissues and wetting of dressings, etc., from the irrigation
Closure with suction-irrigation	Perforated portions of drain tubes are tied together; the ends exit at opposite ends of the closed wound	Inflow (with normal saline) and outflow continuously lavage the closed wound	Wound closures are possible even with heavy bioburden at the time of debridement	Inflows (typically 50 cc/hr) decreased by 10cc/hr each day; tubes removed about the 6th post-op day Inflow and outflow directions changed each hour-i.e., countercurrent effect
Negative Pressure Wound Therapy	Refer to Table 9-11 A contact layer trimmed to wound size is covered with an impervious membrane & connected to a vacuum pump	Removal of secretions Wound contraction Maintains moist environment	Angiogenesis Reduction of bioburden Contact/contraction effects enhance fibroblast activity	Costs about $100/day; cost-effective by eliminating hospitalization Not limited by wound size Contraindications include wounds with necrotic bases & untreated osteomyelitis Rarely discontinued due to pain or skin maceration Changed 2-3 times per week
Surgery	Debridement, revision and/or stabilization Vein surgery	Eliminate bioburden and necrotic tissue Prepare wound for closure/coverage	Switching to simpler dressing agents Control sepsis	Operating room time is expensive Side effects occur with anesthesia; bleeding and other surgical complications

*These are examples with which the authors have had experiences. The list is not intended to be all-inclusive. Consequently, the omission of an item is not intended to deprecate the value of other products or techniques nor suggest that they do not have features equal to or better than those in the above table.

**For more complete descriptions of the products and their costs, information should be obtained from the manufacturers. The internet was found to be a useful starting point for obtaining information to generate this table.

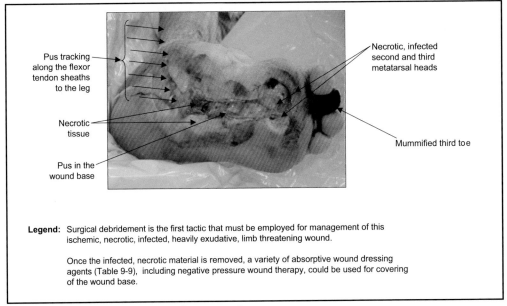

Pus tracking along the flexor tendon sheaths to the leg

Necrotic, infected second and third metatarsal heads

Necrotic tissue

Mummified third toe

Pus in the wound base

Legend: Surgical debridement is the first tactic that must be employed for management of this ischemic, necrotic, infected, heavily exudative, limb threatening wound.

Once the infected, necrotic material is removed, a variety of absorptive wound dressing agents (Table 9-9), including negative pressure wound therapy, could be used for covering of the wound base.

Figure 9-6. Tactics for the heavily exudative wound.

Appearances and Causes of Secretion Producing Wounds

Secretion producing wounds have a variety of appearances and causes (Figure 9-6). They may vary from small to large in size (size assessment on the **Wound Score** from 0 to 2 points). Generally, small-sized wounds generate secretions because of underlying necrotic tissue, ischemia-hypoxia, or foreign material in the wound. In these situations, the assessment of the appearance of the wound base is typically 0 or 1 point on the **Wound Score**. The foreign material may be sutures, retained vascular grafts (Dacron®, Goretex®, Marlex®, allo- or autologous-vessel substitutes), remnants of dressings, or sequestered secretions. Necrotic tissue may include skin, subcutaneous tissue, bone, cicatrix, fascia, joint capsule, ligament, muscle tendon, synovium, or combinations of these. Large wounds produce secretions due to the large surface area they have for the transudation of fluids. Large fluid losses can lead to protein depletion and be an important reason for non-healing of wounds (Chapter 6, nutrition section). The first measure to handle secretion producing wounds is to identify and remove the above listed offending factors (Chapter 7).

Challenges of the Secretion Producing Wounds

For the above reasons, the secretion producing wounds are the most challenging with regard to selection of wound dressing agents. The products available are among the most sophisticated of all those used for wound care. Many are highly promoted, both because of their purported effectiveness as well as economic incentives for the manufacturers. The main function of this group of wound dressing agents, as the section title implies, is to manage secretion producing wounds. Many also have important secondary effects, such as managing the bioburden and moisturization of the wound base. When products to manage secretion producing wounds are evaluated with the criteria used for the moist dressing agents and the wound covering selections, their roll is obvious as the following information demonstrates:

- **Adaptability** - Although there is a range of products available, almost every conceivable wound size can be managed by one or more of these products once the wound base is "cleaned up" (Chapter 7). Negative pressure wound therapy (NPWT) is a technique that has recently become available and has contributed more to the advancement of the selection of the dressing agent strategy than any product since the gauze dressing moistened with normal saline (Figure 9-7).[19, 20] The concept is simple; however, the proper and safe application of NPWT requires training in order to avoid complications and be effective. A foam-like material or gauze interface is trimmed to conform to the shape of the wound. A tube is placed in the center of the interface after a non-permeable adhesive covering is placed over the interface to seal the wound. The tube exits through the seal to a vacuum pump. A vacuum is generated by the pump, which in turn, collapses the interface. The negative pressure draws secretions out of the wound through the porous interface material while contracting the wound. Usually the interface material is changed two or three times a week. The use of NPWT often makes it possible to transfer a patient from the acute care facility to a lower level of care and justifies the cost-effectiveness of this device.[21, 22] Initially, continuous suction may be selected for NPWT for secretion management. After several days, intermittent suction is recommended. Intermittent suction promotes angiogenesis and fibroblast function through micro- and macrostrain tissue deformation.[23] The total contact of the wound base with the interface plus the intermittent negative pressure may also be a signaling device to promote these functions. Different interface materials may be used for special situations such as tracking wounds, wounds with recesses, infected wounds and wounds over critical structures, such as bowel, bone, joint and tendon. Over a dozen NPWT product lines are available, each with various wound interface materials, pressures settings, etc. (Table 9-11). Additionally, hundreds of articles have been published touting the use of NPWT.[24, 25, 26]
- **Availability** - Because the manufacturers of these products are heavily driven by economics, they tend to be well-advertised, actively promoted, and readily available to the wound care practitioner.
- **Costs** - Costs to use these products vary from moderate to expensive. However, when their use facilitates the transfer of patients to lower levels of care with wounds which otherwise would require hospitalization in an acute setting, they can become very cost-effective. This observation is especially apparent when using NPWT for large wounds where it is not practical to use most of the other secretion managing agents.
- **Effectiveness** - These agents generally work well for secretion producing wounds, but it is questionable whether they are more effective than the moist dressing and the use of techniques to partially close the wound in a serial fashion (Chapters 7 and 11).[27] Finally, less expensive techniques (see previous section) can be used for wounds with healthy bases.
- **Versatility** - The products to manage secretion producing wounds especially NPWT are useful for a wide variety of wounds, ranging from cavitary to secretory to vascular based. Contraindications for using these products include necrotic material in the wound base, malignancy in the wound, untreated osteomyelitis, exposed vital organs and non-enteric and unexplored fistulas. In addition, NPWT cannot be used for wounds in locations where a seal cannot be obtained, for example, the perianal/gluteal crease area, around digits, or where the skin is macerated, cellulitic, or extremely friable.

TABLE 9-11. NEGATIVE PRESSURE WOUND THERAPY (NPWT) / SUB-ATMOSPHERIC WOUND DRESSING

Name / Year (Manufacturer)	Interface Material	Pressure Settings (mmHg negative pressure)	Comments
Redon / 1955	Drain	900	Vacuum drainage bottle; pressure decreases as bottle fills
Russian Systems/ 1986 x 2, 1987, 1991 &1998	External funnel device; drain tubes	100-760	Combined with aggressive debridement to significantly reduce bacterial counts in purulent wounds; intermittent; 2-3x day
Chariker, Jeter and Tintle / 1989	Moist gauze	60-80	Flat drain then covered with moist gauze and bio-occlusive dressing; hospital wall suction
Argenta and Morykwai / 1993 (V.A.C.Æ Therapy System, KCI, Inc.)	Polyurethane foam Polyvinyl alcohol foam (varying pore sizes and densities) Change q 48-72 hours	75-125 (continuous or intermittent) 22-24 hours/day	Tegaderm™ drape, bridging available. Multiple reports on efficacy May use silver impregnated dressing, non-adherent gauze or enzymatic debriding agents between wound base and foam depending on the wound characteristics Instillation of topical solutions possible
Invia™ Vario 18 c/i / 2006 Medela Healthcare, Medela, Inc.	Antimicrobial Kerlix^M gauze Non-adherent wound contact layer	0-412.5 Continuous or intermittent	Various dressing sets with flat or round drains covered with moist gauze and transparent film; bridging not specified
Engenex® / 2006 Boehringer™ Laboratories, Inc.	Bio-Dome™ Dressing Change q 48-72 hours	30-75	Bio-Dome™ Dressing is a non collapsible wound surface interface of non woven polyester layers joined by silicon elastomer Polyurethane drape; bridging available
PRO-I™ and PRO-II™ / 2006 Prospera™	Non-adherent wound contact layer; Moist Antimicrobial dressing Change q 48-72 hours	Variable pressure levels oscillate from 40-80 or continuous at 80-200	Oscillating effect reported to increase in comfortable increments providing massage effect Various drain types covered with moist antimicrobial dressing and bio-occlusive film; bridging not specified
V1STA™ 2006 EZCare™ 2007 Smith & Nephew, Inc.	Gauze dressings Change q 48-72 hours	40-80; 200 mmHg Maximum setting 6-8 hours/day Continuous or intermittent pressure	Various drain types covered with moist gauze and bio-occlusive dressing; bridging not specified
Prodigy™ 800 and 800V / 2007 Premco Medical Systems, Inc.	Not available	Not available	Company website did not provide information on specifications
SVEDMAN® / 2007 Innovative Therapies, Inc.	SvampÆFoam Dressing change Change q 12-48 hours	70, 120 or 150 with intermittent options	Polyurethane drape over foam then SpeedConnect^M flange and tubing set; bridging not specified; instillation of topical solution possible
Genadyne A4 / 2007 Genadyne Biotechnologies, Inc.	Antimicrobial sponge; Non-adherent wound contact layer Change q 8-12 hours	50-250 Continuous or intermittent	One of the smallest portable units currently available
Venturi™ / 2008 Talley Group, Ltd.	Antimicrobial Kerlix^M gauze Non-adherent wound contact layer Change q 48-72 hours	Defaults to continuous at 80; can be continuous or intermittent pressure with various vacuum levels	Various wound sealing kits with flat or round drain covered with moist antimicrobial dressing and adhesive gel patch; bridging not specified
Renasys™ EZ/ 2008 Smith & Nephew, Inc.	Foam or gauze dressings Change q 48-72 hours	40- 200 6-8 hours/day Continuous or intermittent pressure	Various drain types covered with moist gauze or foam dressing and bio-occlusive film; bridging not specified
Exusdex® / 2008 Synergy Health plc	Kerlix^M gauze moistened with saline	50-200 Continuous or intermittent pressure	Various dressing kits; bridging not specified
NPD 1000 / 2009 Kalypto Medical.	Non-adherent silver coated wound contact layer	125 continuous	Super absorbing non woven polymer matrix absorbs exudate, hence no canister; semi-permeable wound cover then pressure port connection to pocket sized portable pump

TABLE 9-11. NEGATIVE PRESSURE WOUND THERAPY (NPWT) / SUB-ATMOSPHERIC WOUND DRESSING (CONTINUED)

MoblVac® / 2009 Ohio Medical Corporation	Non-adherent wound contact layer with or without antimicrobial; Change q 48-72 hours	0-200 continuous or intermittent; 24 hour battery mode	Various dressing sets with flat drains covered with moist gauze and transparent adhesive dressing; bridging not specified. Pump provides one of the highest flow rates available, thus providing a quick seal

Note: This listing is believed to be accurate and as comprehensive as possible at the time it was generated by the authors. Even so, new products and changes in product names and manufacturers occurred during the process of generating this table.

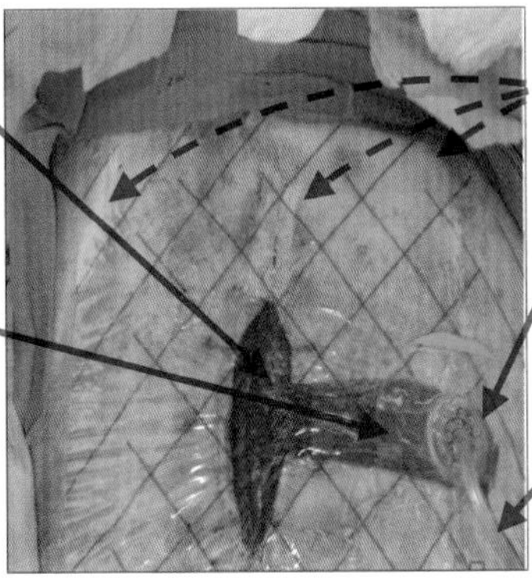

Sponge trimmed to conform to the shape of the back wound

Self-adhesive impermeable membrane (bio-occlusive adhesive drape) to "seal" system

Drain tubing adaptor device to the sponge (perforations allow fluid to be sucked through the bridging sponge and enter the connecting tubing)

Bridging sponge on the skin (acts as a conduit to carry secretions to the drain tubing while avoiding pressure sores from the tubing)

Drain tubing connecting to suction (negative pressure) pump

Wound from dehiscence of a back surgical site

Legend: Negative pressure wound therapy is a relatively new, very useful technique for difficult to manage wounds. The suction created by negative pressure removes secretions through the porous interface packing that is placed into the wound. In addition, the suction helps contract the wound.

The device need only be changed every two to four days which greatly reduces the time caregivers are needed to dress the wound. Techniques of application must be precisely followed in order for the system to work properly and to avoid complications.

Figure 9-7. Negative pressure wound therapy.

GELS, SALVES, OINTMENTS, AND SOLUTIONS WITH ADDITIVES

The number of gels, salves, and ointments with additives used for wound dressing materials is enormous. Generally, these agents are used for small-sized wounds that have healthy appearances. With few exceptions they are selected for convenience, comfort, and ease of use. Many have additives, which make them useful for specific wound indications (Table 9-12, Figure 9-8). Typically, applications are done once a day or less. For these reasons they are ideal for patients whose "problem" wounds can be managed outside the acute hospital care setting. When these agents are evaluated with the criteria used for the other wound dressing selections, their wide scope of applications is appreciated:

- **Adaptability -** Usually gels, salves, and ointments are used for small (grade 2 points on the size assessment of the **Wound Score**) and medium-sized (grade 1 point) superficial wounds. One notable exception is silver sulfadiazine (Silvadene®), a sulfa-based silver impregnated ointment, which is frequently used for burn, blister and superficial abrasion wounds of any size.
- **Availability -** Many of the agents are available without prescriptions, that is, sold over the counter. This tends to make them easily accessible and reduces their costs. Many of the products have similar or overlapping effects so if a specifically prescribed agent is not available, a generic substitute with similar properties usually is.
- **Costs -** The prices of these agents vary from a couple of dollars for a small tube to as much as $500 or more for agents with genetically engineered additives. In general, since the sizes of the wounds tend to be small, by the time these agents are selected, the cost per application tends to be nominal. As mentioned before, these, like the other wound dressing agent tactics, will be ineffective if underlying deformity, persistent infection (osteomyelitis), and/or ischemia/hypoxia are not addressed.
- **Effectiveness -** These agents are effective, especially when selected for the primary functions for which they are designed (next section). Usually, by the time these agents are selected, the infection in the wound is controlled and the base has become vascular. Consequently, they are selected for the three reasons cited before, namely convenience, comfort and ease of use.
- **Versatility -** Because there are more than a half-dozen specific indications for these agents, as a group they are very versatile, ranging in effects from bactericidal to moisturizing and from enzymatic debridement to induction of healing. Many have secondary and tertiary properties, which add to their versatility such as moisturizing and pH regulation. Finally, many of the active ingredients in these wound dressing agents, for example silver, are added to the absorbent agents to combine the desirable mechanisms of two or more of the wound base dressing agent categories.

The following classification of gels, ointments, creams, and salves with additives is based on the primary actions of the additives.

Antimicrobial Agents

There are many antimicrobial agents that use gels, salves and ointments as vehicles for maintaining the agent in the wound site (Table 9-12). Local antimicrobial agents are not a substitute for systemic antibiotics and fungicidal agents, but are a useful adjunct to wound management when bacteria and /or fungus are residing on the surface of the wound.[28] In addition, the vehicles, usually petrolatum based, help maintain a moist environment for the wound base. Some agents are combined with agents that absorb secretions, as mentioned above, which make them doubly effective for infected exudative wounds. Even though these agents' antimicrobial activities are primarily at the wound surface level, systematic side effects can occur. Consequently, these agents are contraindicated for those patients with known allergies to the antibiotics they contain. These agents should be avoided in cavitary, recessed and tract wounds because the vehicles may seal off secretions and drive the infection inward, causing systemic sepsis. In addition, petrolatum based agents may interfere with cleansing of the wound base during dressing changes, leading to less than ideal wound hygiene. Honey is an agent

TABLE 9-12. EXAMPLES OF AGENTS THAT ARE GELS, LOTIONS, OINTMENTS, SALVES, OR SOLUTIONS THAT HAVE ANTIMICROBIAL ACTIVITY

Agent	Special Features	Comments, Side Effects, Costs, Etc.
Bacitracin	Antibacterial agent for gram positive bacteria Moisturizes (petroleum based)	Non-prescription About $6 for a small tube
Bacitracin + Neomycin + Polymyxin (Triple Antibiotic Ointment®)	Improved spectrum of bactericidal activity (Gram positives & gram negatives) Moisturizes (petroleum based)	Non-prescription About $6 for a small tube Nephrotoxicity and ototoxicity concerns from neomycin; restrict to small wounds
Bacitracin + Polymyxin (Polysporin®)	Antibacterial agent for gram positive & gram negative bacteria Moisturizes (petroleum based)	Similar to above
Cadexomer Iodine Gel (Iodosorb®)	Activity against oxacillin resistant staphylococcus and vancomycin-resistant enterococcus; Dries; absorbs secretions	Prescription required Dressing changes every 2 to 3 days; About $40 for a small tube
Chlorhexidine (Hibiclens®)	For removal of colonized oxacillin resistant *Staphylococcus aureus* from skin (cleanser)	Non-prescription Decolonization by daily showering with product over a 3 to 4 day period
Clotrimazole (Lotrimin®)	For superficial fungus infections, best used for macerated skin rather than directly on the wound base	Non-prescription Other agents with similar effects include Tolnaftate (Tinactin®) and miconazole (Micatin®) Cream or lotion formulations
Clotrimazole + Betamethasone (Lotrisone®)	Useful agent when combination of fungus infection and skin inflammation are present adjacent to the wound	Prescription required because of higher strength steroid Generic formulations are relatively inexpensive; Analogous effects achieved with using component agents in combination with each other
Mafenide Acetate (Sulfamyalon®)	Excellent for blister bases, especially burns Silver ion provides bactericidal activity Excellent for large wounds	Prescription required About $20 for a small jar Contraindicated in patients with allergies to sulfa drugs Leads to oxygen toxicity when used with hyperbaric oxygen
Mupirocin (Bactroban®)	Activity against Oxacillin-resistant *Staphylococcus aureus* (ORSA); Moisturizes (petroleum based)	Prescription required About $40 for a small tube
Silver sulfadiazine (Silvadene®)	Excellent for blister bases; similar to Sulfamyalon® Silver ion gives bactericidal activity; Excellent for large wounds Softens debris; facilitates superficial debridements	Prescription required About $20 for a small jar Contraindicated in patients with allergies to sulfa drugs OK to use with hyperbaric oxygen

Notes:

1. These are examples of agents from the gels, salves, solutions, and ointments category that have antimicrobial additives with which the authors have had experience. The list is not designed to be all inclusive. Consequently, an omission is not intended to deprecate the value of a product not listed in the table nor suggest it does not have features equal to or better than those in the table.

2. By using information in this table for comparisons, thoughtful decisions can be made about the merits of products not included above and/or new products as they become available.

3. Similar tables can be generated for the other five groups of additives (drying, enzymatic debridement, growth factor, moisturizing, and steroid/naturopathic agents) to the gels, lotions, ointments, salves, or solutions category of agents used to cover the wound base.

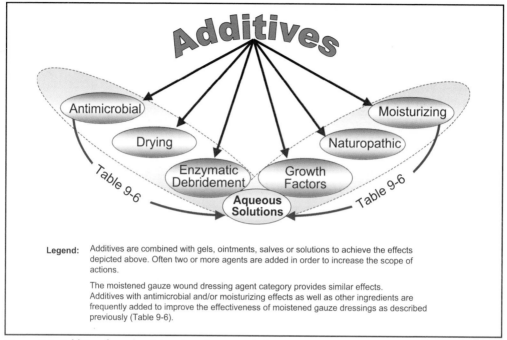

Figure 9-8. Additives for gels, ointments, salves, or solutions.

that has many merits with respect to bioburden management. It is reported to be useful in dealing with infection, inflammation and necrotic tissue.[29] Costs of antimicrobial agents range from less than $5 for a small tube of an over the counter product to more than $50 (Table 9-12). A thin, light application of the agent over the wound base is more effective than thick, totally occlusive applications. Usually a single layer gauze dressing is then placed over the agent for protection of and keeping it in contact with the wound. These considerations make the bactericidal/static agents relatively inexpensive for daily applications on small wounds.

Drying Agents

The need to keep the skin around the wound edges dry and free of maceration is almost as important as is maintaining a moist environment for wound healing. This can be challenging, especially in exudative wounds and may require that dressings be changed three or more times a day. The other use of drying agents is to form a superficial crust over a small, healthy based wound to act as a moisture sealant for the wound. This is the rationale for retaining a dry, thin eschar over a wound to promote epithelialization under the covering (Figure 9-3). Zinc oxide is an agent commonly added to drying agents for its combined desiccating and moisture barrier effects of the peri-wound skin.

Enzymatic Debridement Agents

These agents have substances added that can degrade proteinaceous material. The active ingredients include papain-urea, a cysteine endopeptidase, or collagenase, a proteolyic enzyme that acts on collagens. They are useful in wounds that are covered with a thin layer of necrotic material, such as a fibrinous exudate. These agents are indicated when the necrotic material in the wound base is not amenable to surgical debridement because of its thinness or because it lies over relatively avascular, but important structures such as ligament, tendon or bone. The papain-urea agents are effective over a wide pH range, are selectively active against nonviable tissue, but are harmless to viable tissue. Urea acts as an activator to the papain and a denaturing agent of the nonviable protein. In some of the preparations chlorophyll is added which gives the agent a green color and aids in its wound healing properties. As mentioned previously (Chapter 7) the Food and Drug Administration (FDA) recently instructed manufacturers to stop the production of topical papain products due to a few reported allergic/hypersensitivity reactions. Granulation tissue formation appears to be enhanced by enzymatic debriding agents, perhaps by removal of the barrier effect of the proteinaceous debris. Few side effects are observed, but some patients did not tolerate the papain-urea based preparations because of pain. Whereas a small tube of these agents may cost $50 or more, their once-a-day application and use for small wounds makes them relatively inexpensive per application.

Growth Factors

Agents with growth factor applications were introduced with extensive marketing and great expectations. Unfortunately, the clinical experiences with these agents have not met their expectations. The result is that one of the previous highly marketed and commercialized products (Procuren®, an autologous platelet derived growth factor) is no longer available and another becaplermin (Regranex®) is not being used to the extent it was when first introduced to the wound care community. The reasons for this are probably due more to lack of proper selection of indications than from lack of clinical efficacy. As so frequently reiterated, most "problem" wounds fail to heal due to underlying deformity, uncontrolled infection (osteomyelitis) and/or wound ischemia/hypoxia. When these factors have been addressed with the strategic management approach, and the wound still is not showing signs of improving, growth factor therapy should be considered. Use of these agents is expensive; the retail price is more than $500 for a 15-gram tube. Other than for small-sized wounds, their costs alone would be prohibitive.

Photostimulation and electrical stimulation therapies have also been advocated as a technique to stimulate wound healing. The energy they impart to the tissues is postulated to stimulate the subcellular components of wound healing somewhat analogous to the roles ascribed to growth factors.[30] In our limited observations, the use of these energy imparting techniques have not proven efficacious for the healing of "problem" wounds.

> The appropriate role of growth factor additives for wound healing is in question. One of the challenges that remains is to recognize that multiple growth factors and signaling devices are most likely necessary to achieve wound healing. The products mentioned above incorporate single growth factors.

Moisturizing Agents

This group of agents is hydrophilic; that is, they maintain a moist environment ideal for wound healing. Daily applications are usually sufficient to achieve this goal for the wound base. Since they are water based, rather than petrolatum based, cleansing of the wound with each dressing change is facilitated in contrast to dealing with greasy residuals from hydrocarbon-derived products. These agents are inexpensive, generally only costing a few cents per application for a small-sized wound. Their generic name is hydrogels. Few untoward effects are observed when using these agents for the properly indicated wound. A purified water, liquid paraffin, ethylene glycol mixture with other ingredients (Biafine®), is another agent in this group. The other ingredients are added to its petrolatum base to provide an optimal environment for wound healing and a barrier from harmful bacteria. It is a prescription item and costs about $30 for a small tube. The moisturizing agents are useful for "problem" wounds that are in their final stage of healing with healthy granulating bases, free of significant bioburdens and the remaining step in healing being that of generating an epithelial covering (Figure 9-9).

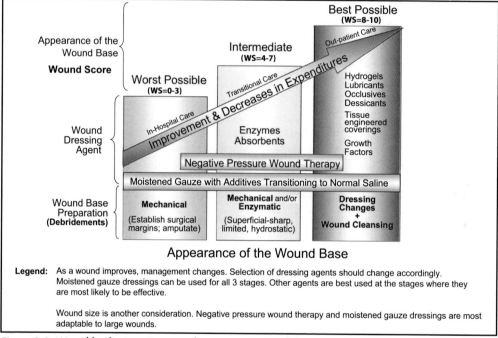

Figure 9-9. Wound healing continuum and appropriate wound dressing agents.

Steroids and Naturopathic Additives

The most well recognized agents from this group are those that have cortisone and cortisone-related compounds added to petrolatum based ointments. They reduce erythema and swelling in the skin around wounds through their anti-inflammatory actions. The steroid ointments are particularly helpful for treating stasis dermatitis that is associated with venous stasis ulcers. Those with low concentrations of hydrocortisone (1% or less) can be purchased over the counter. Prescriptions are required for those with higher concentrations of hydrocortisone or other steroids. Prices range from less than $5 to over $50 per small tube and depend on whether the agent is purchased over the counter or by prescription. Ointments with vitamin E are sometimes used around wounds and on hypertrophic scars for similar reasons.

MYTHS, MISCONCEPTIONS, AND FALLACIES ABOUT WOUND DRESSING AGENTS

Myths, misconceptions, and fallacies were tabulated previously in this chapter (Table 9-4). With the information presented in this chapter, responses to them can now be appropriately addressed as follows:

1. **The moistened gauze wound dressing is archaic.** The moistened gauze dressing is the starting point for the management of most acute "problem" wounds. The more complicated the wound, the more likely the moistened gauze dressing is the dressing of choice. As the wound improves, the moistened gauze dressing can be substituted for less labor-intensive, but probably little or no more effective wound dressing agents. Immediately after debridements, in highly exudative wounds, bloody based wounds, wounds with uncontrolled sepsis and wounds over exposed blood vessels, the moist gauze dressing may be the only choice. Moistened gauze dressings can be applied to any size wound. To improve the effectiveness of moistened gauze dressings, antimicrobial, acidifying and moisturizing agents may be added while achieving the basic requirement of maintaining a moist interface over the wound base.

2. **The more frequent the dressing changes, the better the chances of wound healing.** Dressing changes should be done as frequently as necessary. For exudative wounds, frequent dressing changes are required. Improving wounds need less frequent dressing changes; agents can then be selected that remain effective for longer periods of times as is characteristic of gels, salves and ointments. When the "problem" wound evolves to this stage, increasing the frequency of dressing changes does not speed healing.

3. **One wound dressing agent is ideal for all wounds.** Obviously, with the changing characteristics of wounds as they improve, no single agent is ideal for all situations, but there are situations where a particular agent might not be effective. Of all the wound dressing agents available, the normal saline dressing is the one that comes closest to being the universal dressing agent. The normal saline dressing is the standard for judging cost-effectiveness and cost-benefits of other dressing choices.

4. **Wound size, shape and depth need not be considerations (vs. appearance of the wound base) when making decisions about the selection of wound dressing agents.** These factors, along with the appearance of the wound base, are instrumental in making decisions about which wound dressing agents to use. The **Wound Score** provides objective criteria for which agents to use. For example, "healthy" wounds (wound scores of 8 to10 points) are better managed with the gels, etc., than more complicated to use newer or more expensive agents.

5. **The use of expensive wound dressing agents is the best assurance that wound management will be successful.** Wound dressing agents need to be selected on the basis of the wound's requirements. Usually, the most cost-effective choices are the most cost-beneficial. Use of more expensive agents does not guarantee successful healing. Their use needs to be determined by the particular requirements of the wound. The three major reasons wounds do not heal, that is persistence of deformities, uncontrolled infection (osteomyelitis) and ischemia/hypoxia must always be addressed before seeking a "magic cure" with a wound dressing agent.

6. **When scientific data supporting the benefits of a particular wound dressing agent is reported, it is incontestable.** Unfortunately, bench laboratory studies and patient trials do not always correlate with the clinical realities of wound healing. The benefits of a particular wound dressing agent are only fully appreciated when used in conjunction with the other four components of strategic management of a "problem" wound (i.e. medical management interventions, preparation of the wound base, protection and stabilization of the wound and wound oxygenation). Additionally, correction of the three major reasons a wound does not heal (just reiterated in item 5 above) must be addressed.

7. **Failures with the use of a particular wound dressing agent can always be attributed to lack of patient compliance and/or failure to follow the manufacturer's instructions.** There are many reasons that wounds fail to heal. From the **Wound Score**, failures can be predicted with almost 100% accuracy for the "futile" wound (0 to 3 points on the **Wound Score**). Other failures are due to using the agent for the wrong indications, for example, the use of an occlusive wound covering for an exudative wound. Finally, "problem" wounds may fail to heal and require lower-limb amputations because of new vascular occlusive events, multiple drug-resistant organism infection, irresolvable mechanical problems, co-existent collagen vascular disease and/or intractable pain.

8. **There is only a small range in costs among the different wound dressing agents.** As the preceding information has shown, there is a vast range of costs among the enormous choices for wound dressing agents. The supplies can vary from a few cents a dressing for normal saline, salves, gels and ointments to more than one hundred dollars a day for negative pressure wound therapy. Tissue engineered wound coverings and genetically derived growth factors can likewise be very costly, and in many situations can only be used for the smaller sized wound. The bottom line, in terms of costs, is pairing the cost-effectiveness with the cost-benefits of the wound dressing agent.

9. **If one wound dressing agent is effective, it is not appropriate to change to another even if the wound improves.** As has been discussed, no agent is ideal for every wound. Likewise, no agent is ideal for each stage (Chapter 7 and Figure 9-9) of wound healing. As the wound improves (or worsens), the wound dressing agent should be selected to meet the needs of the wound. Finally, if the wound is not improving with a particular agent, consideration for switching to a different agent with different functions is indicated. In addition, the three primary reasons the "problem" wound is failing to improve (persistence of deformities, uncontrolled infection (osteomyelitis) and ischemia/hypoxia) must be mitigated.

10. **Wound dressing agents that have two or more functions should be avoided. Likewise, the use of two or more agents on the same wound is counterproductive.** Many agents have multiple functions and more than one active ingredient as has been described throughout this chapter. Newer agents are taking advantage of this concept, as is observed in the many wound absorbents that have silver or iodine derivatives added to them. Also, use of two or more agents, such as an absorbing agent to control secretions and a drying agent for the skin margins to prevent maceration, is an example of a technique where two agents work in a mutually beneficial fashion.

CONCLUSIONS

So Many Choices

With "so many choices, so many opportunities" exist. With over 2500 wound care products to chose from, where does one start?[31] First, categorization of the agents into logical groups, as this chapter describes, is imperative. This provides an approach to make rational decisions and evaluate new products as they become available. Cost-effectiveness and cost-benefits are a second consideration. Unfortunately, of the five strategies for managing the "problem" wound, the selection of dressing agents to cover the wound base is the one that is most marketed and the most influenced by the product manufacturers. As highly touted as new products often are, there is only weak evidence of the clinical efficacy of modern dressings compared with the "tried and true" saline and hydrocolloid dressings.[32] Third, healing of the "problem" wound is a dynamic process. As the wound improves, dressing agent requirements change (Figure 9-9). As healing progresses, the requirements are expected to become less costly and less labor intensive. The wound care specialist is remiss in his/her responsibilities if this dynamic process is ignored and dressing agent selections are not modified as the wound changes. Fourth, selection of dressing agents to cover the wound base is but one strategy of the five required for management of the "problem" wound. Without attention to the other four strategies, dressing agents alone will not likely achieve satisfactory results. Finally, when wound healing does not proceed as expected, the three primary reasons "problem" wounds fail to improve, namely persistence of deformities, uncontrolled infection (osteomyelitis), and wound ischemia/hypoxia must be further investigated and resolved.

Summary

The goals of the wound base covering agent selection strategy are threefold: establishment and maintenance of a moist wound base environment, control of the bioburden, and acceleration of healing. The goals are implemented through objective assessment of the wound base and pairing the wound base findings with the appropriate selection of the dressing agent (Figure 9-9). The **Wound Score** provides the mechanism for objectively assessing the wound base. Many choices exist for dressing agents. The four categories of dressing agents introduced in this chapter, namely 1) aqueous gauze dressings; 2) occlusive and semi-occlusive covering agents for healthy wound bases; 3) agents for secretion producing wounds; and 4) gels, salves, ointments, and solutions with or without additives facilitate the selection of the proper dressing for the wound base. As the wound improves, it is appropriate to change the dressing agent from more expensive and labor intensive to less expensive and less frequently applied agents. The main dilemmas for this dressing strategy are determining which agent to use from the enormous number of choices that are available and the infinite variety of wound presentations. Our **Wound Score** assessment and the categorization of dressing agents provide a method to resolve these dilemmas. Finally, while it is virtually impossible to be familiar with all the wound dressing agents available, the wound care provider should be familiar with several options in each category.

QUESTIONS

1. What are the main goals of wound dressing agents?

2. What are the four categories of wound dressing agents?

3. What is the rationale behind the concept of moist wound healing?

4. What problems can be associated with the use of the moistened gauze dressing?

5. What are the advantages and disadvantages of covering agents for healthy based wounds?

6. What are the dressing agent challenges for managing secretion producing wounds?

7. What are the beneficial mechanisms of negative pressure wound therapy (NPWT)?

8. What are the main indications for gels, ointments, and salves in wound care?

9. How do wound size and shape affect decisions about the selection of wound dressing agents?

10. What are some myths, misconceptions and fallacies about wound dressing agents?

REFERENCES

1. Weinstein, ML. Update on wound healing: A review of the literature, Military Med, 1998; 163(9):620-624

2. Field FK, Kerstein MD. Overview of wound healing in a moist environment. Am J Surg. 1994 Jan; 167(1A):2S-6S

3. Chang H, Wind S, Kerstein MD. Moist wound healing. Dermatol Nurs. 1996 Jun; 8(3):174-6,204.

4. Atiyeh BS, Ioannovich J, Al-Amm CA, et al. Management of acute and chronic open wounds: the importance of moist environment in optimal wound healing. Curr Pharm Biotechnol. 2002 Sep; 3(3):179-95

5. Dow G, Browne A, Sibbald RG. Infection in chronic wounds: controversies in diagnosis and treatment. Ostomy/Wound Manage 1999; 45:23-40

6. Wysocki AB. Evaluating and managing open skin wounds: colonisation versus infection. AACN Clin Iss 2002; 13:382-397

7. Edwards R, Harding KG. Bacteria and wound healing. Curr Opin Infect Dis. 2004 Apr; 17(2):91-6

8. Salcido R. What is bioburden? The link to chronic wounds. Adv Skin Wound Care. 2007 Jul; 20(7):368

9. White RJ, Cutting K, Kingsley A. Topical antimicrobials in the control of wound bioburden. Ostomy Wound Manage. 2006 Aug; 52(8):26-58

10. Serralta VW, Harrison-Balestra C, Cazzaniga AL, et al. Lifestyles of bacteria in wounds: presence of biofilms? Wounds. 2001; 13(1):29–34

11. Armstrong H, Price P. Wet-to-dry gauze dressings: Fact and fiction. Wounds 2004; 16(2) 56-62

12. Sloss JM, Cumberland N, Milner SM. Acetic acid used for the elimination of pseudomonas aeruginosa from burn and soft tissue wound. J R Army Med Corps. 1993; 139(3):139

13. Phillips I, Lobo AZ, Fernandes R, et al. Acetic acid in the treatment of superficial wounds infected by pseudomonas aeruginosa. Lancet. 1968 Jan 6; 1(7532):11-4

14. Bennett LL, Rosenblum RS, Perlov C, et al. An in vivo comparison of topical agents on wound repair. Plast Reconstr Surg. 2001 Sep 1; 108(3):675-87

15. Wilson JR, Mills JG, Prather ID, et al. A toxicity index of skin and wound cleansers used on in vitro fibroblasts and keratinocytes. Adv Skin Wound Care. 2005 Sep; 18(7):373-8

16. Ramirez SE, Cardenas LLE, Torres GB, et al. Comparative study of the efficiency of acetic acid vs modified Dakin's solution in the treatment of infections at the insitional [sic] site. Cir Gen. 2000; 22(3):325-328

17. Brown-Etris M, Cutshall W, Hiles MC. A new biomaterial derived from small intestine submucosa and developed into a wound matrix device. Wounds: A Compend of Clin Res Pract. 2002; 14(4):150-166

18. Bello YM, Falabella AF, Eaglstein WH. Tissue-engineered skin. Current status in wound healing. Am J Clin Dermatol. 2001; 2(5):305-13

19. Morykwas MJ, Argenta LC, Shelton-Brown EI, et al. Vacuum-assisted closure: a new method for wound control and treatment: animal studies and basic foundation. Ann Plast Surg. 1997 Jun; 38(6):553-62

20. Argenta LC, Morykwas MJ. Vacuum-assisted closure: a new method for wound control and treatment: clinical experience. Ann Plast Surg. 1997 Jun; 38(6):563-76.

21. Schwien T, Gilbert J, Lang C. Pressure ulcer prevalence and the role of negative pressure wound therapy in home health quality outcomes. Ostomy Wound Manage. 2005 Sep; 51(9):47-60

22. Baharestani MM. Negative pressure wound therapy: An examination of cost-effectiveness. Ostomy/Wound Management 2004: 50(11-Suppl):29S-33S

23. Morykwas MJ, Faler BJ, Pearce DJ, et al. Effects of varying levels of subatmospheric pressure on the rate of granulation tissue formation in experimental wounds in swine. Ann Plast Surg. 2001 Nov; 47(5):547-51

24. Gupta S, Cho T. A literature review of negative pressure wound therapy. Ostomy Wound Manage. 2004 Nov; 50(11A Suppl):2S-4S

25. Jones SM, Banwell PE, Shakespeare PG. Advances in wound healing: topical negative pressure therapy. Postgrad Med J. 2005 Jun; 81(956):353-7

26. Sullivan N, Snyder D, Tipton K. Negative Pressure Wound Therapy Devices. Technology Assessment Report. U.S. Department of Health and Human Services, Agency for Healthcare Research and Quality. March 2009

27. Chaby G, Senet P, Vaneau M, et al. Dressings for acute and chronic wounds: a systematic review. Arch Dermatol. 2007 Oct; 143(10):1297-304

28. White RJ, Cutting K, Kingsley A. Topical antimicrobials in the control of wound bioburden. Ostomy Wound Manage. 2006 Aug; 52(8):26-58

29. Cutting KF. Honey and contemporary wound care: an overview. Ostomy Wound Manage. 2007 Nov; 53(11):49-54

30. Mester E, Spiry T, Szende B. Effect of laser rays on wound healing. Bull Soc Int Chir. 1973 Mar-Apr; 32(2):169-73

31. Fonder MA, Lazarus GS, Cowan DA, et al. Treating the chronic wound: A practical approach to the care of nonhealing wounds and wound care dressings. J Am Acad Dermatol. 2008 Feb; 58(2):185-206

32. Chaby G, Senet P, Vaneau M, et al. Dressings for acute and chronic wounds: a systematic review. Arch Dermatol. 2007 Oct; 143(10):1297-1304

CHAPTER

10 Wound Oxygenation and Hyperbaric Oxygen Therapy

CHAPTER TEN OVERVIEW

INTRODUCTION 255

DEFINITION OF HYPERBARIC OXYGEN, MODES OF
ADMINISTRATION, AND CLINICAL INDICATIONS. 257

HYPERBARIC OXYGEN PHYSIOLOGY: PRIMARY MECHANISMS 263

SECONDARY MECHANISMS OF HYPERBARIC OXYGEN 270

SIDE EFFECTS AND CONTRAINDICATIONS OF
HYPERBARIC OXYGEN THERAPY. 276

CONCLUSIONS 278

QUESTIONS. 281

REFERENCES 282

"So vital...so taken for granted."

INTRODUCTION

Oxygen Tensions and Wound Healing – The roles of oxygen for wound healing and in the control of infections are indisputable. Oxygen tensions of 30 to 40 mmHg are required for biochemical processes in fibroblasts, angioblasts, keratinocytes and white cells to continue and complete the wound healing process (Chapter 2). If extremely low, for example in the 0 to 10 mmHg range, the tissues can die from hypoxia. If in the 10 to 30 mmHg range the tissues may survive, but not function well enough to carry out their metabolic processes. This defines the hypoxic wound (Figure 10-1). Wound healing processes may remain suspended, not improving nor worsening. Any new insult such as trauma, infection or further impairment in perfusion will change the status quo. This may lead to further deterioration of the wound and result in a lower limb amputation (if the wound is in the lower extremity). Conversely, if oxygen tensions are improved, essential biochemical reactions can resume and allow wound healing to proceed. Other factors such as blood viscosity, nutrition, fluid retention, bioburden, age and other comorbidities such as diabetes and collagen vascular diseases influence whether or not healing occurs. This chapter discusses the use of hyperbaric oxygen to improve wound oxygenation. Other interventions such as edema reduction (Chapter 2), use of local and systemic vasodilators, "last resort" revascularizations and rheological agents to improve

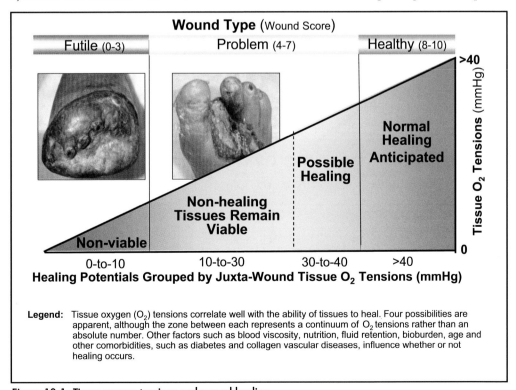

Legend: Tissue oxygen (O_2) tensions correlate well with the ability of tissues to heal. Four possibilities are apparent, although the zone between each represents a continuum of O_2 tensions rather than an absolute number. Other factors such as blood viscosity, nutrition, fluid retention, bioburden, age and other comorbidities, such as diabetes and collagen vascular diseases, influence whether or not healing occurs.

Figure 10-1. Tissue oxygen tensions and wound healing.

wound oxygenation are discussed more fully in the next chapter, the management of the "end-stage" hypoxic wound.

Techniques to Improve Wound Oxygenation – Like the protection/stabilization strategy, wound oxygenation is another of the strategies for managing problem wounds that is most likely to be inadequately managed or totally ignored. It is a paradox that before initiating surgery on the extremities, assessment of circulation to the extremity is customary, but if impaired usually little is done other than noting the patient has poor circulation. Five interventions enhance wound oxygenation (Figure10-2). Improved cardiac function, correction of anemia, and reduction of edema are medical interventions that augment oxygen availability to wounds (Chapter 6). In these situations, improvement in wound oxygenation is a secondary benefit of correcting the underlying medical problem(s). Revascularization, angioplasty, or both result in more oxygen being made available to the wound through enhanced perfusion (Chapter 11). Sometimes tissue hypoxia and non-healing persist after the above techniques. In about one third of patients with "problem" and "futile" wounds, these techniques have already been done, are not feasible due to diffuse vessel involvement and/or there is inadequate runoff to the target area. Hyperbaric oxygen is a therapy that effectively improves oxygen availability to wounds when perfusion is present, but inadequate to deliver enough oxygen to support wound healing. Pharmacological techniques improve oxygen availability through a variety of mechanisms. These will be discussed in the next chapter.

Assessing Wound Oxygenation – Like the other strategies used in the comprehensive management of "problem" wounds, the diagnosis of wound hypoxia can be made by clinical assessment. From the history it is easy to ascertain whether the wound is improving, not changing, or deteriorating. If not improving or deteriorating, wound

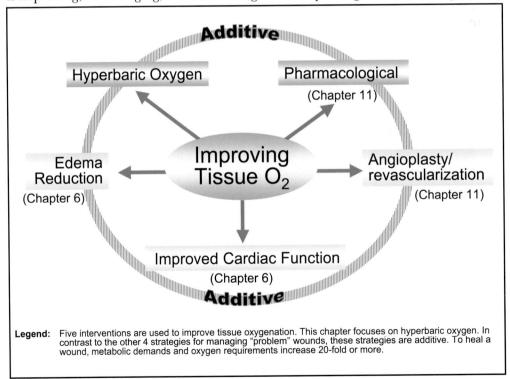

Legend: Five interventions are used to improve tissue oxygenation. This chapter focuses on hyperbaric oxygen. In contrast to the other 4 strategies for managing "problem" wounds, these strategies are additive. To heal a wound, metabolic demands and oxygen requirements increase 20-fold or more.

Figure 10-2. Interventions to improve tissue oxygenation.

hypoxia must be considered as one of the three most likely causes of non-healing, along with underlying mechanical problems (deformities) and unresolved infection (Chapter 2). From the examination, wound oxygenation is determined by the perfusion assessment of the **Wound Score** (Chapter 5). The secondary methods of assessing perfusion, namely capillary refill, skin coloration and skin temperature supplement the evaluation and can be used when wounds, edema, cicatrix or other factors interfere with the detection of pulses. Juxta wound transcutaneous oxygen measurement is a tertiary method to assess wound oxygenation (Chapter 11). From these assessments important information is generated about wound oxygenation. This information is crucial for making decisions about wound management.

Objectivity in Assessing Wound Oxygenation – Juxta-wound transcutaneous oxygen measurements objectively establish the oxygenation status of the wound. In this respect, determination of wound oxygenation status becomes more objective than almost any of the other strategies used for managing the "problem" wound. Criteria for making objective decisions from transcutaneous oxygen and carbon dioxide measurements are presented in the next chapter (Chapter 11). It is ironic that of the five wound strategies, wound oxygenation status is the one that can be most objectively determined, yet is so often not managed to the optimal extent with adjunctive hyperbaric oxygen, pharmacological interventions, and/or revascularization techniques.

DEFINITION OF HYPERBARIC OXYGEN, MODES OF ADMINISTRATION, AND CLINICAL INDICATIONS

Definition and the Monoplace Hyperbaric Chamber – Hyperbaric oxygen (HBO) is a type of inhalation therapy in which patients breathe oxygen at greater than one atmosphere absolute of pressure. This requires that the patient be placed in a sealed vessel (hyperbaric chamber), which is capable of withstanding pressurization. Two chamber types or modes of administration are used for delivering HBO (Figure 10-3). The monoplace chamber is a one-person pressure vessel. It is pressurized with oxygen, which the patient breathes directly from the chamber's atmosphere. Most are made of clear acrylic cylinders with metal bulkheads at each end of the cylinder. A hatch, nearly the width of the bulkhead, allows ingress and egress from the chamber. The patient is transported on a special gurney that has a padded mattress laying on a thin platform on rails. The platform slides into the chamber on rails that meet with rails inside the chamber. The patient usually rests in the supine position during the treatment. Usually oxygen is breathed continuously, that is, there are no air breaks during the one and one-half to two hour treatments in the monoplace chamber.

Multiplace Hyperbaric Chamber – The multiplace chamber is larger than the monoplace chamber, thereby allowing more than one occupant at a time to be treated. It is pressurized with air for several reasons. First, there is too great a risk of fire hazard from the generation of static electricity sparks from movements of the occupants which the more spacious multiplace chamber allows. This could lead to an explosion in the pure oxygen atmosphere, whereas this hazard is markedly reduced in the air atmosphere. Second, the large quantity of oxygen required to pressurize a multiplace chamber would be expensive. Additionally, specialized electronic equipment can be used in the multiplace chamber. In order to achieve hyperbaric oxygen conditions, the patient breathes pure oxygen in a hood or through a facemask when in the multiplace chamber (Figure 10-4). Oxygen breathing periods are usually interrupted with one or two short air breaks of five to 15 minute durations to reduce the chances of oxygen induced

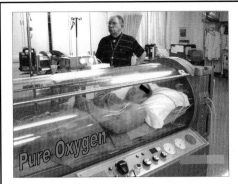

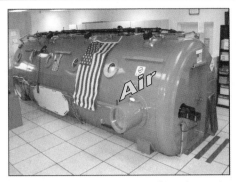

Monoplace Hyperbaric Chamber

Multiplace Hyperbaric Chamber

Legend: The monoplace chamber is a one-person chamber and is pressurized with pure oxygen. The multiplace chamber is pressurized with air. Hyperbaric oxygen delivery is achieved with a hood or mask (Figure 10-4). Two or more patients with an inside tender can be treated at one time in a multiplace chamber.

Figure 10-3. The two types of hyperbaric oxygen chambers.

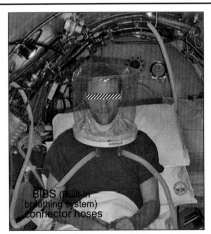

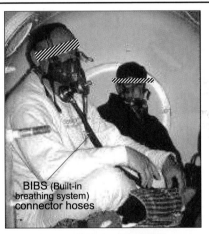

Treatment Hood

Aviator Mask with BIBS

Legend: Oxygen is supplied to the hood or mask through a built-in breathing system (BIBS). About 90 percent of the oxygen inhaled with each breath is then exhaled to the mask or hood. The exhaled oxygen is exhausted to the chamber or by pass throughs in the chamber to the outside atmosphere. If exhausted into the chamber, the chamber must be ventilated frequently in order to reduce the oxygen percentage in the chamber and avoid fire hazards.

Figure 10-4. Oxygen delivery methods for multiplace chamber.

seizure. Air breaks are done merely by removing the mask or hood and breathing the air directly in the chamber. Because of the large hatches now almost a universal feature in the newer, more modern multiplace chambers, patients can enter the chamber by walking in, in a wheelchair or on a gurney. Each chamber type has its own special features, advantages, and disadvantages (Table 10-1).

Dual-type Hyperbaric Oxygen Chamber – For completeness, a third type of chamber is mentioned. It is the dual or hybrid chamber, which combines features of both the monoplace and multiplace chamber. Like the monoplace chamber, it is

TABLE 10-1. COMPARISONS AND CONTRASTS BETWEEN MONOPLACE AND MULTIPLACE CHAMBERS

Item	Monoplace Chamber	Multiplace Chamber
Activity and Movement in the Chamber	Usually minimal activity, typically patients lay supine May move arms and legs, use hands for clearing ears, drinking fluids, etc.	Typically patients sit in a chair; they may move about, but this is discouraged Wheelchairs and gurneys brought into chamber for non-ambulatory patients
Availability for Emergencies	In a unit with two more monoplace chambers, a chamber can always be made readily available to treat an emergency	If an emergency treatment is needed while a treatment is underway, the scheduled treatment may need to be aborted to accommodate the emergency; however several people with emergencies can be treated simultaneously, as with carbon monoxide poisonings
Chamber Entry	Patients atop a gurney which slides-in on rails Treatments are individualized - one patient per chamber; advantages for isolation issues	Patients walk in or are rolled into the chamber and may be treated in the wheelchair or gurney used for transport
Chamber Pressurization and Atmosphere	Pure oxygen usually from a liquid oxygen source. No facemask or hood required.	Air usually from air compressor and storage tank system Hyperbaric oxygen achieved through breathing oxygen with a hood or mask from storage tanks
Chamber Sizes and Costs	Small, 2 to 3 feet wide by 7 to 9 feet in length Prices: $100,000 to $150,000	Large; variable sizes to accommodate 2 to 20 patients and an inside tender Prices: $500,000 to 3 million dollars
Crew Requirements for Emergencies	Staff mobilization for emergencies requires two people including a chamber operator and a physician	Mobilization of chamber crew: inside tender, outside chamber operator and a supervising physician
Emergency Decompression	Possible in 15 seconds or less; Usually a rapid ascent over a 60 second period is done in most emergency situations.	Usually avoided so as not to interfere with the treatment of the other patients in the chamber Emergencies handled by trained inside tenders; physicians and other trained personnel may be present or can be "locked-in" to assist
Depth Limitations	Pressurization possible to 3 ATA (66 feet of sea water) for special conditions such as air embolism, carbon monoxide poisoning, decompression sickness and gas gangrene	Pressurization possible to 6 ATA (165 feet of sea water) in most multiplace chambers—sometimes used for serious cases of decompression illness/arterial gas embolism
Entertainment and Diversion	Patients can watch television, video movies, listen to radio/music, play games (using the speaker system) or read through the clear acrylic chamber tube	Television and video monitors inside the chamber; Reading materials may be taken into the chamber as well as for games like cards, checkers and chess
Management of Critical Care Patients	Possible through in-chamber & remote (that is controlled outside the chamber) systems & monitors including ventilation, cardiac monitors & pacing, blood pressures, intravenous fluid administration, chest tube management & catheters—See Emergency Decompression above	Monitoring can be done essentially to the same extent that can be done in the intensive care unit Ability to manage an acute cardiopulmonary arrest while in the chamber as well as insert a chest tube (these are not feasible in the monoplace chamber)—See Emergency Decompression above
Neurological Assessment	Done remotely through commands via the speaker system—i.e. "move your arms," etc. Checking of pupillary responses possible through the chamber acrylic; Deep tendon reflex testing not possible	Done by the inside tender (or physician if in the chamber) with or without special instructions from the outside medical attendant
NFPA (National Fire Protection Association) **Requirements**	Class C—same as for using respiratory care equipment in a patient's room Gases exiting the chamber must be exhausted to the outside environment	Class A—Multiplace chambers are required to have 1) 3-hour fire protection walls & flooring 2) High pressure sprinkler systems in the chamber 3) Non-conductive flooring
Research Adaptability	Easy to switch from air to pure oxygen atmosphere in the chamber or having the subject breathe with a SCUBA regulator Easy to do sham treatments with pressurization to a few feet of seawater so subjects will experience the need for clearing their ears	Easy to use air or oxygen for the breathing gas in the hood or mask Sham pressure exposures not possible concurrent with patients undergoing hyperbaric oxygen treatments
Special Hazards	Fire risk increased due to the 100% O_2 environment; Utmost precautions to prevent introduction of flammable or spark-inducing clothing & coverings into the chamber—for example clothing is limited to wearing cotton gowns	Decompression sickness in tenders with reports of spinal cord injuries—now tenders are advised to breathe oxygen along with their patients during the latter portions of the treatment
Versatility	Treatment profiles easily modified to accommodate patients' needs, for example slower pressurization for those having difficulty clearing their ears Shorter durations of treatments and shallower depths for infants	Treatment profiles & pressurization rates less versatile than for the monoplace chamber since several patients are treated at one time. Need for myringotomies or ear tubes more frequent in multiplace chambers for this reason

designed to treat one patient occupant at a time. However, there is room for an attendant to sit in a well at the patient's head and assist with patient care during the treatment. The chamber is pressurized with air and hyperbaric oxygen is delivered through a mask if supine or possibly with a hood if the patient sits in the well without the attendant present. In this respect the chamber incorporates features of both the monoplace and multiplace chamber. It can be used as either a single occupant chamber or with an attendant. In either case, the chamber is pressurized in air and hyperbaric oxygenation is achieved through a hood or mask.

Differences in Tissue Gas Exchange between Monoplace and Multiplace Chambers – Are there differences in oxygen delivery to the patient between the monoplace and multiplace chamber? For all practical purposes the answer is no. Hyperbaric oxygen therapy is HBO therapy whether it is given in a monoplace or multiplace chamber. The durations of exposure to HBO are both about 90 minutes. The higher treatment pressures (2.4 ATA versus 2.0 ATA) typically used in the multiplace chamber are somewhat of a "fudge" factor to compensate for the reduced efficiency of using hoods or masks to breathe oxygen as compared to breathing it directly in the chamber atmosphere as done in the monoplace chamber. Are the air breaks necessary and do they reduce the efficiency of the HBO treatment? Answers to these questions are unresolved. Because of the increased activity that is possible in the multiplace chamber and the knowledge that activity increases the likelihood of a seizure in a HBO environment, air breaks appear to be warranted. Vast experiences with monoplace chamber HBO treatments demonstrate that air breaks during a standard treatment are not needed and seizures, while they do occur infrequently, do so at rates no greater than observed in the multiplace chamber. Studies with treatment pressures at 2 ATA show that during air breaks nitrogen rapidly deposits in the tissues because of the gradient, but there is somewhat of a rebound effect such that slightly higher endpoint tissue oxygen levels result by the end of the multiplace HBO exposure.[1,2] For clinical applications, the differences probably have no practical significance. For treatment of decompression sickness where there is already an increased nitrogen load in the tissues, the air breaks may further increase the amount of this gas in the tissues.[3,4,5]

Topox – Topical oxygen treatments, often referred to as Topox, must be differentiated from hyperbaric oxygen therapy. Topical oxygen is a technique in which a wound is enclosed within a plastic bag or similar device, sealed with a rubber fastener or perforated membrane proximal to or around the wound (in the case of indolent hip and presacral wounds) and then slightly pressurized with oxygen (Figure 10-5). This surrounds the wound with oxygen. However, almost no oxygen diffuses through the skin surrounding the wound and the topical oxygen only penetrates to a depth of one millimeter in the wound base.[6] Furthermore, transcutaneous oxygen measurements indicate that juxta-wound oxygen tensions are actually lower during topical oxygen exposures than in room air.[7] This is presumably due to interference with venous return from the constricting effect of the elastic tie or sleeve. In terms of oxygenation, topical oxygen only increases the partial pressure of oxygen about 1/33rd as much as hyperbaric oxygen does (Table 10-2). The Center for Medicare/Medicaid Services (CMS) does not recognize topical oxygen as a reimbursable condition for wound management nor as a variant of hyperbaric oxygen therapy.[8,9]

Clinical Applications of Hyperbaric Oxygen – Hyperbaric oxygen has been used for a variety of clinical problems. Approved uses of HBO is a term that is more a reflection of historical outcomes as well as economics (that is, who will pay for the treatments) than evidence-based indications. The Center of Medicare/Medicaid Services has established a list of conditions for which HBO treatments are considered appropriate and correspondingly will be reimbursed by this agency (Table 10-3).[8] Since a substantial proportion of patients' HBO treatments are reimbursed by Medicare, their approved uses list carries enormous weight and by and large sets the standards for other third party payor reimbursements for HBO therapy. The Undersea and Hyperbaric Medical Society

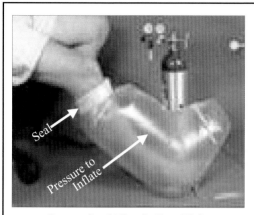
Pressurized Plastic Bag Unit

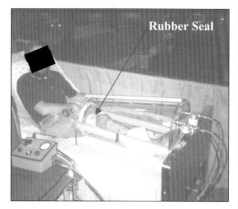
Deluxe Limb Topical Oxygen Unit

Legend: Topical oxygen provides a slightly increased oxygen gradient to the base of a wound. The gradient is equivalent to a pressure of about 0.99 feet of sea water (See Table 10-2). Dehumidified oxygen used with topical oxygen may help to dry secretions and contract the wound.

Figure 10-5. Delivery methods for topical oxygen.

TABLE 10-2. OXYGEN PARTIAL PRESSURE AND PRESSURE COMPARISONS WITH DIFFERENT CONDITIONS

Condition (Commonly Used Pressure Unit)	Pressure (Feet of Sea Water)
Hyperbaric Oxygen (2 ATA)	33
Systolic Blood Pressure (120 mmHg)	5 [33 1/3 times greater]
Topical Oxygen (1.03 ATA)	0.99
Venous Pressure (10 cm H$_2$0)	0.33

Note: HBO increases oxygen partial pressures 33 1/3 times more than topical oxygen

Abbreviations : **ATA** = Atmospheres absolute, **cm** = Centimeters, **HBO** = Hyperbaric oxygen, **mmHg** = millimeters of mercury

(UHMS) has formulated a list of conditions for which HBO treatments are indicated (Table 10-3).[9] This is also a source document for third party payors as well as the United States Food and Drug Administration (FDA). When inquiries are directed to the FDA about the uses of HBO, they use this document to respond whether the condition is an approved (by the UHMS) or an off-label use. Other agencies and organizations have

TABLE 10-3. CONDITIONS "APPROVED" FOR HYPERBARIC OXYGEN THERAPY

CMS/Medicare (ICD-9-CM Codes)	UHMS (Undersea and Hyperbaric Medical Society)	Other Considerations (Medicaid/cal Approved; Off-label Uses)
1. **Actinomycosis** (039.0-039.4, 039.8-039.9)	1. **Air or Gas Embolism**	1. **Complications of Internal Prosthetic Device, Implant and Graft**—Medi-Cal List
2. **Acute Peripheral Arterial Insufficiency**-Thrombotic or Embolic (444.21, 444.22, 444.81)	2. **Carbon Monoxide Poisoning** (In addition carbon monoxide poisoning complicated by cyanide poisoning)	2. **Occlusion of Precerebral/ Cerebral Arteries**—Stroke; Same as above (SAA)—i.e Medi-Cal List
3. **Acute Traumatic Peripheral Ischemia** (902.53, 903.01, 903.1, 904.0, 904.41)	3. **Clostridial Myositis and Myonecrosis** (Gas Gangrene)	3. **Other Peripheral Vascular Disease**—Medi-Cal List
4. **Acute Carbon Monoxide Intoxication** (986)	4. **Crush Injury, Compartment Syndrome & other AcuteTraumatic Ischemias**	4. **Acute Cerebral Edema/Closed Head Injury**– Off-label Use (OLU)
5. **Chronic Refractory Osteomyelitis** (730.10-730.19)	5. **Decompression Sickness**	5. **Acute Myocardial Infarction**--OLU
6. **Crush Injuries—and Suturing of Severed Limbs** (927.00-927.03, 927.09- 927.11, 927.8, 928.00, 928.01, 928.10-928.11, 928.20-928.21, 928.3, 928.8-928.9, 929.0, 929.9, 996.90- 996.99)	6. **Arterial Insufficiencies** - Central Retinal Artery Occlusion - **Enhancement of Healing in Selected Problem Wounds**	6 **Acute Spinal Cord Injury**--OLU 7 **Brown Recluse Spider Bite**--OLC 8. **Cerebral Palsy**--OLU
7. **Cyanide Poisoning** (987.7, 989.0)	7. **Severe Anemia**	9. **Chronic Spinal Cord Injury**--OLU
8. **Decompression Sickness** (993.2,993.3)	8. **Intracranial Abscess**	10. **Enhancement of Healing of Sports Related Injuries**--OLU
9. **Diabetic Wounds of Lower Extremity** (250.7, 250.8, plus 707.10, 707.12, 707.13, 707.14, 707.15, 707.19)	9. **Necrotizing Soft Tissue Infections**	11. **Fatigue and Jet Lag Recovery**--OLU
10. **Gas Embolism** (958.0, 999.1)	10. **Osteomyelitis (Refractory)**	12. **Osteonecrosis**; most frequently of the femoral head--OLU
11. **Gas Gangrene**—Clostridial Myonecrosis (040.0)	11. **Delayed Radiation Injury (Soft Tissue and Bony Necrosis)**	13. **Performance Enhancement in Sports**--OLU
12. **Osteoradionecrosis** (526.89)	12. **Compromised Grafts and Flaps**	14. **Fracture Healing**--OLU
13. **Preservation of Compromised Skin Grafts** (excludes artificial skin grafts) (996.52)	13. **Acute Thermal Burn Injury**	15. **Enhancement of Cognitive Function** (Alzheimer's Disease)-OLU
14. **Progressive Necrotizing Infections**--Necrotizing Fasciitis, Meleney's Ulcer (728.86)		16. **Post-traumatic/Post Ischemic Encephalopathy**-- OLU
15. **Soft Tissue Radionecrosis** (990)		17. **Sickle Cell Anemia Crises**--OLU
		18. **Hepatic Necrosis**--OLU
		19. **Multiple Sclerosis**--OLU
		20. **Severe Sepsis**-OLU
		21. **Stasis or Decubitus Ulcers**--OLU
		22. **Autism** --OLU
		23. **Sensorineural Hearing Loss** -OLU
		24. **Lyme disease** --OLU
		25. **Plastic Surgery Preparation and Recovery** --OLU
		26. **Complex Regional Pain Syndrome/Reflex Sympathetic Dystrophy** --OLU
		27. **Chronic Fatigue Syndrome** --OLU
		28. **Near Drowning** --OLU
		29. **Migraine Headaches** --OLU

Note: 1. UHMS conditions highlighted in yellow denote that they do not have counterparts on the CMS/Medicare List
   2. Medicaid approved conditions vary region by region. The California (Medi-Cal) listings are included as examples of approved conditions for HBO from one Medicaid state.
   3. Abbreviations: **CMS** = Center for Medicare/Medicaid Services, **ICD-9-CM** = International Classification of Disease 9th Edition-Clinical Modification, **Medi-Cal** = California's Medicaid program conditions that are additions to the Medicare listing, **OLU** = Off-label Use, **SAA** = Same as above, **UHMS** = Undersea and Hyperbaric Medical Society

their own approved list of HBO indications. As new information becomes available, the indications lists are modified. Every three to four years the UHMS generates a new HBO committee report with modifications to the list as evidenced-based information warrants it. The Undersea and Hyperbaric Medical Society Hyperbaric Oxygen Committee Report is an excellent source document containing the most up to date references available, peer review guidelines, rationale for using HBO and cost considerations.[9]

HYPERBARIC OXYGEN PHYSIOLOGY: PRIMARY MECHANISMS

Historical Highlights in the Understanding of the Mechanisms of Hyperbaric Oxygen – The physiological effects of HBO, that is, how it works in the human body, are well defined. This information provides the rationale for using it in the conditions previously described (Table 10-3) as well as understanding its side effects. When the mechanisms of HBO are considered, it is useful to divide them into primary and secondary categories. The primary mechanisms are those directly attributable to hyperoxygenation and/or pressurization. Secondary mechanisms occur as a result of tissue hyperoxygenation, but are clear and distinct from hyperoxygenation itself. The modern history of hyperbaric oxygen therapy parallels the understanding of its mechanisms. Confirmation of the hyperoxygenation mechanism occurred in 1960 when Boerma, et al., published their classic paper, "Life without Blood."[10] Through hyperoxygenation they were able to keep piglets alive in the absence of red blood cell transported oxygen. In the 1970's Hunt and his colleagues confirmed what oxygen tensions were required for wound healing and leukocyte killing of bacteria.[11,12,13,14,15] This provides the information to justify using HBO in problem hypoxic wounds. In the 1980 decade, much information was published on the use of HBO for microbiological conditions, including necrotizing soft tissue infections and synergistic bacterial infections.[16,17,18,19] Also during this period, studies confirming the benefit of HBO for edema reduction in traumatic ischemias, appeared.[20,21,22,23,24,25] In the current era, the effects of HBO on reperfusion injury and growth factors have generated much interest.[26,27] Yet to be fully appreciated are the effects of HBO on the blood-brain barrier, severe sepsis and erythrocyte deformation/perfusion through the microcirculation. The following information summarizes the effects of HBO.

Hyperoxygenation – When the mechanisms of hyperbaric oxygen are considered, hyperoxygenation is the quintessence of hyperbaric oxygen therapy. The physics and physiology of hyperoxygenation is the best documented of all the mechanisms of HBO. Objective information from transcutaneous and tissue oxygen measurements confirm its validity.[28,29] Its effects can be observed directly and immediately, such as witnessing improved coloration of dusky colored skin with hyperoxygenation. In simplified terms, hyperoxygenation is the technique of using pressure to force oxygen into plasma and tissue fluids. Normally 97.5 percent of the oxygen carried in the blood stream, termed the blood oxygen content, is carried by the hemoglobin in the red blood cell and amounts to 19.5 volumes percent of hemoglobin carried oxygen for each cubic centimeter of arterial blood (Figure 10-6). The other 2.5 percent, equivalent to 0.5 volumes percent, is physically dissolved in the plasma. Hyperoxygenation increases the amount of physically dissolved oxygen in the plasma.

Hemoglobin Carried and Plasma Transported Oxygen – In the absence of pulmonary disease, the hemoglobin in the red blood cell, after passing through the lung circulation, approaches 100 percent saturation. This means that even with breathing increasing oxygen percentages (that is greater than 20.9%, the amount of oxygen in normoxic air) or breathing pure oxygen greater than one atmosphere absolute pressure (that is hyperbaric oxygen), no additional oxygen can be added to the hemoglobin in the red blood cell. The oxygen carrying capacity in the blood from hemoglobin is only increased through adding more hemoglobin, that is a blood transfusion. This effect is quantified with the formula **Blood Oxygen Content$_{(Hemoglobin)}$ = (1.34 ml O$_2$/gram Hb) X (Hemoglobin$_{(grams/dl)}$)**. In contrast, physically dissolved oxygen in the plasma increases in direct proportion to the partial pressure of the inspired oxygen in the breathing gas. This is a direct application of Henry's law, which states that as the pressure of gas is increased in a system with a gas-liquid interface, more gas is forced into the liquid (Figure 10-7). For each mmHg of inspired oxygen partial pressure, 0.003

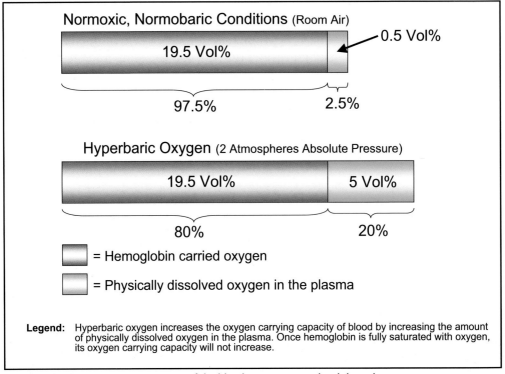

Figure 10-6. Oxygen carrying capacity of the blood in room air and with hyperbaric oxygen.

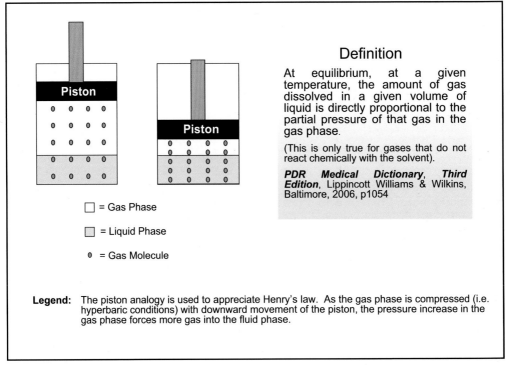

Figure 10-7. Henry's Law.

volume percent of oxygen becomes physically dissolved in the plasma. The formula quantifying this effect is **Blood Oxygen Content**(physically Dissolved) = **(0.003 ml O$_2$/mmHg) X (Partial Pressure Oxygen**(mmHg)**)**. This means that the amount of physically dissolved oxygen in the plasma increases in a linear fashion as the partial pressure of oxygen in the inhaled gas increases.

Dalton's Law – The volume percent of physically dissolved oxygen in the plasma is easily put into numbers when the above information is used with Dalton's law of partial pressures. Dalton's law states that the total pressure of gases in a system is equal to the sum of the partial pressures of the individual gases in the system (**Pressure**(total) = **P**$_1$+ **P**$_2$ +... where **P** equals the partial pressure of each component gas). For air at sea level, the total pressure is one atmosphere absolute (ATA) composed of 0.79 ATA nitrogen, 20.9 ATA oxygen and the remaining 0.1 ATA of water vapor, carbon dioxide and other rare gases in the atmosphere. In summary, hyperbaric oxygen supplements the hemoglobin carried oxygen brought to tissues by increasing the amount of physically dissolved oxygen in the plasma (Table 10-4). The result at the tissue level is that the physically dissolved oxygen in the plasma equilibrates with the oxygen tensions in the tissue fluids to provide an oxygen-enriched environment for tissue metabolism.

Oxygen Transfer from the Capillary to Tissue Fluids – At first inspection, the relatively small, that is, 22.5 percent increase (1.225 fold) in the oxygen content of the blood with HBO at 2 ATA may seem insignificant. However, the real consideration for metabolism is the amount of oxygen available to tissues at the (extracellular-extravascular) tissue fluid level. Normally, approximately five volumes percent of oxygen are off-loaded to the surrounding tissue fluids as the blood passes from the arterial to the venous side of the capillary (Figure 10-8). When breathing room air, 5 volumes percent

TABLE 10-4. BLOOD OXYGEN CONTENT (VOLUMES %) WITH VARYING CONDITIONS

Condition	Hemoglobin Carried	Physically Dissolved (% Increase from Air)	Total (% Increase from Air)
Air at 1 ATA (Sea Level)	19.5	0.5 (Baseline)	20 (Baseline)
Pure Oxygen at 1 ATA	Same as Above (SAA)	2.5 (500)	22 (10)
Air at 2 ATA (33 FSW)	SAA	1.0 (200)	20.5 (2.5)
HBO at 2 ATA (Monoplace Chamber)	SAA	5.0 (1000)	24.5 (22.5)
HBO at 2.4 ATA (Multiplace Chamber)	SAA	6.0* (1200)	25.5 (27.5)
HBO at 3 ATA	SAA	7.5 (1500)	27 (35)
Air at 6 ATA** (165 FSW)	SAA	3.0 (600)	22.5 (12.5)

Notes: *This number is based on the assumption that the mask or hood is 100% efficient in oxygen delivery to the patient.
**This pressure sometimes used for treating arterial gas embolism in a multiplace chamber. Yellow highlighted areas are the pressures most frequently used for wound healing and infection control applications of hyperbaric oxygen.
Abbreviations: **ATA** = Atmospheres absolute, **FSW** = Feet of sea water, **HBO** = Hyperbaric oxygen, **SAA** = Same as above

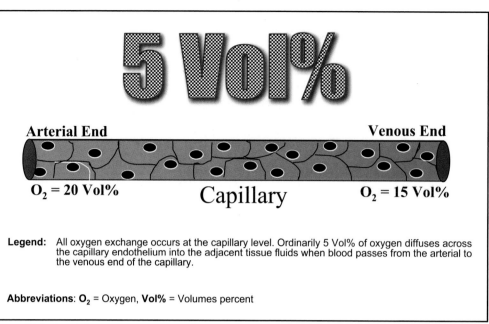

Legend: All oxygen exchange occurs at the capillary level. Ordinarily 5 Vol% of oxygen diffuses across the capillary endothelium into the adjacent tissue fluids when blood passes from the arterial to the venous end of the capillary.

Abbreviations: O_2 = Oxygen, **Vol%** = Volumes percent

Figure 10-8. Arterial-venous oxygen extraction.

Historical Note: In the early 1900's JBS Haldane of Great Britain, an authority on undersea medicine, said that the body, for metabolism purposes, only utilized hemoglobin-carried oxygen. Physically dissolved oxygen in the plasma, even if increased with HBO, was not a utilizable source of oxygen for metabolic purposes. This pronouncement was labeled the "Haldanean Hex" and impeded the clinical development of HBO during the first half of the twentieth century.

In the 1950s Lambertsen, who is universally recognized for his work on oxygen metabolism, challenged the Haldanean Hex. He stated that the body tissues, for metabolism purposes, did not discriminate whether oxygen was supplied by hemoglobin carried or physically dissolved sources, and each could be used equally well to meet tissue oxygen requirements.

This information became known to Boerma, a thoracic surgeon in the Netherlands, who was working on techniques to extend the bypass time for open heart surgeries using heart-lung machines. These factors were the genesis for Boerma's "Life without Blood" study. In the study, piglets were kept alive under HBO conditions after their red blood cells were removed and their blood volumes maintained with Dextran®. This validated Lambertsen's hypothesis, proved the effectiveness of HBO, and dispelled the Haldanean Hex.

of this oxygen is off-loaded from the hemoglobin in the red cell. This is the oxygen that is used by the body's cells for metabolism, wound healing, infection control and other oxidative functions and is termed the arterial-venous (A-V) oxygen extraction or difference. Conditions such as acidosis (the Bohr effect) and increased temperature increase A-V oxygen extraction and serve as protective mechanisms to increase oxygen availability when oxygen availability problems arise. At two ATA, HBO increases the blood oxygen content by almost five volumes percent, which is nearly equivalent to the usual

A-V oxygen extraction. The physically dissolved oxygen in the plasma is as useable an oxygen source for tissue metabolism as is that carried by the hemoglobin. This validates the hyperoxygenation mechanism of hyperbaric oxygen and provides the justification for a multitude of clinical applications of hyperbaric oxygen (Figure 10-9).

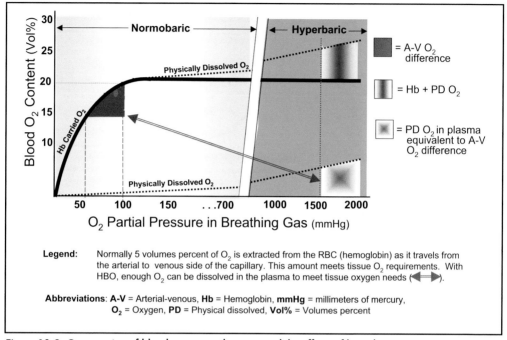

Figure 10-9. Oxygenation of blood, oxygen utilization, and the effects of hyperbaric oxygen

Features of Hyperoxygenation – Hyperoxygenation has several defining features. First, the effects are very rapid. Plasma becomes saturated with oxygen quickly, probably within a couple of minutes of entering the hyperbaric oxygen environment since the time for blood to make one circuit through the blood stream is less than 60 seconds. Tissue fluids saturate more slowly. Their saturations are dependent on the blood flow to the tissues. At rest, non-critical tissues such as muscle, skin, and subcutaneous tissues have minimal perfusion. Studies show that it takes about an hour for muscle and subcutaneous tissue fluids to become saturated with oxygen after starting the HBO exposure (Figure 10-10).[30] Second, the effects are transient. Elevated oxygen levels in the blood stream return to normal within ten minutes after completing the HBO exposure. Oxygen tensions in muscles remain elevated for one and one-half hours while those in the subcutaneous tissues remain elevated for four hours.[30] Third, oxygen tensions in tissues increase in direct proportion to the partial pressure of the inhaled oxygen, as Henry's law predicts. Although it might seem beneficial to increase oxygen tensions to greater than 3 atmospheres absolute, side effects, as will be discussed later in this chapter, occur as oxygen tensions in tissues increase. Finally, hyperoxygenation requires blood flow. If there is no blood flow, it will not be possible for the oxygen physically dissolved in the plasma to get to the capillary where it can diffuse into tissue fluids.

Other Hyperoxygenation Considerations – The physiology of hyperoxygenation has two other special features. First, because oxygen is physically dissolved in the plasma, in contrast to hemoglobin carried oxygen in the red blood cell, oxygen delivery by HBO becomes no more flow dependent than any other substance physically dissolved in the

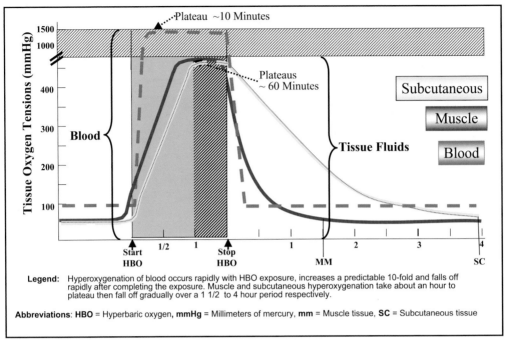

Figure 10-10. Hyperoxygenation pharmokinetics.[30]

plasma. This has important applications in low flow states where the cellular elements in the blood fail to pass through the capillary bed due to stasis, sludging and Rouleau formation while plasma will continue to stream by and be able to meet tissue oxygen requirements. The second feature is that of hyperoxic diffusion. Increased oxygen tensions have a "mass" effect to drive oxygen across relative barriers such as cicatrix and edema and down a concentration gradient. The increase in diffusion is proportional to the oxygen tension and with HBO at 2 ATA is about 3-fold greater through tissue fluids than with breathing normoxic air.[31,32]

Clinical Applications of the Hyperoxygenation Mechanism – Hyperoxygenation has four specific clinical applications (Figure 10-11). First, it is useful in low blood flow conditions where the blood flow is inadequate to meet tissue oxygen demands. This problem is the most frequent indication for HBO and is observed in problem wounds, non-healing wounds, failed amputations and wounds severe enough that major limb amputation is being considered. Problems causing low flow states include atherosclerosis, vasculitis, hypovolemia, compartment syndrome, thromboembolism, hypercoagulable states and trauma with vessel damage and/or transection. The second use of hyperoxygenation is for conditions where relative barriers interfere with oxygen diffusion from the capillary to the tissues. Examples of relative barriers include edema fluid, hematoma, cicatrix, suppuration, radiation injury, sequestered bone, implants and foreign objects. The hyperoxygenation effect of HBO helps drive oxygen across these relative barriers so secondary mechanisms such as angiogenesis, fibroblast function and white blood cell oxidative healing occur. A third use of hyperoxygenation is for its "wash out" effect on toxic substances such as carbon monoxide or inert gas as used for treating decompression sickness. Finally, hyperoxygenation is used for acute blood loss anemia where there is decreased carrying capacity of oxygen in the blood and transfusion is delayed, not possible or refused. This use is a direct clinical application of Boerma's "Life without Blood" study.

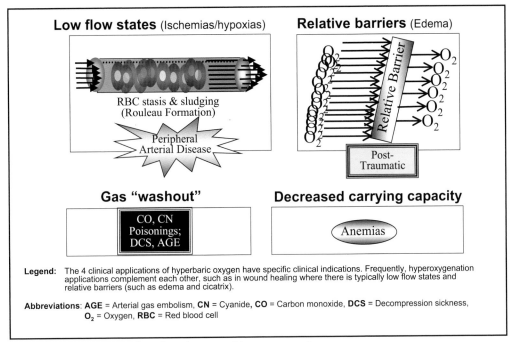

Figure 10-11. Four major clinical applications of hyperoxygenation.

Hyperoxygenation Summary – In summary, the hyperoxygenation mechanism of HBO is its most important. This effect occurs immediately with pressurization. Tissue hyperoxygenation is based on sound physics and physiological principles. At a HBO treatment pressure of 2 ATA, tissue and plasma oxygen tensions increase ten-fold, blood oxygen content increases 22.5% and diffusion distance of oxygen through relative barriers 3-fold (Figure 10-12). Hyperoxygenation's two most important uses for problem wounds are supplementation of hemoglobin carried oxygen in low flow states and improved perfusion of oxygen through relative barriers. More importantly, hyperoxygenation improves the environment, oxygen tension-wise, so the secondary mechanisms of HBO can function, as will be discussed later in this chapter. Consequently, its greatest utilization is in the hypoxic wound or injury. It will not be effective in the ischemic wound or injury where blood flow is insufficient to adequately circulate the plasma.

Bubble Reduction – This primary effect occurs as pressure is increased around an air-filled, flexible walled structure. The effects are defined by Boyle's law, which states that as pressure is increased on a gas at a constant temperature, the volume decreases, that is $(\text{Volume}_1) \times (\text{Pressure}_1) = \textbf{K}$. Bubble reduction occurs immediately upon pressurization of the hyperbaric chamber regardless of the breathing gas; the greater the pressure, the smaller the bubble. However, with each succeeding one ATA increase of pressure, the volume of bubble reduction decreases in a logarithmic fashion. For example, pressurizing a bubble from one ATA (sea level) pressure to two ATA (33 FSW), reduces its original volume by 50 percent. With further pressurization of the bubble from 2 ATA to 3 ATA (66 FSW), its original volume is reduced to one-third, but the change in volume is only 16 2/3% (The difference between 50% and 33 1/3%). The reduction in bubble size is, of course, an important effect of recompression for diving related problems such as arterial gas embolism and decompression sickness, as well as iatrogenic cases of gas embolism, but has no direct applications to problem wounds.

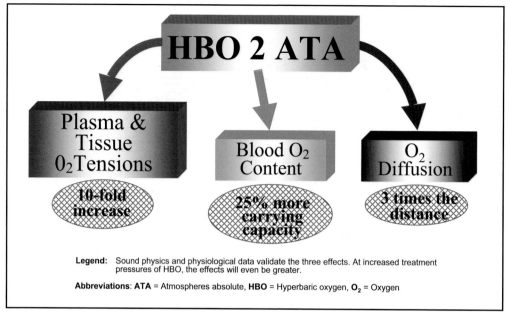

Figure 10-12. The 3 quantifiable effects of hyperoxygenation.

SECONDARY MECHANISMS OF HYPERBARIC OXYGEN

Characteristics of the Secondary Mechanisms of Hyperbaric Oxygen – As stated previously, the secondary effects of hyperbaric oxygen are due to the oxygen enriched environment hyperoxygenation provides to the blood and tissues (Figure 10-13, Table 10-5). Whereas, the effects of hyperoxygenation are transient, the effects of the secondary mechanisms result in permanent changes. Consequently, after the benefits of the secondary mechanisms are realized, hyperbaric oxygen therapy may be stopped. The identification of the secondary mechanisms of HBO parallels the recognition of its value as an adjunctive intervention for managing problem wounds. Host responses and microbiological effects are the most important secondary mechanisms with respect to using HBO as an adjunct to the management of problem wounds. Several of the secondary mechanisms have indirect applications to problem wounds while others are used for problems other than wound healing.

Host Factors – During the 1970's, Hunt and his colleagues demonstrated the necessity of oxygen for wound healing and leukocyte oxidative killing.[11,12,13,14,35,36,37] Adequate tissue fluid oxygen tensions are required for soft tissue as well as calcified tissue healing (bone and calcified cartilage healing). The fibroblast is the cell responsible for soft tissue healing. Three of its functions, migration, proliferation and matrix secretion are oxygen dependent (Figures 2-4 & 2-5). Thirty to 40 mmHg oxygen tensions are required for these functions to occur.[11,12,13,14] If these oxygen tensions are not present; wounds remain in a state of non-healing, although the fibroblasts may still remain viable. Of all the reasons wounds do not heal, hypoxia certainly is one of the most important. This is because it is such a frequent cause (present in over 50 percent of the non-healing wounds we manage), the problem that tends to be the most overlooked in the management of non-healing wounds and the one that can be most objectively documented with use of juxta-wound transcutaneous oxygen measurements. As shown earlier in this chapter, HBO has the potential to increase juxta-wound oxygen tensions 10-fold or more.

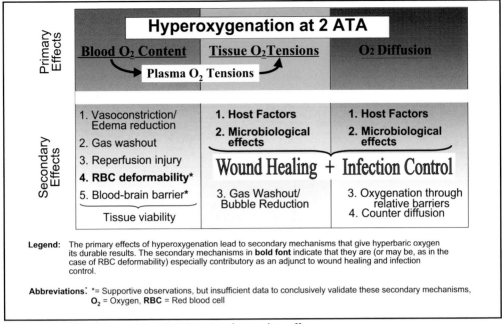

Figure 10-13. Hyperoxygenation: Its primary and secondary effects.

TABLE 10-5. SECONDARY (TO HYPEROXYGENATION) MECHANISMS OF HYPERBARIC OXYGEN

Secondary Mechanisms

• Vasoconstriction	• Gas Washout
• Host Responses	• Counterdiffusion
• Microbiological	• RBC Deformability
• Reperfusion Injury	• Blood Brain Barrier

Whereas **primary mechanisms** are largely responsible for **keeping tissues alive**—a short term effect

Secondary mechanisms are instrumental in **resolving the problem**—the long term result

Note: Secondary mechanisms listed in smaller font indicate that observations support the efficacy of these mechanisms, but there is insufficient information to conclusively validate them

The Oxygen Gradient and Wound Healing – When wound healing models are discussed; the concept of gradient is fundamental (Figure 10-14). While the center of the wound is anoxic, the margins are normally oxygenated. From the adequately oxygenated margins, fibroblasts are able to function to achieve wound healing. This is done through the mechanisms previously described. Angiogenesis, the formation of new blood vessels, at the microcirculation level, is necessary for wound healing. Angiogenesis is dependent on the matrix secreted by the fibroblast. New blood vessels invade the matrix to provide an advancing oxygenated margin toward the anoxic center of the wound. As the oxygenated margins extend, fibroblasts migrate into the newly oxygenated areas to continue their wound healing functions. With the advancing margin of matrix secretion, angiogenesis and fibroblast migration, the anoxic gradient is obliterated. The fibroblast forms collagen, which provides a substrate for the keratinocytes to epithelialize the wound. In addition, fibroblast proliferation is both oxygen and age dependent. With increasing age, the rate that fibroblasts multiply decreases.[33] Hyperbaric oxygen mitigates the age differences in fibroblast doubling times.[33]

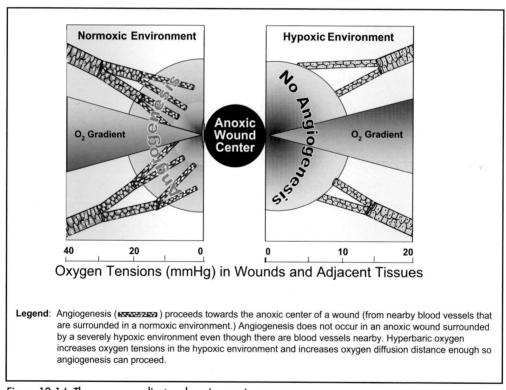

Oxygen Tensions (mmHg) in Wounds and Adjacent Tissues

Legend: Angiogenesis ( ) proceeds towards the anoxic center of a wound (from nearby blood vessels that are surrounded in a normoxic environment.) Angiogenesis does not occur in an anoxic wound surrounded by a severely hypoxic environment even though there are blood vessels nearby. Hyperbaric oxygen increases oxygen tensions in the hypoxic environment and increases oxygen diffusion distance enough so angiogenesis can proceed.

Figure 10-14. The oxygen gradient and angiogenesis.

Angiogenesis – While an oxygenated environment, a direct effect, is needed for angiogenesis, oxygen appears to have a direct effect on angiogenesis also. Vascular endothelial growth factor (VEGF) is an inducer for angiogenesis.[34] Oxygen has been identified as necessary for production of this growth factor in addition to being a signaling device for it. The hyperoxygenation mechanism of HBO increases oxygen tensions in the wound environment and, as a consequence, it may also serve as both a signaling device and a substrate for VEGF when oxygen tensions in the wound are too low for these functions to occur without this adjunct. As noted previously, hyperbaric oxygen also appears to behave as a signaling mechanism for fibroblast proliferation.[33]

Neutrophil Oxidative Killing – Another host cell important in the management of "problem" wounds, the neutrophil (polymorphonuclear leukocyte), also requires oxygen for its function. The neutrophil engulfs bacteria. Once engulfed, the bacteria are killed by oxygen generated radicals, namely superoxides and peroxides. If oxygen tensions are not 30 to 40 mmHg in the fluids surrounding the neutrophil, these radicals are not generated and oxidative killing of the bacteria does not occur. During the respiratory burst when the bacteria are killed in the phagosomes by reactive oxygen species generated by these organelles, oxygen consumption increases as much as 100-fold.[35,36,37] Reactive oxygen species include superoxide, hydrogen peroxide, hydroxyl radical, singlet oxygen, hypochlorous acid, chloramines, nitric oxide and peroxynitrites. Each has its own properties and mechanisms of action; many react with each other to form secondary and tertiary reactive oxygen species products. In summary, adequate oxygen tensions in the wound facilitate bacteria killing by two mechanisms; oxidative killing as just described and by angiogenesis through delivery of antibiotics to the wound site.

Bone Resorption – A third oxygen dependent host cell associated with problem wound healing, the osteoclast, is responsible for resorption of dead and infected bone. The osteoclast is a macrophage, a multinucleated giant cell that has migrated from the blood stream to the vicinity of the bone. It generates acid phosphatases to reabsorb bone. The osteoclast is instrumental in the resorption and remodeling of bone as is required for fracture healing, bone strengthening in responses to mechanical stresses and managing osteomyelitis. Its metabolic activity as reflected by bone resorption is 100 times greater than that of the bone-building cell, the osteoblast.[39] This explains why, of the three cells involved in bone metabolism, the osteocyte, the osteoblast, and the osteoclast, the latter is the most responsive to HBO. Often times resorption of infected bone is observed only after HBO treatments are started (Figure 10-15). Hence, HBO supports

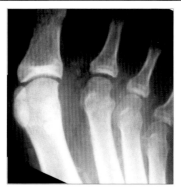
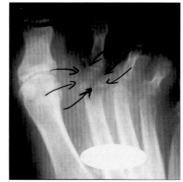

Before Hyperbaric Oxygen   After Hyperbaric Oxygen

Legend: The X-ray of an infected mal perforans ulcer under the right 2nd metatarsal head demonstrated a normal appearance of the bone after 4 weeks of antibiotics and debridements.

Two weeks after hyperbaric oxygen treatments were added, resorption of the second metatarsal head is evident (black arrows).

The improved oxygenation of the wound area secondary to hyperbaric oxygen treatments provided an environment for the osteoclast to absorb the dead, infected metatarsal head.

Figure 10-15 . Hyperbaric oxygen as an adjunct to resorption of infected bone.

a three-pronged approach to manage infections in problem wounds, that is angiogenesis (as a consequence of fibroblast activity) to deliver antibiotics and leukocytes, oxidative killing of bacteria by neutrophils and resorption of infected, dead bone by the osteoclast. These three infection controlling body mechanisms fail to function adequately in hypoxic environments; hyperbaric oxygen is an intervention that addresses all three.

Dosing of Hyperbaric Oxygen – The question of the dose of HBO needed to make the host responses effective remains to be answered with absolute certainty. Elevated oxygen tensions remain in tissue fluids for only one and one-half to four hours (muscle and subcutaneous tissues respectively) after a HBO treatment is completed (Figure 10-10). Yet, only one to two hyperbaric oxygen treatments a day appear to be sufficient to achieve the effects desired from the host factors. In this respect, pulses of HBO, analogous to antibiotic administration, seem to be all that are needed. The current recommendations are once or twice a day HBO treatments for the host factors dealing with fibroblast function, angiogenesis and leukocyte oxidative killing and once a day treatments for the host factors dealing with calcified tissues (bone and cartilage). Usually ten days to two weeks of HBO treatments are sufficient to achieve the soft tissue effects, especially angiogenesis, while one month of daily hyperbaric oxygen treatments may be needed for the calcified tissues.

Microbiological Effects – In addition to the host responses just described that help in the management of infections in hypoxic problem wounds, the hyperoxygenated environment has four direct microbiological effects. First, it has static and cidal effects on microorganisms. Anaerobic organisms such as clostridia, bacteroides and microaerophilic streptococci are the most sensitive to hyperoxia.[40,41,42,43] Actinomycosis is also inhibited by hyperoxic environments.[44] Adjunctive HBO may be beneficial in diabetic patients with zygomycosis.[45,46] Finally, synergistic infections with mixed aerobic and anaerobic organisms and staphylococcus plus streptococcus (which is the flora described in the Meleney's ulcer) are inhibited by the increased oxygen tensions HBO generates in tissue fluids.

Cessation of Toxin Formation – The second microbiological effect is that of cessation of toxin formation. This effect is the primary indication for HBO in gas gangrene.[47] Tissue oxygen tensions greater than 200 mmHg stop *Clostridia perfringens* and other clostridia species from forming the deadly alpha-toxin, a C-lecithinase, which makes this organism so virulent. Third, hyperoxygenated environments inactivate some toxins such as the theta toxin associated with clostridia infections and possibly the toxin associated with the brown recluse spider bite.[48,49] Finally, normalizing oxygen tensions in tissue fluids promotes active transport of antibiotics into microorganisms. The aminoglycosides, amphotericin, vancomycin and possibly other antibiotics require oxygen-dependent transport mechanisms in the microorganism's cell walls to enter the organisms. In hypoxic environments the aminoglycosides are one twentieth as effective as in normoxic environments.[50]

Other Secondary Mechanisms – There are five other mechanisms of HBO that occur as a consequence of hyperoxygenation (Table 10-6). Several such as edema reduction, red blood cell deformability and alteration of the blood-brain barrier may have ramifications for the management of problem wounds. Hyperbaric oxygen reduces vasogenic edema by 20 percent.[21,22,23,24,25,51] This reduces the diffusion distance of oxygen through tissue fluids from the capillary to the cell. The results are improved oxygenation of tissues in hypoxic wounds (Chapter 2) and reduction of pressure in tissue compartments. This latter effect is observed in compartment syndromes where tissue fluid pressures increase to levels greater than the capillary perfusion pressure, cause

TABLE 10-6. CHARACTERISTICS OF THE SECONDARY MECHANISMS OF HYPERBARIC OXYGEN

Mechanism	Physiology	Applications	Comments
Alterations of the Blood-brain Barrier	Hyperoxygenation improves diffusion of agents across the barrier	Antibiotic & chemotherapeutic delivery for CNS infections & tumors	HBO reduces mortality & morbidity in intracranial abscesses
Gas Washout	High O_2 tensions in plasma generate gradients for gases to diffuse into blood & be carried to lungs for exhalation	AGE, DCS & CO poisoning O_2 decompression for long duration and/or deep dives	Justification for HBO recompression for AGE & DCS Speeds removal of inert gas & CO from tissues
Isobaric Counter Diffusion	At constant pressures, gases in tissues & bubbles equilibrate with the gases breathed	AGE & DCS Rationale for using sequential gas mixtures for deep technical diving	Alters bubble composition, e.g. from inert gas to O_2 if breathing pure O_2 O_2 in bubbles diffuse into tissues to reduce bubble size
Red Blood Cell Deformation	The 7.5 " µM in diameter RBC requires O_2 to elongate/pass through the 5.0 " µM diameter capillary and off-load its O_2	Low blood flow states (PAD, frostbite, post-trauma, vasculitities, etc.), sepsis, shock & possibly reperfusion injury	Sepsis & associated stasis (hypoxia in the microcirculation) interfere with the RBC's ability to elongate
Reperfusion Injury	Adhesion molecules in the capillary endothelium become "activated" after blood flow is interrupted Neutrophils attach to the endothelium after flow resumes & release reactive O_2 species that destroy tissues HBO perturbs the attachment	Temporary interruption of blood flow (e.g. stroke, heart attack, thrombo-embolic events, shock, reattachment of body parts, etc.), Possibly prevention of complications from CO poisoning & severe presentations of AGE & DCS	Many potential applications for HBO HBO may also 1) help generate scavengers to detoxify O_2 radicals & 2) prevent conversion of NO (in presence of O_2 radicals) to the very destructive peroxynitrite radical
Vasoconstriction	HBO acts as a vasoconstrictor like an alpha adrenergic agent 20% reductions in vasogenic edema from the reduced flow	Post-traumatic ischemic conditions (e.g. crush injuries, compartment syndromes, CNS trauma, etc.)	HBO maintains tissue O_2 tension in the presence of decreased blood flow In auto-sympathectomized states or calcified vessels, vasoconstriction does not occur

Abbreviations: **AGE** = Arterial gas embolism, **CNS** = Central nervous system, **CO** = Carbon monoxide, **DCS** = Decompression sickness, **HBO** = Hyperbaric oxygen, **NO** = Nitric oxide, **O_2** = Oxygen molecule, **PAD** =Peripheral arterial disease, **RBC** = Red blood cell, **µM** = micrometer (micron)

the capillaries to collapse and lead to ischemia of the tissues in the compartment.[52]

Red Blood Cell Deformability – The 7.5 micrometer in diameter red blood cell (RBC) must deform (elongate) in order to pass through the five micrometer in diameter capillary. In sepsis and hypoxic environments, RBC's lose their ability to deform.[53,54,55] This results in sludging in the microcirculation and bypassing the microcirculation by arterio-venous shunting, as seen in septic shock. Hyperbaric oxygen was observed to protect rats from intra-abdominal sepsis, which was otherwise fatal to the control

Clinical Correlation:

A 62 year old physician became moribund from intra-abdominal sepsis after surgery for a ruptured appendix. In spite of triple antibiotics, intubation with ventilatory support, vasopressors, open drainage of the peritoneum and hyperalimentation, he remained in septic shock and his condition continued to deteriorate. Hyperbaric oxygen was started as a "last resort." Immediately his condition stabilized and then gradually improved to the point of full recovery. After several months of convalescence, he returned to his medical practice.

Comment:

It seems more than coincidental that the patient's improvement began only after starting HBO treatments. What mechanisms of HBO contributed to the improvement? The answer is probably several. However, the one that seems most attractive is that HBO improved RBC deformability so perfusion (and oxygenation) of vital organs could be resumed. This hypothesis is consistent with the observations made in the rat intra-abdominal sepsis model described in the preceding paragraph.

animals.[56] This mechanism of HBO to explain the results observed in this study has not been elucidated. They may possibly be a consequence of increased plasma oxygen tensions providing an oxygenated enough environment for RBC's to regain their ability to deform, pass through the capillary (rather than arterio-venous shunting), off-load their oxygen and thereby correct hypoxia in critical organs such as the liver, spleen and gut which have great abilities to handle bacterial loads as well as alter their blood flows. Matheiu, et al., reported that HBO improved the ability for RBC's to deform.[57]

Alteration of the Blood-brain Barrier – Hyperbaric oxygen has been observed to alter the blood-brain barrier.[58,59] Minimal work has been done on this intriguing subject. Potential benefits of altering the blood-brain barrier include improved antibiotic delivery for central nervous system infections and improved transport of chemotherapeutic agents across the blood-brain for management of tumors. The recent inclusion of "intracranial abscess" as one of the approved uses of HBO by the Undersea and Hyperbaric Medical Society standards is an indirect testimonial to the potential HBO has for altering the blood-brain barrier. In a generic sense, hyperbaric oxygen may be considered "an antibiotic" when the multiple and varied effects this therapy has for mitigating infection are considered (Figure 10-16).[18,60,61]

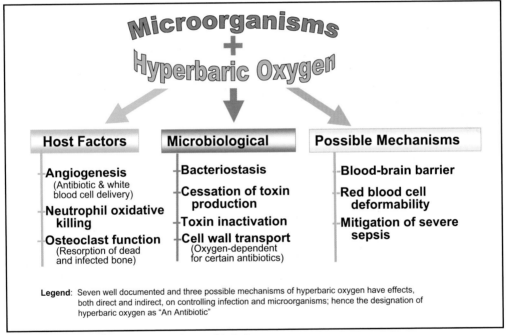

Figure 10-16. Hyperbaric oxygen as "an antibiotic."

SIDE EFFECTS AND CONTRAINDICATION OF HYPERBARIC OXYGEN

Oxygen Toxicity – Hyperbaric oxygen (HBO) has four major side effects. In addition, there are uncompromising safety precautions that must be followed when it is used. Central nervous system oxygen toxicity manifested as a seizure is the most dreaded side effect. It occurs rarely, less than once in every 10,000 HBO exposures.[62] Central nervous system oxygen toxicity is prevented by limiting depths and durations of exposures. It is essential to ascertain whether or not patients have risk factors for HBO associated seizures such as a history of epilepsy, high dose steroid and/or aspirin usage, high fever or acidosis. If these factors are present, remedial measures should be instituted to lower the risk of an oxygen seizure occurring during the HBO exposure. For example, if a history of seizures is present, the patient should be on anticonvulsant medications and blood tests obtained to confirm that the blood levels are in the therapeutic range before starting HBO. If HBO treatments need to be started on an emergency basis, then prophylactic coverage with phenobarbital and/or lorazepam (Ativan®) should be administered before commencing the treatment. If a seizure occurs during a HBO treatment, the breathing gas should be switched to air (which immediately lowers the O_2 concentration by 80%) and the patient brought to the surface over a one to two minute period after tonic phase of seizure activity has ceased. After neurological clearance to rule out other causes of seizures such as hypoglycemia, a cerebral bleed, infection, etc., HBO treatments are usually resumed after 24 hours with a protective umbrella of anticonvulsants.

Ear Squeezes – Middle ear barotrauma is the most frequently observed side effect of hyperbaric exposures. It is associated with pressurization and decompression of the HBO chamber. Minor signs or symptoms of middle ear barotrauma can be detected in about two thirds of the patients during their initial HBO treatments. These problems are usually mild enough that educating the patient in middle ear equilibration techniques, controlling the rate of compression and decompression and use of nasal decongestants is sufficient to handle the symptoms and not interrupt the HBO treatments. In one or two of every 100 patients, middle ear equilibration is not achieved and myringotomy and/or middle ear ventilation tubes need to be inserted in order to continue HBO treatments. In our experiences, intubated, unconscious and/or pediatric patients do not appear to experience higher incidences of middle ear barotrauma than patients who can initiate their own middle ear auto-equilibration techniques.

Claustrophobia – Confinement anxiety (claustrophobia) is a problem that about half the patients experience during their initial HBO exposures. With verbal support, family encouragement and anxiolytics, most patients can continue HBO treatments without interruption. In the motivated patient, even with the severest claustrophobia symptoms, counseling by the HBO staff and gradual increase in the HBO exposure times are remarkably effective in adjusting the patient to the full duration of the HBO treatment. In the occasional patient, psychiatric consultation and major tranquilizers may be needed to continue HBO treatments. Less than one of every 50 patients stop their HBO treatments because of confinement anxieties.

Temporary Alterations in Visual Acuity – After 30 HBO exposures, patients may note a temporary change in their vision such that their near vision improves at the expense of their distance vision. This is attributed to alterations in the shape of the lens from the oxygen exposure. After six weeks to six months, vision usually returns to what it was before the HBO exposures were started. Consequently, patients are informed of this observation and advised not to discard their glasses when they note visual changes with HBO. Hyperbaric oxygen, up to 60 exposures, does not appear to initiate and/or accelerate the formation of cataracts. After 150 to 850 HBO exposures, an increased incidence of cataracts was noted.[63,64]

Fire Hazards of Hyperbaric Oxygen – By and large HBO is a safe medical intervention. The major hazard is that of fire. Whereas, a combustible agent may hardly burn in air, it will burn explosively in the HBO environment. Items that could possibly generate a spark or support combustion such as synthetic fibers, lotions, hair oils, toenail polish, jewelry, and external fixators are removed, or in the case of the latter two items, covered with tape or cotton sheets during the treatments in a monoplace chamber. Cotton gowns, sheets and blankets are the only clothing and covering items allowed in the monoplace chamber. Pillows are feather-filled with cotton pillowcases. In the multi-place chamber, the fire precautions are less stringent, since it is pressurized with air rather than oxygen and in the United States, fire suppressions systems are required. Patients remove their shoes and items that could generate a flame such as lighters, but are allowed to wear scrub suits or jump suits of cotton or cotton-polyester blends and bring reading materials into the multiplace chamber during a treatment.[65]

Contraindications of Hyperbaric Oxygen – Hyperbaric oxygen is a relative contraindication for pregnant women, although reports suggest that for emergency situations such as carbon monoxide poisoning and decompression sickness, it lessens the chances of damage to the fetus from the offending condition.[66,67,68,69,70] Generally, HBO treatments are stopped if patients continue to smoke between treatments since the vaso-constrictive effect of nicotine appears to be additive to that of HBO, and chronic vaso-pathic effects of other substances such as carbon monoxide in smoke lessen the effectiveness of HBO. A few chemotherapeutic agents (e.g. doxorubicin, bleomycin, etc.), interlipids and mafenide acetate (Sulfamyalon®) are contraindications for HBO treatments because their toxicity is exacerbated and/or they lead to oxygen toxicity.[71,72,73] Interestingly, one recent study showed that hyperbaric oxygen therapy does not poten-tiate doxorubicin-induced cardiotoxicity in rats.[74] Finally, critically ill patients who require vasoactive medications such as norepinephrine (Levophed®) or sodium nitro-prusside (Nipride®), impose a relative contraindication for HBO therapy due to their instability and the concerns that their conditions will deteriorate during transport to and from the chamber.[75]

CONCLUSIONS

Medicare Approved Wound Uses of Hyperbaric Oxygen – The Center for Medicare/ Medicaid Services (CMS-Medicare) recognizes and provides reimbursement for hyperbaric oxygen treatments for six problem wound associated conditions. These by and large set the standards that other insurance carriers use for decisions regarding payments for HBO treatments for problem wounds. The six wound associated condi-tions include the following (Extracted from Table 10-3):

- Acute peripheral arterial insufficiency
- Chronic refractory osteomyelitis
- Diabetic foot wound, non-healing
- Gas gangrene
- Preservation of compromised skin grafts/flaps
- Progressive necrotizing soft tissue infections

The most recent addition, the non-healing diabetic foot wound, was added to the list in April, 2003. In many situations, the problem wound encompasses two or more of these diagnoses such as non-healing diabetic foot wound, chronic refractory osteomyelitis, and after surgical interventions, compromised skin graft or flap. The pres-ence of complimentary diagnoses adds justification to using HBO for the management of problem wounds. In a review of 12 published series including three randomized control trials, involving over 1000 patients, wound healing in diabetic patients improved

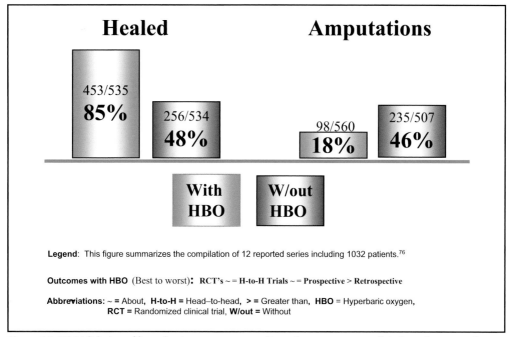

Healed   **Amputations**

453/535
85%
256/534
48%
98/560
18%
235/507
46%

With HBO   **W/out HBO**

Legend: This figure summarizes the compilation of 12 reported series including 1032 patients.[76]

Outcomes with HBO (Best to worst)**:** **RCT's** ~ = **H-to-H Trials** ~ = **Prospective** > **Retrospective**

Abbreviations: ~ = About, **H-to-H** = Head–to-head, **>** = Greater than, **HBO** = Hyperbaric oxygen,
RCT = Randomized clinical trial, **W/out** = Without

Figure 10-17. Validation of hyperbaric oxygen as an adjunct for management of diabetic foot wounds.

from 55 percent to 79 percent when HBO was used as an adjunct to management (Figure 10-17).[76] Lower limb amputations were reduced from 45 percent to 19 percent in the HBO treated group.

Summary – Additional information will be presented in the next chapter with respect to using hyperbaric oxygen as a diagnostic tool as well as a therapeutic agent in the hypoxic wound that is in a transitional stage, based on the **Wound Score**, between a "problem" and a "futile" wound. We have ascribed the label "end-stage" to this group of wounds as well as to other very serious wounds where there is a risk of loss of life or limb from them (Part IV). The importance of oxygen for wound healing is indisputable. It is "So vital...so taken for granted." Wound hypoxia is one of the primary reasons (along with underlying deformities and residual bone infection) problem wounds fail to heal. Deformities and bone infection can be resolved. The patient can live with neuropathy. Hyperbaric oxygen can help to mitigate the wound hypoxia problem and its use integrates well with an algorithm for management of the "problem" wound (Figure 10-18). Once a wound is healed, the juxta-wound metabolic requirements become a fraction of what was required for wound healing (Chapter 2).[77] This is why HBO can be so useful during the angiogenesis and infection control stages of wound healing, but can be stopped after these effects have been achieved. Hyperbaric oxygen is not in competition with the other four strategies for wound healing nor the other techniques used to improve wound oxygenation (Chapters 6 and 11). It is an adjunct to be used with the specific indication of wound hypoxia that is severe enough to interfere with healing. Its immediate effects can be validated by a transcutaneous oxygen measurement during a hyperbaric oxygen treatment.[29]

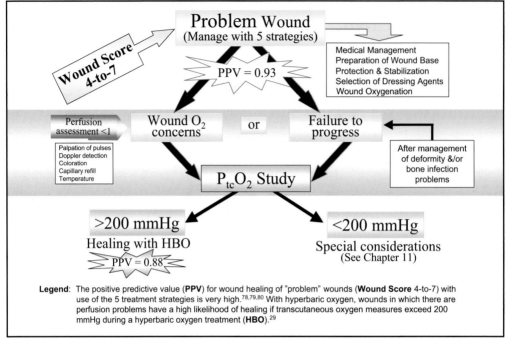

Figure 10-18. The role of hyperbaric oxygen in the management of the problem wound.

QUESTIONS:

1. What techniques are used to improve tissue oxygenation?

2. What are the differences between hyperbaric oxygen therapy and topical oxygen administration?

3. How do the oxygen delivery techniques differ between the monoplace and the multiplace hyperbaric chambers?

4. What are the primary and secondary mechanisms of hyperbaric oxygen and what are their major differences?

5. What are the defining features of hyperoxygenation?

6. What is the role of hyperbaric oxygen in angiogenesis?

7. What are the antimicrobial actions of hyperbaric oxygen?

8. What are the main side effects of hyperbaric oxygen?

9. What are the contraindications for hyperbaric oxygen therapy?

REFERENCES:

1. Hart GB, Wells CH, Strauss MB. Human skeletal muscle and subcutaneous tissue carbon dioxide, nitrogen and oxygen gas tension measurements under ambient and hyperbaric conditions, J Appl Res, 2003; 3(2):187-200

2. Hart GB, Strauss MB. Gender differences in human skeletal muscle and subcutaneous tissue gases under ambient and hyperbaric oxygen conditions, Undersea Hyper Med. 2007; 34(3);147-167

3. Neuman TS, Bove AA. Severe refractory decompression sickness resulting from combined no-decompression dives and pulmonary barotrauma, In AA Bove, AJ Bachrack, LJ Greenbaum, Ed. Underwater and Hyperbaric Physiology IX, Undersea and Hyperbaric Med Soc, Bethesda, 985-992, 1987

4. Neuman TS, Bove AA. Combined arterial gas embolism and decompression illness following no-stop dives, Undersea Biomed Res, 1990; 17:429-436

5. Pearson RR, Goad RF, Delayed cerebral edema complicating cerebral arterial embolism: Case histories, Undersea Biomed Res, 1982; 9:283-296

6. Fischer BF. Topical Hyperbaric oxygen treatment of pressure sores and skin ulcers,, Lancet. 1969; 2:405-409

7. Cotto-Cumba C, Velez E, Velu SS, et al. Transcutaneous oxygen measurements in normal subjects using topical HBO control module. Undersea Biomed Research. 1991; Vol 18:109

8. Hyperbaric Oxygen Therapy, Rev. 48, Issued:03-17-06: Effective/ Implementation Dates: 06-19-06, CMS Manual System, Pub 100-03 Medicare National Coverage Determinations, Transmittal 48, Department of Health & Human Services, Centers for Medicate & Medicaid Services, March 17,2006; Change Request 4278

9. Gessel LB (Ed.). Hyperbaric Oxygen Therapy Indications - The Hyperbaric Oxygen Therapy Committee Report, Undersea and Hyperbaric Medical Society, Durham, NC 2008

10. Borema I, Meyne MG, Brummelkamp WK, Bouma S, Mesch MH, Kamermans F, Stern Half M, Van Aalderen W. Live without blood. A study of the influence of hight atmospheric pressure and hyperthermia on dilution of the blood. J. Cardiovasc Surg 1960; 1:133-146

11. Hunt TK, Twomey P, Zederfeldt B, Dunphy JE. Respiratory gas tensions and pH in healing wounds. Am J Surg. 1967 Aug;114(2):302-7

12. Hunt TK, Dunphy JE. Effects of increasing oxygen supply to healing wounds. Br J Surg. 1969 Sep;56(9):705

13. Hunt TK, Zederfeldt B, Goldstick TK. Oxygen and healing. Am J Surg. 1969 Oct;118(4):521-5

14. Hunt TK, Linsey M, Sonne M, Jawetz E. Oxygen tension and wound infection. Surg Forum. 1972;23(0):47-9

15. Niinikoski J. Effect of oxygen supply on wound healing and formation of experimental granulation tissue. Acta Physiol Scand Suppl. 1969;334:1-72

16. Mader JT, Guckian JC, Glass DL, Reinarz JA. Therapy with hyperbaric oxygen for experimental osteomyelitis due to Staphylococcus aureus in rabbits. J Infect Dis. 1978 Sep;138(3):312-8

17. Bakker DJ. [The treatment of acute skin gangrene (necrotizing fasciitis and progressive bacterial gangrene) with hyperbaric oxygenation] Ned Tijdschr Geneeskd. 1980 Dec;124(51):2164-70. Dutch

18. Knighton DR, Halliday B, Hunt TK. Oxygen as an antibiotic. The effect of inspired oxygen on infection. Arch Surg. 1984 Feb;119(2):199-204

19. Riseman JA, Zamboni WA, Curtis A, Graham DR, Konrad HR, Ross DS. Hyperbaric oxygen therapy for necrotizing fasciitis reduces mortality and the need for debridements. Surgery. 1990 Nov;108(5):847-50

20. Skyhar MJ, Hargens AR, Strauss MB, Gershuni DH, Hart GB, Akeson WH. Hyperbaric oxygen reduces edema and necrosis of skeletal muscle in compartment syndromes associated with hemorrhagic hypotension. J Bone Joint Surg Am. 1986 Oct;68(8):1218-24

21. Strauss MB, Hargens AR, Gershuni DH, Hart GB, Akeson WH. Delayed use of hyperbaric oxygen for treatment of a model anterior compartment syndrome. J Orthop Res. 1986;4(1):108-11

22. Strauss MB, Hargens AR, Gershuni DH, Greenberg DA, Crenshaw AG, Hart GB, Akeson WH. Reduction of skeletal muscle necrosis using intermittent hyperbaric oxygen in a model compartment syndrome. J Bone Joint Surg Am. 1983 Jun;65(5):656-62

23. Sukoff MH, Ragatz RE. Hyperbaric oxygenation for the treatment of acute cerebral edema. Neurosurgery. 1982 Jan;10(1):29-38

24. Nylander G, Lewis D, Nordström H, Larsson J. Reduction of postischemic edema with hyperbaric oxygen. Plast Reconstr Surg. 1985 Oct;76(4):596-603

25. Nylander G, Nordström H, Eriksson E. Effects of hyperbaric oxygen on oedema formation after a scald burn. Burns Incl Therm Inj. 1984 Feb;10(3):193-6

26. Thom SR, Mendiguren I, Hardy K, Bolotin T, Fisher D, Nebolon M, Kilpatrick L. Inhibition of human neutrophil beta2-integrin-dependent adherence by hyperbaric O2 Am J Physiol. 1997 Mar;272(3 Pt 1):C770-7

27. Zamboni WA, Wong HP, Stephenson LL. Effect of hyperbaric oxygen on neutrophil concentration and pulmonary sequestration in reperfusion injury. Arch Surg. 1996 Jul;131(7):756-60

28. Sheffield PJ. Measuring tissue oxygen tension: a review. Undersea Hyperb Med. 1998 Fall;25(3):179-88

29. Strauss MB, Bryant BJ, Hart GB. Transcutaneous oxygen measurements under hyperbaric oxygen conditions as a predictor for healing of problem wounds. Foot Ankle Int. 2002 Oct;23(10):933-7

30. Wells CH, Goodpasture JE, Horrigan DJ, Hart GB. Tissue gas measurements during hyperbaric oxygen exposure, Proceeding of the Sixth International Congress on Hyperbaric Medicine, 1977, G Smith, Ed., Aberdeen University Press, p 118-124

31. Krogh A. The number of distribution of capillaries in muscle with calculations of the oxygen pressure head necessary for supplying the tissue. J Physiol 1919; 52:409-415

32. Peirce EC II. Pathophysiology, apparatus, and methods, including the special techniques of hypothermia and hyperbaric oxygen. Extracorporeal Circulation for Open-Heart Surgery 1969 Charles C. Thomas, Springfield, IL, 84-88

33. Reenstra WR, Buras JA, Svoboda KS. Hyperbaric oxygen increases human dermal fibroblast proliferation, growth factor receptor number and in vitro wound closure. Undersea Hyperb Med, 1998; 25(Suppl):35-36

34. Patel V, Chivukula IV, Roy S, Khanna S, He G, Ojha N, Mehrotra A, Dias LM, Hunt TK, Sen CK. Oxygen: from the benefits of inducing VEGF expression to managing the risk of hyperbaric stress. Antioxid Redox Signal. 2005 Sep-Oct;7(9-10):1377-87

35. Hohn, DC, Hunt TK. Oxidative metabolism and microbicidal activity of rabbit phagocytes: Cells from wounds and peripheral blood, Surgical Forum, 1975, 26:85-87

36. Saiepour D. Glucose and insulin modulate phagocytosis and production of reactive oxygen metabolites in human neutrophil granulocytes, Umea [Sweden] University Medical Dissertations, 2006, pg14

37. Sbarra AJ, Karnovsky ML. The biochemical basis of Phyagocytosis I. Metabolic changes during the ingestion of particles by polymorphonuclear leukocytes; II. Incorporation of C14-labeled building blocks into lipid, protein, and glycogen of leukocytes during phagocytosis, J Biol Chem, 1959; 234(6):1355-1362 and 1960; 235(8):2224-2229

38. Hampton, MB, Kettle AJ, Winterbourn CC. Inside the neutrophil phagosome: Oxidants, myeloperoxidase, and Bactgerial Killing, Blood, 1998; 92(9):3007-3017

39. Johnson LC. Kinetics of osteoarthritis. Lab Invest. 1959 Nov-Dec;8:1223-41

40. Kaye D. Effect of hyperbaric oxygen on Clostridia in vitro and in vivo. Proc Soc Exp Biol Med. 1967 Feb;124(2):360-6

41. Unsworth IP, Sharp PA. Gas gangrene. An 11-year review of 73 cases managed with hyperbaric oxygen. Med J Aust. 1984 Mar 3;140(5):256-60

42. Fredette V. Effect of hyperbaric oxygen upon anaerobic streptococci. Can J Microbiol. 1967 Apr;13(4):423-5

43. Bornside GH. Bactericidal effect of hyperbaric oxygen determined by direct exposure. Proc Soc Exp Biol Med. 1969 Apr;130(4):1165-7

44. Manheim SD, Voleti C, Ludwig A, Jacobson JH. 2nd. Hyperbaric oxygen in the treatment of actino-mycosis. JAMA. 1969 Oct 20;210(3):552-3

45. John BV, Chamilos G, Kontoyiannis DP. Hyperbaric oxygen as an adjunctive treatment for zygomy-cosis. Clin Microbiol Infect. 2005 Jul;11(7):515-7

46. Barratt DM, Van Meter K, Asmar P, Nolan T, Trahan C, Garcia-Covarrubias L, Metzinger SE. Hyper-baric oxygen as an adjunct in zygomycosis: randomized controlled trial in a murine model. Antimi-crob Agents Chemother. 2001 Dec;45(12):3601-2

47. Hart GB, Lamb RC, Strauss MB. Gas gangrene. J Trauma. 1983 Nov;23(11):991-1000

48. Svendsen FJ. Treatement of clinically diagnosed brown recluse spider bites with hyperbaric oxygen: a clinical observation. J Arkansas Med Soc 1986; 83:199-204

49. Bangasser RP. Treatment of the Brown Recluse Spider Bite with Hyperbaric Oxygen Therapy in Hyperbaric Medicine Practice, 3rd Edition (eds Kindwall EP and Whelan HT) Best Publishing Company, Flagstaff AZ, 2008; 975-981

50. Verklin Rn, Mandel Gl. Aleteration of effectiveness of antibiotics by anaerobiosis. J Lab Clin Med 1977;89:65-71

51. Gruber RP, Brinkley FB, Amato JJ, Mendelson JA. Hyperbaric oxygen and pedicle flaps, skin grafts, and burns. Plast Reconstr Surg 1970; 45(1): 24-30

52. Strauss MB, Miller SS. The Role of Hyperbaric Oxygen in Crush Injury, Skeletal Muscle-Compart-ment Syndrome and Other Acute Traumatic Ischemias in Hyperbaric Medicine Practice, 3rd Edition (eds Kindwall EP and Whelan HT) Best Publishing Company, Flagstaff AZ, 2008; 757-790

53. Hurd TC, Dasmahapatra KS, Rush BF Jr, Machiedo GW. Red blood cell deformability in human and experimental sepsis. Arch Surg. 1988 Feb;123(2):217-20

54. Baskurt OK, Gelmont D, Meiselman HJ. Red blood cell deformability in sepsis. Am J Respir Crit Care Med. 1998 Feb;157(2):421-7

55. Powell RJ, Machiedo GW, Rush BF Jr. Decreased red blood cell deformability and impaired oxygen utilization during human sepsis. Am Surg. 1993 Jan;59(1):65-8

56. Thom SR, Lauermann MW, Hart GB. Intermittent hyperbaric oxygen therapy for reduction of mortality in experimental polymicrobial sepsis. J Infect Dis. 1986 Sep;154(3):504-10

57. Mathieu D, Goget J, Vinkier L, et al. Red blood cell deformability and hyperbaric oxygen therapy. (Abstract) HBO Review. 1985;6:280

58. Chambi IP, Ceverha MD, Hart GB, Strauss MB. Effect of hyperbaric oxygen in the permeability of the blood-brain-barrier. Eighth International Congress on Hyperbaric Medicine, Long Beach, CA, 1984

59. Lanse SB, Lee JC, Jacobs EA, Brody H. Changes in the permeability of the blood-brain barrier under hyperbaric oxygen conditions, Aviat Space Environ Med, 1978; 49(7):890-894

60. Hopf HW, Hunt TK, West JM, Blomquist P, Goodson WH 3rd, Jensen JA, Jonsson K, Paty PB, Rabkin JM, Upton RA, von Smitten K, Whitney JD. Wound tissue oxygen tension predicts the risk of wound infection in surgical patients. Arch Surg. 1997 Sep;132(9):997-1004

61. Mathieu D. Role of hyperbaric oxygen therapy in the management of lower extremity wounds. Int J Low Extrem Wounds. 2006 Dec;5(4):233-5

62. Kindwall EP. Contraindications and Side Effects to Hyperbaric Oxygen Treatment in Hyperbaric Medicine Practice, 3rd Edition (eds Kindwall EP and Whelan HT) Best Publishing Company, Flagstaff AZ, 2008; 285

63. Palmquist BM, Philipson B, Barr PO. Nuclear cataract and myopia during hyperbaric oxygen therapy. Br J Ophthalmol. 1984 Feb;68(2):113-7

64. Gesell LB, Trott A. De novo cataract development following a standard course of hyperbaric oxygen therapy. Undersea Hyperb Med. 2007 Nov-Dec;34(6):389-92

65. NFPA 99: Standard for Health Care Facilities, Chapter 20: Hyperbaric Facilities, 2005 Edition. National Fire Protection Association, 1 Batterymarch Park, Quincy MA 02269-9101

66. Hardy KR, Thom SR. Pathophysiology and treatment of carbon monoxide poisoning. J Toxicol Clin Toxicol. 1994;32(6):613-29

67. Thom SR, Keim LW. Carbon monoxide poisoning: a review epidemiology, pathophysiology, clinical findings, and treatment options including hyperbaric oxygen therapy. J Toxicol Clin Toxicol. 1989;27(3):141-56

68. Elkharrat D, Raphael JC, Korach JM, Jars-Guincestre MC, Chastang C, Harboun C, Gajdos P. Acute carbon monoxide intoxication and hyperbaric oxygen in pregnancy. Intensive Care Med. 1991;17(5):289-92

69. Jennings RT. Women and the hazardous environment: when the pregnant patient requires hyperbaric oxygen therapy. Aviat Space Environ Med. 1987 Apr;58(4):370-4

70. Gilman SC, Bradley ME, Greene KM, Fischer GJ. Fetal development: effects of decompression sickness and treatment. Aviat Space Environ Med. 1983 Nov;54(11):1040-2

71. Monstrey SJ, Mullick P, Narayanan K, Ramasastry SS. Hyperbaric oxygen therapy and free radical production: an experimental study in doxorubicin (Adriamycin) extravasation injuries. Ann Plast Surg. 1997 Feb;38(2):163-8

72. Berend N. The effect of bleomycin and oxygen on rat lung. Pathology. 1984 Apr;16(2):136-9

73. Kindwall E. Contraindications and side effects to hyperbaric oxygen treatment. In: Kindwall EP, Whelan HT, eds. Hyperbaric Medicine Practice. 2nd ed. Best Publishing Co;1999:83-97

74. Karagoz B, Suleymanoglu S, Uzun G, Bilgi O, Aydinoz S, Haholu A, Turken O, Onem Y, Kandemir EG. Hyperbaric oxygen therapy does not potentiate doxorubicin-induced cardiotoxicity in rats. Basic Clin Pharmacol Toxicol. 2008 Mar;102(3):287-92

75. Aksenov IV, Asciuto TJ, Strauss MB, Miller SS, Kulkarni VA, Hart GB. Contraindications for Hyperbaric Oxygen Treatments in Critically Ill Patients, American Thoracic Society International Conference, San Francisco, CA, Am J Resp Crit Care Med, 2007, 175: A220

76. Strauss MB. Hyperbaric oxygen as an intervention for managing wound hypoxia: Its role and usefulness in diabetic foot wounds, Foot Ankle Intl, 2005, 26(1):15-18

77. Strauss MB. Diabetic foot and leg wounds: principles, management and prevention. Primary Care Reports 2001;7(22):187-197

78. Strauss MB, Groner-Straus W. Wound scoring system streamlines decision-making. Biomechanics VI(8):37-43, Aug 1999

78. Strauss MB, Borer RC Jr., Borer KM. An algorithm approach to decision making in problem wounds. Undersea Hyperb Med. Vol 27 2000 Supplement pg 35

80. Borer KM, Borer RC Jr., Strauss MB. Prospective evaluation of a clinical wound score to identify lower extremity wounds for comprehensive wound management. Undersea Hyperb Med. Vol 27 2000 Supplement pg 34

PART **IV**

IDENTIFICATION AND MANAGEMENT OF THE "END-STAGE" WOUND

CHAPTER	TITLE	PAGE
11	THE "END-STAGE" HYPOXIC WOUND	293
12	OTHER "END-STAGE" WOUNDS	331

INTRODUCTION TO PART IV

"End-stage" wounds are those that are so serious that healing of the wound or avoidance of a major amputation is only a marginal possibility. The other alternative for wounds of this severity is initiation of comfort care/hospice measures. In other words, an "end-stage" wound is about as serious as a wound can be, yet offers some possibility of healing or avoidance of a lower limb amputation. On the **Wound Score** (0-to-10) continuum, the "end-stage" wound is in the 2 ½ to 4 ½ point range. It represents a transition between the "problem" and the "futile" wound and overlaps each to some extent (Part IV, Figure 1). Management requires the use of the five strategies previously discussed (Part III), plus the utilization of special considerations that are needed for each of the "end-stage" wound types. The "end-stage" wound needs to be differentiated from the "futile" wound in which there is no chance of healing or avoidance of an amputation, and the "problem" wound where there is a high likelihood of healing.

With the "end-stage" wound, an attempt to salvage the limb and/or heal the wound versus recommending a major amputation or comfort care measures only (if the wound is that of a truncal pressure sore) requires subsidiary information. The patient's health status, nutrition, and aspirations must be known before an answer can be given. The **Host-Function Score** (Table 2-4 and repeated in this introduction) provides a "quick and easy" evaluation of the patient's overall health and level of function. As mentioned before (Chapter 2), age, ambulation, cardiovascular/renal status, smoking/steroid history, and neurological deficits are each graded from 0 to 2 with two being best and zero being the worst to generate the **Host-Function Score**. By summating the grades of the five assessments, a 0 to 10 score is established. Information from Chapter 6 can be used to supplement information from the **Host-Function Score** and further support the decision for salvage versus major amputation (and/or initiation of comfort care only measures). In general, in order to recommend salvage of an "end-stage" wound, the **Host-Function Score** should be five points or greater. The nutritional status, the next factor to consider in the decision making process, must be known. As discussed before (Chapter 6), nutrition problems can always be managed using a hierarchy of interventions (Figure 6-6).

The patient's (and family members') desire to salvage the leg (and/or heal the extremity wound or the truncal pressure sore) is also "quick and easy" to determine by using the zero to ten point **Goal-Aspiration Score** (Table 1-3 and repeated in this introduction). A **Goal-Aspiration Score** of five points or greater provides additional support to justify an attempt to salvage the limb and/or heal the wound. Consequently, utilization of the **Host-Function Score** and **Goal-Aspiration Score** and the nutrition assessment provide the basis for making intelligent recommendations for managing the "end-stage" wound. A variety of conditions qualify as "end-stage" wounds that are in the transition zone between "problem" and "futile" wound types. Inadequate perfusion (and oxygenation) to the wound site is the most frequent cause (Chapter 11). Ironically, some "end-stage wounds" such as those associated with Charcot arthropathy and erythromyalgia are a consequence of too much blood supply. Other "end-stage" wounds are due to malnutrition, venous stasis problems, radiation injury, or collagen vascular diseases. Finally, "end-stage" wounds, especially those in the truncal region, are frequently a consequence of intractable joint contractures. The chapters in this part of *MasterMinding Wounds* discuss the conditions that meet the criteria for "end-stage" wounds, describe the considerations essential in decision making for their management, and the interventions used to salvage these wounds when the decision is made to do so.

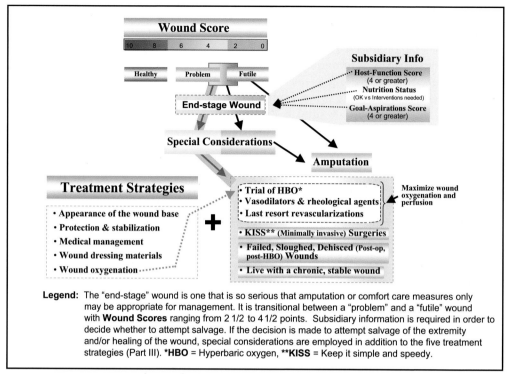

Part IV, Figure 1. Decision making and management of the "end-stage" wound.

PART IV, TABLE 1. THE HOST-FUNCTION SCORE AS A TOOL FOR DECISION MAKING REGARDING THE "END-STAGE" WOUND (Reiteration of Table 2-4)

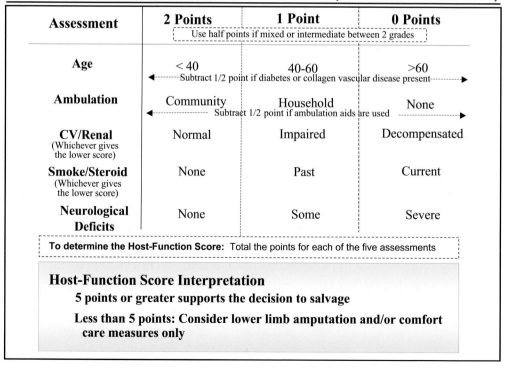

Assessment	2 Points	1 Point	0 Points
	Use half points if mixed or intermediate between 2 grades		
Age	< 40	40-60	>60
	◄------Subtract 1/2 point if diabetes or collagen vascular disease present------►		
Ambulation	Community	Household	None
	◄------ Subtract 1/2 point if ambulation aids are used ------►		
CV/Renal (Whichever gives the lower score)	Normal	Impaired	Decompensated
Smoke/Steroid (Whichever gives the lower score)	None	Past	Current
Neurological Deficits	None	Some	Severe

To determine the Host-Function Score: Total the points for each of the five assessments

Host-Function Score Interpretation

5 points or greater supports the decision to salvage

Less than 5 points: Consider lower limb amputation and/or comfort care measures only

PART IV, TABLE 2. THE GOAL-ASPIRATION SCORE AS A TOOL FOR DECISION MAKING REGARDING THE "END-STAGE" WOUND (Reiteration of Table 1-3)

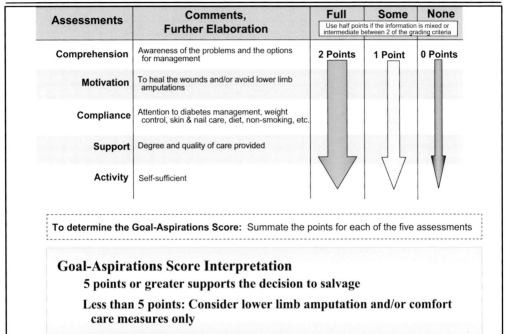

Assessments	Comments, Further Elaboration	Full	Some	None
		Use half points if the information is mixed or intermediate between 2 of the grading criteria		
Comprehension	Awareness of the problems and the options for management	2 Points	1 Point	0 Points
Motivation	To heal the wounds and/or avoid lower limb amputations			
Compliance	Attention to diabetes management, weight control, skin & nail care, diet, non-smoking, etc.			
Support	Degree and quality of care provided			
Activity	Self-sufficient			

To determine the Goal-Aspirations Score: Summate the points for each of the five assessments

Goal-Aspirations Score Interpretation

5 points or greater supports the decision to salvage

Less than 5 points: Consider lower limb amputation and/or comfort care measures only

CHAPTER

THE "END-STAGE" HYPOXIC WOUND

CHAPTER ELEVEN OVERVIEW

INTRODUCTION 295

A TRIAL OF HYPERBARIC OXYGEN 296

PHARMACOLOGICAL METHODS TO INCREASE PERFUSION AND
  THE ONE-TWO-THREE PROTOCOL 300

LAST RESORT DISTAL ARTERIAL BYPASS SURGERY 304

MINIMALLY INVASIVE,
  "KEEP IT SIMPLE AND SPEEDY" SURGERIES 308

SALVAGING THE FAILED, SLOUGHED, DEHISCED, POST-OP,
  POST-HBO WOUND 320

LIVING WITH A CHRONIC,
  STABLE, NON-HEALING WOUND 325

CONCLUSIONS 326

QUESTIONS 328

REFERENCES 329

"It doesn't take much to keep tissues alive;
to achieve wound healing is another matter."

INTRODUCTION

Defining the "End-Stage" Wound – Of all the "end-stage" wounds, the hypoxic wound due to peripheral arterial disease is the most common. It is also the one for which the most alternatives for management exist. Combinations of interventions are usually used. Diagnosis of the "end-stage" wound becomes obvious when profound ischemia is evident from the vascular examination, the wound is not healing in the expected manner, and the other factors that interfere with wound healing have been appropriately managed. A **Wound Score** in the 2 ½ to 4 ½ point range helps to confirm the diagnosis. In the past, the ankle-brachial index (ABI) was used as the standard for vascular assessment of the ischemic foot; however, it is unreliable, especially in the diabetic limb. Spurious readings from transmission of the pulse waveform along the calcified blood vessel may give the impression that perfusion is adequate. Even though there is no substitute for the clinical evaluation, transcutaneous oxygen measurements and Doppler pulse wave assessments should be used as an adjunct to assess circulation and tissue oxygenation and substantiate findings from the clinical exam.

Blood flow and Metabolic Requirements – As mentioned earlier (Chapter 2), in the steady state, non-wound healing situation, blood flow requirements to resting non-critical tissues such as the skin, subcutaneous tissues and connective tissues is minimal.[1] If the steady-state situation for these tissues is assigned a perfusion, metabolic requirement of one, then to meet healing and infection control requirements, they need to increase 20-fold or more.[1] If perfusion cannot meet these increased demands, healing does not occur as is so often observed in the "end-stage" hypoxic wound. Juxta-wound transcutaneous oxygen measurements (coupled with transcutaneous carbon dioxide measurements) provide a simplified decision-making matrix for management options, especially with the adjunctive use of hyperbaric oxygen, and are highly predictable of outcomes (Figure 11-1).[2] If carbon dioxide levels are normal (indicating enough perfusion to carry off carbon dioxide, the major waste product of metabolism), but transcutaneous

> The ability for the blood to transport carbon dioxide away from tissues is about 20 times greater than its ability to transport oxygen to the tissues. This is because of the increased diffusibility and blood carrying capacity of carbon dioxide as compared to oxygen.

oxygen levels are low, hyperbaric oxygen is indicated and highly likely to be effective in correcting the hypoxic condition. Thus, transcutaneous oxygen measurements with hyperbaric oxygen can be diagnostic, help define the end-stage hypoxic wound, and provide objective indications for using hyperbaric oxygen (Figure 11-1). In the "end-stage" wound, transcutaneous oxygen measurements measured in room air are typically less than 20 mmHg, and in the extremely ischemic/hypoxic foot, it is not unusual for readings to be below 5 mmHg. If the transcutaneous oxygen measurements with hyperbaric oxygen do not increase to over 50 mmHg, then wound healing is very unlikely unless perfusion is improved with angioplasty and/or revascularization.

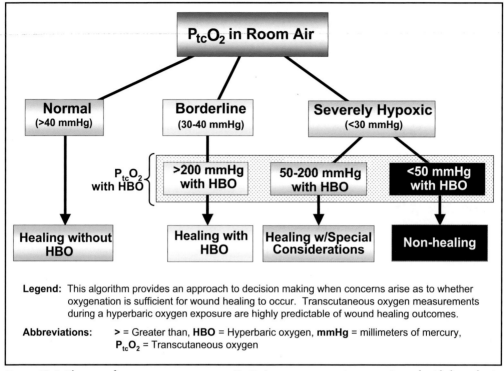

Figure 11-1. The use of transcutaneous oxygen (PtcO₂) measurements in room air and with hyperbaric oxygen (HBO) to make management decisions.

Making Decisions About Management of "End-Stage" Wounds – Unfortunately, in futile situations angioplasty and revascularization have often already been done, but have not resolved the perfusion problem or are not feasible because of the diffuse nature of the disease and inadequate runoff. Nonetheless, at times interventions are performed for the "futile" wound (**Wound Score** less than 4) in attempt to avoid major lower limb amputations. In such situations, information from the **Host-Function Score** and the **Goal-Aspiration Score** is crucial. If one or both scores are low, then limb salvage should not be attempted. If the scores are reasonable, that is, five or above, a concerted effort to heal the wound and salvage the limb is justified, especially if the patient already has a lower limb amputation on the contralateral side. The decision is rarely difficult to make if the **Goal-Aspiration Score** and **Host-Function Scores** are utilized in the decision making process.[3] The remainder of this chapter discusses five techniques that are effective in avoiding major lower limb amputations in the "end-stage" wound and even sometimes in the "futile" wound (providing **Host-Function** and **Goal-Aspiration Scores** justify the care required). Usually for the "futile" wound, the patient and/or their caregivers must decide whether to live with a chronic non-healing wound or undergo a lower limb amputation.

A TRIAL OF HYPERBARIC OXYGEN
Making a Decision for Using Hyperbaric Oxygen for the "End-Stage" Wound – The mechanisms of hyperbaric oxygen that are especially applicable to wounds were described previously (Chapter 10). Since there are both immediate effects from hyper-oxygenation as well as delayed effects that promote wound healing, such as fibroblast

Clinical correlations:

A 19-year-old male sustains a severe open fracture and arterial injury of his left leg. After debridement, stabilization, with revascularization, the patient's limb was in jeopardy of amputation because of marginally viable soft tissues around the exposed fracture site, which had missing bone. The **Wound Score** was three. His **Host-Function Score** and **Goal-Aspiration Score** were both 10. The decision to do everything possible to salvage the limb was easy to make based on his **Host-Function Score** and **Goal-Aspiration Score** and justified using hyperbaric oxygen, doing a microvascular free flap and delayed bone grafting.

A 57-year-old diabetic male with end-stage renal disease, dementia, bedridden and unable to swallow because of residuals of stroke has a necrotic based ulcer on the back of his heel. Even though his **Wound Score** was four (on the 0 to 10 scale), the decision to perform a below knee amputation was made because of very low **Host-Function Score** (2 points) and **Goal-Aspiration Score** (1½ points).

Comment:

The **Host-Function Score** and **Goal-Aspiration Score** provide objective criteria to substantiate decisions whether to attempt to salvage an "end-stage" wound or recommend lower limb amputation.

---

function and angiogenesis, it seems logical that a trial of hyperbaric oxygen is warranted in certain specific situations.[4] This recommendation is based on observations that transcutaneous oxygen readings increase during courses of hyperbaric oxygen therapy.[5,6] These decisions to salvage the wounds arise when the **Wound Score** is less than three, the **Host-Function** and **Goal-Aspiration Scores** are five or greater, the wound is an approved use of hyperbaric oxygen (Chapter 10), and the patient and/or family members want everything possible to be done to avoid a lower limb amputation. Regardless of the initially low transcutaneous oxygen readings during a single hyperbaric oxygen exposure, a trial of hyperbaric oxygen is recommended in these circumstances. Improvements in juxta-wound transcutaneous measurements usually precede and are highly predictive of eventual improvement in the wound. Furthermore, juxta-wound transcutaneous oxygen measurements predict wound healing better than toe and/or ankle Doppler blood pressures.[7]

"End-Stage" Wound Outcomes – Usually, the hyperbaric oxygen treatments are done in conjunction with the other interventions for avoiding amputation in the "end-stage" wound that are discussed subsequently in this chapter. Three outcomes have been observed with this approach. First, the wound deteriorates during the course of hyperbaric oxygen treatments (and other measures to improve perfusion), and the patient requires a lower limb amputation. If the patient refuses the amputation, the consequences of living with the wound may contribute to comorbidities such as anemias, malaise, renal insufficiency, altered mental status, or death from the septic process. Usually if the patient and/or family are satisfied that everything possible has been done and are made aware of what the potential consequences of delayed surgery are, they become willing to accept a lower limb amputation. The second option is that the wound stabilizes after the strategic management interventions, including hyperbaric oxygen, have been done. That is, it does not improve, but likewise it does not continue to worsen. In this stable wound situation, the patient often opts to live with the wound, perform daily dressing changes, and use protective footwear for limited mobility. The third

Clinical correlations:

A 64-year-old male with diabetes and advanced coronary artery disease, requiring an implantable defibrillator, with end-stage renal disease managed with a renal transplant had progressively deteriorating wounds after bilateral trans-metatarsal amputations.

The patient refused to consider lower limb amputations. After a course of 21 hyperbaric oxygen treatments, the open transmetatarsal wounds stabilized enough that with daily dressing changes he was able to remain a limited ambulator using a walkerette and protective footwear. Limited in-office debridements were done at monthly rechecks. Mobility and very positive feelings about "keeping" his feet sustained the patient and even allowed him to travel over a three and a half year period. Thereafter, he died while sleeping, presumably from a new cardiac event.

Comment:

Although the patient and his family were inconvenienced by the wounds and the care they required, he remained independent for his household activities. With his cardiac status as it was, the energy demands of using bilateral leg prostheses would probably have made him wheelchair bound and totally dependent on his family for all activities had he undergone bilateral below knee amputations.

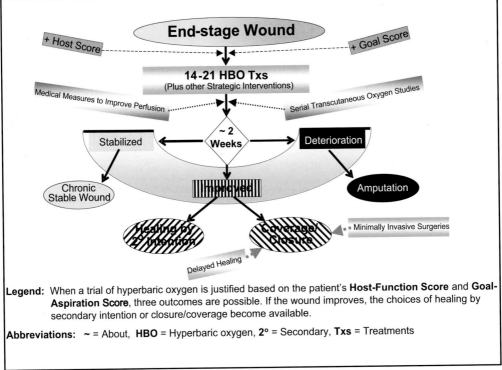

Legend: When a trial of hyperbaric oxygen is justified based on the patient's **Host-Function Score** and **Goal-Aspiration Score**, three outcomes are possible. If the wound improves, the choices of healing by secondary intention or closure/coverage become available.

Abbreviations: ~ = About, **HBO** = Hyperbaric oxygen, **2°** = Secondary, **Txs** = Treatments

Figure 11-2. Outcome permutations in the hypoxic, "end-stage" wound where a trial of hyperbaric oxygenation has been initiated.

Clinical correlations:

A 56-year-old female with diabetes and end-stage renal disease on dialysis acutely developed a gangrenous right great toe. The patient had been a limited community ambulator without the requirement for walking aids even though she had advanced, non-reconstructable peripheral arterial disease. Juxta-toe transcutaneous oxygen measurements, in room air and with hyperbaric oxygen, predicted failure of any amputation distal to the below knee level. The demarcation between the gangrenous hallux and the adjacent forefoot was not sharply defined. A thin exudate covered the transition zone of the non-viable toe and the adjacent forefoot. Even though the foot was very ischemic, pain was easily managed with one or two Vicodin® (acetominophen and hydrocodone) tablets a day.

After options were presented to the patient, she elected to undergo a course of 14 hyperbaric oxygen treatments for the acute peripheral ischemic process involving the great toe. The hallux began to mummify and the demarcation between viable and non-viable tissues became sharp. The exudate cleared. The decision was made to give an additional seven hyperbaric oxygen treatments for its angiogenesis effect, allow the hallux to go onto auto-amputation and permit the patient to continue her ambulatory activities with protective footwear.

Comment:

Although the patient is at risk for complications such as the development of new areas of gangrene in the foot and an ascending necrotizing soft tissue infection into the foot, in the absence of severe pain a lower limb amputation was avoided. The minimal perception of pain in the presence of the profoundly ischemic foot was due to the sensory neuropathy. Even though the hyperbaric oxygen treatments only minimally augmented the transcutaneous oxygen readings, the clinical progress supported the benefit of this modality. Demarcation and mummification were presumably due to improved oxygen availability to the margins of the severely ischemic tissues from angiogenesis induced by hyperbaric oxygen treatments.

option is that the wound improves sufficiently that closure and/or coverage measures can be done with expectations of reasonable outcomes. Typically minimally invasive, "Keep it Simple and Speedy" surgical techniques (soon to be described) are utilized in order to optimize outcomes. Often in this group of patients, the initial closure fails or partially fails. Healing by secondary intention usually occurs if the patient and caregivers are motivated enough (as the **Goal-Aspiration Score** helps ascertain) to manage the post-op failed, sloughed, dehisced wound and carry it through the four stages of delayed healing (as will also be discussed subsequently in this chapter).

Hyperbaric Oxygen Treatment Protocols for the "End-Stage" Wound – If a trial of hyperbaric oxygen is instituted, pre-established protocols should be followed starting with 14 daily hyperbaric oxygen treatments. It is important that the patient and/or the family appreciate the "end-stage" nature of the wound and what the three possible outcomes from the trial of hyperbaric oxygen therapy are, that is, improvement, stabilization, or deterioration (Figure 11-2). Progress is established by clinical observation and/or improvements in transcutaneous oxygen measurements. At this point, especially if progress is verified by the **Wound Score**, an additional seven to 14 hyperbaric oxygen treatments are recommended in conjunction with continuing optimal wound management and antibiotics. If no improvement occurs during the initial course of hyperbaric oxygen treatments, a decision for the patient to live with a chronic wound or proceed to a lower limb amputation is made. If the wound deteriorates during the course of hyperbaric oxygen treatments and the other strategic management interventions, a lower limb amputation is advised.

PHARMACOLOGICAL METHODS TO INCREASE PERFUSION AND THE ONE-TWO-THREE PROTOCOL

Overview – Pharmacological agents provide a second method for augmenting oxygen delivery to the "end-stage" wound. Factors, in addition to blood vessel disease, affect perfusion and oxygen delivery to tissues (Figure 11-3). Many of the factors are remedial; that is, they can be corrected with specific interventions such as giving a transfusion for anemia. This section discusses the agents that affect blood rheology and the microcirculation, or the flow of the blood itself. These agents work through a variety of mechanisms (Table 11-1). While the effects of hyperbaric oxygen for improving tissue oxygenation are quantifiable with transcutaneous oxygen measurements available in "real time" readouts (Chapter 10) and can be verified by transcutaneous oxygen measurements, those for improving blood rheology and flow in the microcirculation are not. Their use is justified by knowing how the agents' mechanisms affect the underlying pathophysiology of these problems. Often, an agent to improve blood flow and oxygen delivery in the microcirculation is used in conjunction with other oxygen augmenting

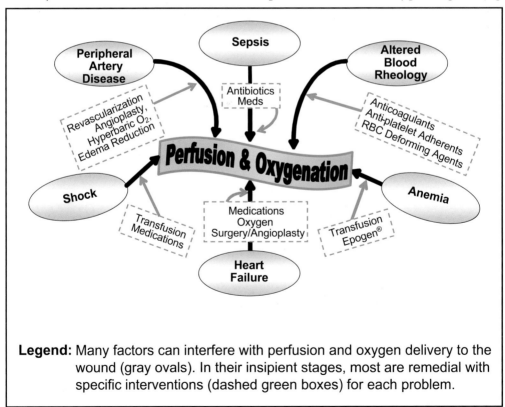

Legend: Many factors can interfere with perfusion and oxygen delivery to the wound (gray ovals). In their insipient stages, most are remedial with specific interventions (dashed green boxes) for each problem.

Figure 11-3. Problems that interfere with wound perfusion and oxygenation—and methods to manage these problems.

TABLE 11-1. AGENTS TO IMPROVE BLOOD RHEOLOGY AND PERFUSION

Mechanisms	Agents (Brand names)	Dose (Duration)[1]	Comments
Anticoagulation	Warfarin (Coumadin®)	4 mg +/-3 mg daily PO (5 days)	Marked individual variations in dosing; monitoring required with INR's; Inhibits vitamin K-dependent coagulation factor synthesis; Reversed with vitamin K and fresh frozen plasma
	Unfractionated Heparin	5,000 units q 6 hrs IV or SQ (6 hrs)	Acts at multiple sites in coagulation process; binds to antithrombin III, catalyzing inactivation of thrombin and other clotting factors; Monitored with PTT; Reversed with protamine sulfate
	Enoxaparin (Lovenox®), low molecular weight heparin	40 mg SQ daily (24-36 hrs)	Mechanism similar to unfractionated heparin, but no lab monitoring required
Anti-platelet Aggregation	Aspirin	81-320 mg daily (5 days)	Not usually monitored; increases bleeding time
	Low molecular weigh dextran (Rheomacrodex®)	500 cc q 12 hrs; (24 hrs)	Same as above
	Clopidrogel bisulfate (Plavix®)	75 mg daily (5-7 days)	Inhibits adenosine diphosphate binding to platelet receptors
	Cilostazol (Pletal®)	100 mg PO BID (4 days)	Inhibits cellular phosphodiesterase
	Ticlopidine hydrochoride (Ticlid®)	250 mg PO BID (up to 30 days)	Inhibits denosine diphosphate-induced platelet-fibrinogen binding
Increased RBC Deformability	Pentoxifylline (Trental®)	400 mg TID (120 day, the lifespan of the RBC, to reach its full effect)	Improves RBC deformability to help the 7.5 micron RBC pass through the 5 micron wide capillary; Also, has anti-platelet agglutination effects
Vasodilation	Nitroglycerin preparations (Nitro-Dur®, Nitro-Bid®)	0.1 - 0.4 mg/hr release from patches daily (24 hours)	Local vasodilation via direct absorption through the skin; may cause headache & hypotension
	Nefidipine (Procardia®)	60 mg SR daily (24 hours)	Inhibits calcium ion influx into vascular smooth muscle and myocardium; side effects include hypotension, bradycardia, dizziness

KEY: Duration indicates the time it takes for medication to reach its full effectiveness and/or be eliminated from the body
Abbreviations: **cc** = cubic centimeters, **INR** = International Normalized Ratio, **IM** = intramuscular, **IV** = intravenous, **mg** = milligrams, **po** = per os = orally ingested, **q** = every, **RBC** = red blood cell, **SR** = sustained release, **BID** = twice a day, **TID** = three times a day, **PT** = Prothrombin Time

Clinical correlations:

A 65-year-old male, non-diabetic without peripheral neuropathy developed gangrene over the tips of several toes of his left foot. These ulcerated and became so painful that optimal wound care was not possible. The gangrene was thought to be due to microemboli (trash syndrome) following a left iliofemoral angioplasty.

As an alternative to a proposed transmetatarsal amputation, hyperbaric oxygen and pentoxifylline (Trental®) were started for the acute peripheral ischemia. Pentoxifylline improves red blood cell deformity as well as reducing platelet adhesiveness, but takes several weeks to become effective. Rapidly, pain issues improved enough that cleansing and bandaging could be done with minimal discomfort for the patient. Hyperbaric treatments were stopped after 21 sessions. The gangrenous portions of the toe tips mummified and went onto auto-amputation. Pentoxifylline was continued.

Comment:

Hyperbaric oxygen appeared to have both immediate and long-standing effects for the patient's ischemia problems of his toes. The immediate effects were those associated with hyperoxygenation resulting in pain relief and making it possible to do wound care. Angiogenesis, a delayed, secondary mechanism, stabilized the condition thereby allowing discontinuation of hyperbaric oxygen. The pharmacological actions of pentoxifylline complemented both effects, taking several weeks to become effective. Once healing became evident and perfusion improved, hyperbaric oxygen was no longer needed, but pentoxifylline was continued.

interventions. Two or more agents that have different mechanisms may be used simultaneously. Their use is often continued after wound healing has been achieved. This is in contrast to hyperbaric oxygen where the number of treatments is usually quite specific and is usually stopped as soon as the wound shows signs of improvement.

Justification for Use of Pharmacological Agents – Although the decisions to use pharmacological agents to supplement wound perfusion are largely empirical, there are some guidelines for their selection. Agents are usually selected for reasons other than to augment perfusion for an "end-stage" wound. For example, warfarin (Coumadin®) may be prescribed by the vascular surgeon after revascularizations, clopidrogrel (Plavix®) by the cardiologist after coronary artery angioplasty, and enoxaparin (Lovenox®) by the traumatologist after surgeries for severe injuries. If a co-existent "problem" wound is present, these agents may coincidentally improve perfusion to it. There are logical reasons for prescribing two agents concurrently to improve blood rheology and the microcirculation for the "end-stage" wound. For example, it seems logical to use pentoxifylline (Trental®) for its effects on red blood cell deformability in conjunction with an anti-platelet medication such as clopidrogrel (Plavix®) or aspirin.

One-Two-Three Protocol – The One-Two-Three Protocol is a technique to determine which agents will most effectively augment juxta-wound transcutaneous oxygen measurements in those "end-stage" wounds where the decision to avoid lower limb amputation has been made. The protocol has four steps:

1. A juxta-wound transcutaneous oxygen measure is obtained in room air and with hyperbaric oxygen. If it is in the "non-responder" range with hyperbaric oxygen, that is, less than 50 mmHg, the One-Two-Three Protocol is initiated with the day one measurements used as a baseline.
2. On day two, a 2 mg/hr nitroglycerin impregnated patch (e.g. Nitro-Dur®) is applied just proximal to the wound, and two to four hours later the juxta-wound transcutaneous oxygen measurements are repeated in room air and with hyperbaric oxygen.
3. On day three, nefedipine (Procardia XL®; 60 mg orally) is taken, and four to six hours later the transcutaneous oxygen measurements are repeated as done for day two.
4. Finally, on day four, both the nitroglycerin preparation and nefidipine are used. Transcutaneous oxygen measurements are repeated as above.

From this information, the permutation that elevates the transcutaneous oxygen the most is used as an adjunct to hyperbaric oxygen treatments. Initial experiences have shown that there are substantial individual variations in the responses to the One-Two-Three Protocol. In about two-thirds of the cases, the combination was not as effective as using either agent alone.[8] Nefedipine was contraindicated in a substantial number of patients because of the concurrent use of other cardiac medications.

> Does it make a difference which calcium channel blocker is used to improve perfusion? The answer appears to be "yes." Calcium channel blockers other than nifedipine (Procardia®) in conjunction with hyperbaric oxygen may generate a capillary leak especially in the pulmonary vasculature. For example, the use of diltiazem (Cardizem®), another calcium channel blocker, was associated with pulmonary edema when hyperbaric oxygen was used in a patient on this medication.

Bleeding Challenges and Surgery – Agents to maintain blood flow either with or without associated revascularization procedures can interfere with other elements of strategic management (Table 11-1). The major concern is that of excessive and/or uncontrolled bleeding when definitive surgeries are done while the patient is on agents to improve blood flow. However, if the definitive surgeries are very distal on the extremity and perfusion to the operative area is still marginal, definitive surgeries such as toe, distal forefoot, and partial ray amputations can usually be done without concerns of uncontrollable bleeding. If bleeding becomes excessive during surgeries, specific interventions are usually successful in controlling it. First, a distally applied tourniquet using an elastic (Ace®) bandage can effectively control bleeding during the actual surgery. Second, whereas electrocautery may not effectively control bleeding, suture ligatures usually do so. Third, packing the wound with an absorbable gelatin sponge (Surgifoam®, Gelfoam®) impregnated with thrombin or other haemostatic agents controls diffuse, oozing type of blood loss as is so often observed in patients on platelet anti-agglutination agents. Finally, if the operative sites cannot be closed primarily due to infection or other reasons, sutures

Clinical correlations:
A 56-year-old male with diabetes required a below-knee amputation because of a non-healing wound in a foot which could not be revascularized. Post-operatively, the patient resumed aspirin and Plavix® because of his history of coronary artery stenting.

On the fifth post-op day, the patient fell onto his stump while attempting an unassisted transfer from his bed to a wheelchair. The wound dehisced totally with marked bleeding from the open stump end. Bleeding could not be controlled with compression dressings.

Gelfoam® and Thrombin® were obtained from the operating room and placed over the bleeding surfaces. Several large sutures were placed in order to partially approximate the flaps and to tamponade the bleeding. These latter two measures controlled the bleeding. Four units of packed red blood cells were transfused to compensate for the blood loss.

The anticoagulants were discontinued. About a week after the accident, the failed below knee amputation site was revised. This healed uneventfully and the patient subsequently resumed ambulation with a prosthesis.

Comment:
This scenario illustrates several points. First, had the patient worn the knee immobilizer as instructed, and had he requested assistance for the transfer as is recommended in the immediate post-op period, this serious complication undoubtedly would not have occurred.

Second, the bleeding had almost reached the point that a tourniquet was required. Because of the diffuse nature of the bleeding, that is, no identifiable vessels to ligate, returning the patient to the operating room would not have offered much more benefit than carrying out the interventions immediately at the patient's bedside.

Third, failure to precisely follow the post-operative protection, the immobilization strategy resulted in a major complication, near disaster. Finally, the use of anticoagulants post-operatively requires added diligence, since complications from them can be as serious as the problems they are trying to prevent.

to partially approximate the flaps will have a tamponading effect to control blood loss. In all situations where post-operative bleeding is a concern, drains should be placed before wound closure to prevent hematoma formation and the complications associated with this occurrence. In addition, post-operative monitoring of hematocrit/hemoglobin should be done and packed red blood cell transfusions given, if indicated.

Managing Chronic Anticoagulation and Surgeries – If major surgeries that are proximal to the foot and/or likely to be of long duration are to be performed, and the patient requires chronic anticoagulation with agents such as warfarin (Coumadin®), aspirin, or clopidrogrel (Plavix®), these agents should be discontinued five to seven days prior to surgery. If necessary, to maintain anticoagulation in the interim, then unfractionated heparin or low molecular weight heparin (enoxaparin - Lovenox®) can be used to maintain anticoagulation until immediately prior (6 hours for unfractionated heparin and 12 hours for enoxaparin) to surgery. These agents can be resumed post-operatively again to provide immediate anti-coagulation protection when post-operative bleeding has stabilized. Concomitantly with post-operative stabilization of bleeding, the chronic anti-coagulation agent is restarted and when at protective levels, the immediate-acting agent discontinued. If immediate surgery is required due to uncontrolled limb threatening infection or acute limb threatening ischemia and the patient is on warfarin (Coumadin®), Vitamin K and fresh frozen plasma should be given prior to surgery to reduce blood losses during surgery. If the patient is on clopidrogrel (Plavix®) and immediate surgery is required, be prepared for blood loss during surgery since no medications are currently available to immediately counteract this anti-coagulant. Preparations include having blood typed and crossed and available in the operating room and being prepared to control bleeding during surgery with the techniques previously described.

Preventing Post-operative Bleeding Complications – Finally, patients with "problem" wounds who also are on anticoagulants have an increased likelihood of post-operative bleeding complications. These include hematoma formation, oozing of blood from the skin flap edges leading to dehiscence, and persistent bleeding from the wound base. Extraordinary operative site protection and wound stabilization measures should be done in order to reduce the chances of these complications. They include utilizing the protection strategies tactics described previously (Chapter 7). For foot and ankle surgeries, at the minimum, post-operative splinting should be done. For knee and leg surgeries, lower extremity (long leg) casts or knee-immobilizing splints should be used. Dressings should be meticulously applied and elastic wraps used to maintain uniform compression without interfering with blood flow.

LAST RESORT DISTAL ARTERIAL BYPASS SURGERY

Revascularization Considerations – The value of arterial bypass surgery, angioplasty, and/or stenting to improve perfusion is without question. However, with the "end-stage" wound, there may only be limited options for revascularization. Vascular assessment of the limb with the "end-stage" wound can be challenging, but an algorithmic approach, as described below, provides a logical approach to the assessment.[9] The vascular surgeon with experience in distal bypass surgeries can be an invaluable asset to the wound team and can often times make the difference whether wound healing is successful or not. Obviously, without adequate perfusion, wound healing is impossible. The challenge is the situation where the perfusion is marginal, but revascularization is not feasible or will only be of limited value. Predictors of failures in lower extremity revascularizations include: 1) impaired ambulation before surgery, 2) chronic kidney disease/end-stage renal disease, 3) hyperlipidemia, 4) gangrene and 5) bypass surgery distal to the inguinal area.[10] Likewise, success of the revascularization should not only be measured by patency of the graft, but also by wound healing, need for re-operation, independent living status and continued ability to ambulate.[10]

Perfusion Work-up – The perfusion work-up of the extremity with an "end-stage" wound is done in a step-wise fashion (Figure 11-4).[9] The assessment starts with the physical exam. Detection of pulses is the hallmark of this exam. As mentioned previously (Chapter 5), the examination for pulses can be supplemented with evaluation of skin temperature, skin color and capillary refill. Step two is the use of the Doppler to detect pulses. Simple Doppler readings may be spurious due to transmitted pulsations through calcified blood vessels. A better technique is the use of a Doppler that displays wave forms. If triphasic or biphasic, perfusion is probably adequate. If monophasic, perfusion is usually inadequate and not sufficient to meet the additional blood flow requirements for healing of a wound and/or controlling infection. Additional perfusion and tissue oxygenation assessments such as angiography and transcutaneous oxygen measurements should be done if healing is not progressing. When perfusion is marginal from the angiography studies, juxta-wound transcutaneous oxygen and carbon dioxide measurements while breathing room air and with hyperbaric oxygen should be obtained. Permutations for interpretation of results are described in the next paragraph. If the perfusion exam demonstrates overt vascular insufficiency and/or rest pain or claudication symptoms are obtained from the history, proceeding directly to angiography is recommended. Although angiography using dye is the gold standard for making decisions about revascularization, there are potential complications associated with this study. Complications include bleeding and hematoma formation around the arteriotomy site, renal shut down from the contrast agent especially in patients with

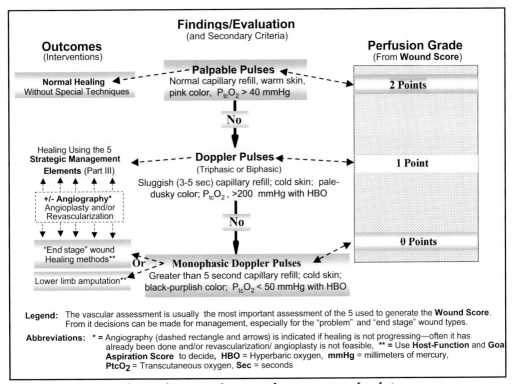

Figure 11-4. Decision making and anticipated outcomes from assessment of perfusion.

chronic kidney disease and allergic reactions to the contrast agent. The magnetic resonance angiogram (MRA) is a newer technique that eliminates these complications, but presently does not provide as precise information about blood flow or blood outflow as an angiogram using intravenous dye. In about half the cases, the MRA provides enough information to proceed with surgery. In the other half, angiograms with contrast agent are needed to arrive at these decisions.

Permutations from Juxta-Wound Transcutaneous O_2 and CO_2 Measurements – A simple four-cell matrix simplifies decision making for oxygen supplementation interventions when transcutaneous oxygen and carbon dioxide measurements are available (Table 11-2). The guideline complements the juxta-wound oxygen tension values from the algorithm used to predict healing of wounds (Figure 11-1).[11, 12] If juxta-wound transcutaneous oxygen and carbon dioxide measurements are in the normal range, wound healing is expected to occur without using adjunctive methods to augment oxygen availability to the wound. If the oxygen readings are low, but carbon dioxide tensions are in a normal range, this suggests the wound is hypoxic, but has enough flow to carry away carbon dioxide, which is 20 times more transportable in the blood than oxygen.[13] This is the permutation where hyperbaric oxygen is indicated. If both are abnormal (i.e. low O_2's and high CO_2's), healing will not likely occur without substantially improving blood flow to the wound site with revascularization, stenting or angioplasty. This permutation describes the situation where flow is so diminished that it is inadequate to carry the highly transportable carbon dioxide away from the wound site. The fourth permutation is the unusual situation where juxta-wound oxygen tensions are adequate for healing, but carbon dioxide tensions are high. This suggests that blood flow is so impaired that it is inadequate to carry away carbon dioxide, while there is a concomitant lack of oxygen utilization. Clinical conditions in which this may be observed include venous stasis and

TABLE 11-2. JUXTA-WOUND TRANSCUTANEOUS O_2 AND CO_2 MEASUREMENT PERMUTATIONS, EXPECTATIONS AND INTERVENTIONS FOR WOUND HEALING

Transcutaneous Measurements	O_2 Measurements	
	Normal (>40 mmHg)	**Low** (<30 mmHg)
Normal (40 mmHg +/- 4 mmHg)	**Healing with Room Air** (Wound healing expected without special interventions such as HBO and/or revascularization)	**Healing with HBO** (Hypoxic wound **with** enough perfusion to carry off CO_2, but inadequate O_2 for healing)
High (> 44 mmHg)	**Special Situations** (Outflow and/or utilization problems such as venous stasis disease, anteriovenous fistulas, compartment syndromes or anaerobic metabolism	Revascularization without enough CO2 not

(leftmost label: **CO_2 Measurements**)

Abbreviations: **CO_2** = Carbon dioxide, **HBO** = Hyperbaric oxygen, **mmHg =** mm of mercury, **O_2** = oxygen, **>** = Greater than, **<** = Less than

other causes of outflow obstruction, arteriovenous fistulas, metabolic conditions where tissue metabolism is impaired such as hypothyroidism, skeletal muscle-compartment syndromes, and possibly where metabolism becomes predominantly anaerobic.

Misconceptions About Augmenting Perfusion – The following summarize misconceptions about revascularizations and angioplasties. First, although they may be technically successful, perfusion may still be insufficient to meet the metabolic demands of healing. The difference in blood flow and metabolic requirements for wound healing and infection control are substantially increased (estimated to be 20-fold or more as previously discussed—Chapter 2) as compared to the steady state situation. Juxta-wound transcutaneous oxygen measurements, before and after angioplasty and/or revascularization, confirm the effectiveness of the intervention. With diffuse peripheral artery disease, perfusion may be improved after angioplasty or revascularization, but not

Clinical correlations:
A 69-year-old male with diabetes and peripheral artery disease developed a 5 cm wide pressure sore behind his right heel. The wound base was pale, consistent with ischemia. A small rim of cellulitis encircled the wound. Pain associated with the wound was absent due to a sensory neuropathy. The Wound Score was 5 ½ (appearance = 1, size = 1, depth = 2, infection =1 and perfusion = ½) consistent with a "problem" wound.

A percutaneous angioplasty was performed on the right superficial femoral artery. Although flow was improved distal to the angioplasty, the foot still remained profoundly ischemic. Hyperbaric oxygen treatments were requested, but the patient was unwilling to undergo treatments due to claustrophobia. Wound care with an enzymatic debriding agent and antibiotics were continued as they were provided pre-angioplasty. The rim of cellulitis resolved, but generation of a granulating base and epithelialization at the margins failed to occur. A trial of bio-engineered skin substitutes was not helpful. The patient opted to live with the wound as apposed to a below-knee amputation.

Comment:
Although the angioplasty was technically successful, blood flow was not increased enough to heal the heel wound. The resolution of cellulitis is attributed to the increased (but inadequate to achieve healing) blood flow. Would hyperbaric oxygen have made a difference? Possibly; the patient's diffuse vascular disease in his right lower extremity did not allow sufficient blood flow to meet the requirements of healing.

The seeming paradox of resolution of the cellulitis, but lack of healing is best explained by the fact that antibiotic delivery is achieved by physical dissolution in the plasma while oxygen delivery is almost entirely dependent of the red blood cell. In low and/or impeded flow states, plasma is expected to stream through the compromised microcirculation while the cellular elements (red blood cells) would not.

Hyperbaric oxygen tends to "equalize" the equation by making oxygen delivery to the wound no more flow dependent than the physically devolved substances in the plasma. Consequently, from a physiology perspective, hyperbaric oxygen would have been a logical intervention.

enough to meet the metabolic demands of wound healing. Second, in about 30 percent of cases, as mentioned above, in patients with profound vasculopathy, angioplasty, stenting, and/or revascularization is not possible due to the diffuse nature of the problem, the lack of run-off, previous revascularization that was unsuccessful, infection/wound adjacent to the surgical site, or combinations of these. Third, the consequence of the inability to perform an angioplasty or revascularization is not always a lower limb amputation. With utilization of the other techniques for managing the "end-stage" wound, healing is observed in enough cases that it justifies using these interventions, in the motivated patient, even if angioplasty, stenting or revascularization are not feasible. Fourth, a successful angioplasty or revascularization that later occludes does not necessarily signify that a lower limb amputation is eminent. If these interventions can maintain flow during the critical healing and infection control phase, the collateral circulation may become sufficient to maintain flow and metabolic needs during the less demanding steady state situation after the revascularized vessel occludes. Finally, a lower limb amputation should not be considered a failure of management, but rather a rational decision based on the circumstances of the case. Often our vascular surgeons will enter the operating room for the "end-stage" wound with a double consent. That is for exploration and revascularization if the exploration indicates that revascularization has a reasonable chance of being successful. If not, then the surgeon will proceed directly to a lower limb amputation.

MINIMALLY INVASIVE "KEEP IT SIMPLE AND SPEEDY" SURGERIES

Surgeries for "End-Stage" Wounds – The fourth technique to improve outcomes with "end-stage" wounds is the use of surgeries that are effective in managing the wound, but minimize the surgical trauma to the patient.[14] We refer to these as MIS (minimally invasive surgeries) or KISS (Keep It Simple and Speedy) surgeries. In order for surgery sites to heal, blood flow and metabolic demands may need to increase as much as 20-fold beyond the steady-state situation (Chapter 2). The failure to meet these requirements results in the non-healing wound which after surgery may be characterized by dehiscence, slough and/or infection. Surgeries designed to be minimally invasive and minimally traumatic reduce metabolic demands for wound healing and the likelihood that these complications will occur. Five generic descriptors encompass the variety of problems that are seen in "problem" wounds in general and "end-stage" wounds in particular. They include ulcers, deformities, surgically generated wounds, amputations and problems associated with special conditions such as Charcot arthropathies. Although these minimally invasive surgeries are summarized in this chapter, they are applicable and highly recommended for almost all problem foot wounds that require surgery. Whereas in-office counterparts have been mentioned previously (Chapter 7) and will be additionally addressed in Chapter 16, counterparts performed in the operating room will be introduced in this section.

Surgical Considerations – The conditions for which minimally invasive surgeries are indicated have similarities as well as differences. Similarities include the triad of findings associated with "problem" wounds that are typically present, namely deformities, ischemia and infection (Chapter 2). One exception to this generalization is that in Charcot arthropathies, as will be discussed in the following chapter, ischemia is not usually a problem. Another similarity is that each of these conditions has counterparts that can be done in the non-operating room setting such as the clinic, private office or

TABLE 11-3. MINIMALLY INVASIVE SURGERIES (MIS) OR KEEP IT SIMPLE AND SPEEDY (KISS) PROCEDURES FOR "PROBLEM" AND "END-STAGE" WOUNDS

Problems	In-office Procedures*	In-operating Room Counterparts
Ulcers	Debridements (See Chapter 7)	Excision of ulcers & debridement of underlying tissues
Deformities	Percutaneous tenotomies of toe tendons (single toes at one time) Joint manipulations with or without splinting or spacers	Limited open tenotomies (multiple toes), especially extensor tendons & ankle tendons Minimally invasive (percutaneous) realignment of depressed metatarsal heads (drill & osteoclasis) Percutaneous Achilles tendon lengthening
Complicated Wounds	Partial wound edge approximations and/or reducing the wound surface area with spanning sutures	Medial and/or lateral ray resections Inside ray resections & forefoot narrowing with mini external fixator Closure of contaminated wounds with suction-irrigation
Amputations	Open amputation of a lesser toe Partial toe amputation(s)	Standard amputations at toe, forefoot, midfoot, ankle or leg levels Open amputations with staged closure surgeries Multi-level amputations requiring creative flaps**
Miscellaneous	Toenail care (trimming, debridement debulking & in-grown nail management) Application of bio-engineered skin coverings	Joint resections and/or fusions Osteotomies to correct alignment Management of "end-stage" Charcot arthropathy wounds with debridement, realignment & fixators

Key : * = Also includes wound clinic and on the hospital ward,
    ** = Implies amputations at 2 levels, e.g. transmetatarsal medially & Lisfranc level laterally

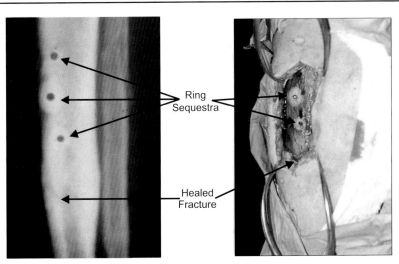

Ring Sequestra

Healed Fracture

Legend: Necrotic bone developed in this diabetic patient's tibia after a power drill was used to insert pins for external fixation of a fracture. Thermal injury from drilling the pin hole resulted in bone necrosis. The white ring sequestra on x-ray are pathognomonic of dead bone from the thermal injury.

During the fracture healing process living bone is reabsorbed, i.e. fracture osteoporosis. This did not occur for the avascular (white rings on photograph) bone. Because of peripheral artery disease, circulation to bone was not sufficient to dissipate the heat generated by the power drill.

Figure 11-5. Ring sequestra secondary to thermal injury to bone.

the hospital ward (Table 11-3). A third similarity is that the procedures are designed to be as minimally traumatic to the tissues as possible. Dissection is kept to a minimum. Definitive incisions are made cutting through multiple tissue planes simultaneously. Most bone work is done with non-heat generating instruments such as ronguers, bone cutters or handsaws. If power saws and rotary burrs are used, the saw blade and burr and the underlying bone are continuously irrigated to minimize thermal injury to bone that can be generated by the power equipment (Figure 11-5). Ischemic tissue, especially bone, is unable to dissipate heat generated by power instruments, as well as normally perfused bone and soft tissue.

"Keep is Simple and Speedy" Surgery Considerations – Not all KISS surgeries are simple and speedy, but the principle of being minimally invasive is a goal for each. There is a continuum of complexities from very simple to highly technical in their implementation. Some KISS procedures are as straight forward as excising an ulcer and debriding the underlying tissue, while others can thoroughly challenge one's ingenuity such as complex flap closures, deformity corrections and/or management of large, open, infected wounds of the legs, ankles and feet. In contrast to most surgical procedures where detailed, step-by-step descriptions are available on how to perform the surgery, detailed descriptions for managing the above three problems are not typically available in articles and texts. Often times special experience by the surgeon such as familiarity with developing and managing flaps, doing unconventional amputations, application of external fixators and intramedullary rodding is required. Fortunately many KISS surgeries, such as tenotomies and percutaneous osteoclases of metatarsal necks, only require minimal post-op care such as protection of the surgical sites, incision hygiene, and suture/staple removal, if used. Other KISS procedures such as deformity correction and wound management with an external fixator require diligent post-operative management and outcomes are highly dependent upon how compliant the patient and their caregivers are with the necessary post-operative care. Other KISS procedures need to be done as staged surgeries that require return to the operating room for second and possibly third-stage surgical interventions. This is frequently the situation with necrotizing soft tissue infections where the initial surgery is debridement; staged closure is performed with flap mobilization or skin grafting when the wound has improved enough for these to be done with reasonable expectations of good outcomes. The following information describes the five generic in-operating room minimally invasive surgeries that may be needed to manage the "end-stage" wound (additional discussion of the in-office, etc. procedures are found in Chapter 16).

1. Ulcers - An ulcer is a term for a wound which can be defined as having the following characteristics: 1) a defect in the integrity of the skin, 2) variable depths from skin level to bone or internal organs, 3) healing typically requires special interventions, 4) invariably associated with uncontrolled infection, underlying deformities and/or ischemia when associated with "problem" and "futile" wounds and 5) comorbidities, especially in those ulcers that are not healing in an anticipated fashion. Ulcer management in the operating room must take into consideration the above characteristics. This is especially true for dealing with the comorbidities and generating a treatment plan (that is, the strategic approach as described in Part III) to manage wound ischemia, deformities and uncontrolled infection.

Ulcer Classification – Ulcerations are classified by many grading systems (Chapter 4). The depth assessment of the **Wound Score** (Chapter 5) is a speedy and easy to use tool for grading ulcers, regardless of the location, and provides insight as to what interventions are required. Pre-ulcer (skin concerns over bony prominences, from shear and/or moisture retention) and superficial ulcerations only involving the epithelium are given a grade of 2 points. If subcutaneous tissues are exposed, the ulcer is given a grade of 1½ points. A grade of 1 point indicates the ulcer depth is to the muscle and/or tendon level. If exposure of the ulcer base is to the periosteum or joint capsule level, a grade of ½ point is assigned to the wound depth. Finally, a 0 point grade indicates that bone, joint or both are exposed. When only the very outer margin of the bone is infected, as is frequently associated with deep presacral and hip trochanteric pressure sores, osteitis is the term used to describe the clinical findings. To successfully eradicate osteitis, the infected cortical bone needs to be debrided. If the central or cancellous (spongy) portion of the bone becomes infected, it is termed osteomyelitis. If osteomyelitis is present in the "end-stage" wound, bone has to be resected to infection free margins in order to eliminate the infection. In the foot, this often times requires amputations.

Medical Management – Before definitive surgery is performed for ulcers in general and "end-stage" wounds in particular, an appropriate database needs to be compiled. The chapter on the medical management strategies (Chapter 6) offers an approach for recognizing and managing comorbidities. Wound cultures should guide antibiotic therapy choices. Information about wound perfusion and oxygenation, as previously described in this chapter, is necessary for making decisions and predicting outcomes of surgical interventions. If adequate, surgical management of ulcers is expected to provide uniformly good outcomes. If marginal, initial failures and delayed healing after surgery is typical.

Wound Excision – The procedure of choice for managing ulcers in the operating room is excision of the ulcer and debridement of the underlying tissue (i.e. EUD). In contrast to most exploratory surgeries where incisions are carried to depth tissue plane by tissue plane, for EUD surgeries, a single incision to the bone level is recommended. If possible, the ulcer is incised in toto by converting the starting incision to an ovoid shape to circumscribe the ulcer. For hallux and fifth toe amputations, racquet shaped incisions and capsulectomies at the metatarsal phalangeal joint levels are ideal. The infected tissue of the wound is removed in a few moments. Traction placed on the edge of the ovoid of excised tissue and/or the end of the toe (with a sharp towel clip or bone tenaculum) facilitates rapid removal of incised tissue and minimizes contamination. This approach keeps the infected tissue from coming in contact with the clean surgical margins. Intuition and creativity are required for wounds in other locations such as around the ankle, the heel and the plantar aspect of the foot. The direction of the incision may be axial, transverse, diagonal, "S" shaped or combinations of these based on the need for exposure and the vascularity of the flaps.

Debridement Goals – Once the deep tissues are exposed, definitive debridement is done. This includes removal of all cicatrix from the under surface of the flaps and poorly vascularized tissue such as bursa, joint capsule, tendon, fibrous tissue and infected granulation tissue from the depths of the wound. A thorough debridement of the cicatrix is appreciated by palpation of a smooth, soft, pliable texture of the tissues in the wound base; visualization is not nearly as precise for ascertaining that the debridement is adequate as is palpation. Next, debridement of bony deformities is done using power saws and rasps, ronguers, and non-power rasps. Five goals should be achieved with the debridement of the tissues: 1) removal of all infected bone, 2) establishment of vascularized margins, 3) obliteration of the deformity, 4) generation of a plantigrade foot position, and 4) sufficient resection of soft and hard tissues to approximate or nearly approximate the flaps. Typically, the achievement of each goal complements the others. Several of the goals must absolutely be met, such as establishing vascularized, non-

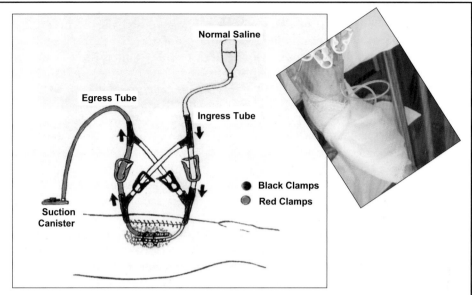

Legend: When concerns arise about residual contamination of soft tissues, but osteomyelitis has been managed, closure with suction-irrigation tubes is a useful technique. The closed system allows the inflow and egress of fluid (red clamps and black clamps) to be changed easily—usually each hour. By changing flow direction, a counter current "washout" effect occurs. Typically, fluid inflow is decreased each day, until after five days, both tubes are placed on suction (i.e. the black and red clamps on the inflow side are closed, and conversely, the opposite clamps are left open). The remark (upper right insert) is a picture of the Synder® directional flow device used for an infected foot wound.

Figure 11-6. Wound closure over suction-irrigation tubes.

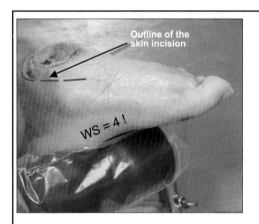 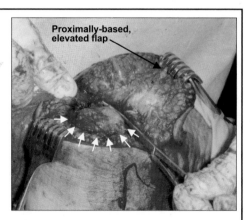

Legend: Because of the size and location of the "end-stage" wound (**Wound Score** = 4 1/2 points ; Appearance of wound base =1 point, Size =1 point, Depth = 1/2 point, Infection/bioburden= 1 point, and Perfusion =1 point), typical excision of ulcer and debridement of underlying bone was not feasible. The fish-mouth incision provided access to the underlying bony deformity (circumscribed with white arrows in right-side photo). After removal of the deformity (ostectomy), the flap healed primarily and the ulcer by secondary intention.

Figure 11-7. A fish mouth plantar incision provides access to a calcaneal deformity, the cause of a non-healing, limb-threatening heel ulceration.

infected, deformity-free margins. Other goals are desirable, but can be achieved with secondary procedures, such as establishing a plantigrade foot position and delayed closure techniques.

Closure Options – There are several closure options for EUD procedures. The most desirable is primary approximation of the flaps without tension. If not possible, then partial closure is recommended with later secondary closure, skin grafting, flap surgery or healing by secondary intention. If concern is raised that there is remaining contamination of soft tissues in the wound, such as flaps with resolving cellulitis, consideration for closing with suction-irrigation or using negative pressure wound therapy (wound vacuum techniques) should be given. With suction-irrigation, the wound is closed over drains (Figure 11-6).[15] Continuous irrigation and suction provide uninterrupted counter-current lavage and washout of contaminated material, debris and transudates. If the wound is left open, then wound base management, as described previously (Chapters 7, 8 & 9) should be employed.

2. Deformities - Management of these problems is crucial in the eradication and prevention of wounds. Deformities in "problem" wounds have two primary sources. Management usually becomes obvious once the deformity is recognized. First are those deformities that arise from muscle imbalances such as clawing of the toes. A second primary cause of deformities is the abnormal shape and/or positioning of bones. Often combinations of these problems are present, with each contributing to the non-healing wound in an additive effect. Wound management usually is enormously simplified once the deformity is corrected. In fact, many times the correction of the underlying deformity results in spontaneous healing of the wound. In order to gain access to plantar heel deformities, fish mouth incisions are particularly useful (Figure 11-7).

Wound Solution from a Deformity – Wounds secondary to deformities typically evolve through a series of clearly defined stages. Initially the body reacts by forming callus over the deformity and hypertrophy of the bursa between the deformity and the overlying skin. These are spontaneous protective measures in response to the increased stresses the deformity imposes on the underlying skin. The second stage is that of ulceration, which indicates that the stresses exceed the skin and the tissues overlying the deformity's abilities to maintain their integrity. Frequently, the ulceration is from inside to out and is usually associated with formation of hypertrophic bursas and/or extensive recesses in association with the ulcer. This is typical of what is observed in the mal perforans ulcer that develops under depressed metatarsal heads. Metatarsal head depression is secondary to clawing of toes from muscle imbalances that arise as a consequence of neuropathy. Shear stresses from muscle imbalances and deformities while walking or transferring contribute to bursa formation and ulceration. If the condition worsens, osteomyelitis is an eventual consequence. Finally, if the wound seals off, the infection becomes enclosed and typically dissects proximally along tendon sheaths to cause tenosynovitis, necrotizing soft tissue infections/fasciitis and systemic sepsis.

3. Wounds - Much has already been discussed about the management of wounds. Special techniques may be needed to manage "end-stage" wounds beyond what was described above for ulcers and deformities. In this context, "end-stage" wounds" require that oxygen and metabolic demands for healing be reduced as much as possible. Previously it has been stated that for wound healing to occur, metabolic oxygen requirements, etc., need to increase 20-fold (Chapter 2). It is obvious that some wound healing techniques and mechanisms require less metabolic and oxygen availability requirements for wound healing than others. For example, epithelialization under a thin crust can occur in an ischemic wound, whereas healing of a deep cavity would not. These examples

TABLE 11-4. METABOLIC, PERFUSION, AND OXYGEN REQUIREMENTS FOR HEALING OF WOUNDS

Requirements	Wound Characteristic	Type of Coverage/Closure
↑ Decreasing / Increasing ↓	Thin, dry, firm **Crust**	**Epithelialization** occurs under crust
	Superficial, healthy **Granulation tissue**	**Skin in-growth** from the wound margins
	Healthy base with **Adequate vascularity**	**Split thickness skin graft** (STSG)
	Incised, **Healthy skin edges**	**Simple approximation,** of skin edges
	Uncomplicated flaps, e.g., trans-metatarsal or below knee amputation	**Flap approximation** usually one or both on proximal based pedicles after bone shortening
	Complicated, complex flaps	Often times challenging **mobilization, rotation and/or Y-V or Z-plasties**
	Exposed bone and/or major soft tissue defect	**Microvascular free flap** (MVFF) with or without a STSG
	Cavitary wounds not amenable MVFF due to peripheral artery disease, location and/or comorbidities	**Healing by granulation tissue formation, wound contraction and/or secondary intention** with or without NPWT, spanning sutures/ dynamic closure devices or reduction of cavity size by narrowing distance between bony elements

Abbreviations: **MVFF** = Microvascular free flap, **NPWT** = Negative pressure wound therapy, **STSG** = Split thickness skin graft

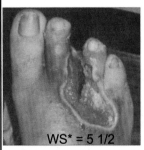
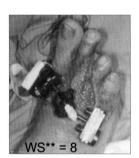
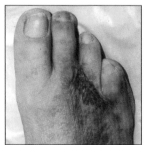

WS* = 5 1/2   WS** = 8

Persistent cavity 6 weeks after partial 3rd ray amputation

Ready for STSG 1 week after forefoot narrowing

Appearance of foot after STSG

Legend: The cavitary wound is the most metabolic, perfusion and oxygen demanding wound in the hierarchy of wound healing (Table 4). By obliterating the cavity, the wound is converted to a type that can be managed by less demanding healing techniques such as skin grafting or healing by epithelialization of the remaining wound.

Abbreviations: **STSG** = Split thickness skin graft, **WS* = Wound Score** (Appearance of the Wound Base = 1 1/2, Size = 1, Depth =1/2, Infection/Bioburden = 1 1/2, Perfusion = 1) , **WS** = Wound Score** after forefoot narrowing (A = 2, S =1 1/2, D = 1 1/2, I/B = 2, P = 1)

Figure 11-8. The obliteration of a non-healing cleft wound by forefoot narrowing and temporary maintenance of the reduction with external fixation.

represent extremes on a continuum of metabolic, oxygen, and perfusion requirements for healing (Table 11-4). The wound care and surgical management for most of the items in the hierarchy are self-explanatory or have been previously discussed, including the use of negative pressure wound therapy and closure with suction-irrigation.

Forefoot Narrowing – One exception that will now be further expanded is the management of deep cavitary or cleft wounds in the forefoot. When a cleft wound is generated in the forefoot after resection of an infected, necrotic middle ray (second, third, or fourth metatarsal and associated toes), obliteration of the cavity converts the wound to one that merely requires superficial skin edge closure, healing by secondary intention or a skin graft (Figure 11-8).[16] Obliteration of the cleft is achieved by placing pins in the first and fifth metatarsals, squeezing these bones together to obliterate the cleft and maintaining tissue approximation with a mini-external fixation device attached to the pins. After three weeks, the fixator is removed. By this time, the soft tissues have adapted to the reduced position as a result of plastic deformation and have had time to heal with the cavity obliterated. Usually a three-week period of walking in a weight-bearing cast follows the fixator removal to allow further maturation of the approximated tissues.

Joint Resection – Intercalary resection of an infected toe or metatarsal phalangeal joint is another technique for managing a special wound type. When one of these joints needs to be resected due to infection, deformity or both and the patient does not want the toe distal to the wound amputated, this type of surgery is an option. Once the infected material is debrided, bone-to-bone contact needs to be achieved to obliterate the cavity. For this, temporary axial alignment with a pin, suture of the tip of the toe to adjacent toe tips or both can maintain alignment until the soft tissues heal. Naturally, the toe will be significantly shortened and the joint converted to an interpositional soft tissue arthroplasty with this technique.

Heal Wound Management Options – Management of heel wounds may require special surgical techniques. The fish mouth flap was described previously in the deformities management portion of this section. For infections of the calcaneous, subtotal resection of the calcaneous may be required. This is achieved with excision of the ulcer, debridement of the underlying, infected bone, and mobilization of the flaps to close or partially close the wound.[17, 18] Creative incisions such as fish mouth, axial, transverse, or splitting of the calcaneous may be required to obtain adequate exposure, eradicate the infection, and optimally mobilize the flaps. When the heel wound is large, it is usually not possible to close it completely. A microvascular free flap is a possibility for achieving coverage of the bone, but associated comorbidities may be a contraindication to this intervention.[19] In these situations, secondary coverage/closure techniques become necessary (Table 11-4). It is desirable to preserve the subtalar joint and the insertion of the Achilles tendon, but limited ambulation in protective footwear (CROW boot—Chapter 15) is possible even with a total calcanectomy.[20] A wedge-shaped filler that conforms to the heel defect can be placed in the footwear device to facilitate ambulation. Although the patient will not be able to walk normally, with aids such as a cane or walkerette, independent ambulation is possible and may be more desirable because of lower energy demands, than walking with a prosthesis.

4. Amputations - Although conventional amputations for the foot, ankle, and leg are sufficiently described in other texts, those needed for "end-stage" wounds are typically unconventional. Amputations are not usually performed as in-office procedures, but minor ablations such as parts or entire toes can be done appropriately in this setting (Figure 11-9). If wounds are already present on the toes, the incision can be extended to encircle the entire toe and the toe disarticulated at the next more proximal joint level by incising the joint capsule. If healthy soft tissue extends beyond the bone, healing by secondary intention, partial closure, delayed primary closure or definitive closure are viable options. The choice depends on the healthiness of the soft tissues at the amputation site. If bone is "proud," that is, extends beyond the soft tissues, it can be debrided to a more proximal level with a ronguer and/or bone cutter. In the patient with diabetes, profound sensory neuropathies usually obviate the need for anesthesia. If sensation is present, local anesthesia at the amputation level, metatarsal block or foot blocks can be done in the office setting to allow the procedure to be performed without discomfort for the patient.

Amputations in the Operating Wound – When amputations are performed in the operating room, several goals must be achieved. First, all nonviable and structurally unsound tissues need to be removed. Second, a structurally sound foot platform or an amputation stump that will accommodate a prosthesis is essential. Third, contractures should be corrected and interventions to avoid future contractures addressed. This is especially important when an equinus contracture is present at the ankle in association

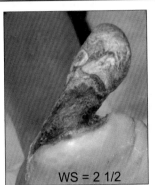 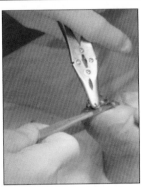 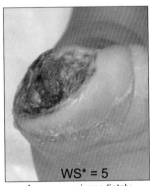

WS = 2 1/2
Presentation

Hallux removed after incision through capsule; articular cartilage being debrided

WS* = 5
Appearance immediately after debridement

Legend: Partial or complete toe amputations in the non-operating room setting are a cost-effective and time-saving option. The amputation itself took less than 10 minutes and the facility charge was a fraction of what it would have been to do the procedure in the operating room. Finally, the surgical fee is the same regardless of the venue.

Abbreviations: WS = Wound Score (Appearance = 0, Size =1/2, Depth = 0, Infection/Bioburden = 1 and Perfusion = 1),
* WS = Wound Score immediately after debridement (A = 2, Size 1, D = 0, I/B =1 P =1)

Figure 11-9. In-office open amputation of a mummified hallux.

with a wound that requires a forefoot or more proximal foot amputation. Prophylactic Achilles tendon lengthening is advised whenever very proximal transmetatarsal or midfoot amputations are required. The reason for this is that with the loss of the lever arm of the forefoot, there is the likelihood that the imbalance between the strong calf muscles and the shortened foot will generate an equinus deformity. If the contracture is severe, it can interfere with walking. In addition, it may lead to skin breakdown with the concentration of weight bearing stresses at the end of the amputation stump. Frequently, this is the site of the suture line for the approximation of the flaps, which makes it even more vulnerable for formation of a new wound when weight bearing is resumed. Temporary pin placement across joints is a useful technique for maintaining

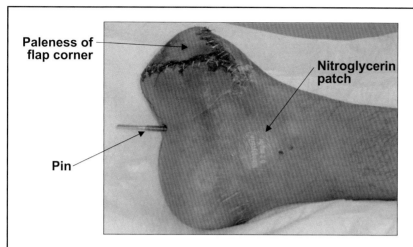

Paleness of flap corner

Nitroglycerin patch

Pin

Legend: Axial directed, threaded Steinmann pin through calcaneous, talus and into the tibia to keep the ankle in neutral position and counteract over-pull of the calf muscles.

The pin optimally immobilizes the operative site (immobilization and protection strategy from management of the "problem" wound, Chapter 8). Because of the "short" amputation, it would be difficult to maintain the ankle in neutral position with casting or splinting.

Note flap concerns exist with paleness of the medial corner of the flap and a narrow eschar along the suture line. The nitroglycerin patch over the posterior tibial artery was applied to promote local vasodilatation. Hyperbaric oxygen therapy was also utilized to promote healing.

Figure 11-10. Percutaneous pin immobilization for an "at risk" midfoot amputation.

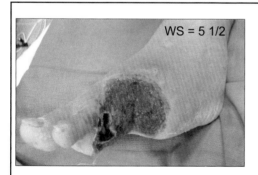

WS = 5 1/2

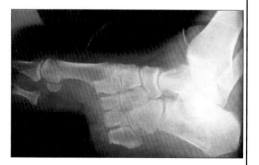

Legend: The left foot is status post amputation of the lateral three rays and intercalary amputation of the second metatarsal

Options include skin grafting the healthy wound base or conversion to an unconventional proximal transmetatarsal amputation with a medial based flap

Although the first ray is ordinarily responsible for 50 percent of the load bearing of the forefoot, the long lever arm without adjacent soft tissue supportive structures would predict early ligamentous failure at the medial ray Lisfranc (tarsal, metatarsal) joint level

Abbreviations: WS = Wound Score (Appearance of wound base = 2, Size = 1/2, Depth = 1/2, Infection/Bioburden = 1 1/2 and Perfusion = 1)

Figure 11-11. Decision making after lateral ray amputation.

> When an axial pin is placed through the heel, utmost precautions are necessary to prevent the patient from loading the pin and driving it proximally into the heel with weight bearing. This can inoculate the calcaneous with bacteria and lead to osteomyelitis.
>
> Even though patients may promise to be non-weight bearing on the pinned extremity, do not expect them to avoid this with transfers, especially if they have difficulty making transfers or the contralateral limb has been previously amputated.
>
> Methods to avoid loading the axial pin include placement of the limb in a lower extremity cast with the knee flexed to 45 degrees or applying an unwieldy type leg cast with a metal outrigger over the exposed pin end.

joints in the neutral (functional) position and preventing the development of contractures during the wound-healing period (Figure 11-10).

Considerations for Foot Amputations – For the goals of establishing viable soft tissue margins and a structurally sound stump end in the presence of complicated wounds, conventional amputation techniques may be inadequate. Ingenuity and imagination may be required in order to achieve a functional amputation in these circumstances. Considerations include doing a multi-level amputation, that is, part of it at one level of the foot and the remainder at another level. Other considerations include using unconventional flaps to achieve closure such as dorsal, medial or lateral flaps when the traditional plantar flap is not available or insufficient to achieve closure (Figure 11-11). Open amputation is a third consideration when definitive amputation and primary closure are not feasible because of unhealthy margins or unresolved sepsis. In the patient who has the potential to walk, enough perfusion that wound healing is possible and the motivation and support (i.e. a high **Goal-Aspiration Score**), the open amputation is an option. Healing is expected to occur by secondary intention or later return to the operating room for revision, flap and/or grafting surgery.

5. Miscellaneous Procedures - Several other minimally invasive procedures are useful for managing the "end-stage" wound or its complications. Not infrequently, after an "end-stage" wound has been controlled, residual deformity, joint instability or combinations of these two problems prevent useful function of the extremity. Initial attempts to control these problems with protective footwear and braces including the CROW (Charcot Restraint Orthotic Walker) boot, are appropriate. If ineffective or inadequate, then specially designed, minimally invasive surgical interventions are indicated. Since the wound problem is or had been "end-stage," it is understandable why any additional surgeries on the foot must be planned to minimize trauma and surgical exposure.

Contracture and Muscle Imbalance Surgeries – For deformities, tendon and joint capsule release surgeries are the first line KISS (Keep It Simple and Speedy) procedures. These problems arise from motor neuropathies from diabetes or other conditions which cause neuropathies. Many times tenotomies for larger tendons can be done with an incision less than two centimeters (about 3/4th of an inch) in length. Usually the offending tendon is easily palpable under the skin because of the deformity. Consequently, exposing and isolating the tendon is straightforward. Simple transection of the tendon is recommended in contrast to step-cut lengthening. This obviates the need for extended exposures and immediate post-operative non-weight bearing protection. Joint capsule releases can be done percutaneously or with small incisions. After distracting the joint, the scalpel blade tip is introduced into the joint cleft and using the cleft as a guide, the contracted part of the joint capsule is incised with a sweeping motion of the blade tip. These minimally invasive procedures work well in the following situations:

- Abduction deformities of the first ray managed by release of the abductor hallucis muscle and, if indicated, the medial capsule of the first metatarsal-phalangeal joint.
- Hallux valgus associated with bunion deformities managed by release of the adductor hallucis muscle and the lateral joint capsule for the first metatarsal-phalangeal joint.
- For corresponding deformities of the fifth ray, analogous procedures can be done for the lateral side of the foot.
- Equinus contracture of the ankle is managed by percutaneous tri-hemisection of the Achilles tendon. After the Achilles tendon release, casting, initially non-weight bearing, then weight bearing is recommended for six weeks.
- Midfoot inversion with ulcer formation on the lateral side of the foot should be initially managed by minimally invasive soft tissue releases, including percutaneous Achilles tendon lengthening plus limited open release of the anterior tibial, and possibly extensors to the great toe and posterior tibial tendons. The latter two releases are usually done if the foot is semi-rigid from glycosylation and conversion of brawny edema into cicatrix and the releases of the Achilles and anterior tibial tendons do not allow the foot to be manipulated into the plantigrade position. Although a consequence of this may be a drop foot, the contracted, semi-rigid joint capsules secondary to the deformity often make bracing unnecessary. If not, bracing for a steppage gait is a preferred option to continuing to walk on the side of the foot and worsening of the ulcer.
- Flexion contractures of the knees managed with limited open releases of the medial and lateral hamstring muscle, tendon insertions. Temporary placement of large, threaded crossed Steinmann pins (one started laterally above the knee

Clinical correlations:

An elderly male with diabetes developed limb-threatening wounds on the lateral aspect of his right foot. The problem was compounded by forefoot splaying and abduction, midfoot inversion, and ankle equinus secondary to neuropathy. Release of the abductor hallucis muscle did not control the deformities. A modified transmetatarsal amputation with complete fifth and partial fourth metatarsal amputations was done because of recurrent wounds. To control the residual deformities, transection of the anterior tibial tendon and percutaneous Achilles tendon lengthening were performed. With the soft tissue releases, the foot rested in the plantigrade position with the forefoot directed straight ahead.

Comment:

It was apparent that the abductor hallucis release alone did not adequately control the deformity. Had the additional tendon surgery have been done at the time of the abductor hallucis release, could the transmetatarsal amputation have been avoided? The answer is not an unqualified "yes," but the scenario illustrates how necessary it is to achieve a plantigrade foot position to avoid development of wounds, especially in the insensate foot.

joint and the second started laterally below the knee joint) will maintain the knee in extension without risk of pressure sore development that could occur from trying to use splints or casts to maintain knee in extension after the releases. The pins are usually removed at the time the skin sutures or staples are removed, and the patient's ambulation or the activity level that existed prior to the development of the contractures is resumed.

• Hip flexion-adduction contractures managed with percutaneous and limited open releases of both the proximal and distal flexor-adductor muscle, tendon groups (Chapter 12).

Joint Alignment and Stability – If stability is a significant consideration, then joint alignment and fusion must be considered. A variety of open techniques are available for these purposes in patients with adequate circulation to the extremity. However, in the presence of the "end-stage" wound, these options may not be possible due to high risks of non-healing and infection. Minimally invasive surgical techniques are an option. Often, the joint can be aligned by percutaneous soft tissue releases and debridement with an arthroscopic shaver. Then maintenance of alignment is achieved with temporary stabilization of the joint done with casting and/or percutaneous pinning. In contrast to patients with normal sensation, a fibroankylosis seems as effective as bony union for patients requiring alignment and stabilization of joints associated with their "end-stage" wounds.

Subtalar Fusion – The hyperpronated, valgus-deformed flat foot is a difficult to manage deformity often associated with "end-stage" wounds. It is most frequently associated with posterior tibial tendon insufficiency, but may also be a component of the foot and ankle with Charcot arthropathy (Chapter 12). If the deformity cannot be controlled with footwear, then fusion of the subtalar joint is needed. Again this can be done minimally invasively with a motorized burr and use of morcelized cancellous allograft bone packed through a small incision that provides access to the joint. This technique can also be used where resorption or removal of bone has led to such severe bony instability of the foot that loading of the extremity for weight bearing is not possible.

Intramedullary Rod Joint Stabilization – Another useful minimally invasive surgical technique is use of the intramedullary ankle rod to stabilize the ankle and subtalar joints (Chapter 16). Although technically demanding, this procedure is the epitome of a minimally invasive procedure. It may be the only option to manage a problem in an "end-stage" dysvascular limb where ankle instability is unmanageable with protective footwear and bracing. The procedure commences with percutaneous debridement of the ankle and possibly subtalar joints with an arthroscopic abrader. For this portion of the procedure, one centimeter incisions are adequate. The intramedullary rod is inserted through a three-centimeter wide incision in the heel and interlocked with screws requiring incisions one centimeter or less. For osteopenic bone, axial alignment is the best choice for maintaining alignment and stability. Post-op protection with casting and/or bracing is advised for a year because of the slow healing anticipated in this patient group.

SALVAGING THE FAILED, SLOUGHED, DEHISCED, POST-OP, POST-HBO WOUND

Initial Surgical Failures – When surgical procedures as described in the previous section are done on "end-stage" wounds, realistic expectations for healing must be given to the patient, their families and/or caregivers. In our experiences, 50 percent of the surgeries done for these types of wounds heal primarily when the management previously described for the "end-stage" hypoxic wound is employed. This is both a reflection of the challenges these types of wounds present and an affirmation how important the **Goal-Aspiration Score** and **Host-Function Score** (Chapter 1 and 2) are in making a decision whether to recommend lower limb amputation (or comfort care measures only as will be described in the next chapter) or attempt to salvage the limb.

> Even though approximately 50% of the surgeries done for "end-stage" hypoxic wounds initially fail, slough or dehisce, 90% of these -- or a combined total of 95% (50% primary healing + 90% of the 50% that initially fail) subsequently heal or stabilize enough to avoid lower limb amputations. Patient selection, that is qualifying Goal-Aspiration and Host-Function Scores and utilization of the techniques described in this chapter are the reasons these outcomes can be achieved.

Justification of Surgeries with High Initial Failure Rates – Can surgeries be justified with primary healing rates of 50 percent? The answer is a qualified "yes" for three reasons: First, even though 50 percent of the wounds fail, slough, or dehisce initially, 90 percent of these eventually heal or go on to a chronic stable wound (next section) that allows the patient to return to his/her pre-morbid level of function.[21, 22] Second, with satisfactory **Goal-Aspiration Score** and **Host-Function Score**, that is, greater than five points on the 0-10 point scale, there is a reasonable expectation that the patient and the other caregivers will provide the necessary day-to-day care that is essential for healing. Third, all of these wounds that initially fail, but eventually go onto heal, pass through four clearly defined stages. When this is explained to the patient and their caregivers and they observe the evolution of wound healing through the four stages, they feel reassured and remain motivated to continue the care.

Healing Stages of Failed Surgeries – Although wound healing is a continuous process, four stages of healing are identifiable for the failed, sloughed, dehisced (FSD) post-op, post-HBO (hyperbaric oxygen) treated wound (Table 11-5, Figure 11-12). Each stage has its own characteristics and special management requirements. The time to evolve through each stage varies widely; from as short as a week to as long as six months or more. Consequently, initial failure in healing of the post-op wound managed with hyperbaric oxygen and the other strategic management elements rarely lead to a lower limb amputation. Hyperbaric oxygen appears to "jump start" the healing process, even though its effects may not have been sufficient to allow primary healing of the surgical site. The explanations for this are two-fold: First, as mentioned previously, primary healing of a surgical site may require 20-fold increases in perfusion, oxygen availability and metabolic substrates. When these demands are not met, the surgical site fails. Healing by secondary means appears to have lesser metabolic demands than primary healing (Table 11-4). Second, hyperbaric oxygen stimulates angiogenesis. The healing responses observed suggest that this is an on-going process and continues, once initiated, after the course of hyperbaric oxygen has been completed.

Deterioration Phase – Initially the FSD (failed, sloughed, dehisced) post-op, post-HBO managed wound passes through a deterioration phase. This occurs from immediately post-operatively until no further deterioration is observed in the wound. Essential management for this stage includes wound hygiene, bed rest, debridement of

TABLE 11-5. STAGES IN THE HEALING OF THE FAILED, SLOUGHED, DEHISCED (FSD) POST-OP, POST HYPERBARIC OXYGEN TREATED WOUND

Stage	1 Deterioration	2 Latency	3 Angiogenesis	4 Epithelialization
Findings	Slough, dehiscence and/or necrosis	No change in wound size	Development of a healthy granulating base	Coverage with skin
Management (Wound base, etc.)	Cleansing of margins, Moist gauze dressings for open portions changed TID, antibiotics debridements, HBO	Enzymatic debridement daily dressing changes, weekly sharp debridements	Hydrogel dressing changes daily; sharp debridements as needed every 3 to 4 weeks	Same as for stage 3
Protection	Cast or splint, rest in hospital of skilled nursing facility	Cast or splint	Removable walker boot	Post-op shoe
Activity	Rest in hospital or skilled nursing facility	Mobilization, but non-weight bearing of affected extremity	Full weight bearing in boot with travel for community activities	Full weight bearing in shoe with unrestricted travel activities
Goals	Demarcation of live & dead tissue	Wound base nearly free of necrotic material	Granulating wound base that is beginning to epithelialize or is ready for a skin graft[1]	Healed wound
Duration[2] (Average)	1 week to 1 1/2 months (~2 weeks)	2 weeks to 4 months (~6 weeks)	1 to 6 months (~2 months)	1 to 6 months (~3 months)

KEY: [1]The majority of patients elect to let the wound heal on its own rather than undergoing skin grafting   [2]Varies with wound size, perfusion, location and depth

Abbreviations: **HBO** = Hyperbaric oxygen, **TID** = Three times a day, ~ = Approximately

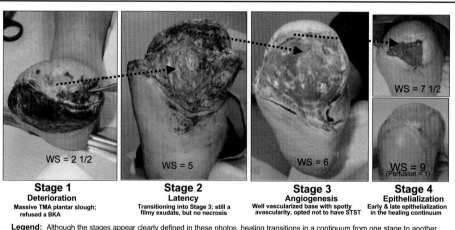

Stage 1 Deterioration	Stage 2 Latency	Stage 3 Angiogenesis	Stage 4 Epithelialization
Massive TMA plantar slough; refused a BKA	Transitioning into Stage 3; still a filmy exudate, but no necrosis	Well vascularized base with spotty avascularity, opted not to have STST	Early & late epithelialization in the healing continuum

WS = 2 1/2   WS = 5   WS = 6   WS = 7 1/2   WS = 9 (Perfusion = 1)

Legend: Although the stages appear clearly defined in these photos, healing transitions in a continuum from one stage to another. Components of adjacent stages are usually observed in this continuum.

For example, the left-sided dotted arrow shows an area covered with a fibrinous membrane & underlying ischemic tissue in both Stages 1 & 2; the middle arrow shows healthy granulation tissue in a portion of Stage 2 & almost 100% of the wound base in Stage 3; the right arrow shows epithelialization at the wound margin in Stage 3 with further skin coverage in Stage 4.

Note the reduction in wound size between Stages 2 and 3; this is due to edema reduction and wound contraction, both signs indicate the increasingly healthy nature of the wound. Note the improvements in the **Wound Score** (WS) with each stage.

Abbreviations: **BKA** = Below knee amputation, **FSD** = Failed sloughed, dehisced, **HBO** = Hyperbaric oxygen. **Op** = Operation, **STSG** = Split thickness skin graft, **TMA** = Transmetatarsal amputation, **WS** = Wound Score

Figure 11-12. Stages in the healing of a FSD post-op, post-HBO wound.

non-viable tissue, antibiotic administration, protective casting or splinting and hyperbaric oxygen. Wound hygiene involves cleansing with normal saline or hydrogen peroxide and moist dressings with acetic acid solution or other antimicrobial additives for the open areas. Dressing changes should be done two to three times a day in order to minimize the bioburden in the wound. Hospitalization or care in a skilled nursing facility is usually needed during this phase. Typically, the deterioration phase continues from less than a week to a month or more. In most of these wounds, demarcation is complete within two weeks.

Debridements During Deterioration Stage – In general, returning the patient to the operating room for surgical debridements to establish healthy margins is not advised during the deterioration phase. Demarcation of viable from non-viable tissues, in these

> Limited local debridements and debulking obviously non-viable tissue (Chapter 7) can be done regularly on the ward or in the office/clinic; usually with minimal or no anesthesia, especially if a sensory neuropathy is present. At this stage the physical therapist can be a very valuable asset to the wound care team by performing hydrotherapy with whirlpool or pulsatile lavage for wound cleansing and softening (hydrophilic effect) the tissues followed by superficial debridements. Adequate precautions must be taken to protect the staff and environment from aerosolized particles that might be spread with the pulsatile lavage.[23]

circumstances, is best accomplished by the body's own healing responses. In contrast, the objective of in-operating room debridements is to establish healthy surgical margins capable of immediate or delayed primary closure. Of necessity, this requires removal of tissue that would otherwise survive if demarcation is achieved by the body's own mechanisms. Often times in order to establish a surgical margin, amputation of a joint proximal to the wound would be required. The exception to this advice, regarding deferring surgical debridements in the operating room, is if the patient remains septic and/or necrosis is ascending proximally from the FSD post-op wound.

Latency Stage – After the deterioration phase, the FSD wound enters a latency period. This latency phase is distinguished by lack of outward progress or improvement. It seems to be a resting period where the wound is mustering resources to go on to complete the healing response. It is likely that during this phase angiogenesis and accumulation of substrates in the wound base are occurring and provide the needed elements for healing to continue. At this time the patient can be managed at home or in an extended care facility. Dressing changes are reduced to daily cleansings and applications of an enzymatic debriding agent. Ambulation may be resumed with walking aids, but the affected extremity should be non-weight bearing, only touching the ground to help with balance. Protection and immobilization of the wound area with a cast or splint is continued. Dependent edema should be controlled with elastic wraps (Ace® bandages) or elastic support hose. Weekly rechecks are advised at which time superficial debridement of necrotic material, fibrin crusts, and fibrinous membranes in the wound base is done with instruments such as a scalpels, forceps, curette and Ronguer (Chapter 7). Antibiotics and hyperbaric oxygen are discontinued during this stage. The latency period ranges from two weeks to four months; most often being complete within six weeks.

Angiogenesis Stage – Angiogenesis is the third stage observed in the healing of the FSD post-op wound. The wound base becoming covered with healthy granulation tissue heralds it. Daily wound cleansing and dressing changes with a hydrogel are advised at this stage. If the wound is of the cavitary type and/or the base edematous due to fluid retention in the lower extremities, use of negative pressure wound therapy is recommended. The patient may be full weight bearing in a removable walker boot at this stage and travel locally as desired. Rechecks are recommended every two to three weeks to assess progress, do minor debridements and encourage the patients to continue with their wound care. The angiogenesis stage may take as long as six months to progress from the appearance of the first buds of granulation tissue until the wound base is fully granulated. Usually it occurs within two months.

Epithelialization Stage – The angiogenesis stage transitions into the fourth and final stage, the epithelialization-coverage stage. The word transition is used because while the base of the wound is granulating, typically epithelialization is occurring at the wound margins. Care is continued as for the angiogenesis stage except for spacing rechecks to monthly intervals. Weight bearing in a post-op padded hard-soled shoe is OK at this stage. The patient may be offered the option of readmission for skin grafting to speed coverage of the wound. Few patients with post-op FSD wounds at this stage choose this option because they prefer not to interrupt their level of activity by the necessary convalescence a skin graft requires. Other considerations include satisfaction with the progress observed with the healing of their wounds and costs which may be five to ten thousand dollars or more for a typical skin graft, which includes surgical charges, anesthesia and hospital stay. In some patients, at this stage, a second latency period is observed. Even though the wound base is granulated, epithelialization around the margins does not seem to be occurring. However, after a two to three month period usually epithelialization begins and proceeds, usually rapidly, to cover the wound. Travel including airline flights and ship cruises is permissible during this stage of the healing FSD wound. Usually epithelialization takes two to three months to complete, but as noted often starts during the angiogenesis phase.

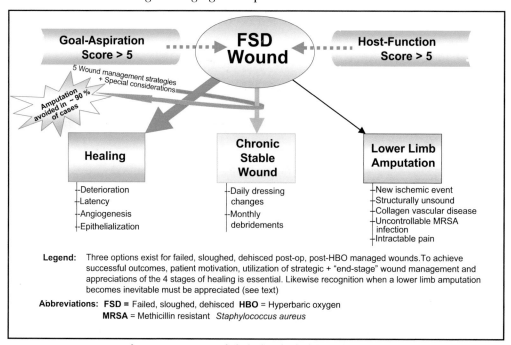

Figure 11-13. Outcomes of post-op, post-HBO failed, sloughed, dehisced wound.

Outcomes with Failed, Sloughed, Dehisced Wounds – Three possible outcomes are anticipated with FSD post-op wounds (Figure 11-13). First, healing is observed in about 90 percent of the cases where the decision is made to try to salvage the "end-stage" hypoxic wound when the five treatment strategies (Part III) are coupled with the special considerations given in this chapter. A very important consideration for justifying management of the "end-stage" hypoxic wound, as mentioned above, is the patient's **Goal-Aspiration Score** and **Host-Function Score**. However, there can be no compromises in employing the management elements described in this chapter. The second outcome is living with a small, chronic, stable wound (next section). The third outcome is that of a lower limb amputation. In almost all cases, this was avoided if the patient's FSD wound was able to progress to the end of the latency and the beginning of the angiogenesis stages. In our experience, lower limb amputations have occurred in five highly predictable circumstances, namely: 1) a new major ischemic event in the extremity, 2) a foot rendered structurally (i.e. mechanically) unstable after control of the infection and establishment of viable margins, 3) co-existing collagen vascular diseases/Raynaud's phenomena where vasculitis and/or vasospasm is a predominant presentation, 4) a subset of patients who have difficulty in eradicating Methicillin resistant Staphylococcus aureus infections in bones adjacent to the wound, and 5) intractable pain from the area of involvement in the lower extremity.

LIVING WITH A CHRONIC, STABLE NON-HEALING WOUND

The Chronic, Stable, Non-healing Wound – Rarely a FSD (failed, sloughed, dehisced) wound that is improving reaches a point that progress with epithelialization ceases. Usually, the remaining open area is superficial, small in size and "so innocent"

Clinical correlations:
A 59-year-old male with diabetes developed a limb threatened infected Charcot arthropathy of his midfoot. With management that included the strategic elements previously described (Part III), a lower limb amputation was avoided.

A small wound persisted on the plantar lateral aspect of his midfoot, hindfoot junction. After three debridements and two attempts at skin grafting after the debridements, the wound persisted. A trial of negative pressure wound therapy irritated the tissues because of the maceration it caused.

The decision was made to use an antibiotic ointment with dressing changes every other day and in-office debridement of hypertropic callus that formed around the wound semi-monthly.

With this management, the patient remained a community ambulator with prescription footwear over a ten-year period. He was able to attend sporting events and social activities. The wound did not prevent the patient from undergoing coronary bypass surgery and participating in the cardiac rehabilitation program.

Comment:
In this situation, eradication of the infection would not likely have resulted in as functional an outcome as occurred by allowing him to live with a chronic, stable wound. The patient's motivation (high **Goal-Aspiration** and **Host-Function Scores**) to keep mobile and preserve his foot was probably the most important consideration for avoiding a lower limb amputation

that it does not interfere with walking activities (Figure 11-14). Typically it occurs in the post-operative foot that has major structural alterations, skin tightly adherent to underlying bone or combinations of these. Further revision surgery would make the foot mechanically unsound and/or subject it to new wound problems should an attempt be made to revise the underlying bony structures and close the defect with a flap or graft. Although the chronic stable wound requires daily wound care by the patient (or caregiver) usually of the simplest type, this outcome is a satisfactory option and allows essentially unhampered ambulatory activity for the patient. Again, the **Host-Function** and **Goal-Aspiration Score** must be sufficient to justify the option of living with a chronic stable wound. Patient compliance requirements include daily wound care such as cleansing, applying a gel or ointment and covering with a thin gauze bandage, repeated monthly or bimonthly follow-up checks and consistent use of prescription footwear to avoid future complications. Follow-up checks are essential to debride callus/keratinized skin around the wound margins that typically occur in these chronic, stable non-healing wounds. During the rechecks, the wound care specialist should ensure that the wound base remains healthy and if not, temporarily switching to enzymatic debriding or bioburden controlling agents and that protective footwear remains in good condition. Occasionally after three or more years of this management, and for reasons totally unexplainable, the chronic stable wound completely heals. This is an additional reason to encourage the active patient to live with the chronic stable wound.

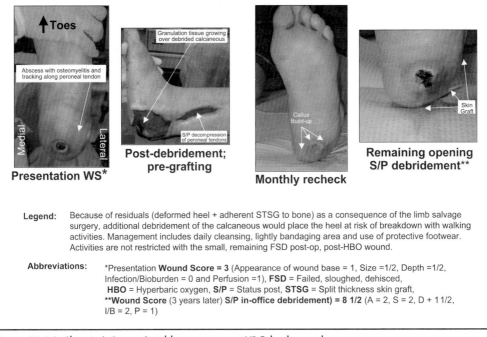

Legend: Because of residuals (deformed heel + adherent STSG to bone) as a consequence of the limb salvage surgery, additional debridement of the calcaneous would place the heel at risk of breakdown with walking activities. Management includes daily cleansing, lightly bandaging area and use of protective footwear. Activities are not restricted with the small, remaining FSD post-op, post-HBO wound.

Abbreviations: *Presentation **Wound Score = 3** (Appearance of wound base = 1, Size =1/2, Depth =1/2, Infection/Bioburden = 0 and Perfusion =1), **FSD** = Failed, sloughed, dehisced, **HBO** = Hyperbaric oxygen, **S/P** = Status post, **STSG** = Split thickness skin graft, ***Wound Score** (3 years later) **S/P in-office debridement) = 8 1/2** (A = 2, S = 2, D + 1 1/2, I/B = 2, P = 1)

Figure 11-14. Chronic (>3 years) stable post-op, post-HBO heel wound.

CONCLUSIONS

Distinguishing Features of This Chapter – In many respects this is the "ultimate" chapter in our text. Not only is it one of the longest, but also more importantly it contains information that is unique and unlikely to be found in any other wound text available. The information in this chapter "pushes the envelope" of limb salvage endeavors. It distinguishes the wound health care providers who are adept at managing the uncomplicated wound from the multidisciplinary wound team with expertise to salvage wounds that place the patient at risk of loss of life or limb. There are few other situations in medicine where the multidisciplinary approach is so essential to achieve good outcomes and avoid major amputations as in the management of the hypoxic "end-stage" wound as described in this chapter.

Factors that Make this Chapter Unique – First, it defines both descriptively and quantitatively (using the **Wound Score**) what an "end stage" wound is. Second, with use of the **Host-Function** and **Goal-Aspiration Scores**, it provides the most objective criteria available for justifying a decision to salvage or recommend a lower limb amputation for the "end-stage" wound. Third, it supplements the five essential treatment strategies (Part III) with five additional "special consideration" interventions. Each of the special consideration interventions is directed by those with the most expertise for the intervention, for example, the hyperbaric medicine specialist for hyperbaric oxygen treatments; medical health care providers for pharmacologically improving perfusion; the vascular surgeon experienced with distal revascularizations for last resort arterial surgeries; and the surgeons dedicated to limb salvage for minimally invasive/keep it simple surgeries. The surgeons dedicated to limb salvage are also the most suited to manage FSD (failed, sloughed, dehisced) wounds and the long term care for chronic stable wounds. Finally, the illustrations, figures and tables used to augment the prose are sui generis (in a class of their own) having been selected specifically to illustrate information in the text and being able to stand alone in conveying the essential information in this chapter.

The Wound Score as a Tool for Evaluation and Management of the "End-Stage" Hypoxic Wound – As quoted at the beginning of this chapter, "It doesn't take much to keep tissues alive; to achieve wound healing is another matter." This statement embodies the sentiment of this chapter. Although hypoxia is the major reason wound healing is not achieved, other reasons exist which will be described in the next chapter. In those wounds where tissues remain alive, but are unable to heal (another definition of the "end-stage" wound) the information presented in this chapter presents an approach and describes predictable outcomes for the hypoxic wound. The **Wound Score** is a useful tool to evaluate, decide on management and document progress in these challenging wounds, as the examples in this chapter demonstrate (Figures 11-7, 11-8, 11-9, 11-11, 11-12, and 11-14). Even though the **Wound Score** improved, the perfusion assessment grades changed little in these examples. Two explanations exist for this observation. First, the limb with the "end-stage" wound frequently has already been revascularized and/or is unable to be re-vascularized and second, even though perfusion is poor, with optimal management even hypoxic wounds can heal as improvements in the remaining four assessments of the **Wound Score** demonstrate. When viability of the hypoxic "end-stage" wound is one consideration and "to achieve wound healing is another matter," the information in this chapter demonstrates how this can be best be achieved.

QUESTIONS

1. What are the roles of the **Host-Function Score** and the **Goal-Aspiration Score** in the process of decision-making regarding amputations?

2. What pharmacological agents augment oxygen delivery?

3. What are possible side effects of pharmacological agents that are used to augment oxygen delivery?

4. What is the One-Two-Three Protocol?

5. What are the predictors of failures in lower extremity revascularizations?

6. What are common misconceptions about revascularizations and angioplasties?

7. What are the goals of "KISS" (Keep it Simple and Speedy) surgeries and minimally invasive surgeries?

8. What are the likely outcomes of surgical and other "end-stage" wound management interventions for the "end-stage" wound?

9. What are the stages observed in the healing of the failed, sloughed, and dehisced wound?

10. What are characteristics of and management for the chronic stable wound?

REFERENCES

1. Strauss, MB. Diabetic foot and leg wounds. Principles, management and prevention. Primary Care Reports 2001; 7(22):187-197

2. Strauss MB, Bryant BJ, Hart GB. Transcutaneous oxygen measurements under hyperbaric oxygen conditions as a predictor for healing of problem wounds. Foot & Ankle Intl. 2002; 23(10):933-937

3. Strauss MB. Problem wounds, practical solutions. J MuscloSkeletal Med. 2006; April:251-262

4. Strauss MB. Hyperbaric oxygen as an intervention for managing wound hypoxia; its role and usefulness on diabetic foot wounds. Foot & Ankle Intl. 2005; 26(1):15-18

5. Sheffield PJ. Measuring tissue oxygen tension: a review. Undersea Hyperb Med. 1998 Fall;25(3):179-88

6. Borer RC Jr., Borer KM, Strauss MB. Prospective serial transcutaneous hyperbaric oxygen challenge measures in problem lower extremity wounds. Undersea Hyperb Med. Vol 27 2000 Supplement pg 40

7. Kalani M, Brismar K, Fagrell B, et al. Transcutaneous oxygen tension and toe blood pressure as predictors for outcome of diabetic foot ulcers. Diabetes Care 1999 Jan;22(1):147-51

8. Strauss MB, Chase P, Kustich N, Nation P. Use of the One-Two-Three protocol to augment HBO managment of dysvascular foot wounds. Annual Scientific Meeting of the Undersea and Hyperbaric Medical Society, 1997

9. Strauss MB, Barry DD. Vascular assessment of the neuropathic foot. J Prosth Ortho. 2005; 17(2) Suppl;535-537

10. Taylor S, Kalbaugh C, Balackhurst D, et al. Determinants of functional outcome after revascularization for critical limb ischemia: An analysis of 1000 consecutive vascular interventions. J Vasc Surg. 2006; 44(4):747-756

11. Strauss, MB; Strauss AB, Borer, KM. Do transcutaneous carbon dioxide measurements predict healing of problem wounds? Undersea Hyperb Med. Vol 27 2000 Supplement pg 40

12. Hartman LA, Strauss MB, Hart GB, Borer Jr RC. Transcutaneous oximetry as predictor of healing in lower-extremity wounds managed with hyperbaric oxygen. Undersea Hyperb Med. Vol 28 2001 Supplement pg 61

13. Guyton AC, Hall JE. O2 Diffusion. In: Textbook of Medical Physiology, 10th ed. Philadelphia, PA: WB Saunders; 2000:454,465

14. Strauss MB. Surgical treatment of problem foot wounds in patients with diabetes, Clin Orthop Related Res. 2005; 439:91-96

15. Wallace DM, Archer P, Roznos K, Peters S, Strauss MB. Use of directional flow irrigation. Ostomy Wound Manage. 1989; Spring; 22:34-40

16. Strauss MB, Bryant BJ, Hart JD. Forefoot narrowing with external fixation for problem cleft wound. Foot & Ankle Intl. 2002; 23(5):433-439

17. Isenberg JS, Costigan WM, Thordarson DB. Subtotal calcanectomy for osteomyelitis of the os calcis: A reasonable alternative to free tissue transfer. Ann Plast Surg. 1995; 35:660-663

18. Smith DG, Stuck RM, Ketner L, et al. Partial calcanectomy for the treatment of large ulcerations of the heel and calcaneal osteomyelitis. An amputation of the back of the foot. J Bone Joint Surg Am. 1992; 74:571-576

19. Del Pinal F, Herrero F, Cruz A. A technique to preserve the shape of the calcaneus after massive osteomyelitis. Brit J Plast Surg. 1999; 52(5)415-417

20. Bragdon G, Baumhauer J. Total calcanectomy for the treatment of calcaneal osteomyelitis. Techniques in Fooot & Ankle Surg. 2008; 7(1):52-55

21. Strauss MB, Futenma CE, Hart JD. Healing in post-hyperbaric oxygen, post-operative failed, sloughed, dehisced foot wounds. Undersea Hyperb Med. Vol 25 1998 Supplement pg 30

22. Strauss MB, Miller SS, Lewis AJ, Aksenov IV. Staging the healing of failed, sloughed, dehisced wounds. Undersea Hyperb Med. 2009 July/Aug; 36(4):282

23. Markagakis LL, Gosgrove SE, Song X, et al. An outbreak of multidrug-resistant acinetobacter baumannii associated with pulsatile lavaage wound treatment. JAMA, 2004 December 22/29 Vol 292, No. 24 3006-3001

CHAPTER

12 OTHER "END-STAGE" WOUNDS

CHAPTER TWELVE OVERVIEW

INTRODUCTION 333

PRESSURE ULCERS/INDOLENT WOUNDS 335

CHARCOT ARTHROPATHY 341

FAILED BELOW KNEE AMPUTATION 346

POST-TRAUMATIC WOUNDS 350

VENOUS STASIS ULCERS 356

SEVERE BURNS 361

CONDITIONS CAUSING OTHER "END-STAGE" EXTREMITY WOUNDS . . 362

CONCLUSIONS 362

QUESTIONS 365

REFERENCES 366

"Time is the ultimate test."

INTRODUCTION

Many other wounds meet the criteria of "end-stage" wounds, that is, wounds that are so serious that lower limb amputation or, if a pressure ulcer/indolent wound, comfort care measures only become a management consideration. **Wound Scores** in the 3 ½ point to 4 ½ point range provide objective confirmation of the seriousness of the wound. Management decisions need to be based on the patient's desires paired with the "reality of the situation." The cognitive status of the patient often is such that the patient lacks decision-making capacity and thus family members, other caregivers, and/or those who have the patient's durable power of attorney must make these life and/or limb threatening decisions. The **Host-Function** (Chapter 2) and **Goal-Aspiration** (Chapter 1) **Scores** provide essential information for appraising the reality of the situation and making crucial decisions whether to salvage, amputate, or in certain situations initiate comfort care measures only.

Comfort care must be differentiated from hospice care, palliative care, and benign neglect.

> Futile care is another term that is sometimes used in this context. Not only does it have a bad connotation, implying that anything that is done for the patient is wasted effort (or futile), but it also implies that it is an ill-advised use of expenditures and health care resources. Naturally, such considerations raise medical ethics and religious moral concerns; discussion of these potentially emotionally charged issues is deferred to other sources.

These interventions represent a continuum of care responses (Figure 12-1). Hospice care is instituted when the realization that death is imminent and the goal is to make the patient as comfortable as possible. Palliative care is the utilization of measures, including surgeries, to make the patient's remaining existence as pleasant as possible. They may include debulking of tumors, implantation of pain management pumps, dispensing high dose analgesics with high addictive potential, and internal fixation of fractures, as well as other measures. Benign neglect care implies that, although death is likely to occur sometime in the future, the decision has been made to reduce care to a minimum, keeping comfort and reduction of resources as primary objectives. In this sense, compassionate care and benign neglect have common elements, but benign neglect implies that there is a treatable problem such as an "end-stage" wound that can be managed with the elements described in the previous chapter. From a "problem" wound perspective, compassionate care is a more appropriate consideration for chronic wound conditions where healing is not an expectation; but conversely, death is not likely to occur as a direct cause of the problem. The patient may live for months or even years with the wound problem.

Three objectives must be realized when initiating compassionate care for the "end-stage" wound. They include: 1) comfort for the patient, 2) ease of care for the caregivers, and 3) maintenance of dignity for the patient. Comfort for the patient is always

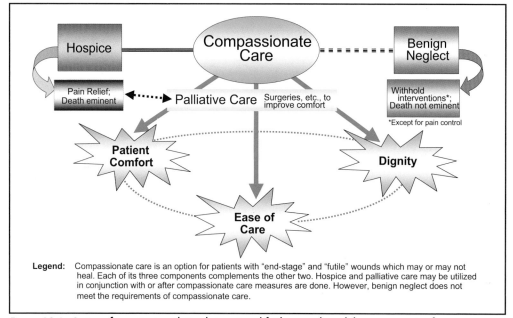

Legend: Compassionate care is an option for patients with "end-stage" and "futile" wounds which may or may not heal. Each of its three components complements the other two. Hospice and palliative care may be utilized in conjunction with or after compassionate care measures are done. However, benign neglect does not meet the requirements of compassionate care.

Figure 12-1. Options for patients with "end-stage" and futile wounds and the components of compassionate care.

the primary objective. Appropriate dressing material selection and reduced frequency of dressing changes can help make wound care as comfortable as possible for the patient and make the wound care as easy as possible for the caregivers. Finally, it is appropriate to do interventions, including surgeries that improve the dignity of the patient, such as releasing contractures so the patient can lie flat in bed. Usually, each component complements the others, as will be described later in this chapter.

Several features of other (than hypoxic) "end-stage" wounds are noteworthy. First, many of these wounds (unlike the hypoxic "end-stage" wound) have a single etiology. That is, the patient does not have significant comorbidities, especially peripheral artery disease. In contrast, usually one or more comorbidities contribute to the "end-stage" hypoxic wound. Second, time seems to favor these types of wounds and is "the ultimate test" of outcomes. With optimal management, most of these "end-stage" wound problems improve, albeit slowly due to their severity. Reasons for this include: 1) Angiogenesis is likely to continue, especially when hyperbaric oxygen is used to initiate this process. 2) Nutritional deficits are remedial (Chapter 6), but take time to resolve.

The above reasons (especially 3 and 4) explain why "Sometimes time is the ultimate test" for deciding the extent of debridement and/or the level of amputation. Although there are strong economic pressures to expedite care, for maximal conservation of tissue and preservation of function in "end-stage" wounds, allowing the time for the wound to demarcate assures the most salvage of tissue at the time of definitive surgery.

This has important functional and economic benefits, such as salvaging the knee with a delayed below knee amputation rather than proceeding directly to an above knee amputation.

3) Demarcation of healthy from non-healthy tissues occurs slowly; the better the demarcation, the easier are the definitive surgeries to cover/close the wound. 4) Wound hygiene takes time to improve in response to wound care and repetitive on-ward debridements; the cleaner the wound and the healthier the surrounding skin, the better the surgical outcomes. 5) Outcomes with surgery are improved when definitive surgery is done during the reparative and remodeling stages rather than the acute, inflammatory stage (Chapter 2); this is especially true with necrotizing soft tissue infections, limb threatening crush injuries, and Charcot arthropathy wounds. 6) Optimization of medical conditions (Chapter 6), if present, such as congestive heart failure, fluid retention, peripheral edema, electrolyte imbalances, respiratory insufficiency, azotemia, etc., takes time. The better the medical condition of the patient, the more successful the outcomes for managing the "end-stage" wound.

Often, higher priority managements such as for cardiac, pulmonary and renal conditions take precedence over definitive surgical management of wounds. Optimal care for wounds associated with purpura fulminans/acute adrenal insufficiency, necrotizing soft tissue infections, and vasculitic ulcers may need to be deferred until the life and/or limb-threatening condition is stabilized. Myocardial infarction, respiratory failure, shock, gastrointestinal bleeding, acute brain insults, and spinal cord injuries are other examples of comorbidities that necessitate primary attention be given to them in deference to the wound. Finally, attention to other surgically correctible problems, such as contractures and deformities, have secondary benefits for wound healing as observed in trochanteric pressure ulcers/indolent wounds, failed below-knee amputations, and foot and ankle wounds that are a consequence of deformities. These may need to be addressed before definitive management of the wound is possible. The remainder of this chapter discusses specific "end-stage" wound types. Each has a different etiology and pathophysiology. Each is reviewed from the standpoints of special features of the wound, pathophysiology, associated comorbidities, management, and compassionate care decision-making.

PRESSURE ULCERS/INDOLENT WOUNDS

Special Features: Pressure ulcers/indolent wounds typically occur in patients with other comorbidities. They occur over bony prominences; most frequently the sacrum, ischial tuberosities, greater trochanters of the hips, and the bony prominences of the knees, ankles, heels, and feet. Most can be managed in their early stages with orthotics, off-loading, and wound care with the expectation of healing. For pressure ulcers/indolent wounds of this level of severity, **Wound Scores** are greater than 4 points. However, a subgroup is nearly impossible to prevent and equally refractory to treatments (Figure 12-2). This defines the "end-stage" pressure ulcer/indolent wound. By definition, **Wound Scores** are 4 ½ points or less. Typically, a constellation of conditions contributes to the development of "end-stage" pressure ulcers/indolent wounds and will be discussed shortly. Even though almost all "end-stage" pressure ulcers/indolent wounds develop over bony prominences, other conditions predispose the skin to ulcerate so problems develop with less than expected perturbations.

Pathophysiology: Pressure ulcers/indolent wounds are complications waiting to happen. Predispositions include atrophy of the skin from age-related changes, malnutrition, moisture control problems, neurological impairments, immobility, peripheral artery disease, shear stresses, and bony prominences. Two mechanisms contribute to pressure ulcer/indolent wound formation. First, direct pressure on the skin over a bony

Although the NPUAP (National Pressure Ulcer Advisory Panel, 1989, 2001— see Chapter 4) staging system for pressure ulcerations is the standard of practice for grading pressure ulcers/indolent wounds, it has deficiencies such as failure to describe the appearance of the wound base (e.g. healthy-vascular versus necrotic), the size of the wound, the bioburden, or perfusion. Also, while the grades may change as the pressure ulcers/indolent wound improves (or worsens) it is not nearly as dynamic in reflecting healing responses as the Wound Score is.

The NPUAP's chief virtue is that it is useful for defining the wound depth. It is no coincidence that it (the wound depth) is one of the five assessments used for generating the **Wound Score**.

A criticism against using the **Wound Score** for grading pressure ulcer/indolent wounds is that usually it is not possible to use pulses to grade the perfusion assessment, especially for pressure ulcers/indolent wounds in the lower trunk and hips. This is a valid criticism, but the answer is to use secondary methods for evaluating perfusion (that is, capillary refill, coloration, and temperature of the adjacent skin.) Rarely is inadequate perfusion the reason "end-stage" pressure ulcer/indolent wounds fail to heal.

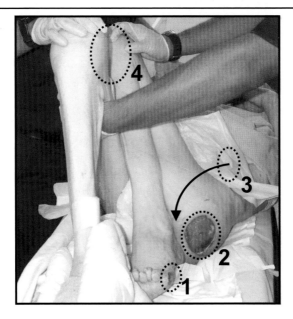

Legend: Multiple pressure sore sites secondary to severe lower extremity contractures: 1) lateral side of left forefoot, 2) left hip greater trochanter, 3) back of left heel, and 4) inside aspects of both knees. The severe contractures render interventions such as off-loading, splinting, muscle relaxants, Botox injections, and physical therapy ineffective. The common denominator in the generation of all these pressure sores is pressure concentrations over bony prominences.

Figure 12-2. Pressure sores secondary to contractures.

prominence causes ischemia of the tissues over the prominence. Even though the patient's systolic blood pressure may be 120 mmHg, the capillary perfusion pressure to the tissues at risk is one fourth of this and may be even less in the patient with peripheral artery disease. Consequently, minimal direct pressure over the bony prominence in the presence of one or more of the above predispositions can quickly lead to devitalized tissue and the development of a pressure ulcer/indolent wound. Observations reveal that direct pressure on impaired skin over a bony prominence for as little as one hour can lead to pressure ulcer/indolent wound formation.[1, 2, 3]

The second condition predisposing to pressure ulcers/indolent wounds is the stretching of skin over bony prominences such as the greater trochanters of the hips. In this sense, the "pressure ulcer/indolent wound" is really a "tension" wound and the pathophysiology is analogous to a Chinese finger trap (Figure 12-3); the more the tension on the skin (or the finger trap), the narrower the lumen and the less perfusion to the skin. In some cases, the bony prominences attenuated the skin enough that they push through the skin from inside out. Consequently, wounds develop even without direct pressure over the area and off-loading the area does not lead to healing. Another consideration is minimal stress to and/or injury of atrophic skin over bony processes from shear stresses. Merely sliding a patient from bed to gurney may generate enough shear stress to disrupt the integrity of atrophic skin over bony prominences.

Comorbidities: The occurrence of pressure ulcers/indolent wounds is almost predictable. Predisposing factors include malnutrition, contractures, and neurological impairment leading to immobility. These three factors are the "terrible triad" of pressure ulcer/indolent wound evolution (Figure 12-4). Neurological impairment as a consequence of strokes, other types of nervous system insults such as multiple sclerosis, Parkinsonism, cerebral palsy, etc., or spinal cord injury is frequently the underlying

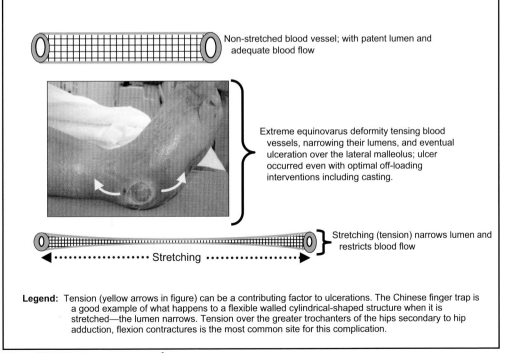

Non-stretched blood vessel; with patent lumen and adequate blood flow

Extreme equinovarus deformity tensing blood vessels, narrowing their lumens, and eventual ulceration over the lateral malleolus; ulcer occurred even with optimal off-loading interventions including casting.

Stretching (tension) narrows lumen and restricts blood flow

Stretching

Legend: Tension (yellow arrows in figure) can be a contributing factor to ulcerations. The Chinese finger trap is a good example of what happens to a flexible walled cylindrical-shaped structure when it is stretched—the lumen narrows. Tension over the greater trochanters of the hips secondary to hip adduction, flexion contractures is the most common site for this complication.

Figure 12-3. Tension as a cause of pressure sores.

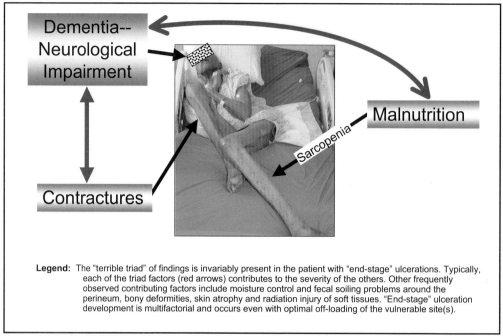

Legend: The "terrible triad" of findings is invariably present in the patient with "end-stage" ulcerations. Typically, each of the triad factors (red arrows) contributes to the severity of the others. Other frequently observed contributing factors include moisture control and fecal soiling problems around the perineum, bony deformities, skin atrophy and radiation injury of soft tissues. "End-stage" ulceration development is multifactorial and occurs even with optimal off-loading of the vulnerable site(s).

Figure 12-4. The "terrible triad" in "end-stage" ulcer development.

problem contributing to pressure ulcer/indolent wound development. Consequences of these neurological conditions are immobility, contractures, and dysphagia. When the factors of the "terrible triad" are present in their severest degrees, pressure ulcers/indolent wounds can almost be impossible to prevent. Although pressure ulcers/indolent wounds are often times ascribed to neglect, neglect may be due to failure to address the underlying global problems of the "terrible triad" rather than the nearly impossible challenge of off-loading the injury site with day-to-day nursing care.

Management: As alluded to above, effective management of "end-stage" pressure ulcers/indolent wounds must be directed at addressing the global problems. Whereas restoration of neurological function is not likely to occur, the other two components of the "terrible triad" of end-stage pressure ulcers/indolent wounds are correctable. Malnutrition is a remedial problem (Chapter 6). The expectation of healing of pressure ulcers/indolent wounds is essentially nil in the presence of severe malnutrition. Invariably, malnutrition is associated with neurological impairment from residuals of stroke and/or deficits in cognitive function. In these situations, alimentation may need to be managed with nasogastric (NG) tube feedings or percutaneous endoscopic gastrostomy (PEG) feedings. Minimal contractures and spasticity may be managed initially with splinting and stretching of the contracted joints. When these problems are of intermediate severity, use of oral baclofen (Lioresal®), an implantable baclofen pump, botulinum toxinA (Botox®) injections, or combinations of these may be sufficient to control the contractures. When severe, surgical release of the contractures is recommended. Although there are numerous references and textbook descriptions of contracture releases in burn, cerebral palsy, and meinigomyelocele patients, there is a dearth of reports about their use in patients with "end-stage" wounds.[4] With minimal invasive surgical techniques (Chapter 16) doing percutaneous and limited open tenotomies at the hip, knee, and ankle levels, contractures can be resolved and amputations avoided (Table 12-1 and Figure 12-5).[5] With nutrition management and contracture releases, progressive worsening of "end-stage" pressure ulcers/indolent wounds is no longer observed; in fact, many begin to improve without changing the wound management. Pain is decreased presumably from release of spastic muscles, positioning of patients facilitated and, in many, the ability to sit can be restored.

TABLE 12-1. MINIMALLY INVASIVE TECHNIQUES FOR LOWER EXTREMITY CONTRACTURE RELEASES

Contracture Problem	Technique	Benefits	Comments
Hip Flexion & Adduction	Percutaneous tenotomies of hip adduction-flexion muscles with an incision <1 cm in length; bleeding is controlled with firm, direct compression in the groin for 10 to 15 minutes. Typically the incision is so small that no closure—or only 1 or 2 staples are used. A compression dressing is strapped across the groin	1. Hip abduction facilitates perineal care 2. Elimination of tension over the greater trochanters of the hips 3. Hip extension complements knee flexion contracture releases to straighten lower extremities 4. Releases counteract lumbosacral spine kyphosis and relieve pressure over the presacral area	The spastic hip flexion-adduction muscles bowstring across the groin as the hip is abducted; this facilities the releases of the percutaneous muscles at their insertions Hip range of motions are usually started one day after surgery
Knee Flexion	Approximately 5 cm incisions are made along the posterior medial and lateral aspects of the knee with the midpoint of the incision at the joint line Tendons are individually "captured" with a curved clamp and brought to the skin surface The tendons (and any associated muscle fibers) are excised with electric cautery The joint is manipulated into as much extension as possible Skin closures are done with staples	1. Knee extension complements release of hip flexion contractures to eliminate the "knees in the chest" deformity 2. Since the hip flexors are biarthroidal (cross two joints) the benefits of releases at the hips and knees complement each other 3. Straightened knees allow techniques to relieve pressure on the posterior aspects of the heels to be easily implemented	If contractures are minimal, extension is maintained with knee immobilizers If moderate to severe, the knee is manipulated into extension and pins placed temporarily (2 to 4 weeks) across the knee joint If the joint capsules are so severely contracted that more than 40 degrees of residual flexion remain, pins are placed in the distal tibial shafts and skeletal traction applied for 1 to 2 weeks to gradually stretch out the joint capsules
Ankle Equinus	Tri-hemisections of the Achilles tendon done with 3 alternating 1/2 centimeter incisions; 2 medially and one laterally starting medially at the tendon insertion on the heel Dorsiflexion pressure is placed on the plantar aspect of the foot to slide the cut portions of the tendons past each other	1. Eliminates ankle equinus and hindfoot varus 2. Allows application of splinting devices to protect the heels 3. Complement knee flexion contracture releases since the gastrocnemius muscles are biarthroidal	Bleeding is controlled with a compression dressing Incisions are small enough that suture or staple closures are usually not needed

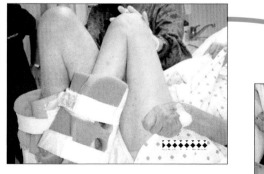
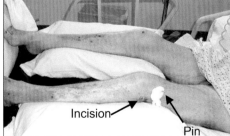

Percutaneous (hips) and limited open (knees) contractures releases

Incision   Pin

Legend: With minimal invasive surgeries (see Chapter 16), much can be gained in those patients with severe lower extremity contractures with or without associated "end-stage" wounds. The improved posturing facilitates optimal positioning of the patient. Pain relief is improved. The releases allow sitting activities and as the patients say, give them a "new lease on life." Temporary pin placement across the knee joint maintains knee extension without use of splints and casts that lead to pressure ulcers/indolent wounds.

Figure 12-5. Immediate lower extremity posturing improvement after minimally invasive contracture releases.

Compassionate Care/Decision Making: If the decision is made to initiate comfort care measures only in deference to achieve healing of the "end-stage" wound, the following five items must be considered:

- Selection of dressing materials that are most comfortable for the patient and do not require inordinate amounts of the caregiver's time. Effective choices include hydrogel and silver impregnated absorptive dressings. Dressings are changed daily, or if the wounds are relatively non-exudative every other day, for these wound dressing materials. Gauze moistened with acetic acid solution is another choice, but usually requires dressing changes twice a day in order to keep the wound base moist. Negative pressure wound therapy (NPWT) is especially useful for cavitary wounds that have viable tissues in the base and are not complicated by underlying bone infection. In convenience to caregivers, they are unsurpassed since dressings changes typically need only be done twice a week. For the ambulatory patient, carrying the NPWT vacuum pump can be a nuisance.
- Optimization of nutrition should be done through oral supplements, tube feeding (NG or PEG), parenteral nutrition (hyper alimentation), or combinations of these (Chapter 6).
- Minimally invasive surgical releases of contractures should be offered as an option to the patients or their health care decision makers. The benefit of contracture releases are several, including: 1) dignifying the patient by making it possible for him/her to lie in bed in the supine position and sit in a chair versus being "rolled-up" in a ball—the so-called "knee chest" position, as is associated with severe hip and knee flexion contractures, 2) improved access for perineal care with release of hip flexion-adduction contractures, 3) ability to off-load presacral, ischial, and hip pressure ulcers/indolent wounds by being able to rotate the patient from side-to-side which is nearly impossible to do effectively with the patient in the knee-chest position. Also, this mitigates pressure concentration over the presacral area from the hyper flexed lumbar spine as a consequence of severe hip flexion contractures; and 4) Ability to relieve effectively relieve heel pressure from the underlying bedding by placement of pillows under the calves or off-loading orthotics that now become possible with straightened lower extremities and elimination of ankle equinus contractures.
- Lower limb amputations are recommended when pressures sores in the feet and ankles are intractable, gangrene is present, and/or they are a source of sepsis. Typically, such problems are associated with "end-stage" wound hypoxia.
- Judicious use of analgesics for pain relief and sedation for agitation is recommended. A fine balance must be achieved between making the patient comfortable and avoiding further depression of already impaired cognitive function.

Decision making for management of "end-stage" pressure ulcers/indolent wounds needs to be based on both subjective and objective criteria. Subjective criteria are based on the patients' and their caregivers' desires. The **Host-Function** and **Goal-Aspiration Scores** (Chapters 1 and 2) help to objectify decision-making for management. The lower both scores are, the stronger the recommendations should be to institute comfort care measures only. Of all the compassionate care measures, the decision for contracture releases is usually the most difficult for those who make decisions for the patient's management. It sounds almost paradoxical to recommend surgical release of contracture as a comfort care measure. However, for the reasons given above, there are justifications for proceeding with these minimally invasive surgical techniques in such situations.

CHARCOT ARTHROPATHY

Special Features: Charcot arthropathy is an enigmatic condition characterized by bone resorption, bone collapse, and ensuing deformities. Its most common presentations are in the foot and ankle. It is invariably associated with neuropathy, and diabetes mellitus is the most common comorbidity associated with Charcot arthropathy. Reported incidents of Charcot arthropathy in the feet of patients with diabetes range from less than one to 37 percent.[6, 7] In our experiences, more than 50 percent of the patients with diabetes we are treating for foot and ankle wounds have neuroarthropathic changes. When wounds are present and complicated by underlying osteomyelitis and major deformities, the condition may rightfully be labeled an "end-stage" wound and lower limb amputation becomes a consideration. Many unanswered questions remain with respect to Charcot arthropathy. For example, what is its cause, why are there so many different presentations, why does it occur in only a small population of patients with neuropathies, and how should it be managed?

A simplified classification system based on acuity, acute or chronic, and the presence or absence of a wound helps in making management decisions (Figures 12-6 a, b).[8] Initially, the acuity must be established. In acute presentations, wounds usually are not present or are only superficial. However, a wound rather than the deformity may be the reason the patient seeks medical attention. Typically, the foot is warm and swollen. If it is acute, then casting evolving to specialized footwear is performed to maintain a plantigrade foot. The potent biphosphonates pamidronate disodium (Aredia®) and zoledronic acid (Zometa®), both useful for prevention of bone resorption and currently approved for the prevention of skeletal related events in patients with bone tumors, should be considered in the acute inflammatory stage of Charcot arthropathy. These medications seem to hasten resolution of the inflammatory response and may lessen the deformity that arises from bone resorption.[9, 10] Surgery rarely needs to be done in the

In the acute inflammatory stage of Charcot arthropathy, it may be difficult to differentiate the physical findings from osteomyelitis. With acute Charcot arthropathy, signs of sepsis such as malaise, fever, chills, leukocytosis, positive blood cultures and dysglycemia are typically absent in contrast to what would be expected with an infection in a closed space.

Plain x-rays of bones and joints with acute Charcot arthropathy often cannot be differentiated from osteomyelitis presentations. However, nuclear medicine scanning with Technetium plus Indium will differentiate inflammation from infection. Interpretations of magnetic resonance studies are usually "over-read" in favor of osteomyelitis with the recommendation made for nuclear medicine studies to establish the diagnosis.

If the diagnosis of Charcot arthropathy versus osteomyelitis is still in doubt, then a bone biopsy for culture and sensitivities under computer tomography guidance should be performed.

acute stage. This is often associated with failed open reduction internal fixation of ankle fractures in neuropathic joints. The hardware is often observed to fail; deformities with open wounds rapidly develop and evolve to bone and joint infections. In all respects, these so-called Charcot fractures (our terminology) qualify as "end-stage" wounds and often lead to lower limb amputations.

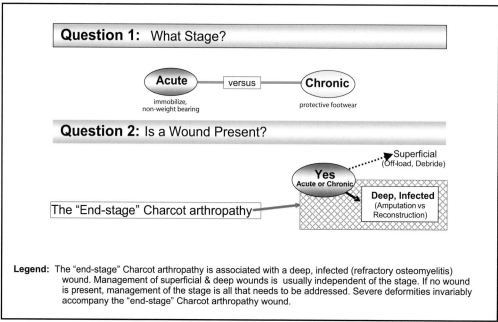

Figure 12-6A. Two questions to ask about Charcot arthropathy and its relationship to the "end-stage" wound.

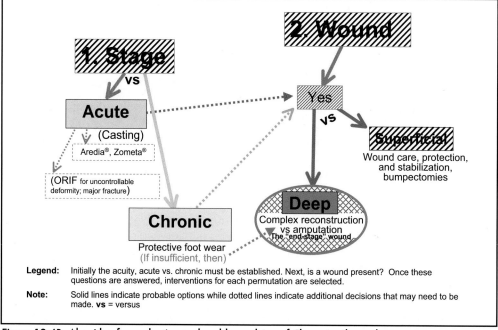

Figure 12-6B. Algorithm for evaluation and problem solving of Charcot arthropathy.

Once the inflammatory (acute) phase transitions into the chronic stage, protective footwear is usually sufficient to allow the patient to ambulate. If not, due to major deformities or deep wounds, complex reconstructions versus amputation are the considerations. The "end-stage" Charcot arthropathy is a chronic condition where a deep wound, usually associated with refractory osteomyelitis and major deformities is present. When treatment interventions such as debridements, antibiotics, and bracing are ineffective and the condition is serious enough that a lower limb amputation is recommended by one or more experts in dealing with this problem, our definition of an "end-stage" wound is met.

Pathophysiology: As mentioned above, the pathophysiology of Charcot arthropathy is unclear. It is invariably associated with a neuropathy, but the perception of pain in the involved area does not rule out its existence. It appears that trauma to the foot or ankle initiates a local hyperemic response. The trauma often goes unrecognized due to absence of pain and/or proprioceptive responses. The consequence of the

The importance of proprioception to protect joints cannot be over-emphasized. Normally, every joint movement is associated with unconscious proprioceptive responses. These responses fine-tune the agonistic and antagonistic muscle activities that move the joint. When disrupted, stresses that usually are mitigated by the protective action of the muscles acting across the joint are directly transmitted to the joint. This leads to bone collapse and resultant deformities. The bones surrounding the joint become increasingly susceptible to collapse due to the osteopenia caused by mineral washout from increased blood flow.

Whereas sensory and motor neuropathies are readily confirmed by the physical examination, proprioception is not. Loss of proprioception is difficult to diagnose and is often only made by deductive reasoning. That is, the diagnosis is made deductively when accelerated joint destruction is observed in the presence of other neuropathy presentations.

increased blood flow is washout of the mineral (calcium) content of the bone. With softening of the bone and absence of protective sensation, bone collapse and joint deformities precipitously develop with usual walking activities. Wounds occur because of repetitive trauma to stress areas generated by the deformities, abnormal mechanics associated with walking using the deformed foot, or combinations of these. Wounds typically progress from superficial ulcers to deep ulcers, then to bone and joint infections. In the presence of deformities, the eradication of bone and joint infections is invariably unsuccessful with usual interventions such as antibiotics and debridements. Deformities are often so severe that they cannot be controlled with bracing.

Comorbidities: As stated above, Charcot arthropathies are invariably associated with neuropathies. Diabetes mellitus is the most common comorbidity found in patients with Charcot arthropathy. Virtually any condition that disrupts innervation to a joint and/or the tissues around a joint can lead to Charcot arthropathy. Other conditions that have been associated with Charcot arthropathy include syphilis, myelodysplasia, trauma, strokes, spinal cord injuries, poliomyelitis, multiple sclerosis, and other demyelinating diseases. Unfortunately, about 50 percent of the patients with "end-stage" Charcot arthropathy are morbidly obese. This substantially complicates management of the "end-stage" wound. Other comorbidities frequently found in patients with

The eponym Charcot arthropathy, the name usually given to this condition, honors Jean Martin Charcot, a French neurologist who first reported its existence. In 1868 he described neurogenic arthropathy associated with Tabes dorsalis (syphilis). Although today syphilis is an extremely rare cause of this problem, the eponym persists and is becoming increasingly recognized as a foot and ankle complication of diabetes mellitus.

"end-stage" Charcot arthropathy include atherosclerotic heart disease with heart failure, low ejection fractions, hypertension and arrhythmias, peripheral artery disease, chronic venous insufficiency, fluid retention, malnutrition, chronic kidney disease, chronic obstructive pulmonary disease, and gastroesophogeal reflux disease.

Management: There are two obvious choices for management of "end-stage" Charcot arthropathy: lower limb amputation, or complex reconstruction of the foot and/or ankle. Selection of the latter choice is contingent on the patient's very strong desire to avoid amputation. The **Host-Function** (Chapter 1) and **Goal-Aspiration** (Chapter 2) **Scores** are useful adjuncts for helping to make decisions about salvage or amputation for management of the "end-stage" Charcot arthropathy. Unless both scores are in the acceptable range, complex reconstruction should not be considered. In addi-

TABLE 12-2. STAGES IN THE MANAGEMENT OF "END-STAGE" CHARCOT ARTHROPATHY

Stage	Management	Duration	Comments
1. Preparation	1. Pre-op optimization of medical conditions and nutrition 2. Antibiotics (if patient septic) 3. Hyperbaric oxygen (HBO) 4. Optimal wound management	2 to 4 weeks	Hyperbaric oxygen (HBO) indicated for chronic refractory osteomyelitis, threatened flaps, mixed synergistic infections, or combinations
2. Surgery	1. Debridement to viable, non-infected bone and soft tissues 2. Correction of deformities with ostectomies, osteotomies, tenotomies-lengthenings and capsulotomies 3. Stabilization of the foot and ankle with ring external fixation (Ilizarov) 4. Complete or partial wound closure 5. Antibiotics based on bone cultures	Surgeries typically require 3 to 4 hours	In general, surgical decisions are based on clinical findings (rather than x-rays) with the goals of eliminating the infection and achieving an aligned plantigrade foot. Whatever needs to be done should be done; for example, partial talectomies, wedge osteotomies of metatarsals, ostectomies, etc
3. Post-op Care	1. Wound care and antibiotics 2. Hyperbaric oxygen 3. Continued rigid stabilization with external fixation	12 weeks (8 weeks minimum time for external fixation)	Premature removal of external fixator may be necessary due to pin tract infections or patient's inability to tolerate the fixator any longer HBO useful to help with flap preservation and healing of a partially closed wound
4. Protection	1. Casting non-weight bearing for 3 months 2. Casting weight bearing for 3 months 3. Ambulation with a walker boot for 3 months	9 months	Cast windows used to provide access to the wound for dressing changes if wounds are still present at this stage
5. Care After Healing	1. Protective footwear including CROW (Charcot Restraint Orthotic Walker) boot if necessary 2. Orthotics 3. Skin and nail care 4. Edema reduction program 5. Prophylactic surgeries, if indicated	Periodic rechecks (for remainder of the patient's life)	Follow-up intervals determined by patient's compliance (as reflected on the **Goal-Aspiration Score**) Frequently, additional surgeries such as toe tendon tenotomies, ankle roddings, ostectomies, etc. are required at this stage

tion, comprehensive management of the patients' comorbidities must be performed to achieve the best possible outcomes. Salvage of the "end-stage" Charcot arthropathy requires a multidisciplinary approach and specific interventions for five clearly definable stages of management (Table 12-2). Convalescence requires a year or more time. Typically one or more additional surgeries, usually minor such as ostectomies (bumpectomies), tenotomies, or osteotomies are required after this time as the patient resumes

Clinical correlations:

A 61-year-old female diabetic was referred for a second opinion regarding a lower limb amputation for an "end-stage" Charcot arthropathy of her right foot. With reasonable Host-Function and Goal-Aspiration Scores, the option of limb salvage was offered. After deliberating on the option for a week, she decided to proceed with limb salvage. Medical management and wound care were optimized over a two-week period. During this stage, shards of infected, non-viable bone, essentially free of soft tissue attachments, were removed with on-ward debridements. These were painless due to the profound sensory diabetic neuropathy in her feet.

At surgery, the wound was debrided of all suspicious infected, non-viable bone based on its clinical appearance. The foot was realigned without the need for osteotomies or ostectomies (other than the debridement). Position of the realigned foot was maintained with a modification of the Ilizarov ring external fixator.

Post-operatively, wound care was required for six months until complete healing occurred by secondary intention as the patient evolved through external fixation, casting and removable walker boot stages. Edema reduction measures and prescription orthopaedic footwear allowed the patient to resume community ambulation walking activity with a cane. In-office tenotomies for clawed toes were done to prevent complications from these deformities.

Comment:

Although the scenario reads as if everything proceeded smoothly, a number of challenges occurred. First, the patient was initially unwilling to devote a year to care and convalescence for the problem, and wanted to proceed immediately with a lower limb amputation. After strong encouragement by the family and review of the expected convalescence with reassurance that at each stage it would be possible to increase mobility, the patient reconsidered. After eleven weeks in the external fixator, the patient was "beside herself" and consequently the fixator was removed one week before the desired 3-month goal.

Post-operatively, the wound was slow to heal. After six weeks in the fixator with no apparent improvement, healing began to occur by secondary intention. This was attributed to the debridement, use of antibiotics, and the "jump start" effect of hyperbaric oxygen.

After the immobilization period, massive foot edema interfered with footwear. An edema reduction program resolved this problem. Superficial ulcerations appeared on the apices of the deformed clawed toe joints when walking was resumed. Prophylactic tenotomies resolved this problem.

In summary, although this scenario was presented as a "relatively smooth" course, multiple challenges that needed immediate and special management were required to achieve the successful outcome.

activities of daily living. Our experiences have shown that lower limb amputation is avoided and resumption of functional ambulation is achieved in about 75% of the cases.

Compassionate Care/Decision Making: In no other "end-stage" wound situation is the importance of information from the **Host-Function** and **Goal-Aspiration Scores** more important in making decisions about selecting management options. For example, if the patient has no potential for resuming ambulation after correction of the problem, an immediate lower limb amputation should be done. Likewise, without strong patient motivation and family support, outcomes for foot and ankle reconstruction are likely to be poor. Since lower limb amputation is a reasonable and acceptable option for managing "end-stage" Charcot arthropathy of the foot and ankle, if a decision is made to salvage the limb, there can be no compromises in the management. When amputation is an option, it is a reasonable compassionate care/decision making choice for the infirm patient who would not likely be able to use the salvaged extremity in a functional way.

FAILED BELOW KNEE AMPUTATION

Special Features: When amputations fail distal to the ankle joint, a concerted effort is frequently made to salvage the foot, especially in the diabetic patient, as was discussed in the previous chapter as the failed, sloughed, dehisced strategy for the "end-stage" wound. In contrast, when a below-knee amputation fails, typically the first consideration is to proceed immediately to an above-knee amputation. In many respects, the failed amputation is an "end-stage" wound. When bone is exposed and necrotic, infected tissue are present in the wound base, the **Wound Score** is invariably in the 2 ½ point to 4 ½ point range, thereby meeting the **Wound Score** point criteria as an "end-stage" wound. In addition, usually the recommendation is made to do a more proximal lower limb amputation, another method of defining an "end-stage" wound.

Much can be said about the benefits of salvaging a failed amputation, especially at

Clinical correlations:
A 67-year-old female underwent a below-knee amputation due to a dysvascular, non-healing, painful foot wound. This amputation failed due to peripheral artery disease and was immediately converted to an above-knee amputation. The patient was strongly motivated to resume independent ambulation. She was fitted for an above-knee prosthesis and underwent rehabilitation to her maximum functional potential.

When the patient was next seen in follow up, she was walking with a walkerette sans her prosthesis. When asked where the prosthesis was she said it was "in the closet." With further questioning, it was learned that the prosthesis was too heavy to use and too difficult to don and remove. She said she did not plan to use the prosthesis ever again and was satisfied to use her walkerette for household activities and a wheelchair for community ambulation.

Comment:
This scenario illustrates the difficulties the older patient with limited activity and energy reserves has in using an above knee prosthesis functionally. One solution is to have the patient evaluated by a physical medicine specialist before prescribing the $15,000 to $20,000 (or even more with computerized knee and special ankle joints) prosthesis to ascertain whether or not the functional and motivational potential exists to justify the expenditure.

the below knee level.[11] In a marginal ambulator, salvage of the distal-level amputation and preservation of independent ambulation may be the difference between continuing in an independent living status versus institutionalization in an assisted living facility. If the patient is an independent ambulator with a foot or below-knee amputation, he or she may not be so with an above knee prosthesis.[12] Not only is the prosthesis more than twice as heavy as the below knee prosthesis, but the energy requirements for walking are more than double those with an above knee prosthesis. If the patient is a functional ambulator with bilateral below knee amputations, conversion of a failed site to an above-knee amputation may exceed the patient's reserve capacity to walk with the above-knee prosthesis. Finally, salvage of a contralateral below-knee amputation in a patient with a non-functional (with respect to prosthesis use) above-knee amputation or the hemiparetic/hemipledgic patient with a below-knee amputation may have significant functional considerations with respect to transfers and mobility. That is, the salvaged below knee amputation will allow the patient to maintain a level of independence for transfers with a below knee prosthesis that would not be possible with an above-knee amputation.

Pathophysiology: Below-knee amputations fail for three main reasons: injury to the stump end, ischemia of the flaps, or severe flexion contracture of the knee (Figure 12-7). The failure is often due to a combination of these reasons. Subgroups of patients with below-knee amputations are particularly susceptible to falls. One group is those patients with impaired cognitive function who do not realize that their limb has been amputated. Typically, the patient gets up at night failing to realize that the leg has been amputated and falls when trying to walk. A second group are those patients with weakness and/or balance problems who fall when the demands of transferring or walking with aids exceeds their functional capacity. In either situation, the trauma of the fall disrupts the closure.

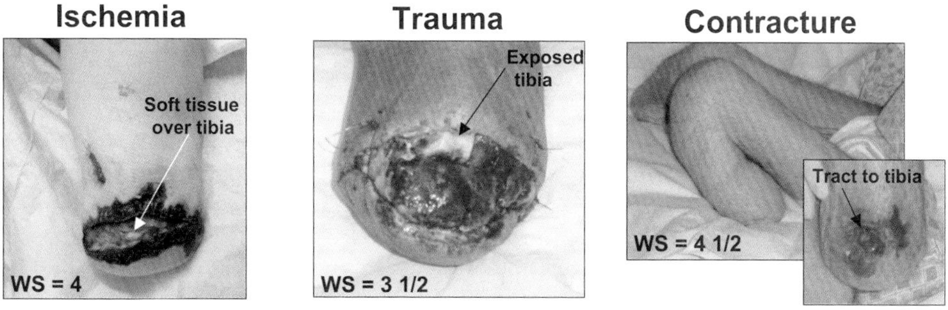

Ischemia

Soft tissue over tibia

WS = 4

Post-op slough secondary to ischemic flaps; patient has multiple comorbidities

Trauma

Exposed tibia

WS = 3 1/2

Dehiscence secondary to a fall; patient decided to use bathroom without assistance. Bleeding required a transfusion

Contracture

Tract to tibia

WS = 4 1/2

Pressure necrosis secondary to knee flexion contracture

Legend: Ischemia, trauma, and contractures are the major causes of early post-op below knee amputation failures. The resultant wounds could be considered "end-stage" because revision to an above knee amputation is an option. The **Wound Score** quantifies the ischemia and contracture related wounds shown above as "end-stage" i.e. 2 1/2 to 4 1/2 point scoring range.

Key: **WS = Wound Score** (see Chapter 5)

Figure 12-7. Early below knee amputation failures leading to "end-stage" wounds.

Since peripheral vascular disease is the most frequent reason for below-knee amputations, the flaps at the below-knee level may be ischemic just as the more distal portions of the extremity were. When flaps fail from ischemia, a typical progression is observed. The progression is from the appearance of threatened flaps with paleness or cyanosis, to dehiscence, to infection of the open wound, to exposure of the transected bone end. Often a combination of minor trauma, such as a bump to the suture line, plus ischemia leads to the breakdown of the amputation site closure.

Knee flexion contractures in the below-knee amputee are particularly pernicious. Causes are post-operative pain, muscle imbalances secondary to neurological conditions, or combinations of these. Typically, the patient with an ischemic leg persistently postures the lower extremity with the knee in 90 degrees of flexion, often dangling the extremity over the end of the bed. The patient does this because it affords the most pain relief. Perfusion to the dependent, ischemic extremity appears to be improved due to the pressure gradient effect on blood flow when the foot is maintained in the lowest possible position.[13, 14] The contracture rapidly becomes fixed due to shortening of the knee flexor muscle lengths and contracture of the posterior capsular structures of the knee. If the knee flexion contracture is not resolved during the amputation surgery, its persistence will place concentrated compression forces on the stump end in the post-operative period. This leads to pressure necrosis and wound dehiscence. If the amputation does heal with persistence of the flexion contracture (due to meticulous off-loading of the stump end), fitting of a functional prosthesis becomes increasing difficult if the knee flexion contracture exceeds 25 degrees.

The immediate post-operative period is the time when the below-knee amputation is at greatest risk of failing. The reasons are several and include 1) the 20-fold or greater metabolic demands for healing a wound as compared to the steady-state/healed situation (Chapter 2), 2) the patient is at the most vulnerable point of his/her convalescence, often times having to deal with residuals of sepsis and/or tissue breakdown products of the infected, necrotic foot before the amputation, then trying to meet the increased metabolic demands of wound healing, 3) minimal tensile strength of the skin flaps immediately after closure,[15, 16] 4) pressure necrosis over the stump end associated with a knee flexion contracture, and 5) over-confidence resulting in falls when the patients thinks he/she can make unassisted transfers for wheelchair ambulation for use of the bathroom.

Late failures of below-knee amputations are usually due to unsatisfactory stump ends with failure of and/or migration of the myofascial closure layer over the end of the tibia. This has been especially noted to occur in myodeses where muscle is sewn into the end of the tibia through drill holes in the bone. The loss of soft tissue padding results in skin being the only covering over the bone end. A knee flexion contracture greater that 25 degrees will make prosthesis fitting difficult and if greater than this, almost impossible. Occasionally bone spurs, neuromas, obesity, and technical problems, such as the fibula being longer than the tibia, are reasons for late failures of below-knee amputations because they cause new wounds, pain or inability to "fit" a prosthesis.

Comorbidities: As indicated above, comorbidities are invariably associated with failed below-knee amputations and contribute either directly or indirectly to the failure. Peripheral arterial disease, venous stasis disease, fluid retention, coronary artery disease and diabetes mellitus contribute to failures due to impaired or inadequate perfusion and oxygenation of the flaps. Patients with residuals of strokes, weakness, and balance problems associated with infirmities, morbid obesity, and impaired cognitive function have a propensity to lose their balance and fall, especially when making transfers. Neurological conditions such as strokes, Parkinsonism, multiple sclerosis, and paraplegia often lead to joint contractures due to spasticity and muscle imbalances. Smoking is another comorbidity/risk factor that is associated with increased failure for healing of all wound types.[17-19]

   Management: There are two obvious choices for management of failed below-knee amputations. The first is re-amputation at a more proximal level, such as through the knee or above-the-knee levels. In those patients who have marginal potential for ambu-

Clinical correlations:

An alert, active, fully independent 69-year-old male required a lower limb amputation due to chronic post-traumatic osteomyelitis involving 75 percent of the leg. The decision was made to do an amputation at the level of the proximal third of the leg. Immediately post-op, the wound dehisced due to infection. With the patient's strong desire to preserve his knee confirmed by high **Host-Function** and **Goal-Aspiration Scores**, the decision was made to salvage the failed amputation. With wound care, on-ward debridements, antibiotics, and hyperbaric oxygen treatments (i.e. strategic management), the infection cleared and the base of the open wound granulated.

At this point, the patient was returned to the operating room for revision of the failed amputation. Closure was achieved by removing the remaining portion of the fibula and shortening the tibia. To optimize post-operative immobilization and maintain the knee in extension, temporary pins were placed across the knee joint.

Even with the above measures, the flaps dehisced. Again, because of the high **Host-Function** and **Goal-Aspiration Scores**, the wounds were managed with the techniques described for managing FSD (failed, sloughed, dehisced) wounds described in the previous chapter. The wounds healed. The patient was fitted with a prosthesis using a neoprene thigh sleeve for attachment. Even though there was only eight cm of remaining tibia, the patient became a community ambulator with the prosthesis without the need for aids and regained over 90 degrees of motion in his knee.

Comment:

Because of the patient's age and moderate obesity, it is unlikely he would have been able to use an above-knee amputation prosthesis. The post-operative complications were consistent with the challenges this scenario presented. The strong **Host-Function** and **Goal-Aspiration Scores** justified the intervention used to preserve the knee joint, and his functional outcome validated the efforts.

lating with a below the knee prosthesis, a higher level amputation with increasing energy demands for walking with the longer length, heavier prosthesis may be the deciding factor for not using a prosthesis. The other choice is salvage of the failed below-knee amputation using the strategic management principles applied to the "end-stage" wound (Table 12-3). Before making a decision to salvage the failed below-knee amputation or move to a higher level amputation, information from the **Host-Function** and **Goal-Aspiration Scores** needs to be considered. The challenges, time considerations, and costs of salvaging the failed below-knee amputation must be weighted against the potential of resuming functional ambulation with salvage of the failed below-knee amputation. The **Host-Function** and **Goal-Aspiration Scores** provide the essential information to make this decision.

TABLE 12-3. MANAGEMENT STRATEGIES FOR THE FAILED BELOW-KNEE AMPUTATION

Interventions	Duration	**Management** (Use Hyperbaric Oxygen with the Wound Care through Early Post-op Care Interventions)
Wound care	2 to 3 weeks	Initial dressing changes are done each 8-12 hours using gauze moistened with acetic acid or similar solutions. When suppuration controlled, switch to daily enzymatic debriding agents (if necrotic tissue remains in the wound) or hydrogels if the wound is clean. Consider negative pressure wound therapy. Wound protection, immobilization, and knee extension are achieved with a knee immobilizer between dressing changes and debridements.
Debridements	Same as above	Debridements typically are done on-ward or in the office. Local anesthetic gels are usually sufficient to provide pain relief for the superficial debridements.
Revision surgery	------------	Major features include debridement of scar tissue, shortening of the tibia, resection of the remaining portion of the fibula (if needed for approximation of the flaps), manipulating the knee into full extension (with hamstring tenotomies if necessary), and placement of pins across the knee joint to keep the knee in extension during the early healing phase.
Early post-op care	Weekly X-2 Alternate weeks X-2	Half the remaining skin closure staples are removed at each visit. Incision hygiene and skin care measures are reinforced. Occasionally, about half the revision surgeries fail, slough or dehisce. However, about 90% of these eventually heal by secondary intention (see failed, sloughed, dehisced wound section in Chapter 11).
Intermediate post-op care	2-3 months	Prosthesis fitting and rehabilitation; skin hygiene (cleansing + lubrication)
Follow-up	Yearly	Typically, prosthetic components wear out. Sockets need to be adjusted as the stump atrophies and changes shape. Prostheses may need to be replaced every 1-3 years depending on the activity of the patient.

Considerations for Compassionate Care: In contrast to hip and presacral pressure ulcer/indolent wound management from a compassionate care perspective, there is a surgical solution for managing the failed below-knee amputation. The solution is, of course, doing an amputation at a higher level. Consequently, strong justification for expending the efforts and expenses to salvage the failed below knee amputation is needed. This justification is precisely what the **Host-Function** and **Goal-Aspiration Scores** provide.

POST-TRAUMATIC WOUNDS

Special Features: Trauma is a major cause of extremity injuries in our highly mobile, vehicle oriented society. Severe injuries, often limb threatening, occur to the extremities because of the enormous transfer of energy to the relatively vulnerable tissues of the body.[20] The consequences are not only fractures, but damage to the soft tissues that surround the bone. The degree of soft tissue injury reflects the severity and is used to grade crush injuries. More often than not, the prognosis for recovery can be determined at the time of the first assessment by the trauma specialist. Several grading systems have been devised to direct management and predict outcomes using the criteria of soft tissue damage for determining the severity of the injury (Tables 12-4a, b and 12-5).[21, 22] The consequences are that limb threatening injuries result from trauma and the management described for other "end-stage" wounds may be needed for obtaining optimal results with crush and similar type injuries.

TABLE 12-4A. GUSTILO* CLASSIFICATION AND OUTCOMES OF OPEN FRACTURE-CRUSH INJURIES

Grade	Findings	Outcomes
1	Puncture-type wound (inside to out) with fracture	Healing ~ 100% of cases
2	Laceration with fracture	~10% infection or delayed healing
3	**Crush Injuries**	**Sub-classifications**
-A	**Sufficient soft tissue to cover bone after debridement**	**Same as for Grade 2**
-B	**Exposed bone remains after debridement**	**~50% infection, non-union complication rate**
-C	**Above findings with concomitant vascular injury**	**>50% complication rate including infections, non-unions and amputations**

TABLE 12-4B. DECISION MAKING FOR SALVAGE AND USE OF HYPERBARIC OXYGEN FOR OPEN FRACTURE-CRUSH INJURIES USING THE GUSTILO CLASSIFICATION PAIRED WITH THE HOST-FUNCTION SCORE

	Healthy	Impaired	Decompensated
1	No	No	Yes*
2	No	Yes	Yes*
3-A	No	Yes*	Yes*
-B	Yes*	Yes*	No**
-C	Yes*	No**	No**

Yes* = Use Hyperbaric oxygen as an adjunct to management

No** = Consider primary amputation

Notes: *Use the **Host-Function Score** (Chapter 2) to help decide whether or not hyperbaric oxygen should be used for limb threatening open fracture-crush injuries (Healthy host 8-10 points; impaired host = 4-7 points & decompensated host = 0-3 points)

**Consider primary amputation for grade 3-B & C injuries in impaired and decompensated hosts

TABLE 12-5. MESS (MANAGLED EXTREMITY SEVERITY SCORE) FOR PRIMARY AMPUTATION OF SEVERELY INJURED EXTREMITIES AND INDICATIONS FOR HYPERBARIC OXYGEN USING THE HOST-FUNCTION SCORE

Assessments	Points	Comments
A. Skeletal/Soft Tissue Injury		
• **Low Energy** (stab, simple fracture, low velocity gun shot wound (GSW)	1	**Variations of Gustilo Grades**
• **Medium Energy** (multiple or open fractures, dislocations)	2	
• **High Energy** (Close range shotgun, high velocity GSW, crush)	3	
• **Very High Energy** (Above + gross contamination, ST avulsion)	4	
B. Limb Ischemia		
• Perfusion normal	0	**Double score if ischemia time >6 hours**
• Pulse reduced or absent, but perfusion present	1	
• Pulselessness, paresthesias, diminished capillary refill	2	
• Cool, paralyzed, insensate, numb	3	
C. Shock (Systolic BP < 90 mmHg)		
• Systolic BP always >90mmHg	0	
• Transient hypotension	1	
• Persistent hypotension	2	
D. Age**		
• <30 years	1	**Can contribute to 25% or more of the MESS score**
• 30-50	2	
• >50	3	

HBO* Indications

Healthy Hosts
MESS scores of 7 or 8

Impaired Hosts
MESS scores of 5 or 6

Decompensated Hosts with scores of 3 or 4

Notes: The MESS score authors recommend primary amputation if the score is 7 or greater.

*The **Host-Function Score** can assist in making decisions when to amputate and when to attempt limb salvage with the adjunctive use of hyperbaric oxygen.

Because age is used in both the MESS and the **Host-Function Score, there is an overlap of these two assessments.

Kinetic energy is the energy of a body due to its motion relative to some inertial frame of reference. From a trauma-to-tissue perspective, the "energy of the body" is the moving vehicle and the "inertial frame of reference" is the extremity. The formula to quantify this exchange is Kinetic Energy = $1/2mv^2$ (where "m" equals mass, i.e. the weight of the object, and "v" equals the velocity, the speed the object is moving). Kinetic energy, as the formula explains, increases geometrically by the square of the velocity, so the damage to tissues is greatly magnified as the speed of the object increases.

Consider the following: a fractured hip may result from fully transferring the kinetic energy of the body weight through stepping down a one foot curb (the velocity is computed from estimating the end-point acceleration) with a resultant transfer of 50 foot-pounds of kinetic energy. In contrast, the energy transferred from a car bumper to a leg (with the car moving at 20 mph) approaches 10,000 foot-pounds of energy—or over a 2000-fold increase of energy transfer compared to that causing the hip fracture.

Pathophysiology: Tissue injury results from both direct and indirect effects of trauma. Components of both types of injuries may occur. Direct damage to tissues is a consequence of the transfer of the kinetic energy of the moving object to the tissues themselves. Death by physical destruction occurs when energy transfer exceeds the capacity of the tissues to maintain their integrity. For example, a kick to the calf during a football game may cause a "pointer" with contusion of tissues, bleeding, soreness, and temporary hindrance of activity. In contrast, a work-related injury involving a fork lift running over an extremity resulting in both the tibia and fibula becoming not only fractured, but smashed into fragments (i.e. comminuted) will undoubtedly damage the soft tissues overlying the bone beyond repair. Typically, there is gradient of injury in crush injuries from tissues damaged beyond repair to those which will survive and normalize with appropriate management to those tissues that are minimally injured and will recover spontaneously to those tissues that are beyond the injury site and are undamaged (Figure 12-8).

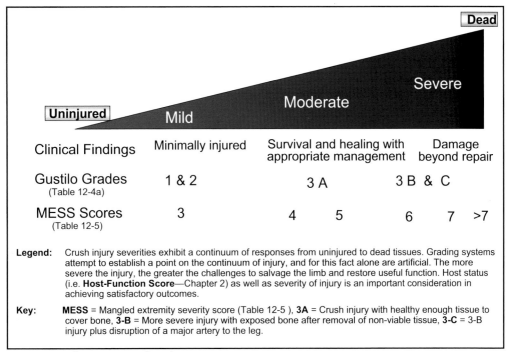

Figure 12-8. The continuum of crush injury severities.

Indirect effects of trauma occur because of damage to the vasculature. Damage from trauma may be at the microcirculatory level or of the major blood vessels supplying the limb. When blood flow is completely arrested, tissues die, just as if they were rendered non-viable by the direct effects of pressure. Frequently, however, at the microcirculation level, there is partial interruption of the circulation such that the tissues are rendered ischemic to the degree that they do not receive enough oxygen, nutrients and leukocytes to carry out their repair and infection control functions even though they do not actually die. Problems associated with partial interruption of the microcirculation include stasis, sludging, arteriovenous shunting, venous outflow obstruction, compartment syndrome, and reperfusion injury. The consequences of impaired flow in the microcirculation lead to secondary complications of crush injuries such as the latent onset of tissue death, non-healing fractures, infection, or combinations of these. This is often a consequence of the self-perpetuating mechanisms (i.e. vicious circle) of edema and ischemia (Figure 12-9). The full extent of the delayed injury may not be appreciated until days after the occurrence. Recognition of the vicious circle of edema plus ischemia and appropriate interventions to mediate its effects are instrumental in minimizing tissue damage and achieving satisfactory outcomes.

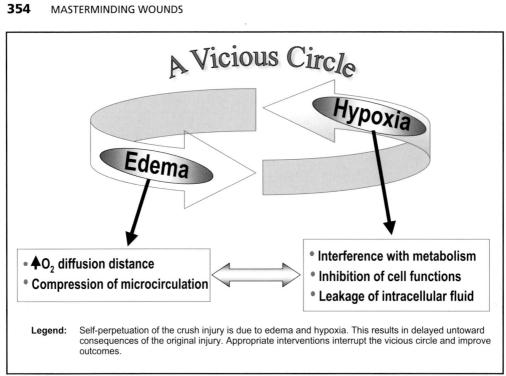

Legend: Self-perpetuation of the crush injury is due to edema and hypoxia. This results in delayed untoward consequences of the original injury. Appropriate interventions interrupt the vicious circle and improve outcomes.

Figure 12-9. The continuum of crush injury severities.

Damage to large blood vessels to the extremity is usually due to laceration of the blood vessel by bone fragments that are displaced at the time of the original trauma or avulsed by dislocations of large joints. Dislocations at the knee joint are particularly vulnerable to vascular injury since perfusion at this level depends on a single vessel, the popliteal artery. Invariably these injuries are a consequence of major trauma—and energy transfer to the tissues with concomitant injuries to bones, ligaments, joint capsules, and tendons. Injuries to major blood vessels need to be recognized immediately and repaired within the four-to-six hour "golden period" that these tissues can withstand cessation of circulation without irreparable damage. The consequences are so dire from crush injury of the extremity with concomitant damage of major blood vessels that complications such as septic non-unions and lower limb amputations are observed in greater than 50 percent of the cases in spite of optimal management.[21-25]

Comorbidities: In contrast to the other "end-stage" wound types, the **Host-Function** and **Goal-Aspiration Scores** are consistently high in this patient group. Typically, traumatic wounds occur in the healthy, active population. Consequently, even with severely traumatized extremities with low **Wound Scores**, concerted efforts are made to salvage the extremity. The MESS (Mangled Extremity Severity Score) provides a guide to when primary amputation of the extremity is indicated and incorporates elements from the **Wound Score** and **Host-Function Score** such as age and perfusion (Table 12-5).[22] In addition, hyperbaric oxygen should be used as an adjunct whenever the extremity is severely traumatized and there are concerns about tissue viability and repair potential (Tables 12-4b and 12-5).

Management: After extrication and attention to CPR and bleeding emergencies at the scene, stabilization and transfer to the emergency department occurs. Upon arrival in the emergency department, after primary and secondary surveys, interventions are

Clinical correlations:

An athletic 46-year-old male sustained a limb threatening, Gustilo grade 3-B (MESS Score = 7) injury to his right leg in a motorcycle accident. The **Wound Score** was 3 points. After debridement and stabilization with external fixation, a large wound with exposed bone remained in the distal third of his leg. The post-operative dressing remained in place until the patient was returned to the operating room for additional debridement and a microvascular free flap 48 hours after the initial debridement.

Post-operatively the patient became septic, the flap sloughed and pus drained from the wound. A staged below-knee amputation was done. It healed with adjunctive hyperbaric oxygen treatments after minor dehiscence and infection in the skin flaps.

Comment:

The patient's high (essentially 10's) **Host-Function** and **Goal-Aspiration Scores** justified attempted limb salvage even though the MESS score (7 points) was high enough to proceed with a primary amputation.

Optimal wound management with frequent dressing changes, on-ward debridements, and hyperbaric oxygen as initial elements of the strategic management of this "end-stage" crush injury were not done before the microvascular free flap.

The premature return to the operating room for the microvascular free flap (before demarcation and edema reduction of the severely injured soft tissues in the gradient of injury was established and wound contamination controlled) probably contributed to the flap failure. If the microvascular free flap had been delayed until the tissues stabilized with support from hyperbaric oxygen, the flap complications and amputation may have been avoided.

directed at stabilizing cardiovascular and respiratory functions, administering antibiotics, determining the circulatory status of the injured extremity, and ascertaining the amount of bony injury (with imaging studies). Emergency surgery has four objectives: 1) exploration to determine the extent of injury, 2) debridement of non-viable tissues up to and including primary amputation, revascularization if indicated and feasible, and 3) stabilization of the bone injuries. If the soft tissue injuries are "end-stage" as established by the **Wound Score** and/or determined to be severe from Gustilo and MESS scores, management utilizing the five treatment strategies (Part III) described for "problem" wounds is essential. Of the five strategies, the use of hyperbaric oxygen is the most overlooked, and is the one that should be started immediately after initial surgical interventions if severely injured soft tissues remain in the wound. After four to seven days, which is usually adequate time for the soft tissues to demarcate themselves as viable or nonviable and edema to be reduced, the patient should be returned to the operating room for additional debridement of the wound and coverage or closure. If bone is exposed, a microvascular free flap may be required to achieve coverage.

Considerations for Compassionate Care: Compassionate care becomes a consideration in patients with severe extremity trauma, when the extremity is salvaged, but the extremity remains functionless due to the extent of injury, the soft tissue loss, chronic infection, non-union, pain or combinations of these. These complications can make the patient an invalid. For the lower extremity, a lower limb amputation becomes the logical compassionate care intervention. Unfortunately, the longer the patient keeps the damaged limb, the less likely an amputation will be accepted. Hence, the recommendation for early amputation should be given. However, not every mangled extremity becomes a liability for the patient. Function and pain are the key determinants in recommending whether to live with an impaired limb or proceed to an amputation.

Clinical correlations

A 29-year old male trucker sustained a severe crush injury to his pelvis and lower extremities after being run over by a fork lift truck. Debridements resulted in removing almost all the soft tissues in his left leg. The foot and thigh segments remained viable. With wound care and hyperbaric oxygen treatments, granulation tissue formed over the periostium of the leg bones. Coverage was achieved with split thickness skin grafts. A fracture of the left ankle and distal tibia was managed with an intramedullary ankle rod. Healing, including the fracture and fusion of the ankle, occurred.

After rehabilitation, the patient became a limited household ambulator with a walkerette and a community ambulator with a wheelchair. Ironically, the left lower extremity became the patient's "good" extremity. The soft tissue injuries to the contralateral right thigh were so severe that the extremity was almost non-functional.

Comment

This scenario demonstrates the results that can be achieved using the "end-stage" wound management interventions. Ironically, the extremity that seemed the more severely injured became the more functional extremity. With ankle fusion, leg muscles are no longer needed to control the foot and ankle. Fortunately neither pain, non-union, nor infection complicated the functional recovery of his left lower extremity. Even with the enormous soft tissue injury, perfusion was sufficient to perfuse the foot and allow healing at the other sites.

VENOUS STASIS ULCERS

Special Features: Venous stasis ulcers present unique challenges. When uncomplicated and managed early, they usually are easily cured. Conversely, when chronic, severe, and associated with other comorbidities, they may qualify as "end-stage" wounds (Figure 12-10). Often, patients with venous stasis ulcers are labeled as being "noncompliant" because they fail to do adequate dressing changes or to use elastic support hose as directed. Caregivers must appreciate that wound care and donning and removing elastic support hose can almost be impossible tasks for patients with impaired mobility, obesity or combinations of these.

Pathophysiology: Venous stasis ulcers usually arise as a consequence of chronic venous insufficiency. Three factors: incompetent valves, insufficient calf muscle pumping action (associated with persistent dependency of the legs), and varicosities trigger venous insufficiency. Decreased intravascular colloid osmotic pressure often associated with malnutrition alters the capillary microfiltration-fluid resorption equilibrium. This generates a gradient for extravascular fluid accumulation resulting in lower extremity edema. Edema contributes to the persistence and refractoriness to treatments of venous stasis

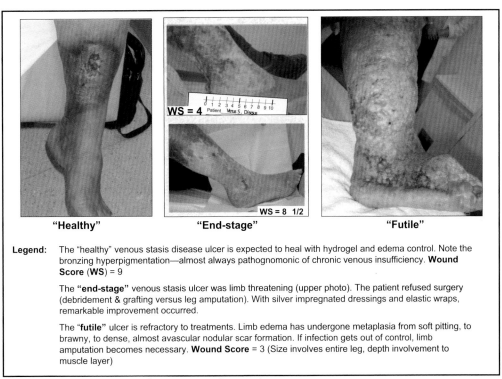

"Healthy"   "End-stage"   "Futile"

Legend: The "healthy" venous stasis disease ulcer is expected to heal with hydrogel and edema control. Note the bronzing hyperpigmentation—almost always pathognomonic of chronic venous insufficiency. **Wound Score (WS) = 9**

The **"end-stage"** venous stasis ulcer was limb threatening (upper photo). The patient refused surgery (debridement & grafting versus leg amputation). With silver impregnated dressings and elastic wraps, remarkable improvement occurred.

The **"futile"** ulcer is refractory to treatments. Limb edema has undergone metaplasia from soft pitting, to brawny, to dense, almost avascular nodular scar formation. If infection gets out of control, limb amputation becomes necessary. **Wound Score = 3** (Size involves entire leg, depth involvement to muscle layer)

Figure 12-10. The continuum of venous stasis disease ulcers

ulcers. Concomitant sclerosis of the lymphatic system is another contributory factor to fluid accumulation. Trauma and phlebitis may be direct or indirect causes of venous stasis ulcers. Minor trauma may disrupt skin already attenuated by hyperpigmentation, venous congestion, age-related atrophic changes, and fluid retention and be the reason that venous stasis ulcerations persist. Phlebitis, another manifestation of venous system pathology, may arise from a combination of factors including valve incompetence from vein wall injury, venous blood flow stasis and/or abnormalities in blood coagulation (i.e. Virchow's triad). This leads to the post-phlebitic, chronic venous insufficiency syndrome with its hallmark signs of chronic edema and bronzing hyperpigmentation of the skin (Figure 12-10).

A consequence of venous insufficiency is fluid leakage from the veins into the subcutaneous tissues resulting in the clinical finding of swelling. Spontaneous, or with minor trauma, ulcerations may develop especially in the distal thirds of the legs. This area is the most vulnerable portion of the leg for ulcer formation because of its minimal subcutaneous and muscle mantle. It is a "watershed" area (i.e. dividing line for the proximal arterial blood supply and the retrograde arterial blood flow from the ankle level) for

In reality, the "end-stage" venous stasis ulcer is really a non-healing wound due to hypoxia, infection, and cicatrix formation in the ulcer base. The cicatrix "barrier" can be so overwhelming that, in a sense, it acts as a chronic compartment syndrome that interferes with perfusion due to scar formation and elevated venous pressures.[26,27] This contributes to their persistence even with optimal management.

perfusion, and it is one of the most persistently dependent portions of the body. The results are slow or non-healing ulcerations usually complicated by secondary infection. The inadequate blood supply often complicated by peripheral arterial disease creates a hypoxic environment. In the presence of hypoxia, the subcutaneous fatty tissues below the ulcer base transform into cicatrix, which becomes an impermeable barrier for angiogenesis and thwarts healing efforts.

Comorbidities: Comorbidities are invariably associated with non-healing, "end-stage," venous stasis ulcerations (Table 12-6). Many times the venous stasis ulcerations are not resolved until the comorbidities are controlled. Morbid obesity is one of the most challenging of the comorbidities. It makes effective venous compression difficult and almost impossible for the patients to do themselves. Other problems can be equally vexing, such as those patients with such impaired lung function or back conditions that force them to sleep sitting up in chairs with their legs continuously in the dependent position. Peripheral artery disease is frequently found in conjunction with venous stasis disease and contributes to the non-healing nature of the refractory venous stasis ulcers. Heart failure, liver disease, malnutrition, chronic kidney disease, and other conditions that cause fluid retention also contribute to the challenges in managing venous stasis ulcers. Lymphedema, often associated with morbid obesity, is another contributing factor to the persistence of "end-stage" venous stasis ulcers.

Management: When dealing with "end-stage" venous stasis ulcerations with or without associated problems (Table 12-6), management goals must be established jointly with the patient and/or the person making the health care decisions for the patient. Information from the **Host-Function** and **Goal-Aspiration Scores** contributes to making appropriate decisions. If the decision is made to allow the patient to "live with the ulcer," the first requirement, in accordance with the precedents of compassionate care, is patient comfort. Uncontrollable pain, when present during dressing changes as well as between dressing changes, is a strong indication for a lower extremity amputation. However, this becomes problematic in the morbidly obese patient where a failed amputation may create wounds more difficult to deal with than the venous stasis ulcerations themselves. The second goal is wound hygiene. Management of the wound base should be done with agents that are the most comfortable for the patient such as hydrogels, antibiotic ointments, or absorbent agents impregnated with silver. The dressing changes should be done as infrequently as is possible, consistent with acceptable wound hygiene. Third, edema reduction measures must be instituted. For reasons previously mentioned, elastic support hose may not be an option. Elastic wraps, sequential segmental elastic bands (Figure 12-11), or elasticized stockinet may be more "user-friendly" for the patient and his/her caregivers. The reduction of dressing changes to as infrequently as possible

> If an amputation is inevitable, the through knee level has desirable features. The soft tissue mantle about the joint and adjacent bones is thinner than in the adjacent leg or thigh, the "hearty" skin over the knee cap provides a durable flap, and once through the skin and subcutaneous layers, the joint capsule, ligaments, and tendons traversing the knee joint are almost avascular.

to maintain satisfactory wound hygiene improves the chances that the patient will be compliant with using limb compression devices. Occasionally, the only option for the patient who is unable to do his/her own dressing changes, nor has others that will help, is to have the patient return to the wound clinic once or twice a week for dressing changes by the clinic staff.

TABLE 12-6. COMORBIDITIES ASSOCIATED WITH "END STAGE" VENOUS STASIS ULCERATIONS

Condition	Associated Problems/Comorbidities	Management Considerations
Diabetes	Associated conditions with diabetes such as hyperglycemia, peripheral arterial disease, heart disease, fluid retention, chronic kidney disease, atrophic skin changes, autonomic nervous system dysfunction, obesity, and limited mobility contribute to the multifactorial problems that interfere with management and healing	Most of these conditions are benefited by medical and surgical interventions; cures are unlikely, but improvements will complement the management of "end-stage" venous stasis ulcers.
Congestive heart failure	Two problems, namely fluid retention resulting in peripheral edema and orthopnea with the need to sit-up continuously with the legs in the dependent position contribute to the refractoriness of venous stasis ulcers	Medical management generally effective in managing congestive heart failure
Morbid obesity	Other conditions found in this table are frequently associated with obesity. Restrictions in mobility make it impossible for the patient to manage their leg ulcers without assistance from others. Limitations in mobility often result in the obese patient sitting with his/her legs in the dependent position during most of their awake hours	Even with help from caregivers, wound care and dressing application can be formidable in the patient with massively obese legs
Vasculitis	This problem is often a consequence of rheumatoid arthritis or other collagen vascular disease such as lupus, scleroderma, mixed connective tissue disorder or dermatomyositis. The requirement for steroids and/or immunosuppressors to manage the primary disease, compounded with vasculitis from the underlying disease processes themselves, interferes with, wound healing and control of infection.	Management is challenging since care of the collagen vascular disease, e.g., the use of steroids, takes precedence over what is "ideal" for healing of the venous stasis ulcer. Cicatrix forms under and around the hypoxic wound. This interferes with perfusion and oxygenation. Without debridement of this relatively avascular fibrotic layer, skin grafting is not likely to succeed.
Chronic obstructive pulmonary disease and/or smoking	These problems are usually related. "End stage" venous stasis ulcers arise when breathing problems are so severe that the patient has to sleep in the sitting position. Dependent edema results and with time the edematous tissues undergo metaplastic changes to fibro-fatty tissue ("brawny" edema) and then to cicatrix. Toxic products of cigarette smoke damage the microcirculation and interfere with gas exchange. Transient vasoconstriction from nicotine interferes with perfusion.	Comfort care measures may be the only alternative for this subset of "end-stage" venous stasis ulcers. With attention to other comorbidities such as obesity and heart failure, these seemingly intractable venous stasis ulcers will respond to treatment. Cessation of smoking can be a major challenge in this group of patients
Post-phlebitic syndrome and post vein stripping complications	Problems arise from interference with venous return and edema formation. Chronically edematous tissues undergo fibro-fatty and cicatrix formation changes as described above. Ulcerations become refractory due to the relative barrier created by the cicatrix to wound oxygenation and angiogenesis.	These wounds tend to be refractory to edema management and wound care measures. Debridement of cicatrix from the ulcer base is a key ingredient for successful skin grafting
Back problems	Occasionally, patients have back problems so severe that they spend all their time, both awake and while sleeping, sitting up. Problems arise as described for the patients with chronic obstructive pulmonary disease.	If pain and wound care become impossible to manage, comfort care measures alone may be insufficient; lower extremity amputation(s) then become a consideration.
Malnutrition	This problem contributes to non-healing of venous stasis ulcers due to edema formation and lack of substrates for healing. It is usually associated with other problems such as dysphagia, malabsorption syndromes, depression and infirmity. Hypoalbuminemia reduces the intravascular colloid osmotic pressure which, in turn, results in fluid shifts from the circulation system to the extravascular spaces, i.e. edema formation.	Although nutrition problems are remedial (Chapter 6), the healing of "end-stage" venous stasis ulcers usually requires more than just the correction of the patient's nutrition status

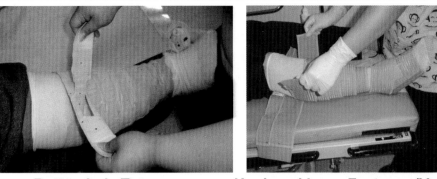

Button-hole Type   **Hook and Loop Fastener (Velcro®)**

Legend: Elastic band or strap-type wraps are effective for edema control in patients who are not able to wear elastic support hose due to leg size, leg shape, underlying bandages, or combinations of these. The posterior portions of the straps are sewn together so they always remain evenly spaced.

With proper instructions, family members or other caregivers can apply the strap-type devices. They may be more effective and "user-friendly" than elastic wraps which often require re-wrappings several times a day due to slippage. Another concern with elastic wraps is a tourniquet effect if the edges of the wraps role and form bands or slide over bony contours and leave some areas uncovered while there is too much compression in the overlap areas.

Figure 12-11. "User-friendly" strap-type edema controlling compression devices.

If the decision is made to heal the venous stasis ulcer, the elements of strategic management (Part III) are instituted. Comorbidities such as vasculitis, heart failure, malnutrition, etc. (Table 12-6) should be controlled to the fullest extent possible. Once the patient's medical condition has been optimized and ulcer bases become healthy, coverage with skin grafting or bioengineered skin substitutes (Tables 9-8 and 9-9) is recommended. An essential ingredient for successful grafting is the debridement of the ulcer base, including the relatively impermeability interface of cicatrix, to healthy vascularized tissue. When the ulcer base is over bony prominences such as the malleoli of the ankle or distal portions of the leg, the debridement may need to be carried down to the periostial layer. Hyperbaric oxygen and/or use of negative pressure wound therapy are useful adjuncts to improve the "takes" of threatened split thickness skin grafts. If feasible, composite closure/coverage techniques may be utilized. For example, the wound may be partially approximated with sutures at its margins to reduce the surface area of the skin graft, rotation flaps may be employed to cover periostium, or combinations of these used.

Considerations for Compassionate Care: Usually the decision for employing compassionate care measures for patients with "end-stage" venous stasis ulcers is obvious; that is, when associated comorbidities are intractable. The more difficult decision is whether to recommend a lower-limb amputation or to "live with" the ulceration. In this situation pain becomes the determinant. If pain is manageable, then amputation should be avoided, especially if the ulcers are bilateral which could make the patient bedridden. The secondary determinant is whether or not wound hygiene is manageable with the care the patient is able to obtain. If not, then a lower limb amputation needs to be considered. Of course, the **Host-Function** and **Goal-Aspiration Scores** add support to which decision is more appropriate.

SEVERE BURNS

Special Features: Burns result from thermal injury to the skin and its underlying structures. Burn wound grading represents a continuum of injury responses as in the other traumatic ischemias. In contrast to crush injuries, thermal energy rather than kinetic energy is the cause of the injury. First-degree burns are characterized by erythema and pain as typically seen in sunburns. They are usually self-limiting, but latent effects lead to premature aging of the skin and skin cancers. Second-degree burns cause partial thickness damage resulting in blister formation and pain. When extensive, fluid losses through the damaged epithelium can lead to fluid and electrolyte complications. Third-degree burns result in full thickness death of the skin and often structures deep to the skin.

The source of the burn injury is important in determining its severity. For example, dry heat burns tend to be less destructive than burns from liquids which have a thousand times or more heat capacitance (specific heat x conductance) than dry air and electricity, which has the propensity to penetrate to deep tissues. Likewise, burns from hot tar, which clings to the skin, can be very destructive. Electrical burns can be surprisingly deceptive with minimal apparent surface injury, yet produce extensive damage to the underlying tissues, including the possibility of bone injury. Often the full extent of the severity of the burn is not appreciated until several days after the injury. Initially, it may be difficult to determine whether the tissues are viable (second-degree burn) or non-viable (third-degree burn) because of the continuum of injury, as is characteristic of all traumatic ischemias (Figure 12-8). Appropriate management of the transitional portion of a burn utilizing the five treatment strategies (Part III) is crucial in establishing the outcome, that is whether the burn evolves to full thickness damages or reverts to second degree involvement.

Pathophysiology: The common final denominator in burn injuries is damage to the underlying vasculature. Burns can rightfully be labeled "ischemic injuries." In first-degree burn injuries, the vasculature is uninjured. Vasodilation occurs as an inflammatory response to the thermal insult. The increased flow dissipates heat and accelerates the normalization of the minimally injured tissues. In second-degree burns, the ischemia injury is superficial enough that only the epithelium is irreparably damaged. Because of underlying vasodilation and loss of the epithelium fluid, losses through the second-degree burn can be substantial. In third-degree burns, the damage tissue is rendered non-viable by the thermal injury. Since there is a continuum of injury, the blood vessels adjacent to the non-viable tissue become non-functional due to stasis, sludging, and edema. There is not only non-viable tissue, but also the vasculature that would ordinarily help in the reparative and infection control processes is so badly injured that it no longer effectively perfuses the tissues that are in greatest need of oxygen, nutrients, growth factors, and leukocytes. The consequence is that these transitionally injured tissues are the most vulnerable to further injury, infection, and death.

Comorbidities: The presence of comorbidities is the exception rather than the rule in most thermal burns. Many burns occur in children from accidental spills of liquid and the working population from work related accidents. When burns are associated with fires in confined spaces, smoke inhalation is always a concern. This injury must be given primary attention, and when coupled with significantly large body surface area burns, has a high mortality rate. Failure to appreciate and manage the enormous fluid losses that can occur from large surface area second- and third-degree burns can lead to shock, renal insufficiency and cardiac problems. Respiratory problems and impaired gas exchange from the smoke inhalation injury compounds these problems.

Management: First and second-degree burns are not "end-stage" wounds. However, third-degree burns, when large in extent, meet the definition of an "end-stage" wound. Fluid and pain management are the first two interventions to be done. Immediate excision of necrotic tissue (escharectomy) and early skin grafting (with autologous skin and/or bioengineered skin substitutes) are contemporary surgical standards of care for managing third-degree burns. Antibiotics are generally withheld unless infection in the injured tissues occurs; then, vigorous organism-specific antibiotics based on cultures and sensitivities are initiated. Finally, hyperbaric oxygen is useful in managing 20-60 percent total body surface area burns and burns of critical areas such as the hands, feet, face, neck, and perineum.[28-32] The immediate initiation of hyperbaric oxygen reduces fluid losses, edema, erythema, and the need for skin grafting by one third. It helps injured transitional tissues, especially between second and third-degree burns, survive. The result is not only better outcomes, but also cost-effectiveness by reducing the requirements for skin grafts and shortening hospital stays when compared to burns of similar severity that did not receive hyperbaric oxygen.

Considerations for Compassionate Care: Only rarely is there a need to consider compassionate care in "end-stage" burns. With greater than 60 percent total body surface area burns, mortality rates are high. In these situations, patient comfort dictates the management. In pernicious burns, especially from electrical injury, the deep soft tissue injury may be so severe that a non-functional, painful scarified extremity results. Amputation and prosthetic replacement may be the best option for the patient in these situations. Scar formation across joints with loss of functional mobility often can be effectively managed with debridement, microvascular free flaps and appropriate splinting during the post-operative period.

CONDITIONS CAUSING OTHER "END-STAGE" EXTREMITY WOUNDS

Other wound conditions can be associated with or evolve into "end-stage" wounds including clostridial myonecrosis, necrotizing fasciitis, refractory osteomyelitis, wounds associated with collagen vascular disease, wounds secondary to coagulopathies, severe burns, erthromelagia, and palmar plantar erythrodysesthesia. Most are the consequences of infection, ischemia, or combinations of these two problems. As in post-traumatic "end-stage" wounds, these conditions tend to occur in the younger patient without other comorbidities or degenerative conditions. Decision-making and management is analogous to the previously described conditions presented in this chapter. These additional conditions are summarized in a table format (Table 12-7). It is noteworthy that for almost all of them, hyperbaric oxygen is a useful adjunct in their management.

CONCLUSIONS

Good judgment is required to make decisions about "end-stage" wounds, whether the wounds are hypoxic or because of the other problems discussed in this chapter. First, the severity of the wound must be ascertained. When a lower-limb amputation is contemplated or a wound fails to heal, the criteria for an "end-stage" wound is met. The **Wound Score** (with scores of 2 ½ points to 4 ½ points) objectifies the clinical impression. The next decision to be made is whether to recommend amputation (or perhaps compassionate/comfort care measures for certain wound types), or to initiate the special considerations (described in Chapter 11) with the goal of limb salvage and/or healing the

TABLE 12-7. OTHER CONDITIONS THAT MAY EVOLVE TO "END-STAGE" WOUNDS

Condition	Special Problems	Pathophysiology	Comorbidities	Management	References
Gas gangrene (Clostridial myonecrosis)	Fulminating course, life threatening sepsis Progression to limb and life threatening within 6-12 hours of symptom onset	Organisms thrive in anoxic environments Prone to develop in devitalized tissues Histotoxic toxins have local (coagulopathy and lytic) and systemic effects	About (~)1/3 of patients without co-morbidities ~1/3 after surgery ~1/3 in compromised hosts (e.g. occult tumors, diabetics)	1-Antibiotics 2-Surgery (often amputation) 3-Hyperbaric O_2 (Stops toxin production; bacteriostatic)	Hart, Lamb and Strauss. 1983 *J Trauma*[33]
Necrotizing Fasciitis (Flesh eating bacteria	May appear to be deceptively benign until debrided Patients may not appear sick	Typically poly flora found in the wound Usually starts from a needle stick (IV drug abuser) or malperforans ulcer Sepsis dissects along tendon sheaths and fascial planes	~50% in IV drug abusers; frequently with hepatitis C, HIV & malnutrition ~50% in compromised hosts; especially diabetics	Same as above; amputations usually avoided with early management. Hyperbaric O_2 reduces tissue loss and returns to the operating room	Jacoby I. Hyperbaric Oxygen Therapy Indications. 2008 UHMS Committee Report[34]
Refractory Osteomyelitis	Infection persists even with optimal antibiotic and surgical management	Infected, dead bone remains isolated from healthy tissue by an avascular interface Recurrences due to multiplication of organisms remaining at the debridement margins	~90% in patients with comorbidities Also observed post-trauma especially with septic non-unions	Hyperbaric O_2 as an adjunct to repeat surgery (debridement and/or stabilization) and antibiotics Limb amputation with severe pain or loss of function	Strauss MB, Miller SS in Hyperbaric Medicine Practice, 3rd edition. Kindwall EP (ed) 2008[35]
Wounds Associated with Collagen Vascular Diseases	Wounds fail to heal even from simple amputations such as a toe tip	Vasculitis reduces perfusion in the microcirculation Usually the most distal portions of the extremities are affected	Steroids and other immunosuppressors interfere with healing and infection control Raynaud's phenomenon often a complicating factor	Adjust immuno-suppressors during the healing period Vitamin C supplements Amputations to levels where healing occurs with hyperbaric O_2	Alivernini S, De Santis M, et al. 2009 *J Am Acad Dermatol*[36]
Wounds Secondary to Coagulopathies	Wound sloughs occur without obvious reasons Problems may be associated with anti-coagulant use	Problems may be due to protein deficiencies (Protein C, Protein S), plasminogen abnormalities, anticardiolipin antibodies, or homocysteine	Usually congenital or acquired defects	Defects detectable by laboratory analyses Cessation of offending agents controls problem Sloughs slow to heal	Nazarian RM, Van Cott EM, et al. 2009 *J Am Acad Dermatol.*[37]
Purpura Fulminans	Accompanied by adrenal failure (Waterhouse-Friderichsen Syndrome), shock, and coagulopathy	Stasis in microcirculation secondary to shock, sludging and/or coagulopathy result in sloughs often so extensive that they are limb threatening	Usually occur in previously healthy patients, often children Invariably preceded by meningitis	Critical care management Hyperbaric O_2 to reduce extent of sloughs, help with demarcation and aid in coverage/ closure	Dinh TA, Friedman J, Higuera S. 2005 *Clin Plast Surg.*[38]
Erythromelalgia (Erythermalgia, Erythralgia)	Extremely rare congenital condition with foot and leg skin erythema, warmth and pain	Wounds develop secondary to the patients' need to continuously immerse feet in cold water to control pain Wounds difficult to manage due to pain	Underlying pathology possibly disordered vasoregulation with uncontrolled blood flow May improve with aging (Hormonal and/or atherosclerosis)	Epidurals and narcotic analgesics may be required to control pain Hyperbaric O_2 observed to help with wound healing	Ley LA. 1985 *Clin Podiatry.*[39]
Palmar Plantar Erthrodysesthesia (Acral erythema or Hand-foot syndrome)	Symmetrical blistering of hands and feet with moist desquamation and severe pain	Idiopathic complication from fluorouracil, capecitabine, etc. used for chemotherapy management of neoplasms	Underlying neoplasm requiring fluorouracil agents	Cessation of chemo-therapy; then resume at lower dose Vitamin B_6 (pyridoxine) Local wound care similar to burn management	*Wasif Saif M, Elfiky AE. 2007 J Support Oncol.*[40]

wound. The **Host-Function** and the **Goal-Aspiration Scores** (Chapters 1 and 2) offer guidelines as to what direction to take. Compassionate care (Figure 12-1) which includes the triad of: 1) comfort for the patient, 2) ease of wound care for the caregivers and 3) dignity for the patient is used when amputation is not feasible or wound healing is not likely to occur. Examples of this are observed in obtunded patients with severe wounds where directives for "do not resuscitate" and "no additional surgical interventions" have been established. Limb amputation is another comfort care consideration and is used to manage the severe extremity wound where salvage is not indicated, but will otherwise meet the three components of compassionate care.

The "end-stage" wounds discussed in this chapter differ from the hypoxic "end-stage" wounds discussed in the previous chapter. All have different, but specific etiologies. In most of these conditions, except for collagen vascular diseases and often necrotizing fasciitis, underlying systemic cardiovascular disease is the exception. Most occur in previously healthy, uncompromised hosts. As in the "end-stage" hypoxic wound, hyperbaric oxygen is a useful adjunct to their management. Gas gangrene, necrotizing soft tissue infections, chronic refractory osteomyelitis, and threatened skin flaps and grafts needed to provide coverage/closure of these wounds are examples of other possible "end-stage" wounds where hyperbaric oxygen is an approved indication. For these wounds, "time is the ultimate test" for establishing seriousness, demarcating viable from non-viable tissues, and for judging outcomes. Finally, once the decision is made to salvage the "end-stage" wound and appropriate management is initiated, almost all improve with time, albeit often requiring weeks or months to reach an endpoint.

QUESTIONS

1. What are the objectives of compassionate care for the "end-stage" wound?

2. What are general features of other than hypoxic "end-stage" wounds?

3. What are the the the pathophysiological mechanisms of pressure ulcers/indolent wounds?

4. What are the predisposing factors for pressure ulcers/indolent wounds?

5. What compassionate care considerations are important for making management recommendations for patients with "end-stage" pressure ulcers/indolent wounds?

6. How does a simplified classification system assist with the evaluation and management of Charcot arthropathy?

7. What are the main causes of failed below-knee amputations?

8. What features of the Gustilo open fracture/crush injury grading system are applicable to "end-stage" wounds?

9. What features make venous stasis ulcerations "end-stage" wounds?

10. What are the roles of hyperbaric oxygen therapy in the management of severe burns?

REFERENCES

1. Gelfen A. How much time does it take to get a pressure ulcer? Integrated evidence from human, animal and in vitro studies. Osteomy Wound Management 2008; 54(10):26-35

2. Gawlitta D, Li W, Oomens CW, et al. The relative contributions of compression and hypoxia to development of muscle tissue damage: an in vitro study. Ann Biomed Eng. 2007; 35(2):273-284

3. Stekelenburg A, Strijkers GJ, Parusel H, et al. Role of ischemia and deformation in the onset of compression-induced deep tissue injury: MRI-based studies in a rat model. J Appl Physiol. 2007; 102(5):2002-2011

4. Cipriano C, Keenan MA. Knee disarticulation and hip release for severe lower extremity contractures. Clinical Orthop Related Res., 2007; 462:150-155

5. Haher JN, Haher TR, Devlin VJ, Schwartz J. The release of flexion contractures as a prerequisite for the treatment of pressure sores in multiple sclerosis: a report of ten cases. Ann Plast Surg. 1983; 11(3):246-24

6. Fabrin J, Larsen K, Holstein PE. Long-term follow-up in diabetic Charcot feet with spontaneous onset. Diabetes Care 2000; 23:796-800

7. Cavanagh PR, Young MJ, Adams JE, et al. Radiographic abnormalities in the feet of patients with diabetic neuropathy. Diabetes Care 1994; 17:201-209

8. Strauss MB, Shields NN. Management of Charcot Arthropathy, 72nd Annual Meeting Proceedings American Academy of Orthopaedic Surgeons 2005; 6:469

9. Jude EB, Selby PL, Burgess J, et al. Bisphosphonates in the treatment of Charcot neuroarthropathy: a double-blind randomised controlled trial. Diabetologia. 2001 Nov; 44(11):2032-7.

10. Anderson JJ, Woelffer KE, Holtzman JJ, Jacobs AM. Bisphosphonates for the treatment of Charcot neuroarthropathy. J Foot Ankle Surg. 2004 Sep-Oct; 43(5):285-9.

11. Miller WC. Measurement properties of the Frenchay Activities Index among individuals with a lower limb amputation. Clin Rehabil. 2004; 18(4):414-422

12. Waters RL, Perry J, Antonelli D, Hislop H. Energy cost of walking of amputees: the influence of level of amputation. J Bone Joint Surg. 1976; 58-A(1):42-46

13. Coni NK. Posture and the arterial pressure in the ischaemic foot. Age Ageing 1983 May; 12(2):151-4

14. Scheffler A, Jendryssek J, Rieger H. Redistribution of skin blood flow during leg dependency in peripheral arterial occlusive disease. Clin Physiol. 1992 Jul; 12(4):425-38.

15. Gamelli RL, Li-Ke H. Model and analysis of wound breaking strength. In Wound Healing Methods and Protocols. (Eds) DiPietro LA & Burns AL, 2003; Humana Press Pg 37-54

16. Lindsted E, Sandblom P. Wound healing in man: Tensile strength of healing wounds in some patient groups. Ann Surg. 1975; 181(6):842-846

17. Silverstein P. Smoking and wound healing. Am J Med. 1992 Jul 15; 93(1A):22S-24S

18. Netscher DT, Clamon J. Smoking: adverse effects on outcomes for plastic surgical patients. Plast Surg Nurs. 1994 Winter; 14(4):205-10

19. Hoogendoorn JM, Simmermacher RK, Schellekens PP, van der Werken C. Adverse effects of smoking on healing of bones and soft tissues. Unfallchirurg 2002 Jan; 105(1):76-81. [Article in German]

20. Strauss M, Miller S. Crush Injury, Compartment Syndrome and Other Acute Traumatic Peripheral Ischemias. In: Hyperbaric Medicine Practice, 3rd Edition. (Eds.) Kindwall EP and Whelan HT. Best Publishing, Flagstaff, AZ 2008:755-790

21. Gustilo R. Management of open factures and their complications. 1982 WB Saunders, Philadelphia PA: 202-208

22. Johansen K, Daines M, et al. Objective criteria accurately predict amputation following lower extremity trauma. J Trauma 1990; 30:568-573

23. Guercio N, Orsini G. Fractures of the limbs complicated by ischaemia due to lesions of the major vessels. Ital J Orthop Traumatol. 1984 Jun; 10(2):163-85

24. Lin CH, Wei FC, Levin LS, et al. The functional outcome of lower-extremity fractures with vascular injury. J Trauma 1997 Sep; 43(3):480-5

25. Cakir O, Subasi M, Erdem K, Eren N. Treatment of vascular injuries associated with limb fractures. Ann R Coll Surg Engl. 2005 Sep; 87(5):348-52

26. Hafner J, Bounameaux H, Burg G, Brunner U. Management of venous leg ulcers. Vasa. 1996; 25(2):161-7

27. Nicolaides AN, Hussein MK, Szendro G, et al. The relation of venous ulceration with ambulatory venous pressure measurements. J Vasc Surg. 1993 Feb; 17(2):414-9

28. Cianci P, Lueders HW, Lee H, et al. Adjunctive hyperbaric oxygen therapy reduces length of hospitalization in thermal burns. J Burn Care Rehabil. 1989; 10:432-435.

29. Cianci P, Lueders H, Lee H, et al. Adjunctive hyperbaric oxygen reduces the need for surgery in 40-80% burns. J Hyper Med. 1988; 3:97

30. Cianci P, Williams C, Lueders H, et al. Adjunctive hyperbaric oxygen in the treatment of thermal burns - an economic analysis. J Burn Care Rehabil. 1990; 11:140-143

31. Cianci P, Sato R. Adjunctive hyperbaric oxygen therapy in treatment of thermal burns: a review. Burns 1994; 20(1):5-14

32. Hart GB, O'Reilly RR, Broussard ND, et al. Treatment of burns with hyperbaric oxygen. Surg Gynecol Obstet. 1974 Nov; 139(5):693-6

33. Hart GB, Lamb RC, Strauss M. Gas gangrene: a collective review. J Trauma 1983; 23:991B1000

34. Jacoby I. Necrotizing soft tissue infections in hyperbaric oxygen therapy indications 12th edition. Gesell LB (ed) The Hyperbaric Oxygen Therapy Committee Report. UHMS 2008; 97-115

35. Strauss MB, Miller SS. The Role of Hyperbaric Oxygen in the Management of Chronic Refractory Osteomyelitis in Hyperbaric Medicine Practice, 3rd Edition. Kindwall EP, Whelan HT (eds). Best Publishing Company Flagstaff, AZ 2008; 677-709

36. Alivernini S, De Santis M, Tolusso B, et al. Skin ulcers in systemic sclerosis: determinants of presence and predictive factors of healing. J Am Acad Dermatol. 2009 Mar; 60(3):426-35

37. Nazarian RM, Van Cott EM, Zembowicz A, et al. Warfarin-induced skin necrosis. J Am Acad Dermatol. 2009 Aug; 61(2):325-32

38. Dinh TA, Friedman J, Higuera S. Plastic surgery management in pediatric meningococcal-induced purpura fulminans. Clin Plast Surg. 2005 Jan; 32(1):117-21

39. Levy LA. Foot and ankle ulcers associated with hematologic disorders. Clin Podiatry. 1985 Oct; 2(4):631-7

40. Wasif Saif M, Elfiky AE. Identifying and treating fluoropyrimidine-associated hand-and-foot syndrome in white and non-white patients. J Support Oncol. 2007; 5:337-343

PART V

PREVENTION OF NEW AND RECURRENT WOUNDS

CHAPTER	TITLE	PAGE
13	WOUND PREVENTION THROUGH PATIENT EDUCATION	379
14	SKIN CARE AND TOENAIL MANAGEMENT	399
15	PROTECTIVE FOOTWEAR	419
16	MINIMALLY INVASIVE PROACTIVE SURGERIES	445

INTRODUCTION TO PART V

The adage "An ounce of prevention is worth a pound of cure" is especially appropriate for wound prevention. This fifth and final part of *MasterMinding Wounds* deals with the prevention portion of the **Master Algorithm** (Figure Part V-1). Although many wounds eventually heal, the real measures of success are durability and restoration of function. In healed "problem" wounds and salvaged "end-stage" wounds, the care given to prevent new and recurrent wounds is a major consideration for long-term good results. Four strategies including: 1) patient education, 2) skin and toenail care, 3) appropriate footwear selection, and 4) proactive surgical interventions are the cardinal ingredients for ensuring lasting successes in these situations (Part V, Figure 2). Each of the four prevention strategies will be discussed in separate chapters to follow.

Several misconceptions exist regarding "problem" and "end-stage" wounds. Some have been mentioned previously, but are repeated here for two reasons: First, to reemphasize their significance and second, to provide additional justification for the care measures that will be subsequently discussed.

- **Misconception:** Difficult to heal wounds inevitably recur after activity is resumed.

  Facts: The reasons for this misconception are the high recurrence rates observed when activity is resumed (after wounds heal with rest and off-loading and malperforans ulcers heal after total contact casting) without attention to the underlying deformities and the other problems that contribute to wound formation.

  With attention to managing deformities, muscle imbalances, wound hypoxia and infection--and initiation of post-wound healing prevention strategies (to be discussed in the four subsequent chapters), wound recurrences rarely occur.

  Furthermore, once a wound is healed, the metabolic demands to maintain the wound site in a healthy condition are a small fraction (previously described as 1/20th in Chapter 2) of what they are for healing and infection control. In the presence of peripheral vascular disease, this reduced demand for blood flow in the healed tissues is usually sufficient to meet the minimal metabolic demands of non-critical tissues. Consequently, with the prevention strategies, healed wounds, especially of the feet and ankles, are observed to remain healed regardless of marginal perfusion to these areas.

- **Misconception:** Preserving the foot has little functional significance in the marginal ambulator.

  Facts: A lower limb amputation in the minimal ambulator who had been independent may increase energy demands for walking with a prosthesis to the point that the patient requires assisted living.

  Energy demands for walking with a prosthesis, as measured by oxygen consumption, essentially double with a below knee amputation and triple with an above knee amputation.[1,2]

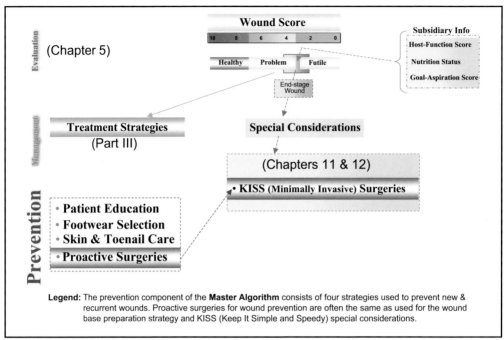

Part V, Figure 1. The prevention component of the Master Algorithm.

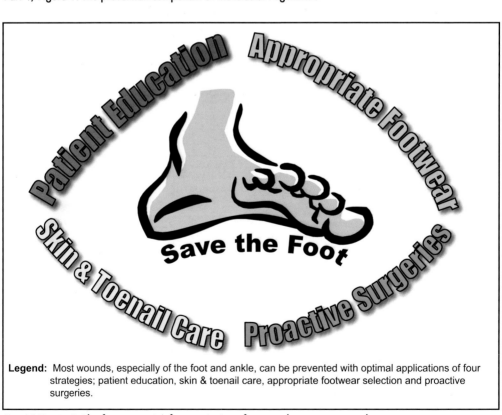

Part V, Figure 2. The four strategies for prevention of new and recurrent wounds.

Furthermore, weakness and arthritic changes in the upper extremities may make donning and removing the prosthesis difficult, if not impossible. In addition, with these comorbidities, use of walking aids such as crutches or walkerettes may be severely restricted.

Rehabilitation and confidence in using a prosthesis may take a year or more to maximize strength, balance, and endurance. In patients with cardiac and pulmonary comorbidities, oxygen consumption demands for walking with a prosthesis may exceed their maximal aerobic capabilities.

Although an amputation may appear to be immediately cost-effective by rapidly moving a patient from the acute setting to a lower level of care, the total expenditures for salvaging a "problem" or "end-stage" wound may not be cost beneficial (Chapter 11). For example, costs for surgery, prostheses, and rehabilitation amount to about $50,000 during the initial 18 months after an amputation.[3,4]

Finally, fitting a prosthesis for the marginal ambulator may be challenging and require repeated adjustments because of stump atrophy, arthritic deformities of the knee joint, and marked variations in stump size due to fluid retention (especially in patients with cardiac and renal impairments).

- **Misconception:** Once a leg is amputated, amputation of the other limb will soon follow.

  Facts: If the lower limb amputation is due to severe, diffuse, bilateral non-reconstructable lower limb peripheral arterial disease, this statement may be valid.

  However, with the wound prevention measures presented in the succeeding chapters, prevention of wounds in the remaining limb usually makes it possible to avoid a second lower limb amputation. The justification for this comment, as discussed previously, is the markedly increased energy demands wound healing and infection control require as compared to the steady state, non-wound healing situation (Chapter 2).

  If the lower limb amputation is due to wounds associated with uncontrolled deformities, such as from Charcot arthropathy or distal leg, ankle fracture non-unions, subsequent amputation of the other extremity is highly unlikely. This is also observed if the lower limb amputation is due to unilateral uncontrolled infection as for example, with chronic refractory osteomyelitis, necrotizing soft tissue infections or gas gangrene.

- **Misconception:** Care of limb threatening wounds is different for the patient with significant comorbidities than in the healthy patient.

  Facts: The severity of the wound is the overriding consideration for making decisions about management of the wound. The **Wound Score** provides a quick assessment for determining the severity of the wound.

If the wound is in the "problem" category, management using the five strategic elements (Part III) is advised regardless of the host status.

If the wound is in the "end-stage" category between "problem" and "futile," information from the patient's **Host-Function** and **Goal-Aspiration Scores** is useful for helping to make a decision whether to amputate or try to salvage the limb. This is especially useful for severe post-traumatic and the other "end-stage" wounds previously discussed (Chapter 12).

If the decision is made to salvage the "end-stage" wound, then special considerations (Part IV) in patient management need to be utilized in addition to the five strategic elements used to manage "problem" wounds. Even though comorbidities may be reflected in the **Host-Function** and **Goal-Aspiration Scores**, once the decision is made to avoid a lower limb amputation, wound management is the same regardless of host status and goal-aspirations.

- **Misconception:** Neuropathy is the major reason wounds fail to heal.

  Facts: As discussed previously, neuropathy is an indirect cause of wounds by delaying diagnosis secondary to loss of sensation, contributing to deformities from muscle imbalances, generating shear stresses with walking from loss of proprioception, making skin prone to breakdown due to autonomic nervous system dysfunction or combinations of these problems.

  The neuropathy itself is not a reason wounds fail to heal. In fact, neuropathy may facilitate wound healing by increasing blood flow through loss of autonomic nerve function controlling vasoconstriction and triggering hyper-perfusion as observed in Charcot arthropathy.

  In some respects, diabetic foot wounds in the presence of sensory neuropathy are the easiest wounds to manage because dressing changes and wound debridements can be optimized since they are not uncomfortable for the patient (Chapter 7).

  Even more convincing information to dispel this misconception is the observation that once foot, ankle, and leg wounds are healed in patients with profound neuropathies, recurrences are the exception in the well-motivated patient who follows the prevention measures described in the four subsequent chapters.

- **Misconception:** It is difficult to predict which patients are prone to wound development in their feet.

  Facts: Generally accepted risk factors for wound development in the feet are easy to recognize (Chapters 5 and 13). Major risk factors include 1) deformity, 2) peripheral vascular disease, 3) history of previous wound, 4) previous amputation and 5) neuropathy.[5-8]

Other risk factors for wound development become apparent from information obtained from the **Host-Function** and **Goal-Aspiration Scores** and will be delineated in the next chapter.

When risk factors are present, special diligence must be exercised by the patient, the caregivers and the medical personnel caring for the patient to prevent wounds from occurring. The best chances for this being successful are achieved by following the prevention measures described in the succeeding chapters.

- **Misconception:** Chronic wounds fail to heal because of inadequate blood supply.

    Facts: Usually problems other than inadequate blood supply are the reasons that chronic wounds fail to heal. The fact that wounds are chronic indicates that there is enough blood supply to keep the tissues alive, but the blood supply is inadequate to meet the increased metabolic demands of wound healing and infection control.

    The two other major reasons chronic wounds fail to heal (in addition to inadequate perfusion/oxygenation) are underlying deformities and unresolved infections—usually of infected, avascular bone (Chapter 7). Often, these problems are related; the deformity causes ulceration and the bone causing the deformity becomes infected from bacteria entering the wound.

    Typically, the bone becomes avascular, especially in the distal tufts of the toes and the metatarsal heads. The blood supplies to these sites are particularly vulnerable to thrombosis because of their small size, and their passing through soft tissue "compartments" that have minimal ability to expand—especially around joints and their end-artery anatomy. Swelling associated with infection and/or trauma increases external pressure around the small blood vessels causing them to collapse (i.e. a compartment syndrome), and further interferes with the already precarious blood supply to the metatarsal heads and distal tufts of the toes.[9]

    Other less frequent reasons chronic wounds fail to heal include immunosuppression from steroids and antimetabolites, morbid obesity which makes non-weight bearing/off-loading of the involved limb impossible, malnutrition, smoking, collagen vascular diseases, chronic liver insufficiency and chronic venous insufficiency/fluid retention.

    Once underlying deformities and infected bone (or in some cases bursa) are removed, healing typically occurs. Juxta-wound transcutaneous oxygen measurements can show whether or not perfusion/oxygenation is adequate to meet the requirements for healing. If not, hyperbaric oxygen therapy should be used as an adjunct to meet these requirements, especially if juxta-wound transcutaneous oxygen tensions increase to over 200mmHg with a hyperbaric oxygen exposure (Chapter 10). If not, but increase to >50mmgHg, then **Host-Function** and **Goal-Aspiration Scores** must be considered to justify doing everything possible to avoid a major lower-limb amputation.

    Although most of the information about wound prevention and avoidance of recurrences after wounds are healed is directed to the diabetic patient population, the care measures presented in the next four chapters are applicable to any patient who has had a serious wound. A serious wound is one where concerns about healing are raised. The 0 to 10 point **Wound Score** provides an even more precise definition, as has been discussed previously, for quantifying the "problem" or "end-stage" wound. As mentioned, the **Wound Score** is also an effective tool for quantifying progress and outcomes using a 2 (healed) to 0 (failed) point grading system (Table 5-5). Once these wounds are healed, it is only sensible that every measure possible must be done to prevent recurrences. The adage "An ounce of prevention is worth a pound of cure" is never more applicable than in this group of patients.

REFERENCES:

1. Waters RL, Perry J, Antonelli D, Hislop H. Energy cost of walking of amputees: the influence of level of amputation. J Bone Joint Surg Am. 1976 Jan; 58(1):42-6

2. Pinzur MS, Gold J, Schwartz D, Gross N. Energy demands for walking in dysvascular amputees as related to the level of amputation. Orthopedics 1992 Sep; 15(9):1033-6; discussion 1036-7

3. MacKenzie EJ, Jones AS, Bosse MJ, et al. Health-care costs associated with amputation or reconstruction of a limb-threatening injury. J Bone Joint Surg Am. 2007 Aug; 89(8):1685-92

4. Mackey WC, McCullough JL, Conlon TP, et al. The costs of surgery for limb-threatening ischemia. Surgery 1986 Jan; 99(1):26-35

5. Boyko EJ, Ahroni JH, Stensel V, et al. A prospective study of risk factors for diabetic foot ulcer. The Seattle Diabetic Foot Study. Diabetes Care 1999 Jul; 22(7):1036-42

6. McNeely MJ, Boyko EJ, Ahroni JH, et al. The independent contributions of diabetic neuropathy and vasculopathy in foot ulceration. How great are the risks? Diabetes Care 1995 Feb; 18(2):216-9

7. Boyko EJ, Ahroni JH, Cohen V, et al. Prediction of diabetic foot ulcer occurrence using commonly available clinical information: the Seattle Diabetic Foot Study. Diabetes Care 2006 Jun; 29(6):1202-7

8. Abbott CA, Carrington AL, Ashe H, et al. North-West Diabetes Foot Care Study. The North-West Diabetes Foot Care Study: incidence of, and risk factors for, new diabetic foot ulceration in a community-based patient cohort. Diabet Med. 2002 May; 19(5):377-84

9. Strauss M, Miller S. Crush Injury, Compartment Syndrome and Other Acute Traumatic Peripheral Ischemias. In: Hyperbaric Medicine Practice, 3rd Edition. (Eds.) Kindwall EP and Whelan HT. Best Publishing, Flagstaff, AZ 2008:755-790

NOTES

CHAPTER

13

WOUND PREVENTION THROUGH PATIENT EDUCATION

CHAPTER THIRTEEN OVERVIEW

INTRODUCTION 381

PATIENT COMPLIANCE 382

DO MAXIMS...385

DON'T MAXIMS 390

SELECTION OF APPROPRIATE ACTIVITIES 394

CONCLUSIONS 396

QUESTIONS...397

REFERENCES..398

"To educate is wonderful, to use what is learned is sublime."

INTRODUCTION

Importance of Prevention Measures– In possibly no other aspect of medicine is the value of prevention as tangible as in the patient with diabetes. This was conclusively demonstrated in the DCCT (The Diabetes Control and Complications Trial Research Group) study.[1] The study showed that with optimal management of blood sugars through glucose monitoring and precise dosing of insulin, diabetic complications were reduced 50 to 75 percent as compared to the control group. Progression of neuropathy and angiopathy were the two complication parameters specifically monitored in the DCCT trial. Observations verify that diabetic foot wound occurrences in particular and virtually all types of problem wounds in general are decreased to a similar extent when wound prevention strategies are employed.[2] Prevention strategies start with patient education (Figure 13-1).

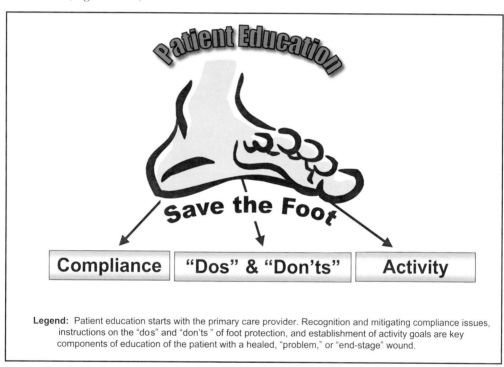

Legend: Patient education starts with the primary care provider. Recognition and mitigating compliance issues, instructions on the "dos" and "don'ts" of foot protection, and establishment of activity goals are key components of education of the patient with a healed, "problem," or "end-stage" wound.

Figure 13-1. The three cardinal components of patient education.

Risk Factors – All patients who are at risk for developing problem wounds, and especially patients with diabetes, require a primary care provider to supervise their medical management. At risk patients are those who have one or more acknowledged risk factor for wound development that include 1) deformity, 2) peripheral artery disease, 3) history of a previous wound, 4) a previous amputation, or 5) neuropathy (Table 13-1). Two considerations dictate the frequency of follow-up medical visits for this group of patients. The first consideration is patient compliance. Once patients are instructed in wound prevention measures, the frequency of follow-up visits is determined by the patient's compliance. As a general rule, the frequency of return visits is inversely proportional to the patient's compliance to health care instructions. This will be further discussed in the next section. The other consideration is the number and extent, that is, the seriousness of the risk factors that are precursors to "problem" wounds. The process starts with the primary care provider since this is the level of care where overall management of the patient is addressed. If new problems arise, such as signs that a wound is developing, the primary care provider typically initiates referral to specialist.

TABLE 13-1. THE FIVE MAJOR RISK FACTORS FOR THE DEVELOPMENT OF EXTREMITY WOUNDS

Factor	Concerns	Examples
Deformity	Concentration of stresses over bony prominences make the overlying skin vulnerable to breakdown.	Erythema over bony prominences, callus formation, clawed toes, mal perforans ulcers, pressure, and tension ulcers/indolent wounds (Chapter 4).
Peripheral Artery Disease	Insufficient perfusion to meet the increased (estimated to be 20-fold) requirements for wound healing and infection control.	Wounds with ischemic bases, scores of 1/2 or less on the perfusion assessment of the **Wound Score** and low transcutaneous oxygen measurements.
History of Previous Wound	This indicates that the patient is at risk for developing wounds. Usually other wound factor concerns co-exist with this risk factor.	This risk factor is especially significant in those wounds that occurred spontaneously or without apparent injury.
Previous Amputation	Same concerns as listed above for history of previous wound.	Amputations on contralateral extremity from toes to hip disarticulations as well as ipsilateral minor amputations of toes fingers, partial feet, or hands.
Neuropathy	Failure to recognize impending problems or delay in the diagnosis of frank wounds. Vulnerability to wound development due to skin dryness, atrophy, and muscle imbalances leading to joint deformities and contractures.	Loss of sensation, ulcerations over apices and tips of clawed toes, mal perforans ulcers, and autonomic dysfunction.

PATIENT COMPLIANCE

Compliance Measures – Patient compliance is an expression used to indicate how well patients follow physician and physician-extender's instructions. The following can be used as objective parameters to reflect patient compliance:

- **Weight management -** obesity as well as malnutrition can be indications of poor compliance. The likelihood of wound-related complications increase in direct proportion to the severity of these conditions.
- **Adherence to instructions for medication usage.**
- **Monitoring of diet and blood glucose measurements**, if diabetic; Hemoglobin A1c monitoring can assist in monitoring the patient's compliance to this parameter.
- **Addressing foot skin and toenail care issues** (Chapter 14).
- **Observance of the dos and don'ts** of wound prevention--described subsequently in this chapter.
- **Implementation of healthful exercise activities** and elimination of inappropriate ones.

Primary Care Provider Roles – The primary care provider should use observations from these findings to recommend the frequency of return visits, whether or not home health nursing interventions are required, or if the patient needs homemaker's services. For example, after wound healing follow-up, visits for compliant patients may only need to be done once or twice a year. Conversely, if there are concerns about the patient's compliance, weekly or biweekly visits with interim home health nursing visits may be needed in order to prevent new or recurrent medical and/or wound problems.

Clinical correlations:
A 49-year-old female with diabetes and sensory neuropathy, but otherwise in apparently good health, developed a wound over the back of her heel associated with footwear. As a marketing specialist she traveled frequently. The medical management of her diabetes had been haphazard at the best and non-existent at the worse.

Initially the wound was transitional between "healthy" and "problem" types with a **Wound Score** of 7 ½ points. Even with strong admonitions about possible consequences of not adhering to all aspects of diabetes and wound management, the patient did not alter her lifestyle and continued to work, travel, socialize, and give minimal attention to her diabetes and wound problems. At this point, her **Goal-Aspiration Score** was 3 points.

Progressive deterioration was noted when the patient returned for weekly rechecks. During one of her travels, the foot became septic with involvement of the entire hindfoot. The **Wound Score** had decreased to 3 points, consistent with an "end-stage" wound. With no other options, the patient agreed to hospitalization. Because of the above events and the objectivity the **Wound Score** and **Goal-Aspiration Scores** provided, a below-knee amputation was recommended.

The patient refused, but during the course of her care gained new insight as to what was expected of her if an amputation was to be avoided. With debridements, skin grafting, and delayed healing of a failed, sloughed, dehisced portion of the skin graft, the wound healed.

She became a "model" patient with respect to managing her diabetes and following wound prevention strategies. Her **Goal-Aspiration Score** increased to 10 points. After this, recheck visits were decreased to semi-annually.

Comment:
The **Goal-Aspiration Score** (as well as the **Host-Function Score**), in contrast to the **Wound Score**, typically changes little, if any, with time. However, in this patient's case, the **Goal-Aspiration Score** improved remarkably. Undoubtedly, the shock of potentially losing her leg apparently was the motivating factor to change the overwhelming denial mechanisms that she used in the past and was the incentive to become compliant in all aspects of her diabetes management and foot wound prevention strategies.

Although management recommendations could have been made without the use of the **Wound Score** and **Goal-Aspiration Score**, they provided objective information for decision-making and, after healing, determining the frequency of return visits.

Family and Caregiver Roles – The patient's family and/or home caregivers have a crucial role regarding compliance, especially if the patient is unable to care for him/herself. This is especially true in the debilitated patient who requires assistance for almost all activities of daily living and those patients with other infirmities such as blindness, residuals of strokes, and mobility restrictions. It is not appropriate to label patients with these conditions as non-compliant. Rather, the primary care provider should provide guidance for preventing new wound problems. The patient's comorbidities, medication requirements, and mobility must be balanced with available resources. Potential resources include family members, social services, home health nursing, homemaker assistance, care by friends or neighbors, and/or assisted living facilities, etc. Most hospitals with active diabetes services provide diabetes education classes. This is an example of a resource which the primary care provider should be aware of and be used to optimize a patient's diabetes care.

Use of the Goal-Aspiration Score to Measure Capacity to Follow Instructions and Gauge Follow-up Visits – The **Goal-Aspiration Score** (Chapter 1, Table 1-3) provides easily measurable criteria for determining the patient's capacity to follow wound prevention measures and for establishing the frequency of follow-up visits (Figure 13-2). This score not only grades compliance as full, some, or none using the 2 point (best) to 0 point (worst) assessment system, but also considers patient comprehension, motivation, support, and level of independence using the same format. From the summation of the grades of the five assessments, a 0 point (worst possible situation) to 10 point (optimal) range of scores is generated.

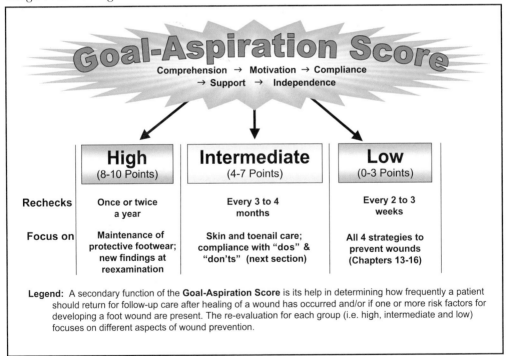

Figure 13-2. Use the Goal-Aspiration Score (Chapter 1) to gauge the frequency of return visits.

If the scores are in the 8-to-10 point range and the wound site is healed, follow-ups need only be infrequent. These scores indicate that the patients will follow the instructions of their caregivers and immediately seek medical help on an as needed basis if anything changes with respect to their health and/or wound site status. Scores in the 4-

to-7 point range indicate the need for regularly scheduled follow-up evaluations and re-enforcement of wound prevention measures. For this group, follow-up evaluations with the physician, wound specialist, or other care provider need to occur every three to four months. Finally, for those patients with **Goal-Aspiration Scores** in the 0-to-3 point range, constant supervision is necessary to prevent new or recurrent wound complications. Return visits to the physician may be required every two to three weeks for patients with these **Goal-Aspiration Scores** if new problems are to be avoided.

DO MAXIMS

Which Patients Need to Adhere to Prevention Maxims – There are a number of maxims regarding wound prevention and recurrences that all patients who have had serious wounds and/or have significant risk factors for wound development need to follow. Most are logical, easy to follow, and only take a moment's time to do (Figure 13-3, 13-4, 13-5). They are as important to wound prevention as blood glucose monitoring and insulin dosing are for preventing complications in diabetes. It is important for the primary care provider and the other caregivers who have helped with management of the wound to appreciate this analogy and impress it upon their patients. Is it necessary for every patient to follow the maxims of wound prevention after the healing of all serious wounds? Obviously, the answer is no. In healthy patients, for example after complete healing of traumatic wounds, no additional attention to the injury area may be necessary. For well-motivated, compliant patients (i.e. a high **Goal-Aspiration Score**), after healing of "problem" wounds, physician follow-ups may only need to be done on an occasional basis and perhaps not at all by the surgeon, especially if the surgical site has healed. Conversely, the lower the **Goal-Aspiration Score** is, the more closely the patient needs to be followed and reminded of the maxims.

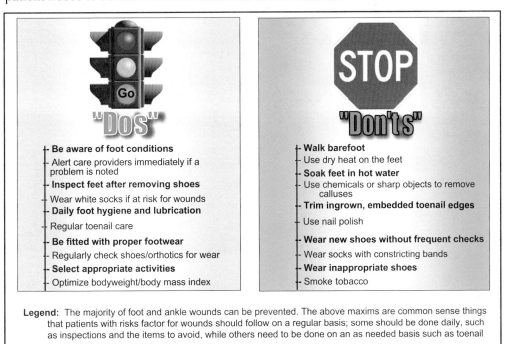

Legend: The majority of foot and ankle wounds can be prevented. The above maxims are common sense things that patients with risks factor for wounds should follow on a regular basis; some should be done daily, such as inspections and the items to avoid, while others need to be done on an as needed basis such as toenail care.

Figure 13-3. Maxims for patients to follow to avoid new and recurrent foot wounds.

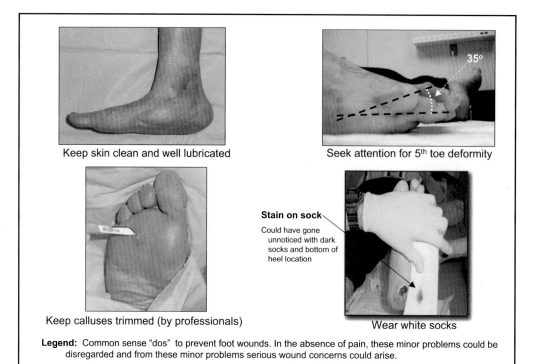

Keep skin clean and well lubricated

Seek attention for 5th toe deformity

Keep calluses trimmed (by professionals)

Stain on sock
Could have gone unnoticed with dark socks and bottom of heel location

Wear white socks

Legend: Common sense "dos" to prevent foot wounds. In the absence of pain, these minor problems could be disregarded and from these minor problems serious wound concerns could arise.

Figure 13-4. Some dos to prevent new and recurrent foot wounds.

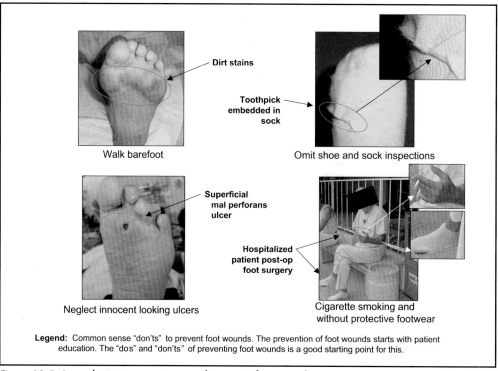

Dirt stains

Walk barefoot

Toothpick embedded in sock

Omit shoe and sock inspections

Superficial mal perforans ulcer

Neglect innocent looking ulcers

Hospitalized patient post-op foot surgery

Cigarette smoking and without protective footwear

Legend: Common sense "don'ts" to prevent foot wounds. The prevention of foot wounds starts with patient education. The "dos" and "don'ts" of preventing foot wounds is a good starting point for this.

Figure 13-5. Some don'ts to prevent new and recurrent foot wounds.

Levels of Responsibility for Patient Education – There are several levels of responsibility for patient education in these matters. First, the primary care physician should make patients with risk factors for wound development aware of the vulnerability of their feet for problems to occur and the need to be notified immediately if any changes are noted. Second, the nurse educator should teach and review the "dos" and "don'ts" of foot health care (as described in the next portions of this text) and wound prevention with each patient.[3] Third, responsibility for surgeries, follow-up surgical care, orthotics, and prescription footwear rests with the foot specialist (namely orthopaedic surgeons specializing in foot and ankle problems, podiatrists and general, vascular, and/or plastic surgeons attending wound clinics). Naturally, the team approach is recommended with each member of the team providing management in their own areas of expertise. The following "dos" should be followed by all patients who have had a "problem" or "end-stage" wound, have other risk factors for wound development, and/or have **Host-Function Scores** less than 7 points:

1. **Be aware of the risk factors that are predispositions to foot problems:**
   1) deformities, 2) peripheral artery disease, 3) history of a previous wound, 4) prior amputation, and/or 5) neuropathy.

   Rationale: Self-awareness and self-reliance are fundamental to maintaining good health, and the prevention of foot problems is no exception.

   Remember: The time the patient spends with a physician or health care provider is almost infinitesimal compared to the time between visits. What the patient does in the time between visits in terms of following health care provider instructions, care measures, and inspections largely determines success. If the patient does not bring a wound problem or potential wound problem to the attention of the health care provider or other caregivers, it will not likely be checked.

   Most foot problems are remedial and the sooner they are addressed, the easier they are to manage. Many problems, when first recognized, can be managed in the office setting with proper protective footwear and/or simple surgical procedures (Chapter 16).

   Any time there is a break in the skin of the feet or legs in a patient with risk factors for amputation, medical attention should be sought. The early removal of a foreign object or necrotic material from the wound and the starting of antibiotics may prevent limb threatening complications.

2. **Make your primary care physician aware of your intentions to keep your feet healthy and your desire for immediate referral to a foot specialist if and/or when needed.**

   Rationale: In the majority of cases, management of foot problems that have the potential to become wounds can be done before serious problems arise with the care measures discussed in the succeeding three chapters.

   Remember: With time constraints and the need for efficiency, the foot exam or questions about the healthiness of the feet may be overlooked unless concerns are specifically expressed to the primary care physician.

3. Inspect each foot and healed wound site daily after removing shoes.

Rationale: The earlier a wound or potential wound is recognized, the easier it is to manage and the faster it can be resolved.

Remember: Use good lighting, wear glasses if needed for viewing small objects, and a mirror if you have problems with positioning to see the bottoms of your feet. Check for red spots (pressure areas), irritated areas ("rubs"), calluses, dry skin, scaling skin, plaques, cracks (especially between toes), fissures in the skin surfaces, blisters, corns, and deformities.

4. Inspect socks daily for stains, and if risk factors for foot wounds are present, always wear white socks.

Rationale: With sensory neuropathy, the first sign of an impending wound problem, namely pain, may not be appreciated. Stains such as expected to occur with blister formation or a wound may be the first clue that something is wrong. Almost any stain will be noted on white socks.

Remember: Stains on socks are a sign that the skin integrity of the foot has been disrupted. To disregard this sign is tantamount to denial that a problem exists. The cause of the stain must always be identified and the problem addressed.

5. Practice good foot skin hygiene daily.

Rationale: The skin is the first "line of defense" for the prevention of foot wounds. The healthier the skin is, the more it can resist insults that lead to wounds. Simple skin cleansing and lubrication measures (Chapter 14) are a first step to insure the health of the skin of the feet.

Remember: As mentioned before, attention to extremity skin care is as important for preventing skin complications of the feet and other segments of the extremity as blood sugar management is to preventing complications of diabetes. In addition, the quality and consistency of foot care is a measure of patient compliance.

6. Perform appropriate toenail care.

Rationale: Toenail problems are commonly present in patients who have risk factors for developing wounds in their feet and will be discussed comprehensively in the next chapter (Chapter 14). Toenail care can be used as another measure to judge patient compliance.

Remember: Only the simplest of toenail care measures should be done by the patients themselves, especially if the toenails are diseased, neuropathy is present, agility problems (that is, enough flexibility to position toes adequately to trim the toenails) exist, and/or vision is impaired.

7. **Wear appropriate protective footwear for your foot problems.**

   Rationale: The more severe the foot deformities, the more specialized the protective footwear requirements are (Chapter 15).

   Remember: Appropriate prescriptions for footwear require knowledge of the underlying problem. Hence, the more complicated the problem, the greater the need is that the footwear prescription is written by a physician with expertise in foot problems.

8. **Check shoes and orthotics periodically for signs of wear or poor fit.**

   Rationale: Prescription protective footwear and orthotics lose their stabilizing ability with activity. In addition, the shape of the patient's foot may change with time. With loss of effectiveness, recurrent, or new wound problems, stress fractures and/or new deformities may arise.

   Remember: Examination of the patient's shoes, footwear, and orthotics should be an integral part of the foot exam for any patient who has risk factors for developing wounds.

9. **Walking and other exercise activities should be selected based on the patient's functional capabilities.**

   Rationale: Exercise has many benefits including improving cardiovascular conditioning, enhancing stamina, promoting weight reduction, augmenting mobility, preventing osteoporosis, and perhaps stimulating angiogenesis.

   Remember: Exercise is not feasible for everyone. When prescribed, it needs to be modified to meet the abilities of the patient, as will be discussed later in this chapter.

10. **Optimize body weight/body mass index.**

    Rationale: Obesity complicates almost every medical problem a patient may have. With respect to foot problems, each additional pound of added weight multiplies stresses across the foot by a factor of three when walking. Wound care can be very difficult in the morbidly obese patient. Casts and orthotics may be difficult, if not impossible, to fit. Non-weight bearing on the injured extremity, even for transfers, may be impossible.

    Remember: Weight reduction is a challenging problem. The primary care physician should initiate recommendations with help from a nutrition specialist. Recently developed minimally invasive surgical techniques add a new dimension for surgical management of obesity.

DON'T MAXIMS

Things Patients With Risk Factors for Wounds Should Avoid – Just as there are maxims the patient should follow in order to prevent wounds, there are, likewise, things the patient should avoid (Figure 13-3 & 13-5). Many of the "don'ts" specifically address problems that can arise when sensory neuropathy interferes with the warning signs of impending injury. All patients who have risk factors for wounds and/or have had a serious wound, especially in the feet, should follow the following instructions.

1. Don't walk barefoot.

Comment: Sharp objects or rough surfaces can cause wounds in the feet. Foreign objects like needles may enter the foot. The injury may go unnoticed until drainage, odor, or both are noted. Sensory neuropathy may disguise the pain.

Factors which interfere with infection control such as peripheral artery disease, collagen vascular diseases, atrophic skin, and deformities may allow infections to develop, whereas they would not occur in people without these problems.

2. Don't use heat on the feet.

Comment: Two factors make the patient with risk factors for wounds particularly susceptible to burn injuries. First, a sensory neuropathy may interfere with the patient's recognition of the magnitude of the heat stress and initiation of immediate measures to interrupt the exposure.

Clinical correlations:
A 39-year-old female patient with diabetes, profound sensory neuropathy, and moderate peripheral artery disease was a passenger in a car on a hot day when the car overheated. To help dissipate the engine heat and continue driving, the driver turned on the car heater.

After reaching their destination, the patient had the perception that her shoes felt tight although no pain was noticed (due to the sensory neuropathy). After removing her shoes and socks, she observed large blisters over the dorsal skin surfaces of the toes and both feet.

With these findings and concerns that she might lose her feet, she presented herself to an emergency department where the diagnosis of second and third degree burns was made. The burns required hospitalization for management.

Comment:
This scenario illustrates the vulnerability of the feet of patients with diabetes to occult injury. The sensory neuropathy masked the pain that normally would be experienced with this amount of heat exposure. In addition, heat transferred to the skin surface from the exposure was probably not dissipated to the same degree that it would be in a person without peripheral artery disease.

Second, heat exposures, which would not ordinarily cause burns, may lead to burns in patients with peripheral artery disease. These patients do not have the ability to dissipate heat at the same rate (via blood circulation) as patients with normal perfusion.

For these reasons, strong admonitions need to be given to patients who use heating pads or hot water bottles to warm their feet because of "poor circulation." If these devices are used, patients should be instructed to use only low temperature settings or water temperatures. For added safety, the electrical devices should have timer switches to limit the durations of exposure.

3. Don't soak the feet in hot water.

Comment: This "don't" is a corollary to the preceding one. Although we recommend skin hygiene measures that start with cleansing with soap and water or soaking in warm water, the exposures should be of limited durations to avoid maceration of the skin (Chapter 14). Water used for these purposes should be warm, not hot.

After the soak, attention must be given to thoroughly drying the feet, especially the skin between the toes in order to eliminate an environment conducive for fungus infection to thrive.

4. Don't use chemicals or sharp objects to trim calluses.

Comment: These items may cause wounds. Because they are not sterile, there is a propensity for infections to develop if the skin is penetrated. Chemicals harsh enough to eradicate calluses will cause damage to the adjacent skin should they come in contact with it.

Furthermore, with impaired agility and/or vision, difficulties in adequately trimming the callus (or applying the chemical debriding agent) may occur. Too little trimming will not be adequate to off-load the underlying deformity. Too much trimming will penetrate the underlying skin surface.

Debulking calluses by "sanding" with a pumice stone, although not recommended, is generally acceptable for patients to do themselves. They should be cautioned not to be overzealous, that is, debulking to the degree that the underlying skin is injured. The patient should be told to do minimal, frequent (at weekly intervals), debulking of calluses rather than the occasional "heroic" effort to remove the callus completely.

5. Don't trim the edge portions of toenails that are embedded into the skin.

Comment: The embedded ends (medial and lateral portions of the distal margins) of toenails, especially the hallux nails, thicken, accumulate debris, and grow into the underlying soft tissues. This becomes one of the precursors for in-grown toenails and paronychia (infection of the toenail margins from the edges of the toenail).

Expertise in toenail care and appropriate instruments are required in order to manage debris accumulation at the toenail margins (Chapter 14).

6. Don't use toenail polish if there has been a previous history of toenail problems.

Comment: Toenail polish, lacquer, or acrylic generates an impermeable barrier over the toenail. The polish may not only hide underlying toenail problems that require special care, but also prevent air from getting to the toenail surface. The drying effect of air may prevent toenail infections since fungus infections thrive in a moist environment.

7. Don't assume a new pair of shoes, even if from a protective footwear prescription, will fit perfectly.

Comment: Even though protective footwear may be specially prescribed, they do not always fit perfectly. In addition, a period of adjustment to new shoes should always be recommended in those patients who have neuropathy in their feet. In such situations, the new shoes should only be worn for a few minutes initially; then the feet should be inspected for pressure areas, blisters, and erythema.

Typically, there is a "break-in" period for new shoes where the shoe materials stretch and accommodate to the wearers' feet. This is why a "go slow" admonition should always be given to each patient who gets a prescription for new protective footwear, and the old shoes not discarded until the new shoes are fully adjusted.

In about half the patients with new protective footwear prescriptions, subsequent adjustments to the footwear are required. This is not a sign of an improper prescription, but rather it reflects the challenges that these feet present.

8. Don't wear constricting bands around the feet and ankles or rings on the toes.

Comment: These devices may interfere with circulation. More commonly, the constricting bands interfere with venous and lymphatic return, resulting in swelling distal to the constriction. Consequences may lead to pressure areas with shoe wear, leading to blisters and ulcerations. If the swelling is severe, it may also interfere with the arterial blood supply and can lead to gangrenous changes, especially in the patient who already has poor circulation.

Indentations from the elastic bands at the proximal margins of socks suggest the bands are too tight. Corrective measures include wearing socks with uniform compression or cutting the elastic bands at the top of the socks. If indentions are observed with sock wear, it is an indication to wear elastic support hose.

Socks that are too tight over the toe areas may cause pressure on the toenails. This can contribute to the development of ingrown toenails.

9. Don't wear inappropriate shoes.

Comment: Shoes with pointed toes, as some people think are fashionable, narrow the forefeet. Acutely, this can lead to pressure sores. With extended use, deformities such as hallux valgus and bunions are prone to develop.

Likewise, high heel shoes should be avoided. These concentrate pressures in the forefeet, especially the metatarsal heads with weight bearing. Consequences are the development of calluses under the metatarsal heads, pressure atrophy of the metatarsal fat pads, hyper-extension of the metatarsal-phalangeal joints of the toes, proximal retraction of the toes on the dorsum of the forefoot, pressure concentrations on the toenails, and shortening of the heel cord.

10. Don't smoke tobacco.

Comment: The harmful effects of smoking tobacco in general and for wound healing in particular have become well-publicized. There are over 4,000 harmful substances in tobacco smoke. Nicotine causes narrowing of the arteries. Other substances such as carbon monoxide and tars cause damage to blood vessels.

Studies show that patients who smoke tobacco have double the complication rates from surgeries, as do non-smokers. Many surgeons, especially for elective cosmetic procedures, refuse to operate on patients who smoke tobacco.[4]

Since smoking tobacco interferes with oxygen delivery to tissues, it is particularly important for patients with risk factors for foot wounds and/or those that have wounds in the process of healing not to smoke cigarettes.

Smoking Considerations – The subject of smoking tobacco deserves additional discussion. There is incontestable evidence that smoking tobacco is an antecedent to medical problems such as chronic lung disease, cardiovascular disease, cancers, and strokes.[5] Premature aging of skin and skin wrinkle formation is another undesirable effect observed from cigarette smoking.[6, 7] This is attributed to the 4,000 toxic products that have been identified in cigarette smoke including nicotine, cyanides, carbon monoxide, acroleins, amines, phenols, tars, etc. Because of double the surgical complication rates observed in cigarette smokers, many surgeons, especially for elective cosmetic surgeries, will not operate on cigar/cigarette smokers. These complications include wound sloughs, wound dehiscences, infections, non-unions of fractures, delayed healing, and excessive scarring.[8, 9] All these problems are encountered in "problem" and "end-stage" wounds even in non-smokers, but are more likely to occur in tobacco smokers.

Nicotine Effects From Smoking – The nicotine in cigarette smoking appears to be a "double-edged sword." Its undesirable effects include vasoconstriction and addiction.

However, the vasoconstriction effect from nicotine after smoking a cigarette appears to be transient, lasting an hour or so. After this, a rebound vasodilation occurs, thereby increasing blood flow. After acute cessation of smoking, juxta-wound transcutaneous oxygen measurement doubled while breathing room air and quadrupled when breathing hyperbaric oxygen at two atmospheres absolute as compared to the values obtained while the patient was still smoking tobacco.[10] It appears that the long-term harmful effects of cigarette smoking are due to damage to the capillary endothelium from chronic carbon monoxide and other harmful toxic product exposures in the smoke, rather than from nicotine itself.[11] Obviously patients with "problem" and "end-stage" wounds should not smoke tobacco. If addicted to smoking, presumably from the nicotine in cigarette smoke, intermittent use of nicotine patches or other methods to provide nicotine (to utilize the rebound vasodilation effect of nicotine) versus continuous application of the patches may be a compromise.

SELECTION OF APPROPRIATE ACTIVITIES

Paring Activity With Function – The third component of the patient education triad is the selection of appropriate activities for the patient's level of function. It is essential to consider the patient's capacity for activities when prescribing an activity program. Activity potential can be placed on a continuum from unlimited, such as world class sports performances, to zero where the patient is totally bedridden and requires help for all life maintenance measures. For simplicity purposes, the ambulation assessment of the **Host-Function Score** (Table 2-4, Chapter 2) can be used as a guideline for making specific activity recommendations for patients who have risk factors for "problem"

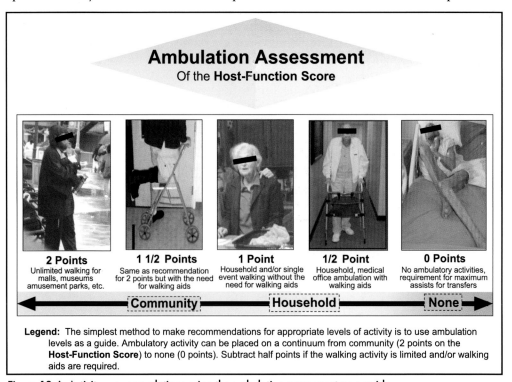

Legend: The simplest method to make recommendations for appropriate levels of activity is to use ambulation levels as a guide. Ambulatory activity can be placed on a continuum from community (2 points on the **Host-Function Score**) to none (0 points). Subtract half points if the walking activity is limited and/or walking aids are required.

Figure 13-6. Activity recommendations using the ambulation assessment as a guide.

wounds (Figure 13-6). Other components of the **Host-Function Score** provide supplemental information for the activity prescription. For example, patients with impaired cardiac function may have to limit activities to those that do not significantly elevate their heart rates. Patients with neurological deficits such as paraplegia may be limited to exercise that only uses their upper extremities. Patients with foot deformities and/or profound sensory neuropathies should be advised against using running activities for exercise.

Assessing Mobility From the Wound Score – Mobility assessment is based on the patient's ability to ambulate and is graded from 2 points (best - i.e. normal walking ability) to 0 points (worst - i.e. bedridden). The optimal situation (grade = 2 points) is unrestricted community ambulation without the need for walking aids. Ambulation restricted to the household level encompasses the intermediate situation (grade = 1 point). Inability to ambulate represents the worst situation (grade = 0 points). Half-point intermediate scores are used where the grade is intermediate between two findings such as limited ability to ambulate at the community level (grade = 1 ½ points), or the need for ambulation aids such as a paraplegic might require for unrestricted community ambulation using a wheelchair (also grade = 1 ½ points). From this simplified approach, rational, rapid, easily documented recommendations for activity level and exercise can be offered to the patients with risk factors for wounds.

Components of an Exercise Program – Naturally there is more to exercise and activity than ambulation level alone. Patients with risk factors for wounds and/or impaired **Host-Function Scores** who are capable of exercising should be encouraged to do so. The three cardinal components of an exercise program include 1) muscle stretching and joint ranges of motion, 2) exercises to increase strength (resistance training activities), and 3) cardiovascular conditioning, often referred to as aerobics and typified by high repetition/low resistance training to improve stamina and endurance (Table 13-2). A comprehensive review of exercise programs are covered much more extensively in other texts. The exercise prescription should be determined in conjunction with the primary care physician. Execution of the program often is best handled by a physical therapist. Caregivers and family members should then be instructed in the procedures so they can be continued after the supervised course of therapy is completed.

TABLE 13-2. THE THREE CARDINAL COMPONENTS OF AN EXERCISE PROGRAM

Component	Goals	Methods	Examples	Concerns
Stretching	Improved mobility, agility, and flexibility	Range of motion (ROM) activities of joints Gentle stretching beyond endpoints	Assisted and active assisted ROM's Passive ROM and stretching	Muscle tears Joint subluxations, dislocations
Strengthening	Improved muscle tone and strength	Resistance training activities	Weight training using barbells/ dumbbells/elastic bands Pull-ups, sit-ups, push-ups, etc.	Muscle strains, tears and ruptures Joint injuries leading to arthritis Bursitis
Cardiovascular Conditioning	Stamina and endurance	High-repetition, low-resistance efforts	Walking, treadmill, swimming, jogging, etc.	Cardiac events, e.g. ischemia, infarction Stress fractures

For the severely infirmed, muscle stretching and joint ranges of motion in bed may be the only component of the exercise program that is feasible to do.

Return of Functional Wound Healing – After extended periods of immobility, return of functional activities may be so slow that it appears no progress is being made. The older the patient and the lower the **Host-Function Score**, the longer it will take for the patient to reach their plateau of maximum function. This needs to be recognized by the patient's caregivers. Even though progress may be protracted, patients should be encouraged to do what they can. Typically after a total joint arthroplasty or a lower limb amputation, the patient's level of function will continue to improve for a year after the surgery is completed. However, the most rapid improvements are expected within the first three months. In patients with risk factors for wounds or healed "problem" and "end-stage" wounds, similar periods of convalescence are expected. By using guidelines such as these, reassurances and accurate predictions of functional outcomes can be offered to patients and their caregivers.

CONCLUSIONS

Putting Patient Education in Perspective – Patient education is fundamental for the prevention of wounds. Perhaps there is no other medical situation where understanding of the predispositions and utilization of prevention measures is so effective in preventing problems as in wounds. Whereas a patient may spend 15 minutes with his physician every two weeks for management of a healing wound and a similar amount of time every three months for education and encouragement to prevent recurrences or new problems, in reality this is only a miniscule portion of time in the total perspective. This observation amplifies the sentiment expressed in the quotation "To educate

> Fifteen minutes of contact with a physician every two weeks represents 0.074 percent of the total time in this interval, whereas a visit once every three months represents only 0.012 percent of the time.
>
> These computations are presented to emphasize the crucial nature of what happens between medical checks is largely the determining factor for success or failure in wound management and prevention.

is wonderful, to use what is learned is sublime" that introduces this chapter. The real success stories in problem wound management and prevention are those where the patients and their caregivers apply what has been taught to them.

Explaining Rationale Rather Than Just Directing Care – The "common sense" approach to patient education is strongly advocated. Rather than telling patients and their caregivers what and what not to do, it is better to explain the reasons for the advice. A starting point for this is the rationale, things to remember, and comments that accompany the "Dos" and "Don'ts" maxims provided earlier in this chapter. Certainly not every patient will understand and remember this information. The 0-to-2 point comprehension assessment of the **Goal-Aspiration Score** provides a starting point for how successful the physician and other educators will be in educating their patients on wound prevention. Sublimity (of outstanding and/or exalted worth and value) in terms of wound prevention may be equated to the state where the patient and their caregivers understand and fully comply with the patient education provided by their physicians and other medical caregivers.

QUESTIONS

1. What are some objective parameters that can be used to reflect patient compliance on this assessment of the **Goal-Aspiration Score**?

2. How can the **Goal-Aspiration Score** aid in wound prevention through patient education?

3. What are some of the "Do" maxims which should be followed by patients who have had a "problem" or "end-stage" wound and/or have risk factors for wound development?

4. What are some "Don't" maxims for the patients with risk factors for wound development?

5. How does smoking cigarettes affect wound healing?

6. How can the **Host-Function Score** be used as a guideline for making specific activity recommendations for patients?

7. What are the three cardinal components of an exercise program?

8. What exercise type activities are appropriate for a bed-ridden patient?

9. Why is what the patient does in the time between doctor or other caregivers' visits so important in wound prevention?

REFERENCES

1. The Diabetes Control and Complications Trial Research Group. The effect of intensive treatment of diabetes on the development and progression of long-term complications in insulin-dependent diabetes mellitus. N Engl J Med. 1993; 329:977-986

2. Singh N, Armstrong DG, Lipsky BA. Preventing foot ulcers in patients with diabetes. JAMA. 2005 Jan 12; 293(2):217-28

3. Meulepas MA, Braspenning JC, de Grauw WJ, et al. Patient-oriented intervention in addition to centrally organized checkups improves diabetic patient outcome in primary care. Qual Saf Health Care 2008 Oct; 17(5):324-8

4. Chang LD, Buncke G, Slezak S, Buncke HJ. Cigarette smoking, plastic surgery, and microsurgery. J Reconstr Microsurg. 1996 Oct; 12(7):467-74

5. Husten CG, Thorne SL. Tobacco: health effects and control. In: Public Health and Preventive Medicine (15th ed.), R.B. Wallace and N. Kohatsu, (Eds), McGraw-Hill, New York, New York (2008), pp. 953–998

6. Morita A. Tobacco smoke causes premature skin aging. J Dermatol Sci. 2007 Dec; 48(3):169-75

7. Freiman A, Bird G, Metelitsa AI, et al. Cutaneous effects of smoking. J Cutan Med Surg. 2004 Nov-Dec; 8(6):415-23

8. Frick WG, Seals RR, Jr. Smoking and wound healing: a review. Tex Dent J. 111 (1994), pp. 21–23.

9. Jorgensen LN, Kallehave F, Christensen E, et al. Less collagen production in smokers. Surgery 123 (1998), pp. 450–455.

10. Strauss MB, Winant DM, Strauss AG, Hart GB. Cigarette smoking and transcutaneous oxygen tensions: a case report. Undersea Hyperb Med. 2000 Spring; 27(1):43-6

11. Hart GB, Strauss MB. Effects of cigarette smoking on tissue gas exchange during hyperbaric exposures. Undersea Hyperb Med. 2010 March/April; 37(2):73-87

CHAPTER 14
SKIN CARE AND TOENAIL MANAGEMENT

CHAPTER FOURTEEN OVERVIEW

INTRODUCTION 401

PREDISPOSITIONS FOR SKIN AND TOENAIL PROBLEMS 402

HYPOXIA 402

DEFORMITIES 403

NEUROPATHY 404

METABOLIC/IMMUNE SYSTEM PROBLEMS 405

EVALUATION AND MANAGEMENT OF
  SKIN HYGIENE AND MOISTURIZATION 408

EVALUATION AND MANAGEMENT OF TOENAIL CONDITIONS 410

DOS AND DON'TS PERTAINING TO SKIN AND TOENAIL CARE 416

CONCLUSIONS 416

QUESTIONS 417

REFERENCES 418

"What you see tells you a lot."

INTRODUCTION

The skin and its appendages - Not only is the skin and its appendages, including nails and hair, the largest organ system in the body, it is the one that has the most contact with the external environment. Consequently, this organ system is the first line of defense in protecting the body from agents in the external environment that could possibly damage the internal contents of the body (Figure 14-1).[1] In addition, this organ system is a window to disease states within its contents, as will be discussed in the next section. Many predispositions cause problems that make the skin and toenails vulnerable to injury and disease. These predispositions include some categories such as neuropathies, deformities, ischemic conditions, infections, metabolic problems and congenital disorders. Some of the information discussed in this chapter, especially with regard to the pathophysiology of skin and toenail problems, has been presented in previous chapters. However, the information in this chapter, as well as the remaining chapters in Part V, are designed to "stand alone," to be complete enough to be used as a monograph on each subject. Hence, the decision was made for repetition of information to meet this goal. Finally, after patients and their caregivers are instructed in skin and toenail care in the lower extremities, inspection of these areas provide objective evidence as to patient compliance. This information can be used as criteria for determining the compliance assessment of the **Goal-Aspiration Score** (Table 1-3) and help gauge the frequency (Figure 13-2) of return visits to the health care provider caring for the patient's foot conditions.

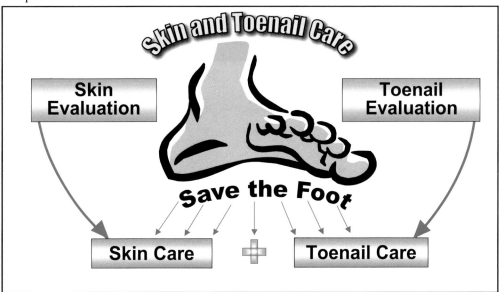

Figure 14-1. Foot wounds and other wounds usually start when the skin and its appendages are no longer able to maintain their protective functions. Skin care and toenail care are the body's first lines of defense for maintaining these protective functions.

Skin and Toenail Wound Paradox - The skin and toenails present challenges with respect to the development of wounds that are almost paradoxical. On one hand, these areas are particularly prone to wound problems, especially if one or more of the risk factors for wound development and/or limb amputation [a) deformity, b) peripheral artery disease, c) history of previous foot wound, 4) previous amputation, and 5) neuropathy] are present. This is because the skin is always in contact with the external environment, even though covering devices may provide partial barriers and the skin of the foot transmits the most concentrated forces, with standing and walking, of any region of the body. On the other hand, with simple evaluations and managements, as will be presented in subsequent sections of this chapter, much can be easily and effectively done to prevent foot skin (as well as other portions of the body) and toenail problems from occurring.

PREDISPOSITIONS FOR SKIN AND TOENAIL PROBLEMS

Comorbidities - Skin and toenail problems are particularly prone to develop in selected patient groups such as those with diabetes mellitus, peripheral artery disease, collagen vascular diseases, vitamin and mineral deficiencies, fluid retention, dehydration, and aging. Problems secondary to these conditions are usually associated with the following predispositions, most of which have been discussed in previous chapters from different perspectives.

HYPOXIA

Consequences of Atherosclerosis - This problem is most frequently a consequence of atherosclerosis. At rest, non-critical tissues such as the skin and its underlying supportive tissues have very low metabolic demands. When these tissues are in a healthy state, the minimal blood supply the atherosclerotic vessels are able to deliver is adequate to meet their metabolic demands. However, with minimal trauma and the need to repair the injury, the blood supply may be inadequate to meet the increased demands (Chapter 2) and problem, non-healing wounds arise. The atherosclerosis process is especially associated with diabetes, but there are many other causes of ischemia and wound hypoxia (Table 14-1). Collagen vascular diseases with associated Raynaud's phenomena profoundly effect perfusion to the most distal portions of the extremities. Wounds in these areas in patients with collagen vascular diseases are notorious for non-healing and often result in the need for more proximal amputations. Fluid retention (edema) creates a relative barrier to tissue oxygenation by increasing the diffusion distance from the capillary to the cell. Impaired perfusion from cardiac causes is another cause of tissue hypoxia.

Oxygen Requirements - Problems arise when the oxygen demands for fibroblast function, angiogenesis, and leukocyte oxidative killing are insufficient to meet the skins' and underlying tissues' demands for repair and controlling infection. The consequences are non-healing and persistence of infection. Of course, in the total absence of perfusion, such as after thrombotic occlusion of a blood vessel, tissues become ischemic and necrotic. If the occlusion is localized to arteries large enough for thrombectomy, angioplasty, or bypass surgery, perfusion can be restored. Unfortunately, in the situations previously described, perfusion problems usually are also present at the microcirculation level, so these techniques may only have limited success. For the majority of

TABLE 14-1. ISCHEMIA RELATED PROBLEMS ASSOCIATED WITH WOUND HEALING CHALLENGES

Problem	Presentations	Management	Comments
Atherosclerotic vascular disease	Localized occlusion, diffuse involvement, or combinations	Angioplasty and/or revascularization for localized occlusions Methods to improve wound O_2 for diffuse, non-correctible involvement	Diffuse vessel disease frequently associated with "problem" wounds
Thrombosis	Abrupt onset of ischemia with a cold, pulseless, pale limb	Thrombectomy and/or thrombolytic (with medications) therapy	
Venous stasis disease	Hyperpigmentation, bronzing of skin Venous stasis ulcers	Compression, elevation and vein ligation; most resolve with these measures Challenges occur when venous stasis ulcers are complicated by arterial ischemia	Hyperbaric oxygen, bio-engineered dressings, negative pressure wound therapy, and skin grafting are useful adjuncts for the most difficult ulcers
Vasculitis	Painful, non-healing wounds in association with collagen vascular diseases Raynaud's phenomena	Rheumatological interventions including steroids, disease-modifying anti-rheumatic drugs, and anti-metabolites to supplement wound care	Healing difficult due to terminal involvement of the microcirculation
Fluid retention	Stasis dermatitis and ulcerations associated with massive peripheral edema	Measures to reduce edema including diuresis, elevation, and compression wraps Hyperbaric oxygen and fasciotomy if associated with a compartment syndrome	Oxygen diffusion decreases as capillary to cell distance increases due to edema
Miscellaneous including heart failure, obesity & malnutrition	Findings associated with the primary problem All contribute to wound susceptibility and wound healing challenges	Correction of primary problems in conjunction with wound management When voluntary weight reduction fails, consider bariatric surgery referral as an adjunct for managing morbid obesity.	Once these problems are resolved, the management interventions listed above for the other problems usually effectively resolve the wound problem

"problem" and "end-stage" wounds of the feet and legs, perfusion is impaired, but by utilizing the five elements of strategic management and special considerations (Parts III and IV), healing and arrest of infection can occur in the majority of the patients.

DEFORMITIES

The Deformity Problem - Deformities are a primary problem in the genesis of wounds. Deformities in weight bearing areas or other areas subject to contact stresses transfer increased pressures to the skin. If the stresses are acute and localized, a blister forms as a result of walking activity associated with new or ill-fitting footwear. If the pressures are intermittent or sub-critical (that is below a threshold where primary damage occurs to the skin), the skin and underlying tissues react in several ways. First, calluses form over deformities. This is a protective response to the stress manifested by thickening and keratinization of the epithelium. Second, the tissues below the skin over the deformity generate a bursa. With chronic, repetitive stresses, a third response occurs, namely hypertrophy of the bone at the apex of the deformity. This appears on x-rays as periostitis and spurring (eburnations, exostoses and osteophytes).

Secondary Problems from Deformities - With continuation of the pressure stresses, secondary problems arise from the reactive processes. If moisture accumulates under the callus, the skin macerates. If the process is not interrupted by debriding the callus and exteriorizing the macerated area, erosion of the skin and introduction of bacteria can occur. If the firm callus cracks or develops a fissure, a pathway is provided for bacteria and moisture to accumulate between the callus and the skin. This provides an environment conducive for bacterial multiplication, development of cellulitis, ulceration, and a pathway for deeper infection to occur. The other problem is the generation of a mal perforans ulcer. This problem is an ulceration that arises from inside to outside due to continued pressure stresses the deformity transfers to the overlying skin. A mal perforans ulcer is characterized by a tract from the skin to the soft tissues immediately overlying the bone. If this protective envelope is breeched, bacteria have direct access to bone and osteomyelitis is a possible consequence. The bacteria may multiply, generate an abscess, and then result in the infection dissecting along tissue planes and/or tendon sheathes. The consequences can lead to a progressive necrotizing, limb-threatening, soft tissue infection. Proactive measures need to be initiated immediately (Chapter 16) to manage deformities where ulceration is a risk due to their presence.

NEUROPATHY

Indirect Effects of Neuropathy - This problem contributes indirectly to skin and toenail problems. Peripheral neuropathies are especially common in patients with diabetes, but can be associated with other problems such as spinal cord injury, parkinsonism, strokes with residual neurological deficits, multiple sclerosis, trauma, and congenital disorders. As mentioned previously, peripheral neuropathies have three presentations that are a factor in the genesis of "problem" wounds. Neuropathy affecting the autonomic nervous system results in dryness of the skin. Early manifestations are scaling and loss of the normal elasticity of the skin. The debris from scaling may

The terms dynamic and static should also be considered when describing abnormal posturing of joints. Dynamic deformities indicate that the contractures are due to muscle activity imbalances such as observed early in the course of disease in patients with cerebral palsy, strokes with residual neurological deficits, multiple sclerosis, etc. The contractures are not fixed. With physical therapy, splinting, medications and tendon surgeries, the deformed joints can be corrected and maintained in nearly normal position.

Static deformities imply that the contractures are fixed; that is, they are not correctible with the measures mentioned above to manage dynamic contractures. Because of the persistence of the deformities, joint capsules become contracted, muscle-tendon units shortened, and joints arthrodesed. To correct fixed/static joint contractures, surgery is invariably required.

accumulate to form crusts and plaques. Dry skin is less able to tolerate shear and contact pressure stresses than normally moisturized skin, thereby making it subject to breakdown with normal activities. Evaluation and management of skin problems associated with autonomic nerve dysfunction are discussed in the next section.

Impairment of Motor Function - Motor neuropathies cause imbalances in muscle activities. Initially, these cause non-fixed positional deformities of joints. With persistence, the positional deformities become fixed, resulting in contractures (i.e. permanently stiff and/or malaligned joints). Common deformities observed in the feet because of muscle imbalances include clawed toes, hammer toes, mallet toes, hallux valgus/bunions, and equinus contractures. With solitary muscle weakness or dysfunction, other manifestations are observed such as midfoot hyperpronation from posterior tibial muscle-tendon dysfunction and drop foot from peroneal nerve palsy. Peroneal muscle weakness is manifested by foot inversion, resulting in overloading of the lateral bony prominences of the foot such as the fifth metatarsal base and the lateral aspect of the fifth metatarsal head. Early attention to these problems with protective footwear, orthotics and surgeries will be discussed in subsequent chapters.

Loss of Sensation - Sensory neuropathy is a third neurological problem that can indirectly contribute to foot and toenail problems. With loss of protective sensation, impending injury to the skin and toenails may not be appreciated and treatment delayed until more complicated problems develop from the injury. Generally, sensory perception below the "protective sensation" level puts the patient at risk of occult injuries occurring

> If wounds, calluses, or toenail problems are already present, a simplified clinical grading system analogous to the other 0-to-2 point assessments used in this text is recommended. A grade of 2 points indicates normal sensation, and anesthesia is needed for debridements and all other in-office procedures other than toenail trimming and callus paring. A grade of 1 point indicates patients perceive pain with procedures on wounds and toenails, but the procedures usually can be done with no or only locally applied anesthetics. A grade of 0 points indicates a total loss of sensation and in-office procedures can be done on the foot without anesthesia (Table 2-5). If findings are mixed or intermediate between two grades, half points may be used to reflect the transition.

to the skin and toenails without appreciation of pain. Protective sensation is ascertained by testing with a monofilament that bends when approximately five grams of pressure is applied to it. The monofilament is placed on the skin and pressure is applied. If the patient perceives the monofilament touching the skin before it bends, then protective sensation is present. In order to be valid, the testing should be repeated at the same and different sites. If calluses or other signs of impending wounds or obvious wounds are observed during the exam and the patient walked into the office with no apparent discomfort from the sites, the clinical inference can be made that protective sensation is lacking regardless of monofilament testing.

METABOLIC/IMMUNE SYSTEM PROBLEMS

Problems Associated with Metabolism and Immunity - These problems are, in particular, associated with diabetes. However, a number of other metabolic, immune system, and related conditions may be predispositions to skin and toenail wound problems (Table 14-2). Elevated blood and tissue fluid glucose provide a more favorable environment for bacterial multiplication and wound infection than in patients with normal glycemic levels. Atrophy of protective fat pads under metatarsal heads is another finding associated with diabetes. Whether this is a consequence of diabetes, ischemia, or a combination of the two is uncertain. The result is less protection of the skin over the metatarsal heads and increased susceptibility to ulcer formation. Hyperglycemia in patients with diabetes causes increased oxidative stress; increased expression of redox-regulated, proinflammatory genes, and transcription factors; changes to the composition of the extracellular matrix and functional deficits of proteins.[2] Some of the changes affect function of mitochondria, suppress cellular immune defense, and alter elasticity of blood vessel walls.[3, 4] Consequences include microangiopathy, polyneuropathy and changes in connective tissue composition.[2] Tissue stiffness that has been described in patients with diabetes makes tissues less resilient to sheer and compression stresses.[5] Loss of elasticity in tendons, ligaments and joint capsules may contribute to joint contractures and deformities.

Problems Associated with Connective Tissue Diseases - Lupus, dermatomyositis, scleroderma, seropositive arthropathies, and mixed connective tissue disorders, although not usually classified as metabolic disorders, have metabolism-related problems and are notorious for being associated with "problem" and "end-stage" wounds. Vasculitis, a common feature in these disorders, occurs at the microcirculation level and

Clinical correlations

A 46-year-old female with a diagnosis of mixed connective tissue disorder on steroids developed a paronychia secondary to an ingrown great toenail. This was managed with surgical decompression and antibiotics. The wound failed to heal and the distal portion of the toe became necrotic. A partial toe amputation was performed. Primary healing appeared to be occurring, but when the sutures were removed, the wound dehisced and subsequently developed a necrotic, infected base.

An amputation of the toe at the metatarsal phalangeal joint level was performed. Hyperbaric oxygen was given as an adjunct to healing of threatened flaps even though foot pulses were palpable and transcutaneous oxygen measures were normal. This surgical site also failed to heal, and the wound site deteriorated so badly after a couple of months that a more proximal partial first ray amputation became necessary.

When the partial first ray amputation subsequently failed over a period of months, a metatarsal amputation was then performed, but gradually dehisced and the wound base showed no signs of healing. Subsequently, a below-knee amputation was done which went onto primary healing. Unfortunately, a wound developed on the opposite foot which eventually ended-up in a below knee amputation on that side.

Comment

This scenario demonstrates the wound healing difficulties that some patients with collagen vascular diseases may encounter. The distal vasculitis problems in the microcirculation appeared to be so severe that perfusion may only be adequate enough to maintain the steady state, but unable to increase enough for wound healing to occur. Palpable pulses and normal transcutaneous oxygen measurements are no guarantee that wound healing will occur in this patient group.

TABLE 14-2. CONDITIONS THAT MAY BE PREDISPOSITIONS TO SKIN AND TOENAIL WOUND PROBLEMS

Condition	Problems	Comments
Age	Slower metabolism, increased doubling times for fibroblasts, impaired circulation, blunted immunological responses, atrophic changes of the skin, etc.	Age is one of the five assessments for ascertaining the **Host-Function Score**
Androgen deficiency	Observed in catabolic states associated with trauma and nutrition problems	Consider androgen supplements when these conditions exist
Anemia	Compromises oxygen delivery to healing and infection fighting tissues	Anemias associated with other wound healing problems such as chronic infection, kidney diseases and malnutrition
Ehlers-Danlos syndrome	Connective tissue disorder with many presentations Non-healing wounds and difficult to control infections observed following "clean" surgeries	Problems probably related to defective fibroblast function
Gout (Hyperuricemia)	Uric acid precipitates form crystals (tophi) in tissues vulnerable to trauma, especially over bony prominences	Uric acid level should be checked, especially in patients with wounds over bony prominences
Hypercoaguable states	Hypercoaguable conditions include protein C deficiency, anticardiolipin antibodies, Factor V Leiden deficiency, protein S deficiency plasminogen activator inhibitors, homocystein disease, high lipoprotein a, warfarin induced skin necrosis, etc.	Work-ups for these conditions are required when seemingly unexplainable skin sloughs (usually massive & multiple) occur
Hypothyroidism	Slowing of metabolism Dry, pale, cold, scaling skin and brittle nails observed	Thyroid function should be assessed in patients on thyroid medications who have wounds
Liver disease	Deficiencies in the formation of protein, growth factors, cytokines, and immunological factors Hepatitis is a comorbidity in some problem wounds	Blood liver function tests and hepatitis studies indicated in patients with chronic wounds
Malnutrition	Inability to form protein and immunological factors needed for wound healing and infection control	It is essential, regardless of the patient's weight, to ascertain nutritional status when "problem" and "end-stage" wounds exist
Medications	Medications such as steroids, non-steroidal anti-inflammatory drugs, immunosuppressors, and disease modifying anti-rheumatological drugs interfere with the inflammatory response	These medications coupled with wound healing problems from the underlying diseases (such as collagen vascular diseases) complicate wound healing
Purpura fulminans	Intravascular coagulopathy, usually secondary to life threatening infection, cause widespread thromboses in the microcirculation and often result in massive sloughs and even limb losses	No effective treatment known to manage the stasis in the microcirculation. Hyperbaric oxygen aids in the demarcation of viable and non-viable tissues and in wound healing
Renal insufficiency and end-stage renal disease	Metabolic waste products create an environment adverse to wound healing. Usually other problems such as diabetes, anemias, and vascular disease co-exist, which compound wound healing problems	Wound healing is challenging, but possible, in many situations with strategic management and special wound healing considerations (Parts III and IV)
Trauma	Acute problems such as nutrition, blood supply, and infection interfere with healing Chronic problems such as scar formation, deformities, and altered blood supply are precursors to the development of new "problem" wounds	Once wound healing has occurred, proactive measures to prevent new problems including orthotics, special footwear, and proactive surgeries may be required

can interfere with perfusion enough to arrest healing of even the most minor wounds. Protein complexes and antibodies cause atrophy and fibrotic changes in the skin and subcutaneous tissues as well as other parts of the body such as the esophagus and the lungs. Calcium deposition in the subcutaneous tissues (calciphylaxis) serves as a nidus for skin ulceration and infection. The etiology for this is not well-established, but may be due to tissue hypoxia, altered acid-base states, abnormal protein complexes, or combinations of these. Raynaud's phenomenon with intermittent, severe ischemia of the fingers and toes often precipitated by cold exposure or localized trauma may be mediated by the sympathetic nervous system. Consequences of Raynaud's include soft tissue atrophy, acrosclerosis (ends of the digits become pointed), and non-healing ulcerations of the finger tips–probably after occult trauma. Finally, use of immunosuppressors (steroids, anti-metabolites, non-steroidal anti-inflammatory agents, and disease modifying anti-rheumatoid drugs) interfere with wound healing and the ability to control infection.

Multiple Predispositions - Multiple predispositions are a frequent finding in the development of "problem" wounds. Deformities are associated with neuropathies. Soft tissue atrophy is related to wound hypoxia and glycosylation. Elements of collagen vascular disease contribute to wound hypoxia. Contractures with clawing of the toes pulls the fat pads under the metatarsal heads towards the heel so they no longer offer protection for the metatarsal heads. Dorsal subluxation of the proximal phalanges of the toes at the metatarsal phalangeal joints (with proximal retraction of the toes in association with the claw toe deformities) forces the metatarsal heads plantarward. These problems combine to make the areas under the metatarsal heads more vulnerable to ulceration. Hypoxic environments interfere with white blood oxidative killing of bacteria while hyperglycemia fosters an environment for bacteria growth.

EVALUATION AND MANAGEMENT OF SKIN HYGIENE AND MOISTURIZATION

Grading Skin Condition - Skin assessment is essential for preventing wounds. For those "at risk" groups, as previously discussed, checking the skin for precursors of wounds should be done daily. A simplified, objective assessment method based on a 0-to-2 point grading system (similar to the assessment approach used in generating the **Wound Score**, **Host-Function Score,** and **Goal-Aspiration Score**) is useful for evaluating and documenting skin hygiene and moisturization (Figure 14-2). From this grading system, immediate decisions become obvious for appropriate management of the skin. For example, if the skin has a healthy appearance and is moist and pliable (skin assessment grade = 2 points), the patient and/or their caregivers should be complimented and encouraged to continue the same care they have been doing.

If the skin is dry and scaly and in need of lubrication (skin assessment grade = 1 point), the patient (or caregivers) should be instructed in foot and leg skin care measures (Figure 14-3). These include the following four steps:

Moisturization and Cleansing: This is done by showering, bathing, soaking the feet in a basin, or wrapping the feet and legs with a warm, moist towel. Warm, not hot water should be used. The skin should be gently cleansed of debris using a soft cloth and a mild soap or skin cleanser during the moisturizing period. Contact with water should be for periods less than ten minutes in order to prevent maceration of the skin.

Drying the skin: This is done with a soft towel or cloth. Additional debris on the skin may be removed while drying the skin. The skin between the toes should be care-

Grade (If mixed findings or intermediate between two findings, use half points)	Example	Findings	Management
2 (Optimal, normal)	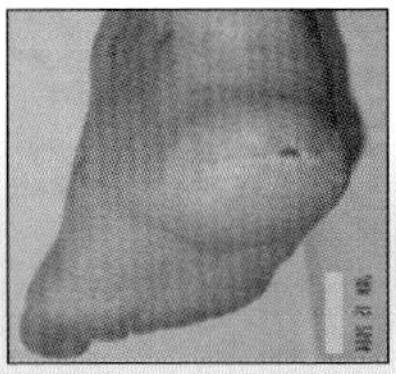	Soft, pliable, well-moisturized, clean skin Free of scaling and plaques	Compliment patient and/or caregivers Continue the same management as before
1 (Sub-optimal, marginally satisfactory)	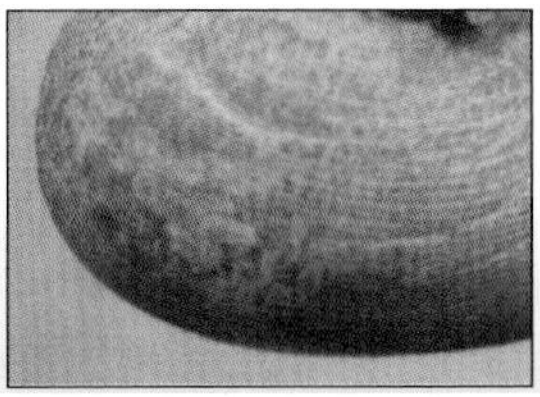	Dry, scaly skin Skin in need of cleansing and lubrication	Instruct and demonstrate to patients and/or caregivers skin care measures (see text)
0 (Unsatisfactory, in need of immediate attention)	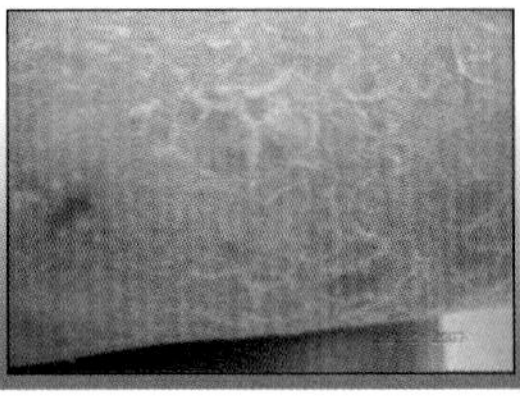	Crusts, plaques, eschars, scaling, desquamated skin, debris and/or maceration	Debride in-office or clinic Skin moisturization and cleansing Skin lubrication

Figure 14-2. Assessment of skin hygiene and moisturization using a 2 (best) to 0 (worst) grading system.

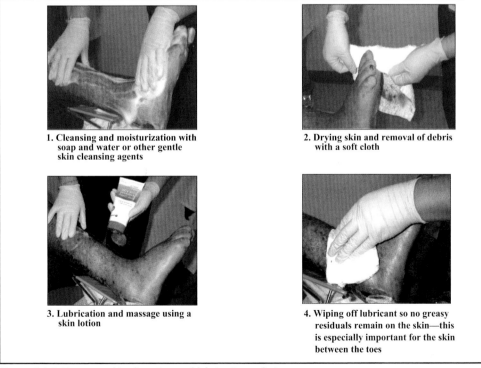

1. Cleansing and moisturization with soap and water or other gentle skin cleansing agents

2. Drying skin and removal of debris with a soft cloth

3. Lubrication and massage using a skin lotion

4. Wiping off lubricant so no greasy residuals remain on the skin—this is especially important for the skin between the toes

Figure 14-3. Four-step skin cleansing and lubrication technique.

fully dried and cleansed of debris to prevent fungus infections. If fungus infection is apparent with findings of redness, fissures, dead skin, localized scaling of the skin and/or odor, an over the counter fungicidal agent [e.g., tolnaftate (Tinactin®), clotrimazole (Lotrimin®), miconazole (Micatin®), etc.] should be used for application to the affected areas after skin care is completed.

Lubrication and massage: After the skin is dry, it should be lubricated and massaged with a lubricating agent. The active lubricating agent in most skin lotions is either a petrolatum/glycerin, lanolin, or silicon-based product. A multitude of products are available (Table 14-3 and Figure 14-4). Usually lubrication and massage only take a couple minutes of time since the moisturized skin tends to readily absorb the lubricating agent.

Removal of residuals of the lubricating agent: This should be done with a soft cloth or towel. Once this step is completed, the skin should feel soft and pliable without a greasiness feeling or visible residuals of the lubricating agent on the skin. Care should be given to removing residuals of the lubricating agents from skin creases and between the toes where moisture accumulation under the agent could lead to maceration and fungus infection.

Zero Point Skin Grade - If plaques, scales, or coatings are present on the skin (skin assessment grade = 0 points / Figure 14-2), skin care should be done in the office. Plaques and scales may be debrided with a scalpel. If the skin is severely in need of

> For efficiency's sake in the office setting, the abbreviations FSC (Foot Skin Care) and TLC (Tender Loving Care) are useful. For example, when it is ascertained that FSC (including the legs, if necessary) needs to be done in the office, the patients are informed that we plan to do TLC for their skin and in the process teach them how to do FSC in the home setting. Usually when they hear the words "tender loving care" they feel they are getting special attention. The use of these abbreviations also saves time for documentation of the treatment plan.
>
> Another situation where TLC is effectively used is for cleansing and lubrication of the skin after cast removal. When this is done, the patients feel that they are getting an additional "extra measure of care."

cleansing and debridement, a finding frequently noted after cast removal, a whirlpool treatment is desirable. While plaque and callus removal is usually done by the physician, the four-step foot and leg skin care measures are usually done by assistants helping the physician. While performing the initial skin care for the patient, the assistants teach the patients how to do the four-step skin care protocol. How well they follow these instructions becomes apparent at the next return visit, reflects patient compliance, and is a criterion for how often the patient needs to return for follow-up care.

EVALUATION AND MANAGEMENT OF TOENAIL CONDITIONS

Toenail Evaluation - Toenail care deserves equal consideration to foot and leg skin care as a prevention strategy for wounds. Any patient who has risk factors for wounds (deformity, peripheral vascular disease, history of previous wound, previous amputation and neuropathy) should have his/her toenails inspected each time the feet are examined. Although many conditions cause toenail abnormalities, four findings are most frequently associated with "problem" wounds (Figure 14-5). Usually two or more findings are present and include the following:

TABLE 14-3. TYPES OF COMPONENTS OF SKIN LUBRICATING AND CLEANSING AGENTS

-------------------Categories of Products -------------------	
Lotion	A liquid preparation applied to the skin—usually with dissolved drugs in it.
Cream	A thick, oily emulsion with suspended drugs in it.
Ointment	A semi-solid preparation that softens, but does not melt when applied to the body with or without added drugs.

---------------Lubricants/Moisture Retainers---------------	
Hydrogels (Hydrosols)	A colloid in which the particles are the external or dispersion phase and water is the internal or dispersed phase.
	This is an excellent choice for maintaining a moisturized environment for the healing of a healthy based (8-10 points on the **Wound Score**) wound.
Petrolatum (Petroleum jelly)	An intermediate product in the distillation of petroleum with excellent skin lubricating properties. Used as a base for many ointments; prevents evaporation of moisture from the skin.
	Greasy residues after application must be wiped off the skin to prevent moisture retention and bacteria multiplication under the film, especially in regards to the toes.
Glycerol (Glycerin)	A fluid obtained by the saponification of fats and vegetable oils. Used as solvent or skin emollient and as a transport vehicle for other agents. Also, prevents evaporation of moisture from the skin.
Lanolin	A fatty substance produced from glands in sheep skin that is water insoluble, has barrier properties, blocks contact with water products such as urine, and prevents evaporation of skin moisture.
Silicones	Polymers of organic silicon oxides which may be liquids, gels, or solids depending on the extent of polymerization; can be used as greases or sealing agents.

-----------------------------Cleansers -----------------------------	
Soaps	The sodium or potassium salts of long-chain fatty acids used as an emulsifier for cleansing purposes.
Medicinal soft soaps	Soaps made with vegetable oils, potassium hydroxide, oleic acid, glycerin, and purified water used as a cleansing agent and stimulant in chronic skin diseases.
Hydrogen peroxide	An unstable compound readily broken down to water and oxygen that loosens and cleanses debris and acts as a mild antiseptic.
Alcohols	A series of organic chemical compounds used as a cleanser, rubefacient (i.e. causes erythema of the skin), coolant, and disinfectant.
Solvents	Liquids that hold other substances in solution; organic solvents are cleansing agents useful for removing adhesive residuals, oils, fats, etc., but are harsh to the skin and should only be used on a one time basis.

---------------------------Additives ----------------------------	
Fragrances	Provide pleasant odors, often helping consumer to identify the product; masks unpleasant odors.
Colorants	Enhance visual appeal of the product; camouflages unpleasant appearances of other ingredients.
Thickening agents/vehicles	Improve consistency, e.g. corn starch, talc, hydroxyethel cellulose, xanthan gum, essence of oats, etc. Thickening agents bring the product to a specified quantify—i.e. a "filler" such as mineral oil, petrolatum, cetyl alcohol, and propylene glycol.
Keratolytic agents	Useful for removing thickened, hypertrophic, desquamated, and callused skin and skin debris; e.g. dimethicone, papain ureas, collagenases, etc.
Antipruritics	Control itching, e.g. diphenhydramine, steroids, zinc oxide, iron oxide, tacrolimus.
Anti-inflammatories	Reduce inflammation; helps to control itching, e.g. hydrocortisone, betamethasone, diclofenac.
Pain relievers	Reduce pain; e.g. local anesthetics (lidocaine, benzocaine), analgesics (salicylates, menthol, capsaicin, camphor), topical narcotics.
Anti-aging agents	Decreases fine skin lines by removing dead skin; e.g. tretinoin, moisturizers, estrogens, Vitamin E ointment.
Anti-infectives	Kill bacteria or fungi; e.g. single/double/triple antibiotic products, antifungals (clotrimazole, nystatin, tolnaftate), phenols, menthol, etc.
Moisture barriers	Physically block moisture contact with skin, e.g. zinc oxide ointment, lanolin, petrolatum, etc.
Sun blocks	Prevent ultraviolet rays A and B from skin penetration, e.g. octocrylene, octylmethoxycinnamate, etc.

Comments:	Although this list is extensive, it is not all inclusive: Hundreds or perhaps thousands of additives can be found in skin lubricants and cleansers. These generic categories help the user to understand the roles of the ingredients. Some over-the-counter skin agents have 30 or more ingredients.

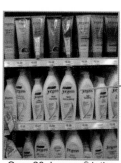

Over 20 Jergens® lotion
options alone

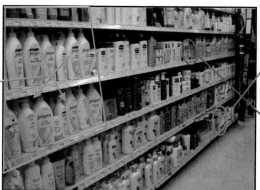

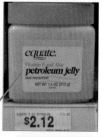

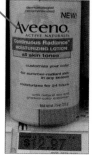

**Options available from a large
discount variety store**

Crème de Corps with Pump	16.4 oz	44.50
Crème de Corps	8.0 oz	26.00
...s Nurturing Body Washing Cream	6.8 oz	17.50
Callus Treatment and Moisturizer	3.4 oz	22.50
Ultimate Strength Hand Salve	5.0 oz	19.50

"Designer" products from
an "upscale" boutique

Over a 6-fold
variation in prices

Legend: Innumerable skin cleansing and moisturizing agents are available. Choices differ by addition of colors, perfumes, anti-aging agents, sun protection factors, smoothing and firming products, etc.

Figure 14-4. Skin and cleansing lotion choices.

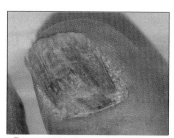

Dystrophic, fissures, laminated,
irregular end

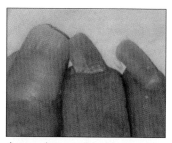

Long, dysmorphic (dome-shaped)

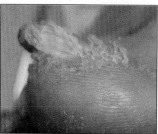

Thickened, fungus-infected,
embedded debris

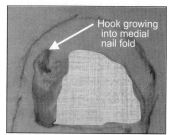

Hook growing
into medial
nail fold

Ingrown (hook) of medial nail fold
which can lead to a pyogenic
granuloma or paronychium

Legend: These examples are among the most frequent toenail problems encountered in a wound healing center. They should be always be documented and managed appropriately.

Figure 14-5. Common toenail problems.

Dysmorphic toenail changes: This finding indicates that the shape of the toenail is abnormal. The toenail end may be curved like the shape of a spoon, vaulted like a cathedral ceiling or curled like a ram's horn. Usually, dysmorphic changes are due to abnormalities in the nail bed from underlying bony deformities or from pressure effects from footwear. When the toenail edges are curved, debris often becomes embedded between the curved toenail edge and the underlying skin.

Dystrophic toenail changes: These problems are reflected in abnormal growth of the toenail and usually arise from problems in the nail matrix from circulation, disease, trauma, toxic substances, or congenital problems. Presentations include thickened, furrowed, discolored, and hypoplastic toenails.

Fungus infected (onychomycosis): Although fungus infection may be a primary problem of toenails, in patients with sensory neuropathy, occult trauma may also be a cause. With occult trauma in these patients, the toenail may be partially avulsed from the nail bed without being recognized. This may allow moisture to accumulate under the toenail and provide an ideal environment for the fungus to grow. Fungus infected toenails become discolored, thickened, friable, honeycombed, and/or laminated (layers of infected toenail and debris).

Ingrown toenail: Direct trauma or contact pressure from shoe and sock wear may force the edge of the toenail into the recess between the nail bed and the nail fold. This may introduce bacteria and cause a localized cellulitis or abscess (paronychia) or pyogenic granuloma. Another way bacteria are introduced into the skin is when the distal edge breaks off or is trimmed off leaving a hook shape to the edge of the toenail. As the toenail grows outward, the hook end of the toenail grows into the adjacent skin.

Grading Toenail Condition - As in the skin grading system, a simple, quick to use 0-to-2 point grading system is recommended for evaluation and management of toenail problems (Figure 14-6). Management of toenails in patients with risk factors for wounds becomes obvious when the grading system is used (Figure 14-7). If the toenails are the proper length and normal in appearance (nail assessment grade = 2 points), the patients should be complimented on their toenail care and encouraged to continue the same care they have been giving to their toenails. If the toenails are long and/or the ends of the toenails are jagged (nail assessment grade = 1 point), but otherwise normal in appearance, two options exist. If the patient is agile and his/her vision is OK or the caregivers are conscientious, they may trim the nails straight across. More preferable, especially if sensory neuropathy is present, is to have them use a disposable nail file to keep the nails at the proper lengths with frequent filings. If the patient and/or caregivers are unable to care for the toenails, then they should be trimmed with nail cutters in the office setting by care providers properly trained in toenail care.

If the toenails are dysmorphic, dystrophic, fungus-infected, or ingrown (nail assessment grade = 0 points—Figure 14-5), toenail management should be done by podiatrists, orthopaedic foot surgeons, or health care providers trained in toenail care

A small rotary craft tool with a cylindrical sanding attachment very effectively debulks and contours thickened toenails. Personnel who use the tool should be gloved, gowned, capped, and masked in order to protect themselves from the flying debris that arises from this technique. A new sanding cylinder needs to be used for each patient. The flying debris generated by the rotatory sander should be simultaneously vacuumed as it is produced.

Grade (If mixed findings or intermediate between two findings, use half points)	Example	Findings	Management
2 (Optimal, normal)		Healthy-appearing, appropriate length toenails Note:*Toenail polish should not be used if risk factors for foot wounds exist	Compliment patient and/or caregivers Continue the same management as before
1 (Sub-optimal, marginally satisfactory)		Long and/or irregular ends of trimmed toenails	Trim toenails with sterilized surgical quality nail clippers in the office/clinic Instruct patients in trimming techniques including use of a nail file to contour and shape toenail ends
0 (Unsatisfactory, in need of immediate attention)		Diseased toenails (Figure 14-5) in need of immediate management	Debride, debulk with sterilized surgical quality nail clippers File and contour with a nail file or rotating sanding drum Teach patient and/or caregivers toenail filing techniques

*Risk factors for wound development include: deformity, previous amputation, peripheral artery disease, previous wounds, and/or neuropathy.

Figure 14-6. Assessment of toenails using a 2 (best) to 0 (worst) grading system.

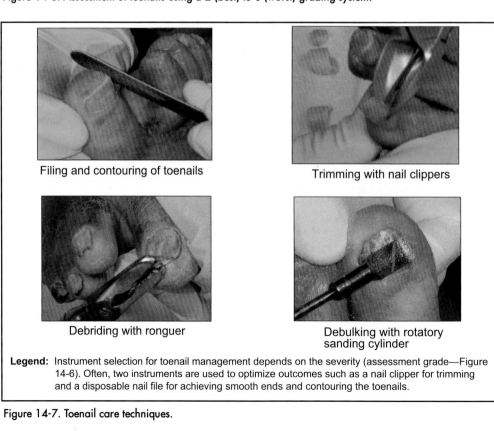

Filing and contouring of toenails

Trimming with nail clippers

Debriding with ronguer

Debulking with rotatory sanding cylinder

Legend: Instrument selection for toenail management depends on the severity (assessment grade—Figure 14-6). Often, two instruments are used to optimize outcomes such as a nail clipper for trimming and a disposable nail file for achieving smooth ends and contouring the toenails.

Figure 14-7. Toenail care techniques.

using sterilized nail instruments specifically designed for these purposes. Embedded material at the nail margins should be debrided. The hooked ends of ingrown toenails should be trimmed proximally to achieve a smooth nail edge. This may require trimming the nail edges almost to the proximal nail fold and result in a curved rather than straight-across toenail end (Figure 14-8). Thickened, fungus infected toenails should be thinned until they are tissue paper thickness. Toenails that are no longer attached to the underlying nail bed should be debrided proximally until the location where they are attached to the nail bed. This usually eradicates the infected portion of the toenail. In this situation, a sensory neuropathy can be a boon to toenail care since very complete toenail care can be done without requiring local anesthetics or the patient experiencing pain. Once this toenail care is completed, the edges of the toenail and the recesses should be painted with an iodine containing disinfectant for infection prophylaxis.

Zero Point Toenail Grade - The above approach to complicated toenail problems (nail assessment grade = 0 points) exemplifies the surgical perspective, that is, aggressively eliminate the problem using appropriate instruments. The time required to achieve this goal is measured in minutes. The other approach when fungus infection of the toenail (onychomycosis) is present is the medical one using fungicidal agents. The

> In the United States it is estimated that 35 million people are affected with toenail infections. About one billion dollars a year is spent on medications trying to eradicate them.[6, 7]

more severe the involvement, the less likely fungicidal agents will be effective. At best, they cure the infection in 40 to 70 percent of the cases.[8] In the USA, over a billion dollars is spent each year on oral and topical agents that are used to treat toenail infections.[9] Furthermore, medical management of infected toenails may take months or more to

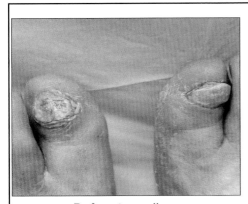

Before toenail care

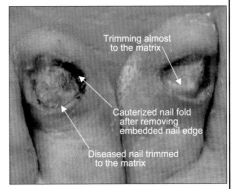

Trimming almost
to the matrix

Cauterized nail fold
after removing
embedded nail edge

Diseased nail trimmed
to the matrix

After toenail care

Legend: Appropriate toenail care to eradicate fungus disease and ingrown margins may require trimming the nail to the matrix and removing embedded debris and ingrown portions from the nail fold. If bleeding occurs, a silver nitrate applicator effectively cauterizes the bleeding site. Because of the extent of the debridement, the toenail and adjacent nail folds should be "painted" with an iodine solution or equally effective disinfectant.

Figure 14-8. Establishment of healthy margins for severely diseased toenails.

cure the problem, if indeed it cures it at all, and monitoring of toxicity from the agent with liver function tests is often required. Once initial debridement of the complicated toenail problem is done, the patient is usually asked to return in a couple of weeks to

> Laser treatment of fungus-infected toenails is currently being investigated (not yet approved by the Food and Drug Administration). The treatment with lasers costs $1000 or more and has reportedly been observed to be effective in 50% to 75% of cases.[9]

"fine tune" the toenail appearance, by hand filing and further contouring the toenails.

"DOS" AND "DON'TS" PERTAINING TO SKIN AND TOENAIL CARE

The previous chapter presented a list of "dos" and "don'ts" that should be taught to patients with risk factors for foot wounds. A number of them are pertinent to skin and toenail care. For this reason, those that apply to foot skin and toenail care are now repeated in tabulated form in this section.

- "Dos" with Respect to Preventing Skin and Toenail Problems
  - Inspect feet daily
  - Practice good foot hygiene, including skin lubrication
  - Perform appropriate toenail care
- "Don'ts" to Prevent Skin and Toenail Problems
  - Don't walk barefooted
  - Don't use heat on the feet
  - Don't soak the feet in hot water
  - Don't use chemicals or sharp objects to trim calluses
  - Don't trim corners of toenails
  - Don't use toenail polish, especially if risk factors for foot wounds exist

CONCLUSIONS

The skin of the feet and the toenails are windows to the interior of the body. That is why the quotation "What you see tells you a lot" is so apropos for this chapter. The major problem is not taking the time to look into the window to examine the skin of the legs and feet and inspect the toenails. The other benefit that examination of these areas reveals is how well these patients follow instructions and are compliant with recommendations. When risk factors for wound development in the feet and legs are present, the skin and toenails are without question the first line of defense for their prevention. Fortunately, as this chapter shows, evaluation and management of skin and toenail problems can be objective as well as quick and easy to accomplish.

QUESTIONS

1. Why are the foot skin and toenails "windows" to the interior of the body?

2. Why are the foot skin and toenails a paradox with respect to developing wounds?

3. What are some predispositions for developing foot skin and toenail problems?

4. How does neuropathy affect wound healing?

5. What are the four steps to manage skin hygiene and lubrication?

6. What are advantages of using the simplified (2 points, 1 point, 0 points) foot skin and toenail evaluation and management system?

7. How are the terms Foot Skin Care (FSC) and Tender Loving Care (TLC) applicable to skin care and toenail management?

8. What considerations should be given to allowing a patient to do his/her own toenail care or have it done by a foot care specialist?

9. Compare and contrast the surgical versus medical management of fungal infected toenails (onychomycosis).

REFERENCES

1. Strauss MB, Miller SS. Addressing foot skin and toenail concerns in diabetics, J. Musculoskeletal Medicine 2007; 24(7):312-319

2. Wolhrab J, Wolhrab D, Meiss F. Skin diseases in diabetes mellitus. J Dtsch Dermatol Ges. 2007; 5: 37-53

3. Wautier JL, Guillausseau PJ. Advanced glycation end products, their receptors and diabetic angiopathy. Diabetes Metab. 2001; 27: 535–542

4. Obrosova IG. Increased sorbitol pathway activity generates oxidative stress in tissue sites for diabetic complications. Antioxid Redox Signal 2005; 7: 1543–1552

5. Buckingham BA, Uitto J, Sandborg C, et al. Scleroderma-like changes in insulin-dependent diabetes mellitus: clinical and biochemical studies. Diabetes Care 1984 Mar-Apr; 7(2):163-9

6. Elewski BE, Charif MA. Prevalence of onychomycosis in patients attending a dermatology clinic in northeastern Ohio for other conditions. Arch Dermatol. 1997 Sep; 133(9):1172-3

7. Roberts DT, Taylor WD, Boyle J. Guidelines for treatment of onychomycosis. British Association of Dermatologists. Br J Dermatol. 2003 Mar; 148(3):402-10

8. Gupta AK, Ryder JE, Johnson AM. Cumulative meta-analysis of systemic antifungal agents for the treatment of onychomycosis. Br J Dermatol 2004 Mar; 150(3):537-44

9. Singer N. False start on a laser remedy for fungus. The New York Times March 20, 2009; p 20

CHAPTER

15 PROTECTIVE FOOTWEAR

CHAPTER FIFTEEN OVERVIEW

INTRODUCTION 421

SHOE COMPONENTS AND SOCK CHARACTERISTICS 422

PROTECTIVE FOOTWEAR OPTIONS. 424

MAKING SENSE OF ORTHOTICS 433

MEDICARE THERAPEUTIC FOOTWEAR BENEFITS 439

DOS AND DON'TS PERTAINING TO PROTECTIVE FOOTWEAR 441

CONCLUSIONS 441

QUESTIONS. 443

REFERENCES. 444

"If the shoe fits, don't always wear it."

INTRODUCTION

The Second Line of Defense - Protective footwear is the second line of defense after skin and toenail care for prevention of new and recurrent wounds (Figure 15-1).[1, 2] Any patient who has one or more of the conditions recognized as risk factors for wound development (namely deformity, peripheral vascular disease, history of a previous wound, previous amputation and/or neuropathy) and is ambulatory, requires intelligent decision-making for the selection of protective footwear. This line of defense is so import that in 1993 Medicare (Center for Medicare/Medicaid Services) under the direction of Congress initiated the "Therapeutic Shoe Bill" benefit for diabetic Medicare beneficiaries with risk factors for wounds. Undoubtedly this decision was based on the assumption that the potential benefits to prevent diabetic foot problems outweighed the costs (that is cost-effective plus cost-beneficial) to provide protective footwear.[3, 4] The bottom line is that it is less expensive to prevent a diabetic foot problem from arising by providing therapeutic footwear than it is to treat the complications that arise from not using appropriate footwear. In recognition of these facts, benefits for protective footwear for diabetic patients were established and will be delineated later in this chapter.

Footwear Selection - Selection of protective footwear is not a matter of fashion. It requires knowledge, insight, and experience. There are a large number of options to

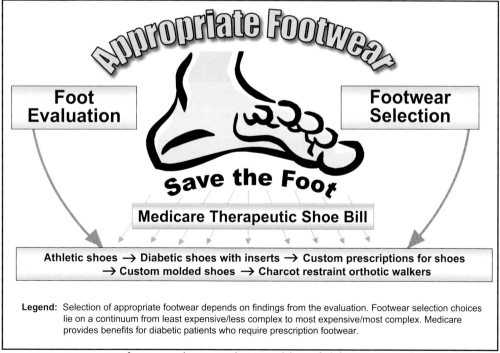

Legend: Selection of appropriate footwear depends on findings from the evaluation. Footwear selection choices lie on a continuum from least expensive/less complex to most expensive/most complex. Medicare provides benefits for diabetic patients who require prescription footwear.

Figure 15-1. Appropriate footwear selection is the second line of defense against developing new or recurrent foot wounds.

consider when recommending and prescribing an individual's protective footwear including one or more personalized adjustments such as wedges, fillers, lifts, orthotics, cut outs, relief areas, bars, or other modifications. To simplify matters, the selection of protective footwear can logically be placed in a hierarchy from least complex to most complex (Figure 15-2). Factors that determine complexity include availability ranging from off-the-shelf to custom molded and modifications from simple inserts to specifically placed reliefs and pads. As the complexity increases, the costs increase proportionately. The hierarchy has five levels: 1) quality walking or athletic shoes, 2) off-the-shelf diabetic shoes with cushioned plantar inserts, 3) custom prescriptions added to off-the-shelf diabetic shoes, 4) custom molded diabetic shoes, and 5) Charcot restraint orthotic walkers (CROW boots).

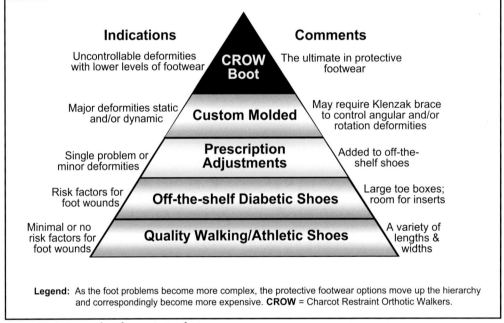

Legend: As the foot problems become more complex, the protective footwear options move up the hierarchy and correspondingly become more expensive. **CROW** = Charcot Restraint Orthotic Walkers.

Figure 15-2. Hierarchy of prescription footwear.

SHOE COMPONENTS AND SOCK CHARACTERISTICS

Shoe Components - In order to appropriately prescribe protective footwear, it is helpful to be aware of the various components of a shoe, its functions, what alternatives exist for each component, and what complications may arise from them. Surprisingly, many options also exist for sock choices. The following is a summary of major shoe components and sock compositions.

1. **Covering Materials (Outer Portions) -** are what the outer component of the shoe is made of, give the shoe above the sole portion its shape, and often give the shoe its common name such as leather, house, tennis, athletic, boot, etc. Common components include leather, cloth, netting comprised of various materials, canvas, rubber, synthetic fibers (rigid or flexible), or plastic. Multiple combinations may be used, as is often found in tennis shoes. Leather is desirable for its durability, breathability, and malleability to accommodate deformities. Flexible synthetic fibers are desirable because they accommodate changes in foot size due to swelling and are pliable enough to avoid pressure concentrations. Rigid plastic coverings, such as used in the Charcot restraint orthotic walkers (CROW boot), require padded inner linings.

2. **Fasteners** - are the devices that help to keep the shoe on the foot. There are three basic choices: 1) string ties, 2) elastic bands, and 3) Velcro® straps. String ties tend to be more secure, but require agility and good proprioception in order to tension properly and tie. If the knot becomes untied, the shoe may loosen subjecting the patient's skin to shear stresses and the foot and ankle ligaments to sprains. Another hazard of string ties is they can become untied and can cause the patient to trip over a shoelace. Elastic bands or Velcro® straps are more user-friendly and the preferred choice for many patients with comorbidities such as arthritis, obesity, hemiparesis, etc. In patients who retain fluids, the elastic bands may indent the edematous skin and interfere with venous return.

3. **Heels** - are elevations that may be added to the back thirds of the shoe sole (discussed below). They may be thick, thin, wedged on either side, extended medially (Thomas heels), or absent depending on the perceived needs of the hind foot. Whereas some of the heel modifications are of dubious value, those used to counteract equinus deformities and position the ankle during Achilles tendon healing are, without question, of value.

4. **Heel Counters** - are the parts of the shoe that come in contact with the back of the shoe wearer's heels. They may be low profile, hardly covering the back of the patient's heel or high enough to extend proximal along the back of the Achilles tendon. The higher the heel counter, the greater the control of the hind foot. The inside portion of the heel counter may be padded with foam or soft cloth or merely lined with cloth or leather to provide a cosmetic appearance for the shoe covering material. Semi-rigid plastic inserts may be placed between the layers to add increased rigidity to the heel counter and control of the hind foot.

5. **Inner Linings** - may or may not be present. They may increase the cushioning properties of the shoe, absorb moisture or help with the fit of the shoe. In stylish shoes, most are thin leather and only added for their cosmetic effect. In addition to leather, lining materials may be cloth or various types of foam.

6. **Lasts** - refer to the shape of the sole portion of the shoe. Usually the last is slightly concave along its medial aspect. For angular deformities (especially metatarsus adductus in children) the lasts may be straight or reversed, that is convex along their medial border.

7. **Shanks** - are devices inserted into the sole portion of the shoe to control flexibility. Most often they are rigid steel bars and used for specific occupational needs rather than as modifications for protective footwear.

8. **Shoe Heights/Upper Portion** - designate the portion of the shoe that is attached to the sole and extends over the foot, ankle or leg. Low cut shoes, such as moccasins and flats, may only cover the bottom half of the foot. Consequently, they provide minimal support and stability. Intermediate cut shoes, the most frequently prescribed protective footwear, enclose the feet and extend to just below the level of the ankle malleoli. High-top shoes extend above the malleoli with boots being a good example of this type of footwear. Naturally with increasing height of the upper portion of the footwear, protection, support, and stability increase. Conversely, the greater the height of the upper portion of footwear, the more difficult it is to don, fasten, and remove the shoe. Velcro® straps help to mediate the difficulties of tying the shoes. Specially designed footwear, such as CROW boots, help to mediate the difficulty of donning and removing the shoe.

9. **Shoe Soles** - are the part of the shoe that makes contact with the ground or floor. They may be rigid or flexible. They are typically flat with or without the

addition of a heel portion. Materials used for the soles of shoes include leather, plastic composite materials, wood, and rubber. The rocker bottom sole is a modification that facilitates walking in the presence of severe deformities or joint mobility problems.

10. **Shoe Tongues** - may or may not be present in protective footwear. Tongues, when present, are usually a separate component that attaches to the toe box (described next). Tongues serve several purposes including providing protection between the laces and the top of the foot, and improving fit and comfort. Tongues may or may not be padded. Shoes that do not have tongues usually have overlapping flaps secured with Velcro® straps. These make the shoe easier to don and remove.

11. **Toe Boxes** - are the portions of the shoe top that cover the forefoot. For most protective footwear, the toe boxes are spacious enough to prevent pressure sores developing from clawed toes and other forefoot abnormalities. Of course, the antithesis of the large toe box is the pointed toe shoe. In comparison to protective footwear, pointed toe shoes have many undesirable features that contribute to bunion deformities, hallux valgus, hyperpronation of the great toe, varus plus supination deformities of the little toes, and cross-over toes. In conjunction with high heels, pointed toe shoes contribute to clawed toe deformities, hyperextension contractures of the toes at the metatarsal-phalangeal joint levels, proximal migration of the forefoot fat pads, as well as calluses, bone spurs, and ulcerations under the metatarsal heads. When toes or a distal portion of the foot are absent, a filler (or spacer) is usually inserted in the toe box to help with shoe fit and prevent shearing stresses on the skin with movements of the foot.

12. **Sock Options** - should not be overlooked in conjunction with footwear selection. Knee-length compression stockings with 20-to-30 mmHg tensions are recommended for all patients who have had foot surgeries, lower extremity edema, mobility problems, venous stasis disease, or spend extended periods of time with their feet immobile in the dependent position (Chapter 12). Sock fiber choices include cotton, wool, acrylic, polyester, polypropylene, or combinations of these fibers. Cotton socks are the least expensive, do not provide very good padding, and manage moisture poorly. Wool socks provide good insulation and manage moisture fairly well. Acrylic socks fit well, reduce shear, cushion well, and handle moisture well. The other synthetic fibers manage moisture well, but do not provide good padding. Blends of these fibers can combine the desirable features of several fiber types. White stockings are especially desirable for those patients with risk factors for wound development since a stain on a white sock will not likely be ignored, as it might be if the patient was wearing dark colored socks (Figure 13-4). Finally, stocking cleanliness is desirable, preferably with changes being done daily. Socks from synthetic fibers tend to retain odors and pile with repeated wear.

PROTECTIVE FOOTWEAR OPTIONS

Footwear Choices - Although nearly a dozen components, as just described, may be considered when prescribing protective footwear, choices can be reduced to five principle types in a hierarchy that ranges from off-the-shelf, least expensive to custom-molded, most expensive (Figure 15-2). Knowledge of the footwear options and what needs to be achieved with the patient's footwear requirements should always be determinants when prescribing protective footwear. Considerations include:

- The patient's functional capacity (amplified with information provided by the **Host-Function Score**)
- The characteristics of the foot problem
- The modifications available for the five principle protective footwear choices
- The patient's goals (supported with information obtained from the **Goal-Aspiration Score**)

In most circumstances this information, except for knowledge of the available modifications, is already available from the patient's initial evaluation or becomes readily obvious with the re-evaluation preceding the footwear prescription. The actual protective footwear selection, addition of modifications and fitting should be done by the pedorthotist or orthotist, who is the health care professional most knowledgeable in this aspect of protective footwear. The following information describes the five principle choices for protective footwear in the hierarchy of complexity and costs. For each upward step in the hierarchy, the costs increase two to three-fold.

Level 1 - Quality walking or athletic shoes: These shoes can be purchased without a prescription and usually do not qualify for Medicare Therapeutic Shoe Bill benefits. They are the least expensive and the best-looking of the footwear options (Figure 15-3). Not only is the construction of the highest quality, but also they usually are available in a variety of lengths and widths to accommodate a wide range of foot sizes. The insides of these shoes are typically well-padded and the soles fairly rigid. The shoes are generally secured by lace-up ties or Velcro® straps. Many choices have large toe boxes that provide room for clawed or hyper-extended toe deformities. This footwear choice is ideal for patients without foot deformities and/or who have only minimal, if any, risk factors for wound development. Prices of quality walking or athletic shoes range from $100 to $200 dollars.

Level 2 - Off-the-shelf diabetic shoes with cushioned plantar inserts: As the name

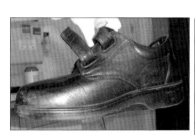

Walking shoe with quality construction, a large toe box, Velcro® fasteners and a thick sole

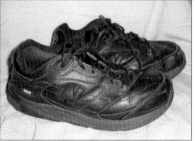

An athletic shoe with analogous features; it is E width to accommodate the patient's wide foot

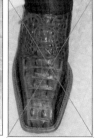

A beautiful shoe… but not for the patient with risk factors for foot wounds

Legend: Quality walking and athletic shoes can be stylish as well as functional, but contrast markedly with the shoe in the right hand figure, which has pointed toes, a thin sole, compressed toe box, and slip-on (moccasin style) fixation to the foot.

Figure 15-3. Quality walking and athletic shoes versus a high fashion shoe.

implies, these are production model (i.e. mass produced) shoes that generally are available in most well stocked specialty footwear and orthotic-prosthetic shops. The shoes are similar to the descriptions given above for quality walking or athletic shoes with the major difference being that there is enough room to accommodate extra-depth inserts (Figure 15-4). Although these shoes with the prescribed orthotics can be purchased without a prescription, a prescription by a physician is necessary for patients with diabetes to receive Medicare Therapeutic Shoe Bill benefits. There are advantages in obtaining these shoes from salespeople trained in the fitting of protective footwear including: 1) improved likelihood of proper size selection, 2) experience with the choices available to comply with the footwear prescription, 3) recognition and management of special needs such as different sized shoes for each foot, 4) preparation and fitting of multi-density inserts (Table 15-1), 5) ability to stretch and relieve pressure areas that are noted after using the shoes (Figure 15-4), and 6) recourse such as exchanges or refunds if the patient is not satisfied with the footwear that was selected.[5] In general, patients who enter the footwear selection hierarchy at this level have minimal deformities although they have risk factors for the development of foot wounds.

Durability of Level 2 Protective Footwear - For household and limited community ambulation needs, off-the-shelf diabetic shoes should remain effective for approximately a year. At the time of publication of this text, the Medicare Therapeutic Shoe Bill allows for shoe replacement yearly. With use and time the shoes stretch, become easier

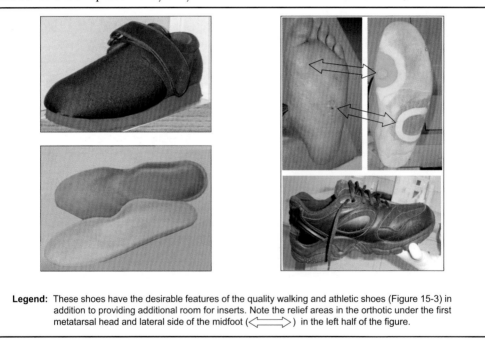

Legend: These shoes have the desirable features of the quality walking and athletic shoes (Figure 15-3) in addition to providing additional room for inserts. Note the relief areas in the orthotic under the first metatarsal head and lateral side of the midfoot (<———>) in the left half of the figure.

Figure 15-4. Off-the-shelf diabetic shoes with cushioned plantar inserts.

to don and remove and, according to the patients, feel more comfortable. Unfortunately, these may be clues that it is time to replace the shoes. Other signs of shoe deterioration include wearing down of the heels or soles so they no longer keep the foot plantigrade, shifting of the upper portion of the shoe on the sole, wearing away of the inner linings especially over bony prominences, separation of seams and excessive wear and tear of the upper portions. Consequently, if the shoe fits, it does not always mean it should be

TABLE 15-1. MATERIALS COMMONLY USED FOR SHOE INSERTS AND/OR ORTHOTICS

	Material	Characteristics	Comments
Natural Varieties	Cork	Porous, lightweight; distributes forces over entire surface, but relatively firm	Often used with leather to provide padding plus durability
	Felt	A firm woven cloth of wool or cotton with excellent pressure off-loading and distributing characteristics; often used in total contact casting Poor durability; retains odors; difficult to clean	Sliding effect of fibers under pressure areas off-load these areas without cut-outs or reliefs
	Leather	Durable, malleable, relatively rigid; long-wearing just as leather soles and upper portions of shoes are Non-cushioning	More difficult to mold and contour than foams and felt. Useful for lifts and wedges for shoes
Synthetics	Polyethylene	Closed-cell foam; soft; poor cushioning due to bottoming out quickly Moldable with low heat	Useful as padding with more rigid materials
	Polypropylene	Rigid, moldable with heat usually after making a plaster foot mold	Often padded with a soft foam
	Polyurethane	Soft foam with good elastic properties (i.e. does not bottom out); poor durability and resistance to tearing	Excellent as a skin-contact padding material over more rigid materials
	Silicone	A polymer of organic silicon oxides which may be a liquid, gel, or solid depending on the degree of polymerization	Excellent padding and skin contact material (especially for prostheses) Gel states excellent for off-loading pressure areas

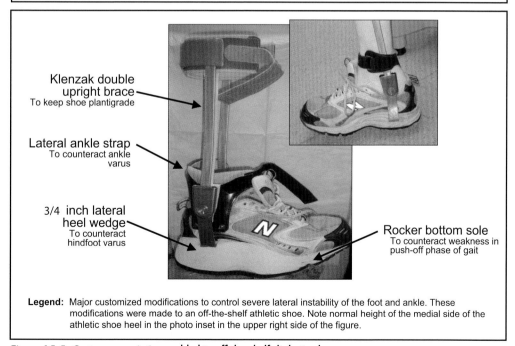

Klenzak double upright brace
To keep shoe plantigrade

Lateral ankle strap
To counteract ankle varus

3/4 inch lateral heel wedge
To counteract hindfoot varus

Rocker bottom sole
To counteract weakness in push-off phase of gait

Legend: Major customized modifications to control severe lateral instability of the foot and ankle. These modifications were made to an off-the-shelf athletic shoe. Note normal height of the medial side of the athletic shoe heel in the photo inset in the upper right side of the figure.

Figure 15-5. Custom prescriptions added to off-the-shelf diabetic shoes.

worn. Multi-density inserts quickly lose their cushioning ability with use. The Medicare Therapeutic Shoe Bill provides for replacement inserts as frequently as every four months if they are no longer effective. Prescription footwear with inserts usually cost about two to three times as much as quality walking or athletic shoes or in the $300.00-$500.00 range.

Level 3 - Custom prescriptions added to off-the-shelf diabetic shoes: This is the third level in the footwear selection hierarchy (Figure 15-5). This step of the hierarchy is typically associated with a single fixed (static) or dynamic deformity of the foot or ankle. Generally, shoes from the previous level are used as the foundation for the prescription modifications. A large number of options exist; essentially every shoe component previously discussed can be modified in one way or another (Table 15-2). When shoe modifications are prescribed, several requirements need to be met. First, the modification should address the structural deformity. The deformity can be as simple as mildly depressed metatarsal heads that require placement of a simple metatarsal pad to as complicated as deformities associated with Charcot arthropathies.[6] Second, the modification needs to provide a stable platform for the bottom of the foot in order to transfer the patient's body weight to the underlying walking surface. Third, the modification needs to reduce focal areas of pressure as typically found over deformities. Fourth, the modification needs to eliminate shear stresses. For example, the indication for prescribing a filler or spacer for the forefoot after a transmetatarsal amputation (Figure 15-6).

Bracing for Protective Footwear - Another prescription addition that may be required at this level of protective footwear is the use of the metal double upright brace (Klenzak). Whereas plastic AFOs (Ankle Foot Orthoses) have many desirable features such as lightness and ease of application, they do not control angular and rotation deformities very well. They are most suitable for drop foot (peroneal nerve palsy) problems where a single (i.e. lack of foot dorsiflexion), non-angular deformity is present. In addition, in the presence of sensory neuropathies of the feet, AFO's are a cause of ulcerations. The Klenzak brace with its distal insertion into a high quality shoe (frequently with prescribed adjustments) can control angular, rotation, static and dynamic deformities simultaneously. In this respect, in spite of its weight and unattractiveness, it is a valuable asset in the armamentarium of protective footwear alterations.

Successful use of Protective Footwear - Although prescription modifications may be the logical choice for the problem observed in the foot and ankle, they are not always successful. Maintaining the ability to walk and the prevention of new wound problems confirm successful use of the footwear. This is only achieved in conjunction with patient education (Chapter 13) and proper skin and toenail care (Chapter 14). Revisions (i.e. "fine tuning") and adjustments are often needed in order to make the protective footwear function optimally. Even then, they may only be able to maintain the status quo, to prevent the wound from worsening while maintaining the patient's mobility such as described in the chronic, stable, "end-stage" wound (Chapter 11). A second corollary of successful protective footwear modifications is that they may require on-going adjustments. Frequently, the shape of the foot changes with time. This is especially noted with Charcot arthropathies, posterior tibial tendon insufficiencies, and motor neuropathies. The third corollary is to establish whether or not the deformity is static, or present even when not weight bearing or dynamic, or it is present only with weight bearing. In general, static deformities are harder to control with prescription adjustments than dynamic deformities. However, prescription adjustments for dynamic deformities have a propensity to generate shear stresses when walking and thus are more prone to cause skin ulcers. Shoe

TABLE 15-2. FOOT PROBLEMS MANAGEABLE BY FOOTWEAR MODIFICATIONS

Problems (Examples)	Modifications	Comments
Foot inversion/eversion, heel varus/valgus, midfoot hyperpronation	Molded arch supports with or without wedges added to edges of the orthotics (or soles of the shoes)	When these problems are severe and have dynamic components, double upright braces (Klenzak) attached to the shoes may be required
Bony deformities (Spurs, bunions, depressed meta-tarsal heads, bunionettes)	Extra-depth inserts; relief areas of pressure concentration by filing-down, off-loading with pads and/or cutting out portions of the shoe	When bony deformities are not controlled with footwear modifications, surgical correction is indicated
Partial amputations (Toes, rays, transmetatarsal, midfoot, partial heel)	Fillers/spacers; usually constructed of "memory" foams such as polyethylene	Usually attached to a full foot insert Lamb's wool is an effective filler
Rocker bottom and/or hypermobile foot segments	Conforming inserts with rigid rocker bottom shoe soles typically 2 to 4 cm thick to equalize limb lengths	Thickness needed to compensate for collapses of foot and ankle bones and provide a rocker bottom platform
Proximal midfoot (Chopart and Boyd) **amputations**	Slipper-like inserts with fillers/spacers attached to them; often with cosmetic appearance to the fillers (e.g. simulated toes)	If inadequate to support foot, then high-topped shoes or orthotics that resemble a prosthesis devoid of the foot/ankle portion
Equinus contractures	Heel wedges for shoes or if mild, added to inserts inside the shoe	Stress concentrations occur on meta-tarsal heads; extreme precautions required for the neuropathic foot
Abduction/adduction deformities of the forefoot	If flexible, straight and reverse last shoes may control problem, especially in children	When uncontrollable, forefoot/midfoot fusions may be required

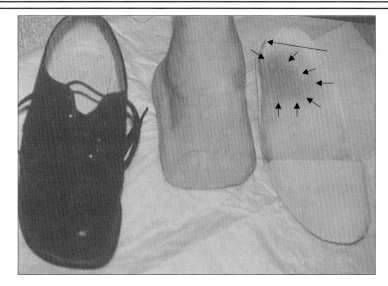

Legend: Extra-depth Plastazote® insert plus filler for missing forefoot added to an off-the-shelf diabetic shoe that has a large toe box. The filler prevents the shortened foot from sliding forward in the shoe when walking.

Note the slight ridge at the heel portion (long black arrow) of the insert. This helps stabilize the heel. Also, note the darkened spot on the heel portion of the insert. This "dirty" area confirms that the patient has been an active ambulator with the prescription protective footwear.

Figure 15-6. Custom prescription for a transmetatarsal amputation.

Clinical correlations:

A 34-year-old male developed an infected bursa over the lateral side of his right fifth metatarsal head due to walking on the side of his foot secondary to sensory and motor neuropathies from diabetes. Other comorbidities included obesity, post-phlebitic syndrome, coronary artery disease, and peripheral artery disease.

The bursa was debrided and the underlying bone of the fifth metatarsal head decompressed. The wound was slow to heal. Even with prescription protective footwear, callus reformed with walking activities over the operative site because of the fixed and dynamic components of the pervasive eversion posturing of the foot.

At this point a Klenzak (double upright brace attached to the shoe) was prescribed. This kept the foot plantigrade when standing and walking, allowing him to ambulate without developing a new wound.

Comment:

Whereas non-fixed dorsal and plantar deformities of the foot and ankle may be controlled with lifts and/or ankle orthoses, they are unable to control adequately marked rotation and angular deformities of the leg, foot and ankle.

modifications/adjustments are another provision of the Medicare Therapeutic Shoe bill for diabetic patients. In general, adding prescription modifications to off-the-shelf shoes triples the costs of the unmodified shoes.

Level 4 - Customized molded protective footwear: This is the fourth level in the hierarchy of footwear options and is especially suited for patients with multiple deformities that have dynamic as well as static components (Figure 15-7). These shoes, as the title implies, are custom molded to accommodate unique foot and ankle deformities. Common features of these shoes are their unattractive appearance, their high-topped lengths, and their asymmetry with the opposite shoe. Typically the deformities are unilateral and so severe that the footwear selections from the first three levels of the selection hierarchy are not able to protect (from new ulcerations) and maximize function of the foot and/or ankle. Examples include Boyd amputations (all the foot bones are removed

Clinical correlations:

A 60-year-old man with diabetes and severe peripheral artery disease developed a major slough on the plantar aspect of his foot. After revascularization and a microvascular free flap, the patient resumed community ambulation. However, with progression of his vascular disease and the development of new foot wounds, the patient eventually ended-up with a modified Boyd (preservations of the calcaneus sans the other foot bones) amputation.

High-topped, custom molded asymmetrical footwear with a shoe insert and filler for the missing portion of the foot allowed the patient to remain a limited community ambulator and gainfully employed. Eight years later, the patient died from causes unrelated to his foot condition.

Comment:

This scenario illustrates how compound deformities (i.e. fixed and static) may require several prescription footwear adjustments to control.

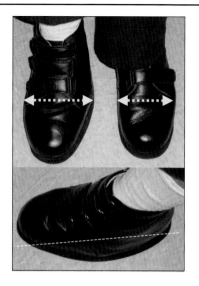
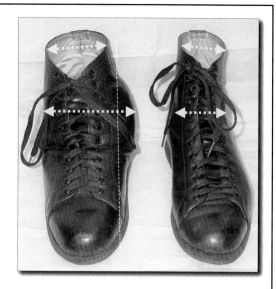

Legend: Custom molded shoes to manage major deformities of the feet and ankles. Note the asymmetry of the shoe lasts and upper portions. Regardless of the appearances of the shoes, the patients were thankful that these protective footwear devices allowed them to remain ambulatory and gainfully employed while not developing new wounds.

Figure 15-7. Custom molded protective footwear.

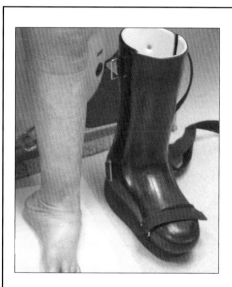
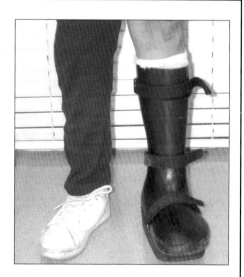

Legend: The CROW boot is at the apex of the protective footwear hierarchy. Features include a thick rocker bottom sole, a rigid posterior-plantar shell, an injected molded rubberized foam lining that conforms to the patient's foot/ankle deformity, a padded anterior splint that mates with the posterior shell, and Velcro® straps.

Figure 15-8. Charcot restraint orthotic walker (CROW boot).

except for the talus and calcaneus), rigid foot deformities where the majority of the foot bones have fused into a solid mass, and the splayed forefoot where the medial and lateral toes and rays are widely divergent. These shoes are two to three times more expensive than shoes from the previous level of the hierarchy. The costs of custom fabricated shoes and/or double upright braces attached to prescription shoes is in the $1,000 to $1,500 range or two to three times the costs of shoes with prescription adjustments.

CROW (Charcot Restraint Orthotic Walker) Boots: The CROW boot represents the ultimate in the hierarchy of prescription footwear. When multiple fixed and dynamic deformities are present in the foot and ankle, uncontrollable by other means and the leg is at risk of a below knee amputation because of them, a CROW boot is indicated (Figure 15-8). The CROW boot consists of a rigid posterior foot and leg shell that is filled with an injection molded rubberized foam material that conforms to the foot and ankle deformities. The patient "steps into" the posterior shell with the rubberized lining conforming exactly to the shape of the foot and leg. A padded anterior splint is placed over the front aspect of the foot and leg to "close" the boot and completely encircle the extremity. The anterior portion of the boot is held securely to the posterior shell with three Velcro® straps. With the uniform contact of the foam lining material, dynamic rotational problems between the foot and leg are controlled. With the elasticity of the lining material and the leeway the Velcro® straps provide in closing the CROW boot, leg swelling from fluid retention can be accommodated. The sole of the CROW boot has a rocker bottom shape to facilitate walking with its rigid construction.[7] Typically it is three to four centimeters thick so a thick-soled shoe may be needed on the other foot to equalize lower extremity lengths.

Indications for a CROW Boot - A CROW boot is usually not prescribed until other levels of the footwear hierarchy have been tried and found to be unsuccessful. However, with the most severe foot and ankle deformities such as those associated with severe deformities from Charcot arthropathy, a CROW boot becomes a first line defense to

> Usually the deformities that are found in conjunction with the Charcot arthropathy shorten the foot and ankle so much that the thick sole of the CROW boot equalizes the lower extremity lengths with regular thickness shoe soles on the other foot.

prevent new and recurrent foot wounds and maximize the patient's walking ability. Clinical judgment is required to make the decision. If the patient has little or no potential for ambulation, there is little indication to order a CROW boot. In this situation, the ambulation goal would be mobility with a wheelchair. If the deformity is controllable by cast wear and the cast makes it possible for the patient to do limited walking, a CROW boot is indicated. As with the other levels of the protective footwear hierarchy, the CROW boot may require adjustments and replacements with time and use as the foot shape changes and the device wears.

Considerations Re: CROW Boots - As desirable as the CROW boot is as a functional device for ambulation in patients with the severest of foot and ankle deformities, it has undesirable features. These include its appearance, weight, and contraindication for wear when any but the smallest wounds are present. CROW boots cost $1500 to $2000. Even when CROW boots are prescribed with the indications given in the previous paragraph, about one fourth of the patients do not use them. Reasons in addition to those mentioned above include worsening infirmities that may negate walking and development of new wounds. When sizable wounds are present and/or new wounds develop, then last resort surgical options such as complex foot reconstruction (Chapter 12) or lower limb amputation must be considered.

MAKING SENSE OF ORTHOTICS

Orthotic Considerations - In the previous section, orthotics were mentioned as a prescription item added to off-the-shelf footwear to control alignment of the feet and ankles. Simply stated, orthotics are devices that improve or straighten the alignment of body parts. They can be as simple as a heel pad added to a shoe or as complicated as a total control lower extremity brace. Orthotics play an important role in prescription footwear since deformities so frequently are a precursor to foot wounds and so many patients with feet at risk for wounds have deformities. The three largest user groups for orthotics are children with foot concerns articulated by their parents, athletes, and others who experience foot pain with activities and patients who have neurological impairments (especially patients with diabetes). Much confusion exists as to what orthotics do and when they are needed (Figure 15-9).[8] The consequences of this are over utilization, inappropriate applications and needless expenditures for these devices. The following information discusses seven misconceptions and/or fallacies pertaining to orthotics. The

> A good example of the effective use of an orthotic is in the situation of a shortened limb. The shortening will cause a person to limp and lean to the side when standing unless compensatory measures are done such as bending the opposite knee or the spine. This puts an extra strain on the muscles and joints controlling these body parts and likely becomes a source of pain.
>
> The easiest solution is to add a lift to the shoe of the shorter extremity to equalize the extremity lengths. This will correct the alignment and prevent the extra stresses and strains placed on the body parts used to compensate for the limb length discrepancy.
>
> Comment:
> This exemplifies the principle of using an orthotic. In the case of the foot at risk with deformities, the role of orthotics is to prevent wounds.

goals are twofold: to make sense of their use, and to delineate their indications for foot conditions at risk for wounds (Table 15-3). Indications for prescribing and using orthotics are different for those patients with risk factors for developing wounds (deformity, previous amputation, previous wound, peripheral artery disease, and/or neuropathy) versus those using orthotics to manage symptoms that are associated with walking and running.

Misconception/Fallacy 1 - A minimal discrepancy or deformity, for example mild flattening of the feet or tilting of the heels, never needs an orthotic.

Fact - The answer to this question is tricky. If the problem causes symptoms, for example pain, stiffness, soreness, swelling, etc. with activities or signs of irritation of the skin are observed at the deformity site, it should be managed with orthotics (or other off-loading techniques). The question is tricky because if the person can do the activity without symptoms, as is often the case in athletes or children, orthotics are not needed. However, if the foot is at risk for wound formation, everything possible

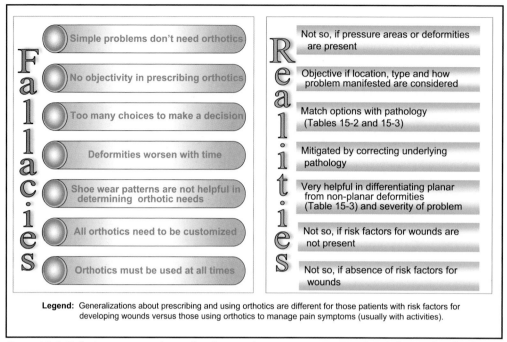

Legend: Generalizations about prescribing and using orthotics are different for those patients with risk factors for developing wounds versus those using orthotics to manage pain symptoms (usually with activities).

Figure 15-9. Fallacies versus realities of orthotic indications in patients with risk factors for developing wounds.

including orthotics (and other off-loading measures) should be done to prevent a wound from developing due to the multiplier effect of repetitive sub-threshold (i.e. below the severity to generate an acute ulceration, but enough to generate erythema, callus formation and/or pain) stresses.

Misconception/Fallacy 2 - There is little objectivity in deciding what situations require an orthotic.

> If a deformity, albeit minor, places extra work on muscles and joints or places extra stresses on the skin, problems from repetitive stresses, such as occurring with walking, have a multiplying effect.
>
> For example, a problem that requires a muscle to contract only 1/16th of an inch more than normal may have to move an extra 27 ½ feet with walking a mile (assuming a stride length of 12 inches) than muscles not having to work as hard during the mile walk. In the situation of contact pressures to the skin, 1/16th of an ounce more weight to the skin with each step subjects the skin to over 300 pounds of summated extra contact pressures over the deformity with the mile walk.

Fact - Objectivity in prescribing orthotics is afforded by pairing the patient's symptoms with the following signs:

- **Imbalances -** refer to alterations in muscle control that lead to abnormal posturing of joints. Some muscles may become overactive while others may be so weak that they cannot counteract the antagonist muscles' activities. Diabetes, nerve injuries/spinal cord injuries, strokes, Parkinsonism, and hereditary conditions are the most frequent causes of muscle imbalances. With time, contractures arise and joints become permanently deformed (next two paragraphs).

TABLE 15-3. FREQUENTLY OBSERVED FOOT DEFORMITIES AND THEIR ORTHOTIC MANAGEMENT

Problems	Type/How Manifested*	Orthotic Management
Location: Primarily the Forefoot		
Metatarsus adductus (In-toeing, adduction)	Planar/static with dynamic components	Straight or reverse last shoes Lateral heel +/- medial sole wedges; pronator pads (all of questionable benefit; usually improves spontaneously with time)
Metatarsus abductus (Out-toeing—abduction, "skew" foot))	Same as above (SAA)	Medial heel and/or lateral sole wedges; pronator pads (all questionably effective)
Toe deformities (Mallet, hammer, claw, angulated or rotatory)	Most are planar and static with dynamic components	Toe separators, lambs wool between toes, shoes with large toe boxes
Forefoot supination (Inversion)	Non-planar/static with dynamic components	Lateral forefoot wedges for inserts and or soles of shoes; if due to Charcot arthropathy, consider CROW (Charcot restraint orthotic walker) boot
Forefoot pronation (Eversion)	SAA	Medial forefoot and/or sole wedges
Location: Primarily the Midfoot (Arch portion of the foot)		
Flatfoot (Pes planus)	Planar/dynamic, but accentuated with loading	Arch supports; if asymptomatic, leave untreated
Hyperpronation (Usually with hindfoot valgus + flat feet)	SAA	Custom molded arch supports with medial heel wedges
Cavus foot (Abnormally high arches)	Planar/static	Custom molded arch supports supplemented with forefoot and heel pressure relief pads
Congenital vertical talus	SAA	Custom shoes; generally not manageable with footwear and orthotics; surgery usually required
Location: Primarily the Hindfoot (Heel portion of the foot) **and Ankle**		
Varus heel (Inward tilting, supination)	Non-planar/static	Lateral heel wedges; frequently in association with forefoot and midfoot supination management
Valgus heel (Outward tilting pronation)	SAA	Medial heel wedges; usually in conjunction with midfoot hyperpronation management
Equinus contracture	Planar, non-planar (with hindfoot varus/Static)	Heel lifts; Klenzak brace; management of heel varus; Frequently Achilles tendon lengthening required
Location: Combinations (Involvement of 2 or more foot and ankle components)		
Clubfoot (Heel varus, forefoot adduction + ankle equinus	Non-planar/static	Casting, Achilles tendon lengthening; custom orthotics as needed
Charcot arthropathy (Multiple presentations, see Chapter 12)	SAA	The hierarchy of prescription footwear; see Figures 15-2 through 15-8
"Zig-zag" (Planar deformities in 2 or more directions**)**	Planar/static	Custom molded shoes

Notes: * **Type** refers to plane of the foot; **plana**r indicates it is flat, while **non-planar** means it is tilted (e.g. varus vs valgus; pronation vs supination; inversion vs eversion, etc.)

How manifested refers to whether it is **Static,** that is the deformity is presented when the foot is unloaded or **Dynamic,** that is it occurs with loading, muscle contraction and/or walking.

- **Contractures** - arise in joints when imbalances persist or joints are positioned in the wrong position for sustained periods, such as with casting. Joint stiffness and decreased range of motion are findings associated with contractures. A joint contracture is defined when the loss of motion becomes fixed. For example, an equinus contracture from shortening of the Achilles (calf) tendon/muscle group. When this occurs, the ankle can no longer be brought to the neutral position.
- **Deformities** - are structural changes in the anatomy of the foot and ankle such as bunions, Charcot arthropathy, forefoot adductus, hindfoot varus, or depressed metatarsal heads (the precursor of forefoot mal perforans ulcers). Deformities arise from muscle imbalances as observed with clawing of toes, loss of ligament support, bony overgrowth from repetitive pressure/shearing stresses, and structural abnormalities of bone (e.g. spurs, malalignment after fractures, congenital anomalies, collapse associated with Charcot arthropathy, etc). Many deformities are amenable to management with orthotics as will be described in the third fallacy in this section.

When orthotic selection is addressed from these three perspectives, logical decisions become obvious. When sensation is absent, as is so frequently observed in patients with problem wounds, the decision for orthotic selection is made from the above signs. When these problems are not manageable by orthotics, then surgical interventions, many of which are minimally invasive and can be done in the office setting (Chapter 16), are needed. This is in contrast to athletes where pain symptoms are the indication for obtaining orthotics.

Misconception/Fallacy 3 - So many deformities can occur in the foot and/or ankle that it difficult to make decisions as to what orthotic is appropriate.

Fact - Although more than a dozen deformities may be ascribed to the foot, they can be readily understood if considered from the following elements (Table 15-3): 1) location (forefoot including toes, midfoot, hindfoot or combinations), 2) type (such as primarily a) planar—the foot remains flat such as with abduction, adduction and equinus) or b) non-planar—the normal flat surface of the foot is tilted as observed in hyperpronation-eversion-valgus or supination-inversion-varus deformities), and 3) how manifested

From the above information, some terms refer to specific locations while other terms overlap. Varus and valgus type deformities imply a single location such as the heel, forefoot or ankle. Pronation type deformities are generally ascribed to the midfoot. Often hindfoot valgus occurs in association with midfoot pronation. Abduction and adduction deformities are used to describe forefoot abnormalities. External and internal rotations refer to the foot position with respect to the leg. Supination, eversion and inversion are terms implying involvement of the entire foot.

Static manifestations refer to the deformity being present without loading. Dynamic deformities become apparent with muscle activity, loading and movement. In general dynamic deformities in non-neurologically impaired individuals do not require orthotics when they are present in the absence of pain. In contrast, dynamic deformities in the patients with neuropathies require interventions, initially with protective footwear, and if not successful, surgery. This is because this latter group of patients is prone to develop pressure ulcerations from their deformities with activity, but not recognize them until the wounds have already occurred.

(dynamic implies that the problem occurs with activity whereas static means the problem is fixed and present whether at rest or with activity). Each problem may be due to a single element or compound consisting of two or more of the above elements.

Misconception/Fallacy 4 - Foot deformities invariably worsen with time; hence, orthotics should be used as soon as a problem is recognized.

Fact - Judgment is essential for making decisions about when to prescribe orthotics. The majority of foot deformities in children such as in-toeing, flat feet and toe walking resolve spontaneously as the child matures. In the presence of neurological impairments (e.g. cerebral palsy, myelodysplasia, polio, etc.), spontaneous correction is not likely to occur. Orthotics and/or surgical interventions should be utilized early to prevent worsening deformities. For adults with asymptomatic, non-progressing deformities, orthotics are not indicated. For adults who develop new deformities such as hyperpronation of the midfoot (e.g. secondary to posterior tibial tendon dysfunction), especially those with risk factors for developing foot wounds, orthotics and protective footwear are indicated as soon as the problem is recognized. The goals are to prevent the deformity from progressing and/or the development of wounds that could require surgery in the future.

Misconception/Fallacy 5 - Shoe comfort and wear patterns are not reliable indicators of the need for orthotics

Fact - Shoe comfort and wear patterns provide important clues for decision making about orthotic selection. In the normal foot, shoe wear is first noted along the lateral edge of the heel and the center portion of the toe-ward end of the sole. As the shoe wears, the upper materials may stretch to accommodate a deformity, and in the absence of sensation, the patient may not complain of pain in the shoe as it is stretched out. Obviously, pressure areas are deforming the shoe and can evolve to ulcerations at the deformity site. If the shoe is uncomfortable, explanations are needed and proper adjustments made. Shoe wear patterns also provide helpful information. For example, if the upper, medial portion of the sole of the shoe has excessive wear, pronation (eversion) is usually the explanation. Excessive medial heel shoe wear indicates excessive hindfoot valgus. These problems need to be recognized and managed with orthotics if the patient has risk factors for developing foot and ankle wounds and/or the deformities are a source of pain.

Misconception/Fallacy 6 - If orthotics are indicated, they need to be customized.

Fact - Many conditions for which orthotics are indicated can be managed by simple corrections such as adding a padded insert, an off-the-shelf metatarsal pad, a heel pad, a toe separator, a donut pad or similar devices.[9] Many of the padded inserts have additional features such as padding to counteract pronation and gel inserts to provide extra heel or forefoot padding. The off-the-shelf devices usually cost a fraction of custom molded orthotics. If they relieve symptoms and off-load pressure areas, more costly customized orthotics are not indicated. Two guidelines are recommended for prescribing custom molded orthotics. First, in patients with normal foot sensation, they should be obtained after a trial of less expensive off-the-shelf versions have been tried, but the off-the-shelf choices provide only partial or no relief of symptoms. Second, in patients with sensory neuropathy and associated deformities, prescription orthotics and footwear are usually indicated even without a trial of off-the-shelf devices.

Lamb's wool is a very effective padding/off-loading device. It is used by ballet dancers to protect their toes en pointe (i.e. toe dancing) because it does not compress and concentrate forces as pressure is applied to it. Additionally, it does not lose its form and function from moisture. For these reasons, patients with pre-ulcerative lesions on their toes or in need of a filler for missing toe parts, can use lamb's wool as an effective, inexpensive toe separator or pressure distributor and/or filler in their shoes.

Like other fabric materials, it will become soiled with use and retain odors so the lambs wool padding must be changed on an as needed basis when these are observed.

Misconception/Fallacy 7 - If orthotics are obtained, they need to be utilized 100 percent of the time with footwear.

Fact - For patients with normal sensation, orthotics may only need to be used for repetitive stress activities such as running. Running activities multiply and replicate the stresses through the feet more than three times the person's body weight, somewhat analogous to driving a nail into a board. If symptoms are not noted with standing or walking, orthotics need not be used for these activities. In patients subject to foot or ankle ulcerations because of sensory neuropathy or other risk factors for wounds, the

Driving a nail into a board is a good analogy when considering what happens with repetitive multiplier forces. The hammer, merely resting on the nail, will not drive the nail into the board. However, with each strike, the force of the hammer head is multiplied many-fold (i.e. its kinetic energy), thereby driving the nail into the board.

Clinical correlations:

A 38-year-old healthy male began to experience unilateral left mid-calf pain during running activities. Typically, symptoms did not occur until five miles into a 7 to 10 mile run. Although concern was raised that the patient may have a chronic exertional compartment syndrome, examination demonstrated a hypermobile left forefoot and his symptoms were attributed to a chronic, overuse calf muscle strain with running activities.

The insertion of a quarter inch heel lift into his running shoes eliminated his pain symptoms with long runs. The lift was not used for regular walking activities.

Comment:

By reducing the excursion of the left calf muscles with the quarter inch heel lift, the summated repetitive forces to the calf muscle were substantially reduced over a seven mile run (1/4 inch less excursion with each step <> multiplied by the patients 180 pound body weight <> multiplied three-fold with stance phase loading <> times 2000 foot stance phase loadings—assuming a three foot running stride—for each mile <> times 7 miles summates to over a million foot pounds force reduction for the left calf muscles with the lift during the run).

orthotic is used to prevent a wound from occurring and consequently should be utilized with all standing and walking activity.

Prescribing Orthotics - In summary, the decision to prescribe orthotics should be based on the patient's complaints, the problems (e.g. muscle imbalances, contractures or deformities) found during the exam, and what is the most cost-effective way of managing it. For patients with normal sensation, many orthotic requirements can be met with off-the-shelf devices. Custom made orthotics should be prescribed by physicians familiar with the evaluation, management and prevention of foot and ankle problems and obtained through pedorthotists and podiatrists familiar with the options and available applications. In patients with neurological impairments, associated deformities, and the other risk factors for foot and ankle wound occurrence, custom prescribed orthotics and protective footwear are advised since this is the at risk group for developing problems.

MEDICARE THERAPEUTIC FOOTWEAR BENEFITS

The Therapeutic Shoe Bill - It is no coincidence that Medicare (Center for Medicare/Medicaid Services) provides funding for diabetic footwear. In 1993 the "Therapeutic Shoe Bill" benefit became a Medicare entitlement for diabetic patients.[10] This policy exemplifies the goals of preventive medicine. It provides a mechanism for diabetic patients with risk factors for developing foot wounds to obtain protective footwear. Most significantly, this benefit is proactive (in contrast to many of the other Medicare entitlements), providing a means to prevent a problem from occurring rather than the much more expensive alternative of treating it after it has already arisen. This entitlement provides tangible benefits with protective footwear rather than only education as in smoking prevention, need for exercise and weight reduction programs.

Stipulations of the Therapeutic Shoe Bill - The "Therapeutic Shoe Bill" benefit has several stipulations. First, the beneficiary must have Medicare Part-B (physician services) coverage. Second, the beneficiary must have a certifying statement from the prescribing physician that therapeutic footwear is required, which includes the following four statements.

- The patient has diabetes mellitus
- The patient has one or more of the following conditions involving either foot:
  - History of partial or complete amputation of the foot
  - History of previous foot ulceration
  - History of pre-ulcerative callus
  - Peripheral neuropathy with evidence of callus formation
  - Foot deformity
  - Poor circulation
- The prescribing physician is treating the patient under a comprehensive plan of care for his/her diabetes
- The patient needs special shoes (extra-depth or custom-molded shoes), inserts, or modifications because of his/her diabetes

Third, the prescription for therapeutic footwear is written by a qualified physician, someone knowledgeable about protective footwear and inserts. Finally, the therapeutic footwear must be supplied by a pedorthotist or other qualified individual or a retail store that sells footwear approved by the "Therapeutic Shoe Bill."

Replacements and Costs - Medicare therapeutic footwear benefits are provided yearly. Shoe benefits include one pair of off-the-shelf shoes and three pairs of multi-density inserts over a one-year period. If footwear higher up on the protective footwear hierarchy is required, two alternatives exist. 1) The beneficiary may receive one pair of off-the-shelf shoes with modifications (such as fillers, lifts, wedges, relief for pressure areas, etc.) plus two pair of multi-density inserts, or 2) One pair of custom-molded shoes plus two pairs of multi-density inserts each year. Eighty percent of the amount designated as the "allowable" will be reimbursed by Medicare. This amount will vary from state to state.

> This means that the patient or the patient's secondary insurance is responsible for paying the remaining 20 percent of the bill at the time the shoes and/or inserts are dispensed if the supplier accepts the Medicare assignment. If not, the patient needs to pay the supplier and submit the paper work directly to Medicare for reimbursement.

By the footwear/insert provider accepting the assignment, it is understood that the charges for the protective footwear will conform to what Medicare considers reasonable and customary.

Alternatives to the Therapeutic Shoe Bill - Although the Medicare "Therapeutic Shoe Bill" applies specifically to diabetic patients, do other alternatives exist for patients with "problem" wounds or risk factors for developing "problem" wounds who do not have Medicare Part-B benefits? The answer is a somewhat qualified yes. Many state Medicaid programs have provisions that parallel the Medicare guidelines. Private insurance companies may or may not have provisions for protective footwear. However, if the footwear is indicated, a "letter of petition" by the prescribing physician to the insur-

> Clinical correlations:
> A 25-year-old male metal worker sustains a crush injury to his left foot when a one thousand pound plate falls on his foot necessitating a modified (the lateral two rays removed to the level of the cuboid) transmetatarsal amputation.
> Although his insurance benefit provides a prosthesis for a below-knee amputation, they specifically exclude providing off-the-shelf shoes with modifications.
> A "letter of petition" was submitted to the insurance company explaining the necessity for protective footwear for the patient. The letter included three major arguments. First, without the prescribed protective footwear, the patient was at risk of developing new problems that could result in costly hospitalizations and an even higher-level amputation. Second, with the prescription footwear, there would be a high likelihood that the patient could return to his previous level of work without restrictions. Third, other insurance providers, including Medicare, have provisions to address this problem.
> With the "letter of petition," the request for protective footwear was approved for the patient.
>
> Comment:
> Insurance carriers are more likely to respond to out of network benefits, when the benefit is cost-beneficial, allows the patient to return to his/her usual and customary activities, and is a provision provided by Medicare or other third party carriers.

ance carrier describing the problem, the justification and the predicted cost-benefits for protective footwear is often sufficient to obtain reimbursement for the footwear. A third alternative is for the patient to pay for the protective footwear/inserts himself/herself. Charges for similar items often vary considerably from one supplier to another and/or discounts are given for paying cash. For non-wound prevention considerations, such as pain relief with running, the patient may have to pay for the custom orthotics "out of pocket." Finally, less costly alternatives such as using lambs wool for fillers and toe separators, off-the-shelf inserts, shoes with built-in pronation inserts, casts, etc. can be used as an interim measure when it is not possible to obtain custom protective footwear.

"DOS" AND "DON'TS" PERTAINING TO PROTECTIVE FOOTWEAR

A list of "dos" and "don'ts" that should be taught to patients with risk factors for foot wounds was previously presented (Chapter 13). As with prevention of skin and toenail problems (Chapter 14), several are pertinent to protective footwear. For this reason, those that apply to protective footwear are now repeated in tabulated form in this section:

- "Dos" with Respect to Protective Footwear
  - Wear appropriate footwear for your foot and ankle problems
  - Check shoes and orthotics frequently for signs of wear or poor fit

- "Don'ts" to Prevent New or Recurrent Foot Wounds
  - Don't walk barefooted (use protective footwear at all times when out of bed)
  - Don't assume a new pair of shoes, even if provided from a footwear prescription, will fit perfectly. "Break them in" slowly, initially wearing the shoes for only for a few minutes at a time and then removing them to inspect the skin for pressure areas or signs of rubbing
  - Don't wear inappropriate shoes for fashion reasons or because they feel comfortable (such as house shoes and slippers)

CONCLUSIONS

The selection of protective footwear is both an art and a science. The science is reflected by the wealth of information available about the components of footwear, the variety of choices available for protective footwear and orthotics, and the ability to confirm by examination and imaging studies what the structural problems are. The selection of protective footwear is also an art. Decisions have to be made as to what level of the protective footwear hierarchy is appropriate for the patient. Foot and ankle problems are frequently unique and require individual modifications for the shoe as foot problems change, so what is appropriate initially may require alterations in the future.

It is obvious that "if the shoe fits, don't always wear it." This has several implications. First, patients may prefer to wear their old, worn, deformed shoes because they feel so comfortable instead of their new or replacement footwear. Second, newly prescribed footwear often requires modifications to fit properly. The more complicated the problem, the more likely modifications will be required. In our experiences, about 50 percent of the footwear prescriptions we write require additional modifications by the pedorthotist or certified footwear provider as the patient begins to use the footwear.

Third, there may be delays in the patient's appreciation of new foot and ankle problems with their new footwear due to sensory neuropathy. Fourth, patients with risk factors for developing foot and ankle wounds often have on-going, progressively worsening deformities, peripheral artery disease and neuropathy. The changes associated with these may require expedient revisions in footwear and/or surgical interventions.

Listen to the patients and hear what they like about their old shoes and what they do not like about their new protective footwear. Then pair this information with the science that is needed to meet their prescription footwear needs. As stated previously, protective footwear is the second line of defense (after skin and toenail care) for preventing problems in patients with risk factors for foot and ankle wound formation. If protective footwear is appropriately prescribed and the patient is instructed in the philosophy behind the quotation "if the shoe fits, don't always wear it," new wound problems can usually be prevented. When protective footwear cannot accomplish these goals, then surgery, the first line of offense, may be required (Chapter 16).

QUESTIONS

1. What are the major components of shoes?

2. What are the advantages and disadvantages of different sock compositions?

3. What are the important considerations for prescribing protective footwear?

4. What are the main five levels or selection choices for protective footwear?

5. When are CROW (Charcot Restraint Orthotic Walker) Boots indicated?

6. What do orthotics do and when are they needed?

7. Are shoe comfort and wear patterns reliable indicators of the need for orthotics?

8. What provisions must be met to receive benefits from Medicare's Therapeutic Shoe Bill?

9. What must be considered with the maxim "If the shoe fits, don't always wear it"?

REFERENCES

1. Cavanagh PR, Owings TM. Nonsurgical strategies for healing and preventing recurrence of diabetic foot ulcers. Foot Ankle Clin, 2006; 11(4):735-743

2. Strauss MB, Miller SS. Diabetic Foot Problems: Keys to effective, aggressive prevention. Consultant. 2007; March:245-25

3. Sugarman JR, Reiber GE, Baumgardner G, et al. Use of the therapeutic footwear benefit among diabetic Medicare beneficiaries in three states. Diabetes Care 1998; 21:777-781

4. Wooldridge J, Moreno L. Evaluation of the costs to Medicare of covering therapeutic shoes for diabetic patients. Diabetes Care 1994; 17:541-547

5. Paton J, Jones RB, Stenhouse E, Bruce G. The physical characteristics of materials used in the manufacture of orthoses for patients with diabetes. Foot Ankle Int, 2007; 28(10):1057-1063

6. Hastings MK, Mueller MJ, Pilgram TK, et al. Effect of metatarsal pad placement on plantar pressure in people with diabetes mellitus and peripheral neuropathy. Foot Ankle Int. 2007; 28(1):84-88

7. Brown D, Wertsch JJ, Harris GF, et al. Effect of rocker soles on plantar pressures. Arch Phys Med Rehabil. 2004; 85(1):81-86

8. Janisse DJ, Janisse E. Shoe modification and the use of orthoses in the treatment of and ankle pathology. J Am Acad Orthop Surg. 2008; 16(3):152-158

9. Groner C. Orthosis Symbiosis: Clinicians are finding a middle ground in the debate over custom versus prefab foot orthoses. BioMechanics 2005, 12(5):22-33

10. Janissee DJ. The Therapeutic Shoe Bill: Medicare coverage for prescription footwear for diabetic patients. Foot Ankle Int. 2005; 26(1):42-45

CHAPTER

16

MINIMALLY INVASIVE PROACTIVE SURGERIES

CHAPTER SIXTEEN OVERVIEW

INTRODUCTION 447

CALLUSES, CRUSTS, AND BLISTERS 449

TOE DEFORMITIES 456

MALPERFORANS ULCERS OF THE FOREFOOT 463

SURGICAL WOUND MANAGEMENT 466

CONCLUSIONS 477

QUESTIONS 480

REFERENCES 481

"An ounce of protection...a stitch in time."

INTRODUCTION

The First Line of Offense - Proactive surgeries are the first line of offense in patients that have surgically correctable problems in association with risk factors (e.g. deformities, peripheral artery disease, history of a previous wound, prior amputation, and/or neuropathy) for developing wounds (Figure 16-1).[1] It is an offensive strategy because it represents "an assault" on a problem before it has reached the point where a serious wound develops, and urgent, often major ablative surgery becomes necessary. In other words, most proactive surgeries are done to correct deformities, muscle imbalances, or minor wounds before they evolve into serious wounds. Fortunately, many of the proactive surgeries can be done with minimally invasive surgical techniques that are appropriate for the office setting. There are many advantages for doing proactive, minimally invasive surgeries, especially in patients who have risk factors for developing wounds. These include:

- Minimal skin trauma with percutaneous techniques (e.g. for tendon releases and scoring bone for a controlled osteoclasis/fracture)
- Minimal trauma to tissues with decisive incisions to the wound base negating extensive dissection and forceful retraction of tissues
- Negligible blood loss that almost always obviates the need for a tourniquet or the requirement to discontinue the use of anticoagulants

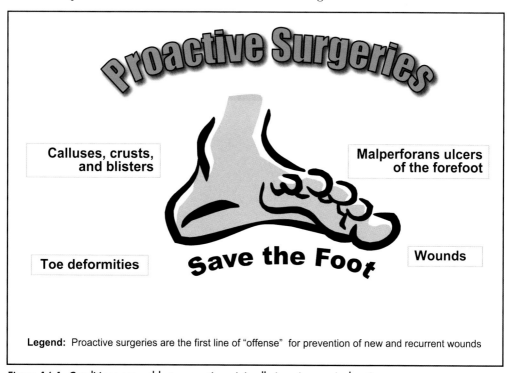

Legend: Proactive surgeries are the first line of "offense" for prevention of new and recurrent wounds

Figure 16-1. Conditions amenable to proactive minimally invasive surgical options.

- Brief operative times are a convenience to the patient and a boon to the operating surgeon; when done in the office setting, they a take a fraction of the time that is needed to do them in the operating room
- Decreased likelihood for post-operative complications in patients with high risks for developing complications
- Minimal post-operative morbidity; in the majority of situations, patients resume their pre-operative level of activity the day after surgery
- Substantial cost-benefits, especially if the procedure is done in the office setting

No group of surgical procedures is so appropriate for and better exemplifies the MIS/KISS (Minimal Invasive Surgery/Keep It Simple and Speedy) principle than the proactive surgeries used to prevent serious foot and ankle wound problems.

Importance of MIS/KISS Interventions - Although minimally invasive surgical techniques for shoulders, knees, and hips receive much attention, such techniques for toe, foot, and leg problems are almost never mentioned in instructional courses, texts, or journal articles. Ironically, minimally invasive surgeries for the foot and ankle are probably of even greater relative importance than those at other sites. This is because minimally invasive surgeries may be the only option to manage a problem in an impaired or severely compromised host (Chapter 11) with reasonable expectations for healing. This contrasts to doing minimally invasive surgeries at other sites where open surgical techniques are an alternative and/or be a back up if the MIS techniques are not effective. Problems such as peripheral artery disease, poor skin quality, pre-existing wounds, or combinations of these result in high risks for healing complications in the patient where proactive MIS/KISS management are most appropriate. This is especially a concern when standard surgical procedures are used for patients with these comorbidities. Minimally invasive surgical techniques can be the "great equalizer" in such situations. These techniques make it possible to achieve satisfactory outcomes even with coexisting serious comorbidities and where other approaches to surgery would generate unacceptably high risks for complications and/or failures.[2]

The Main Reasons Wounds Fail to Heal - The three main reasons for non-healing wounds (deformity, hypoxia, and infection) were discussed previously (Chapter 7, 11, and 12). Whereas the majority of proactive minimally invasive surgeries are done because of deformities, wound hypoxia secondary to ischemia is usually the most likely to accompany a problem present in this group of patients. If the deformity problem has evolved to a wound, colonization of the wound base, likely with multiple drug resistant organisms in the compromised host, adds additional challenges for wound healing. Typically, an impending wound site, due to an underlying deformity, progresses with time and as activity is continued. Hence, proactive minimally invasive surgeries should be done at the insipient stage of the problem rather than waiting until there are no other alternatives.[3] By the time the wound has reached the "no alternative stage," minimally invasive surgeries may no longer be adequate to manage the problem. In the presence of comorbidities, especially hypoxia and infection, wound healing may not occur with surgeries other than those that are minimally invasive. This concept cannot be more succinctly expressed than in the adage, "A stitch in time will save nine."

Justification of Repetition - Many of the procedures discussed in this chapter were mentioned or described in Chapters 7, 11, and 12. We justify this, as in other chapters in Part V that contain information that was introduced in earlier chapters, as follows: First, this like the other chapters in Part V is designed to "stand alone"– the information contained in this chapter is complete enough that reference to previous chapters in this text is not needed. Second, the surgical procedures in this chapter are described from a proactive perspective, that of non-emergency surgeries that will prevent more serious wound problems in the future. This contrasts with Chapter 7, where the procedures need to be done on an urgent basis for "problem" wounds and Chapters 11 and 12, where the surgeries usually need to be done on an emergency basis because of limb threatening conditions. Finally, with only a few exceptions, almost all the proactive surgeries described in this section can be done in a clean office room or clinic setting.

CALLUSES, CRUSTS, AND BLISTERS

Development of Calluses - Calluses develop because of chronic, repetitive, sub-threshold pressure and/or shear stresses over bony prominences. They are also observed to form around ulcerations (usually with underlying infected tissues), chronic wounds, or combinations of these. Callus formation is an inherent reactive response of the skin characterized by keratinization (development of a horny layer) of the epithelium when subjected to the above stresses. Keratin is a protein product that forms the intermediate filaments in epithelial cells. There are at least 20 different types of keratin that are identified by their molecular weights. This gives calluses many characteristics such as dry

> The exuberant callus formation that develops around chronic wounds is often much greater and faster to reappear after debridements than would be expected from pure repetitive (especially if site is off-loaded or padded with protective footwear) pressure or shear stresses.
> Chronic wound and/or persistent infection may alter gene expression and increase the development of exuberant, recurrent, callus formation.[4]

and firm, corn-like, waxy, papillated, pebbled, soft, clear, blood-stained, and moist/macerated. When dry and firm, callus is usually benign and serves as a protective mechanism to prevent ulcer formation over bony prominences. When the stresses are greater than the skin's ability to resolve them gradually with callus formation or the calluses become so thick that they act as a deformity themselves, wounds then develop.

Etiology of Calluses - The first question that needs to be asked when a callus occurs is, "What is its etiology?" (Figure 16-2). The first answer is an underlying bony prominence or deformity resulting in vulnerable skin being interposed between "a rock and a hard place." The "rock" is represented by the deformity, and "the hard place" is represented by the point of contact from the shoe or underlying support structure such as a bed or wheelchair. The second answer is the occurrence of shear stresses with repetitive activities such as walking. Factors in addition to pressure and shear are often found to be associated with callus formation and make the callus lesions especially subject to evolving into wounds. These include:

- Malnutrition
- The other risk factors, in addition to deformity, that predispose patients to wounds including peripheral artery disease, previous amputation, previous wounds, and sensory neuropathy
- Age-related atrophic changes of the skin and subcutaneous tissues
- Loss of skin elasticity and subcutaneous padding associated with scar formation from wound healing, glycosylation, cigarette smoking, collagen vascular diseases, etc.

- Motor neuropathies that cause contractures and other anatomical changes, such as migration of fat pads from under metatarsal heads

All these predispositions have been addressed in preceding chapters.

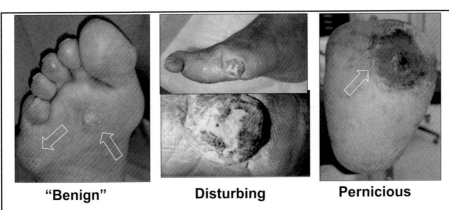

"Benign"   **Disturbing**   **Pernicious**

Legend: Calluses appear in a variety of forms, and all can have worrisome consequences and indicate underlying problems. Consider the following:

"Benign": These seemingly innocent calluses under the second and fifth metatarsal heads are the body's responses to increased pressure under the these structures. This is the first stage in malperforans ulcer formation. Notice the clawed toes with the "hidden (flexor) crease" signs which contribute to the problem.

Disturbing: The thick hyperkeratosis is a consequence of shear and pressure stresses over the end of the partial ray resection. If moisture gets under the callus, bacteria will multiply leading to an infection.

Pernicious: Pressure concentrations from the rocker bottom foot deformity of the midfoot amputation has led to a massive callus. The central portion (red arrow) is soft and necrotic tissue tracts to bone.

Figure 16-2. An array of hyperkeratotic (callus) lesions and their concerns.

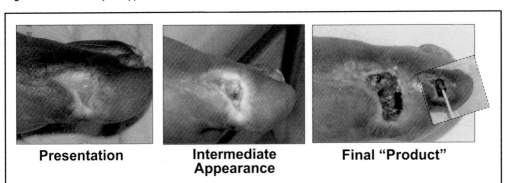

Presentation   **Intermediate Appearance**   **Final "Product"**

Legend: Relatively "benign" appearing ulceration covered with a biofilm on medial aspect of left great toe. The underlying deformity was a bone spur on the medial side of the base of the proximal phalanx.

Presentation- Both firm and soft calluses surround the ulceration. The surrounding skin does not appear erythematous or indurated, suggesting the underlying bony deformity is not infected.

Intermediate Appearance- Notice the rim of soft (white) callus around the periphery of the ulcer that came into view with debridement of the firm callus. Most of the biofilm has been removed from the ulcer base. The moist callus is undesirable because it provides an environment for bacterial proliferation.

Final Product- The moist callus has been "shaved" down to an underlying rim of healthy, pink skin surrounding the ulcer. The ulcer base has been debrided to the subcutaneous tissue level. This eliminates the bioburden and results in a healthy appearing vascular based wound. Note the thin black crusts on the ulcer base as a consequence of using silver nitrate (insert photo) to cauterize bleeding.

Figure 16-3. Debridement of peripheral callus around a toe wound.

Management of Calluses - Calluses should be managed in a two-step fashion. The first step is debridement (paring) of the callus, an in-office procedure (Figure 16-3).[5] A single use, sterile disposable scalpel with a large flat blade (#10 or #21) is recommended. The flat blade facilitates paring the callus parallel to the underlying skin and avoiding cutting into the skin. This works well for dry, firm calluses. Management of moist, papillated, pebbled, and macerated calluses is more problematic (Figure 16-4). These types of calluses usually indicate that there is an infection focus in the underlying tissues such as bursa or the bone. A forceps in addition to the scalpel will facilitate debriding these types of calluses. The moist callus should be pared down to the thinnest possible layer and flat with the adjacent healthy skin. The lowest layer of the epidermis should not be violated. However, as often happens, the bases of these problematic calluses are uneven and punctate sites of bleeding occur. Usually, the bleeding can be easily controlled by cauterization with a silver nitrate tipped applicator. If not, a tightly wrapped compression dressing held in place for ten to 15 minutes, then a dry gauze padded dressing will usually suffice. Even if the patient is anticoagulated, callus debridement can be done without excessive bleeding using these techniques. Removal of biofilms and fibrous membranes in the wound base by sharp dissection or curette should be done in association with debridement of the peripheral callus around the wound base.

> Moist and papillated calluses around superficial ulcerations, although very suggestive of an underlying chronic infection focus, are not an absolute indication for surgical removal. These problems can often be adequately managed with biweekly or monthly debridements, as discussed in the "living with a chronic stable wound" section (Chapter 11). If the wound site were to be eradicated with surgery, the consequence could be a mechanically unsound foot or an amputation.

Off-loading of Calluses - The second step in callus management is off-loading the area of pressure concentration and elimination of shear stresses with prescription protective footwear (Chapter 15). This may require relieving the areas of pressure contact in the shoe, incorporating fillers to prevent shear after partial amputations, use of donut-shaped pads, incorporation of gel pads, or combinations of these. When wounds that require debridement of callus are in other locations, for example the leg (Figure 16-4), elastic compression devices to control edema are an essential component of the management.

Surgical Management of Calluses - When the above measures are not successful in controlling the callus formation or the tissue under the callus begins to ulcerate, surgical management, usually in the operating room, becomes necessary. The generic surgical procedure for this is excision of the ulcer and debridement of the underlying tissue (abbreviated for convenience EUD where E = Exploration, U = Ulcer and D = Debridement). The type of problem and where it lies determines the approach to the wound site and the depth of debridement. The depth assessment (i.e. skin or subcutaneous tissue, muscle or tendon and bone or joint) of the **Wound Score** (Chapter 5) provides a useful guideline for determining and documenting the depth of the EUD. Often the depth of the debridement is superficial, such as done when a hypertrophic bursa lies directly over a bony prominence or cicatrix. If surgery is performed, the underlying bony deformity (and its overlying bursa) should be eliminated even if the bone is not infected.

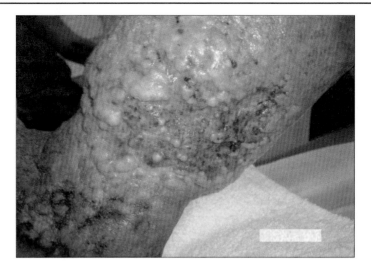

Legend: This "end-stage" (i.e. leg amputation is an option) wound began as a venous stasis ulcer. Note the mammillated appearance of skin surrounding the wound and the biofilm covering the wound base. These findings are consistent with underlying infected cicatrix and micro abscesses.

Debridement of the irregular papillated projections, some covered with moist callous, and the biofilm will improve the hygiene of the wound. Bleeding is controlled with silver nitrate cautery and a compression dressing. In order to obtain an optimal outcome, edema reduction of the leg using elastic compression devices is required.

Figure 16-4. Metaplasia of callus around a chronically invested venous stasis ulcer.

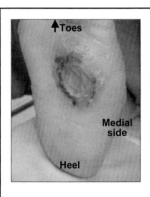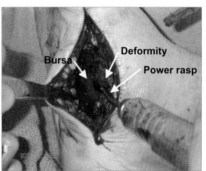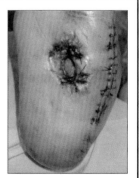

Legend: With a medial approach to the deformity, the plantar ulceration wound does not need to be enlarged to provide access for debridement.

After removing the infected bursa under the ulcer, the round shape of the ulcer is converted to an ovoid and the toe-ward and heel-ward portions of the wound approximated with non-absorbable sutures. This immediately reduced the surface area of the plantar wound by 75 percent.

Because the medial side incision that provided access to the deformity is in a less vulnerable area for healing problems than the plantar wound (which would have to be enlarged to expose the deformity), primary healing of the medial exploratory incision is anticipated regardless of its length.

Figure 16-5. Medial approach to debridement of a bony plantar deformity.

Surgical management of plantar ulcers and their underlying bony deformities are prone to dehisce and persist as chronic non-healing wounds. This is especially the situation when excision of the ulcer and debridement of the underlying bone are done directly from a plantar approach.

To avoid this problem, the deformity should be approached from the lateral or medial side of the foot through an incision long enough to expose the deformity (Figure 16-5). Once access is obtained, the deformity is removed with ronguer, osteotome and/or use of a power rasp. The plantar wound, usually round, is converted to an ovoid shape, the underlying bursa debrided and then the ovoid wound partially approximated with non-absorbable sutures.

Although this approach is not always successful in immediately eliminating the plantar wound, slow progressive healing is observed with removal of the deformity and the infected bursa. Often, periodic debridements of marginal callus and thin biofilms in the wound base are required. If there is concern that the bony deformity contains osteomyelitis, the middle third of the medial or lateral incision to approach the deformity is left open to heal by secondary infection with accompanying wound care (wicking using gauze moistened with normal saline, acetic acid solution or Dakin's solution) and antibiotics.

When the ulceration is to the bone and joint level, osteomyelitis is usually a consequence. Induration around the ulcer margins and a papillary appearance of the callus around the wound margins are indicators of underlying osteomyelitis.

Blister Formation - Acute super-threshold pressure and shear stresses lead to frank disruption of the skin with blisters and ulceration (Figure 16-6). The blister signifies superficial skin involvement, whereas an ulceration indicates full thickness damage of the skin to the subcutaneous or deeper level. Blisters are typically filled with serous fluid. If the injury is severe enough or the patient has a propensity for bleeding, the blister can be filled with blood. The worst situation occurs when the serous fluid becomes infected, resulting in a purulent material filled blister. Although some recommend allowing the blister to rupture and decompress spontaneously, the better choice is to unroof the blister with sterile instruments such as scalpel or scissors and forceps, trim all non-adherent skin and then use an antibiotic impregnated gauze or silver-containing cream to cover the wound base (Table 16-1).[6]

Removal of blisters of second degree burns may interfere with epidermal growth, fibroblast migration, and collagen synthesis as well as increase the likelihood of bacterial colonization of the blister base.[7-9]

Usually the blister base normalizes within a few days with daily cleansing and dressing changes.

Management of Crusts - Of the three problems discussed above: calluses, blisters and crusts, the latter is the least problematic (Figure 16-6). Most frequently, crusts arise from desiccation of serum oozing from the wound or incision line. Usually they are dry, firm and clear. If mixed with blood they may become hemosiderin stained. Eschars are thin crusts that cover wounds. They may arise from desiccation of overlying necrotic

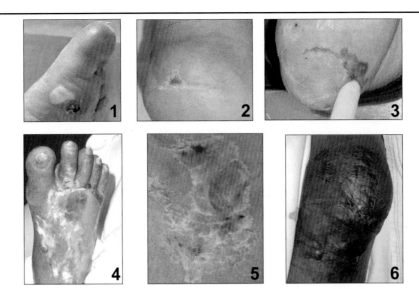

Legend: 1. Small forefoot serous-filled blister from shoe pressure 2. Benign serous crust from minute dehiscence of heel incision 3. Shear-induced blood blister from heel motion in shoe 4. Pus-filled blister secondary to burn wound in a diabetic foot 5. Thin serous crust over and surrounding a small plantar foot ulcer 6. Worrisome appearing blood filled blisters over knee from too tight of wrap in patient on anticoagulants. All (except perhaps the serous crust i.e. #2) should be managed with debridement, then appropriate dressings.

Figure 16-6. Crusts and blisters from minor considerations to major concerns.

TABLE 16-1. UNROOFING VERSUS NOT DISTURBING (I.E. "TO POP" OR "NOT TO POP") BLISTERS WITH SPECIFIC REFERENCES TO BURN BLISTERS[5-8]

Inflammation and Infection	Healing	Patient Comfort (Mobility)	Aesthetics
Advantages of Unroofing & Debriding Blistered Skin			
Inflammatory mediators increase capillary permeability, size of blister and pressure on surrounding tissue; leads to ischemia and deepening of the wound Prostaglandins, thromboxanes and free radicals in blister fluid impair the microcirculation Immunosuppressive action of fluid leads to lymphocyte repression, decreased phagocytosis, and decreased oposonization (for Pseudomonas). Some studies show systemic immune compromise Non-viable tissue in wounds are a medium for bacteria; (intact blisters have lower colony counts—see below) Colonization (versus infection) may be advantageous for floral balance and wound debridement.	Improves moisture balance; may have growth-promoting benefits Avoids maceration of partial thickness epithelial blister bases Augments healing	Helps patient return to activity earlier Better to remove blistered skin in a controlled environment than allowing them to rupture spontaneously Allows application of temporary skin substitutes for comfort, moisturization and protection Eliminates discomfort that is associated with pressure or traction on large blisters	Cytokines in blister fluid (e.g. TGF-β) may contribute to increased contraction, pigment changes and hypertrophic scarring Bullae are unattractive and may give the impression that mysterious illnesses are the cause
Disadvantages of Debriding Blistered Skin			
Desiccation of unroofed blister base may allow conversion of the wound to a full thickness slough Bacterial colonization highest in exposed wounds, intermediate in aspirated blisters and least in intact blisters[7]	Desiccated blister base interferes with epidermal migration Fibroblast and collagen synthesis stimulated by blister fluid[8] Keratinocyte growth stimulated by blister fluid[5]	Blisters offer comfort over exposed nerve endings	

KEY: TGF-β = Transforming growth factor-Beta

skin, fibrinous membranes, serum (i.e. crusts), or blood coagulums. As long as they remain firm and dry, they act as a biological dressing—i.e. "nature's own Band-Aid®." Of the hierarchy of coverage/closure techniques (Chapters 7 and 11), epithelialization under a crust or thin eschar is the least metabolic demanding of any technique and may be the best alternative in the patient with severe peripheral artery disease. Consequently, a dichotomous approach is recommended for managing crusts and eschars. When dry and firm, they should remain as a biological dressing for wound coverage with the margins regularly trimmed to allow for wound contraction and epithelialization at the margins of the skin to occur. When loose and/or partially separated from the underlying tissues, they should be debrided to prevent moisture accumulation and bacterial proliferation under the crust (Figure 16-7).

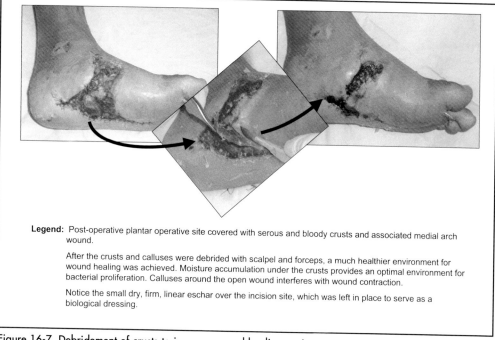

Legend: Post-operative plantar operative site covered with serous and bloody crusts and associated medial arch wound.

After the crusts and calluses were debrided with scalpel and forceps, a much healthier environment for wound healing was achieved. Moisture accumulation under the crusts provides an optimal environment for bacterial proliferation. Calluses around the open wound interferes with wound contraction.

Notice the small dry, firm, linear eschar over the incision site, which was left in place to serve as a biological dressing.

Figure 16-7. Debridement of crusts to improve wound healing environment.

Reimbursements for Debridements - For reimbursement purposes using the Medicare RB/RVS (Resource-Based/ Relative Value System) guidelines, only the depth of the debridement is considered, as has been tabulated previously (Table 7-3). For blisters and calluses, this equates to a partial or full thickness depth and is independent of the surface area of the debridement. If the ulcer base is debrided in conjunction with the callus or crust debridement, then the depth is appropriately documented as subcutaneous level. The 2009 reimbursement rates from the Southern California region, for example, range from \$47.91 for a partial skin thickness debridement to \$376.64 for debridement to the bone level. In addition, debridements should be documented by the sophistication of the instruments (Table 7-4) used and the size of the wound (size assessment of the **Wound Score**) with operative reports generated, especially for the deeper depth wounds. Most debridements for "problem" wounds meet the MIS/KISS (Minimal Invasive Surgery, Keep It Simple and Speedy) criteria and can be performed expediently in the office setting. When an EUD procedure requires the equipment avail-

Obviously in terms of efficiency and cost-effectiveness, it behooves the surgeon to perform these procedures in the office setting since reimbursements are the same for the surgeon. The costs for bringing the patient to the operating room for even a same day surgery for the procedure would be ten to fifteen times greater than doing the procedure in the office setting.

Time considerations are likewise illuminating. Even though the actual time to do the surgery will be similar, preparation time, patient movement, documentation, order writing, and travel time will require four to six times more of the physician's time than doing the procedure in the office setting.

able in an operating room (i.e. power instruments, suction, cautery, intra-operative x-rays, etc.) because of its size, depth, or location, reimbursements are still based on the RB/RVS depth criteria.

TOE DEFORMITIES

Challenges of Toe Deformities - Toe deformities are paradoxical. Frequently, they are overlooked or intentionally disregarded until a problem arises. Conversely, they usually are so obvious and the pathomechanics so easy to appreciate that is hard to understand why proactive measures are not done as soon as a problem is recognized. Any patient with one or more risk factors (deformity, peripheral vascular disease, history of previous foot wound, previous amputation or neuropathy) for wound development who has toe deformities should have the toe problems managed with minimally invasive surgical techniques. Ten or more toe deformities can lead to wounds (Table 16-2). Toe deformities may arise from a variety of causes with neuropathy leading to muscle imbalances and contractures, trauma and congenital anomalies being the most frequent etiologies. After a toe deformity develops, factors that contribute to evolution of toe problems include footwear choices, muscle imbalances, toe joint contractures, toenail disease, skin health, and activity.

Management of Toe Deformities - Once the etiology of the toe deformity is ascertained, management usually is obvious. In most situations, resolution of the problem is possible with minimally invasive surgical techniques. For many of the problems, especially when abnormal muscle and tendon activity cause clawing of the toes, percutaneous tenotomies are effective. A percutaneous tenotomy is the quintessence of a minimally invasive prophylactic foot surgery (Figure 16-8).[10] The stepwise procedure is as follows:

1. Selection of the site. For the extensor tendon, select a site on the dorsum of the foot proximal to the metatarsophalangeal joint—preferably where the tendon is most prominent, either by palpation or direct observation. For the flexor tendon, select a site at about the level of the metatarsal head.

2. If anesthesia is required (this step can be omitted in patients with profound sensory neuropathy), after cleaning the skin with an alcohol swab, instill about 2-5 cc of 1% lidocaine subcutaneously just proximal to the tenotomy site.

TABLE 16-2. TOE DEFORMITIES AND THEIR POTENTIAL WOUND PROBLEMS

Deformity	Description	Pathomechanics (Etiology)	Wound Concerns
Mallet toe	Flexion contracture at the distal interphalangeal joint	Overactivity of the flexor digitorum longus muscles	Ulcerations at the toe tip and over apices of the IP joint; toenail injury
Hammer toe	Flexion contracture at the proximal IP joint	Overactivity of the flexor digitorum brevis muscles and loss of toe intrinsic muscles	Same as above
Combination hammer and mallet toe*	Flexion contracture at both the IP joint levels	Combinations of the mallet and hammer toe etiologies	Same as above plus "kissing" lesions between phalanges
Dorsiflexed toe	Hyperextension posturing of toe at the metatarsal-phalangeal joint level	Overactivity of the long extensor tendons to the toe	Nail matrix and dorsal distal phalanx wounds from pressure contact with the toe box of the shoe
Claw toe	Hyperextension contracture at the MTP joint and flexion contractures at the PIP and DIP joints	Loss of toe intrinsic muscle function plus over activity of toe flexor and extensor muscles. MT heads displaced plantarward	Wounds over IP joints and tips of toes; malperforans ulcers under metatarsal heads from metatarsal head displacements
Angulated toe	Toe deviated in abduction or adduction from their axial alignment with the MT	Disruption of tendon pulley and/or forefoot malalignment; also post-traumatic, shoe wear, or congenital causes	"Kissing" wounds with adjacent toes; Pressure sores on medial aspect of hallux or lateral aspect of little toe from contact with the shoe toe box
Curved toe (Clinodactyly)	Bent toes at the IP joint level	Disruption of collateral ligaments; other causes as for angulated toes	Same as above for angulated toes
Rotated toe	Pronation (internal rotation) or supination (external rotation)	Mechanical problems in foot especially in association with hallux valgus or little toe varus; often secondary to inappropriate footwear or congenital	Same as above
Hypertrophic condyles and juxta-articular spurs	Bony deformity at the IP joint levels	Congenital; osteoarthritis; abnormal toe mechanics from toe malalignments or repetitive pressure stresses	Same as above
Combination deformities	Two more of the above such as bunion + hallux valgus + hyperpronation	Combinations of the above pathomechanics, footwear, or congenital causes	Wounds over IP joints and tips of toes; malperforans ulcers under metatarsal heads from metatarsal head displacements

Note: *Since the hallux has only a single interphalangeal joint, a flexion deformity at this level may be named either a hammer or a mallet toe

Abbreviations: DIP = Distal interphalangeal, **IP** = Interphalangeal, **MT** = Metatarsal, **MTP** = Metatarsalphalangeal, **PIP** = Proximal interphalangeal

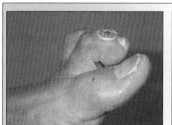 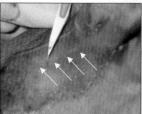 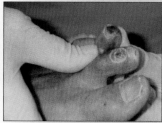

| Hyperextended second and third toes at the metatarsalphalangeal joint with associated flexion contractures at the interphalangeal (IP) joints | Extensor tendon of second toe visible (at tips of arrows) in subcutaneous tissue of distal forefoot | Manipulation of the contracted second and third toes into a straight position |

Note pre-ulcerative callous over the distal IP joint of the 2nd toe

Legend: In-office management of clawed toes can be done with minimally invasive surgery. With a #11 scalpel blade, the tendon can be released with a two to three mm incision (see text). Typically, no closure is required for the small incision, and bleeding is easily controlled with a few minutes of direct compression (even if the patient is on anticoagulants). After this "Keep It Simple and Speedy" in-office procedure, the patient is able to leave the office as he/she walked in.

Figure 16-8. Release of extensor tendon to manage hyperextension deformity of toes.

3. Prep the skin. Usually a 2-½ cm by 2-½ cm area around the intended incision site is sufficient using Betadine® or a similar disinfectant—three swabbings are recommended.

4. Tauten the tendon. Have the patient forcefully dorsiflex or plantarflex the toe in the direction of the action of the tendon to be cut. Then the surgeon or an assistant places counter pressure at the distal portion of the toe in the opposite direction.

5. Insert a #11 scalpel blade through a two to three mm incision so the tip is deep to the tendon (for the flexor tendon this may to the depth of the metatarsal head).

6. Sweep the tip of the scalpel blade across the tendon in a pendulum-like fashion using the skin as a pivot point; with release of the taut tendon, audible and palpable sensations are observed—similar to the "twang" observed when cutting a taut bow string. By using the entry point in the skin as a pivot point, the entrance incision is not enlarged.

By using such a small incision, there is no need to suture, staple, or Steri-Strip™ the operative site.

7. Manipulate the contracted joint by passive stretching.

8. Apply direct pressure over the operative site with a gauze sponge for ten minutes to ensure hemostasis, then cover it with a small compression dressing.

Anticoagulation is not a contraindication for doing this minimally invasive surgery. In the rare situation where there is still some residual bleeding at the end of the ten-minute compression period, compression should be continued longer and then a more firm compression dressing applied at the time the patient leaves the office.

9. Resume pre-operative level of activity including walking out of the office; however, the patient is instructed to minimize walking activities until the next day.
10. A short course (typically one to three days) of oral antibiotics is prescribed for prophylactic purposes.

Even though the percutaneous tenotomy is the epitome of a minimally invasive procedure, a short course of antibiotics is recommended for several reasons. First, the patients for which this is done are frequently compromised hosts with peripheral artery disease, diabetes and neuropathy. Second, even though the tenotomy is done with a sterile disposable scalpel, the procedure is done in the unsterile (as compared to an operating room) office setting. Third, the patients are not restricted in their post-op activities after the day of surgery.

Other Caveats for Managing Toe Deformities - Several other caveats should be remembered when doing percutaneous or limited opening toe tenotomies.

First, it is recommended that the tendons of only one toe be done at a time to eliminate complications such as infection, wound healing problems, or excessive bleeding. If other sites are needed, they can be done at weekly intervals.

If the offending extensor tendons of the toes are not easily palpated through the skin, it is recommended that the limited open technique described below be performed in the operating room.

Often the extensor tendons are obscured by forefoot soft pitting edema, brawny edema, cicatrix, hidebound skin, surgical scars, etc., so it may be difficult to palpate the extensor tendon and successfully release it through a minute percutaneous incision.

In addition, anatomical variations with tendon crossovers and bridgings may be the reason the single extensor tenotomy does not correct the hyperextension deformity completely.

Second, if the patient prefers all tenotomies be done at one time, he/she should be scheduled for the procedures to be done in an operating room and post-operative activity should be minimized for a week or so. The technique for tenotomies done in the operative room is modified slightly. For the extensor tendons, a two-centimeter incision is made between the tendons of two adjacent toes. Blunt dissection with a curved hemostat is done through the subcutaneous tissues to the extensor tendon level. The tendon is then brought out through the skin incision with a curved hemostat and incised under direct vision. The tendon to the adjacent toe is identified and managed in a similar fashion through the same incision. The skin incision is approximated with sutures or staples. In a similar fashion, the extensor tendons to the next two toes are released. A separate excision directly over the extensor hallucis longus tendon is made should this tendon also need to be released. The contracted toe joints should be manipulated to as straight positions as possible while the patient is still under anesthesia.

Clinical correlations:

A 72-year-old male patient with diabetes with severe clawing of the toes (motor neuropathy) and associated moderately severe sensory neuropathy (level 1/2 on the 0-to-2 neurological impairment assessment component of the Host-Function Score) developed a pressure sore over the apex of the right second toe proximal to the interphalangeal joint. The pressure sore was partial thickness through the epithelium. Circulation to the forefoot was poor with cool temperature and sluggish capillary refill.

At the initial examination, in-office flexor and extensor tenotomies of the toe were recommended. This was done percutaneously with a small amount of local anesthesia (two cc 1% xylocaine to each site). The contracted joints were manipulated after the tenotomies so the toe rested in the straight position. The patient walked out of the office.

At the recheck one week later, the pressure sore was healed. Prophylactic releases of the other contracted toes were recommended. Rather than doing these serially at weekly intervals, the patient opted to have the remaining tenotomies done all at one time as an outpatient surgery. This was done with intravenous sedation using two cm incisions between adjacent metatarsals on the dorsum of the foot and percutaneous tenotomies for the flexor tendons. Prophylactic antibiotics were prescribed for three days and the patient was instructed to minimize walking activities to household ambulation until the first post-operative check in one week.

Post-operatively, the dorsal incision wounds in both feet partially dehisced. These eventually healed over a two-month period with wound cleansing, small compression dressings and oral antibiotics.

Comment:

This scenario illustrates several salient points. First, the patient was obviously a compromised host with only marginal perfusion to his distal forefeet. While healing the percutaneous in-office tenotomies occurred without difficulties, complications arose from the slightly larger dorsal incisions done in the operating room. This demonstrates the philosophy and benefits of minimally invasive surgical procedures, especially for the compromised host.

Second, it is more difficult to do these procedures percutaneously without the patient actively extending the toes to make the tendons taut. This was not possible when the patient was asleep with IV sedation.

Third, the cost-benefits of doing serial in-office tenotomies are substantial. The total charges for doing the procedures on a one-time basis in the operating room are estimated to be ten times greater than doing the procedures serially in the office setting.

Finally, was it justified to correct the deformities of the other toes even though pressure sores from the contractures had not developed? The answer is an unequivocal "yes." If more severe ulcerations developed in the remaining clawed toes with open joint infection and/or osteomyelitis, toe amputation may be the only option. With the complications observed with healing of the small dorsal incisions, toe amputation flaps might fail to heal, necessitating more proximal amputations of the foot. In addition, the clawed toes lead to other problems, especially malperforans ulcers under the metatarsal heads (next section).

Third, flexor tendons are managed percutaneously in the operating room as described above for the office setting. However, without the patient actively flexing his/her toes (as would be the rule in the office setting flexor tenotomy with the patient awake), it is more difficult to achieve a successful release. Actively flexing the toes tautens the flexor tendons and when successfully released, there is a very conspicuous sensation of the toes becoming flaccid.

> Surprisingly, patients rarely complain about loss of active toe movements after tenotomies to correct deformities. This is explained by the fact that the contracted toes have little if any function in walking or balance.
>
> Consequently, the issue remains whether the patient wants inactive straight toes that are not likely to develop wounds after tenotomies or nonfunctional contracted toes that are subject to developing wounds.
>
> After explanations of the benefits and risks of the minimally invasive tenotomy surgeries and the expected outcomes, most patients invariably opt for the straight toe option.

Minimally invasive, limited open techniques have also been recommended for the flexor tendons.[11]

Fourth, anatomical variations of the toe tendons, joint anklyoses and, rarely, re-anastomosis of the incised tendons (often observed in children), may cause persistent or recurrent toe deformities. Should this occur, then repeat tenotomies and/or joint resections are indicated.

Hammer and Mallet Toe Deformities - Hammer (proximal interphalangeal joint) and mallet (distal interphalangeal) toe contractures can occur without the metatarsal-phalangeal joint hyperextension component. They can also be managed with in-office flexor tenotomies (Figure 16-9). If ulceration develops over the end of a bone, a partial toe amputation or debridement is required. Once the distal tuft of a distal phalanx of a toe becomes infected, it usually becomes avascular and removal of the infected bone is necessary. Contractures of the interphalangeal joints at the apex of clawed toe deformities can also be managed with minimally invasive techniques. If the joint is open, the joint and the adjacent bone on either side can be debrided with a ronguer through the dorsal wound in the office setting. If needed, local anesthesia is used. This readily corrects the deformity. A couple of small sutures placed at the margins of the wound will partially approximate the void created by the debridement, help maintain the toe in the straight position, and still allow access to the wound site for wicking-type dressing changes. In the operating room, the principles and techniques are slightly different. Frequently, the deformity correction is done "electively" as an add-on to some required surgery on the foot and the deformity has not yet caused an ulceration. In this situation, an oval incision is made over the apex of the joint on the dorsal aspect of the toe. The joint is resected with a ronguer and the incision is closed with sutures or staples. The geometry of the ovoid incision results in approximation of the bony surfaces and maintenance of the toe in the straight position. This obviates the need for temporary intramedullary pinning and the inherent complications, especially in the compromised host, and activity restrictions that are associated with this stabilization technique.

Toe amputations - Finally, partial or complete toe amputations can be done in the office setting (Figure 16-10). If the demarcation is sharp between mummified and

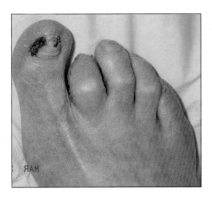
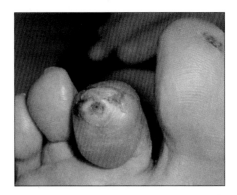

Legend: The bruising and superficial ulceration at the tip of the right second toe occurred because of the downward pressure concentration on the toe with walking. Fortunately, the ulceration did not track to the underlying distal phalanx.

With an in-office percutaneous tenotomy and manipulation of the proximal interphalangeal joint, the hammer toe deformity was corrected. With resolution of the deforming flexor forces on the toe, the bruising resolved and the ulceration healed.

Had this intervention been delayed, the likely outcome would have been ulceration to the distal tuft, infection of the bone, and a toe amputation.

Figure 16-9. Consequences of a severe hammer toe deformity.

May be done in an in-office setting

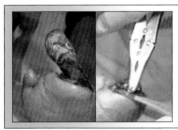
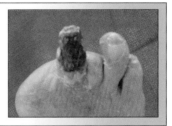

Requires toe amputations, explorations, and debridements in the operating room

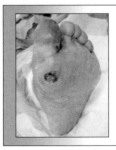
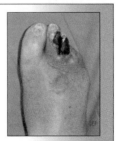

Legend: With dry gangrene and sharp demarcation between healthy and mummified tissues (upper two photos), amputation can be done through the joint capsule without power instruments. The findings in the lower two photos are in direct contrast, with wet gangrene, poor demarcation, ascending cellulitis, and associated wounds. For these amputations, all the resources of an operating room are required.

Figure 16-10. In-office versus in-operating room toe amputations.

healthy tissue, the joint capsule next proximal to the line of demarcation can be incised after making the skin incision. A scalpel is the only instrument required. Flaps can be approximated with adhesive-strips or sutures or the amputation site left to heal by secondary intention. Usually debridement of bone (with a ronguer) is required to shorten the bone proximal to the edges of the skin flaps. If demarcation is not sharp, the patient is septic and/or there is evidence of ascending tenosynovitis, hospital admission and formal exploration, debridement, decompression tenosynovectomy and ablative surgery needs to be done in the operating room with appropriate anesthesia and equipment.[12] Additional discussion of toe amputations is provided in the wound management section of this chapter.

MALPERFORANS ULCERS OF THE FOREFOOT

Wounds Under Bony Prominences - A malperforans ulcer is a generic term for a wound that appears under or over a bony prominence. When the malperforans ulcer occurs in the forefoot, clearly defined causes and obvious stages of progression are identifiable. Management incorporates the techniques just described for pre-ulceration, callus and toe deformity managements. The causes of forefoot deformities have been described previously (Chapter 7). In the patient with risk factors (deformity, peripheral vascular disease, previous foot wound, previous amputation and neuropathy) for wound development in the foot, the depressed metatarsal head is usually the underlying cause of the malperforans ulcer. However, there is usually a well-defined progression of pathomechanical problems.

Clawing of Toes - Initially, clawing of the toes arises from muscle imbalances secondary to the motor neuropathy. This causes the toes to sublux dorsally and move proximally onto the dorsum of the foot at the metatarsophalangeal joints leading to two problems (Figure 16-11): First, the metatarsal heads are driven downward and second, the protective fat pad under the metatarsal heads is pulled forward on the forefoot. When this occurs, the toe tips no longer touch the floor when standing and the plantar flexor creases of the toe interphalangeal joints are not visible (i.e. the "hidden crease" sign). Initially the body reacts to the abnormal mechanics and anatomy by forming callus under the metatarsal head secondary to pressure stresses placed on the metatarsal head with standing and walking. With progression, an ulceration develops under the metatarsal head now more vulnerable to such because of the loss of protective padding from the displaced metatarsal fat pad. With further progression, the ulceration becomes a tract to the metatarsal head. The endpoint of the progression is infection of the metatarsal head and/or sepsis dissecting proximally along the fascial and tendon planes of the foot.

Stages of Malperforans Ulcer Under Metatarsal Heads - From this information, progression of the malperforans ulcer under the metatarsal head can be divided into four stages, with clearly indicated interventions for each (Figure 16-12). For the first three of the four stages, minimally invasive surgeries usually resolve the problem and interventions used for each stage are additive. The stages, their findings, and interventions are as follows:

> **Stage 1: Callus**
> **Findings -** Pre-ulceration and/or callus formation under the metatarsal head in association with clawing of the toes
> **Interventions -** Periodic debridement of the callus and protective footwear to off-load the area(s) of pressure concentration under the metatarsal head

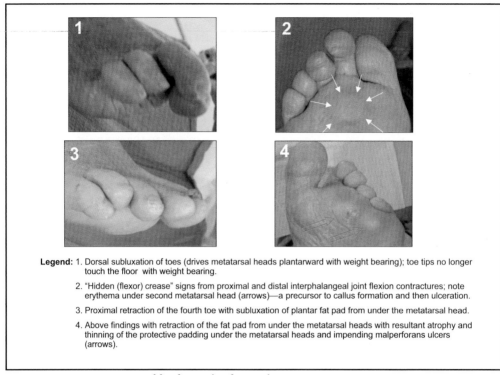

Legend: 1. Dorsal subluxation of toes (drives metatarsal heads plantarward with weight bearing); toe tips no longer touch the floor with weight bearing.

2. "Hidden (flexor) crease" signs from proximal and distal interphalangeal joint flexion contractures; note erythema under second metatarsal head (arrows)—a precursor to callus formation and then ulceration.

3. Proximal retraction of the fourth toe with subluxation of plantar fat pad from under the metatarsal head.

4. Above findings with retraction of the fat pad from under the metatarsal heads with resultant atrophy and thinning of the protective padding under the metatarsal heads and impending malperforans ulcers (arrows).

Figure 16-11. Incipient stages of forefoot malperforans ulcers.

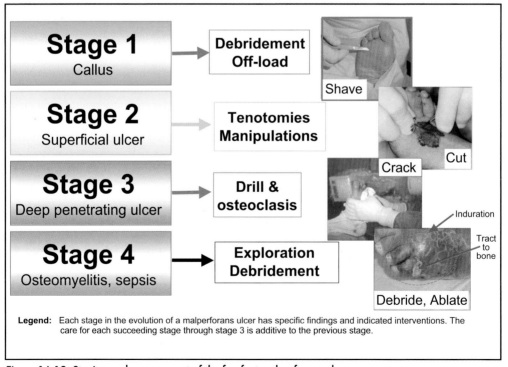

Legend: Each stage in the evolution of a malperforans ulcer has specific findings and indicated interventions. The care for each succeeding stage through stage 3 is additive to the previous stage.

Figure 16-12. Staging and management of the forefoot malperforans ulcers.

Stage 2: Superficial Ulcer
Findings - Superficial ulceration with moist or firm callus formation around the margins of the ulcer
Interventions - Correction of the claw toe deformity (i.e. tenotomy & manipulation of the contracted joints) plus the above interventions

Stage 3: Deep Penetrating Ulcer
Findings - Deep penetrating ulcer to the soft tissues covering the metatarsal head
Interventions - Realignment of the metatarsal head plus the above management

Realignment of the metatarsal head is another minimally invasive surgery that exemplifies the "Keep It Simple and Speedy" principle. In the operating room, or an equivalent sterile surgical area, the metatarsal neck of the offending metatarsal head is localized using mini-fluoroscopy equipment.

A 0.62 mm Kirshner wire with a power drill is used to score (make multiple drill holes in) the metatarsal neck. The drill holes provide a stress risor for a controlled fracture (osteoclasis) through the drill holes. The osteoclasis is done by forcefully pushing upward on the metatarsal head while counter pressure is placed on the metatarsal shaft in the downward direction. The osteoclasis is verified by an audible "crack" sound and the palpable sensation of being able to push the metatarsal head upward. Antibiotics are prescribed post-operatively for three days.

Post-operatively, the patient is immediately encouraged to walk in a post-operative rigid-soled shoe. With the weight bearing activity, the fractured metatarsal head settles in a position that can load share with the other metatarsals as fracture healing occurs. Usually, because of associated sensory neuropathy, pain does not interfere with post-operative walking activity.

With correction of the deforming force, the malperforans ulcer heals amazingly rapidly, usually within two or three weeks. Because the metatarsal head is load sharing with the other metatarsal heads, transfer lesion malperforans ulcers are less likely to occur than if the metatarsal head is removed. In addition, the only violation of the skin is the single puncture wound for the Kirshner wire to score the bone. Consequently, wound healing is almost never a problem, even in the presence of severe peripheral arterial disease.

Stage 4: Osteomyelitis, Sepsis
Findings - Osteomyelitis of the metatarsal head and/or ascending infection proximally along the tissue planes in the foot with associated sepsis
Interventions - Debridement of the metatarsal head, incision drainage, debridement, and amputation, depending on the severity of the infection

Proactive MIS/KISS Surgeries for Malperforans Ulcers versus Total Contact Casting - As stated previously (Chapter 8), the minimally invasive surgical approach for managing stage 2 and 3 malperforans ulcers is strongly recommended in contrast

For metatarsal head removal, a dorsal incision is recommended. Once the metatarsal head is removed and the infected tissue debrided, the plantar wound may be excised and closed while the dorsal incision is left to heal-in by secondary intention. This approach is less likely to lead to wound healing problems than enlarging the plantar wound to provide exposure.

If infection dissects along tendon sheaths, then they need to be explored and decompressed. For the dorsal (extensor) tendons, this can be done by extending the dorsal incision. For the plantar (flexor) tendons, exploration and decompression should be done in the medial arch, and if infection has extended proximal to this level, then at the tarsal tunnel. If the tendon tract is easily probed with a tonsil clamp, then decompression is necessary. The tip of the tonsil clamp should be used to push out the skin thereby serving as a guide where to make the decompression incisions in the arch and tarsal tunnels sites, and thereby avoid injury to the neurovascular structures.

Non-weight bearing, wound care, and antibiotics are required during convalescence. Naturally, this amount of surgery no longer qualifies it as minimally invasive. Since the metatarsal head is removed, load sharing is lost and transfer lesions to the other metatarsal heads can be a consequence.

to the total contact casting method. It hardly makes sense to heal a wound when an underlying deformity persists and will likely lead to recurrence of the wound once regular activities are resumed after the casting period, even with protective footwear. Furthermore, an understanding of the pathomechanics of the malperforans ulcer and the simple staging system used above makes the management logical and objective.

SURGICAL WOUND MANAGEMENT

MIS/KISS Proactive Wound Management Techniques - Even though the subject of management of the wound base has been discussed at length in previous chapters (Chapters 7, 11, and 12), several techniques keeping with the MIS/KISS principles apply to proactive surgeries. It sounds paradoxical that proactive surgeries would be appropriate for wounds that already exist. However, if they speed healing or prevent wound complications, they meet the MIS/KISS criteria. The first proactive surgical goal is to make the wound base as clean and healthy as possible. Debridements with instruments appropriate for an office such as scalpels, forceps, scissors, curettes, and ronguer can achieve this goal in a few moments, in contrast to what may take weeks to achieve with dressing changes with or without enzymatic debriding agents.

In Office Debridements - Proactive in-office debridements and their operating room counterparts are the first of five proactive wound management techniques described in this section. In the "end-stage" wound especially, it may take weeks for the wound base to become healthy enough to consider closure/coverage options. Repetitive in-office debridements preserve the most possible tissue, since there is no requirement to establish clean surgical margins with each debridement, as there would be if the surgery were done in the operating room. As a corollary to this, excision of the biofilm, which often covers the wound base and fosters continuation of infection, is expediently removed with a scalpel in contrast to almost total ineffectiveness of enzymatic and anti-

Biofilms are receiving increasing attention as an impediment to wound healing. It is an amorphous glycocalyx of organic matter produced by bacteria that is almost impenetrable to antibiotics, disinfectants, phagocytes, and enzymatic debriding agents. The glycocalyx consists of proteins, glycoproteins and carbohydrates. It protects the bacteria colony producing it from the environment including the agents used to clean, debride and disinfect the wound.

Antibiotics may be 1/1000 as effective when a biofilm is present. Hence it behooves the wound care provider to eliminate the biofilm to the fullest extent possible when debriding the wound base (Figure 16-4).[13,14]

Clinical correlations:

A 75-year-old male patient with diabetes and severe peripheral arterial disease, whose status is post left below-knee amputation, required a similar amputation of the opposite leg because of uncontrolled infection and gangrene of the foot. Post-operatively, a massive slough of the posterior flap occurred. The patient was reluctant to undergo amputation at a more proximal level.

Biweekly in-office debridements using scalpel, scissors, and forceps complemented the patient's slow but progressive angiogenesis response, resulting in a fully vascularized wound base in three months. The debridements were well tolerated due to the patient's sensory neuropathy. The biofilm covering the wound base was managed by sharp debridement with each office visit, but progressively decreased as the wound base vascularity improved.

Unfortunately, the end of the tibia protruded 1½ cm beyond the healthy wound base. Because of insurance approval considerations, it was not feasible to return the patient expediently to the operating room. Consequently, a sterile power saw was borrowed from the operating room and the protruding tibia osteotomized in the office. Because of the visible progress and treatment authorization request approval challenges, the patient did not want to consider the option of covering the stump end with a skin graft. Over the next six months, the stump end epithelialized completely and the patient became a limited community ambulator with bilateral prostheses and a walking aid.

Comment:

Whether the in-office debridements are considered proactive or reactive; the MIS/KISS principles were followed, resulting in a satisfactory outcome. Had a debridement (rather than converting the below-knee amputation to an above-knee one) been done in the operating room, it is doubtful that healing would have occurred any more rapidly since the ultimate outcome depended on the patient's ability to generate vascularity in the wound base. Furthermore, a couple of weeks after the in-operating room wound debridement, the wound base (with re-accumulation of the biofilm) would probably have looked no different than it would have looked two weeks after an in-office debridement.

septic solutions for managing this problem. Second, in the presence of sensory neuropathy, debridements can be done without anesthesia, which saves time, money, and the need to do the procedure in the operating room with an anesthesiologist. Third, repetitive in-office debridements save time. Whereas it may take only a few minutes to debride the patient as an outpatient, the surgeon can anticipate several hours of peri-operative "lost time" for doing an analogous procedure in the operating room. Finally, it is appropriate for non-surgeon wound care trained physicians and nurse specialists to perform debridements in the office; whereas, because of credentialing requirements, this would not be possible in the operating room. All debridements should be documented appropriately with specific reference to the type of instruments used, the size of the wound and the depth of the wound (Table 16-3 and 7-4).

Principles Regarding MIS/KISS Debridements - The following principles, many of them introduced previously, should be followed when debridements and other aspects of wound management are done in the operating room:

1. Use ovoid incisions to excise the ulcer. If the flaps are mobile enough, the ovoid incision can be approximated more easily than a round incision. If not, the distal and proximal thirds of the ovoid incision can be partially approximated to reduce the surface area of the wound while the middle third is left open for post-operative wound care.
2. Carry the incision to the bone level, when possible, with a single passage of the scalpel through skin, subcutaneous tissue, muscle, tendon and/or bursa.
3. Excise all poorly vascularized tissue such as cicatrix, tendon, ligament, joint capsule, plantar plate, etc. Likewise, remove all tags, strands, and pendant-like tissue since there is a high likelihood they are avascular and will serve only to add to the necrotic, ischemia tissue burden in the wound.
4. Debride the bony deformity with power saws, rasps or burrs, ronguer, osteotomies or combinations of these with minimal disruption of the periosteum (and blood supply to the bone) except for the actual portion of the bone removed.
5. Mobilize flaps so they can be approximated with minimal or no tension.
6. Use a small to medium sized drain if the wound is closed, should any concerns be raised that hematoma formation may occur or a potential cavity may fill with fluid after the closure.
7. Close wounds with a single layer of simple or vertical mattress retention-type sutures with further approximation of the skin edges with staples.
8. Use a compression dressing to lesson the chances of post-operative bleeding, swelling and fluid accumulation in a potential dead space created by the debridement. This is especially important when intercalary or partial ray bone resections are done.
9. Splint or cast to reduce movement at the operative site.

Once the deformity is corrected and the wound healed, the wound prevention measures previously described (Chapters 13-16) are employed.

Partial Wound Closure - Serial partial approximations of a wound is a second MIS/KISS proactive surgical technique (Figure 16-13). Again it may be questioned whether this is a proactive measure to prevent a wound or merely another wound

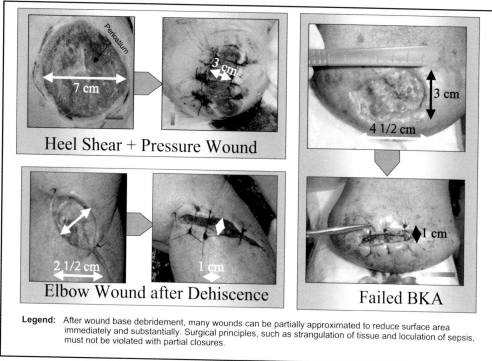

Heel Shear + Pressure Wound

Elbow Wound after Dehiscence

Failed BKA

Legend: After wound base debridement, many wounds can be partially approximated to reduce surface area immediately and substantially. Surgical principles, such as strangulation of tissue and loculation of sepsis, must not be violated with partial closures.

Figure 16-13. In-office partial wound approximations.

The more pliable the tissues around the wound, the easier it is to reduce the size of the wound by partial approximations. Consequently, this technique complements the effects achieved by serial debridements of scar and other non-pliable tissues just described.

Edema reduction and resolution of cellulitis also help to make the tissues more mobile and facilitate partial wound approximations.

Sensory neuropathy facilitates placement of sutures and partial approximation of wounds without the patient experiencing pain. If sensation is present, the intended suture tract can be infiltrated with local anesthesia before placing the suture.

In no way should partial approximations be considered a "sterile" surgical technique. Obviously, sterile suture materials with swaged on needles are required.

The skin through which the suture is passed should be cleansed of debris and prepped with a disinfectant. The wound base itself is, at a minimum, colonized with bacteria. No attempt is made to sterilize this surface. With partial approximations, in contrast to complete closures, of colonized or infected wounds, dressing changes can be continued and loculation of sepsis avoided.

When wound margins are firmly attached to underlying bone, partial wound approximations are not feasible. In these situations, other approaches such as debulking the bone, skin graft, flap coverage, or healing by gradual epithelialization of the wound margins are the options.

closure/coverage technique. The result is that it illustrates the adage that "a stitch in time saves nine." Partial approximations of a wound may eliminate the need for later more complicated surgeries such as rotation flaps or large skin grafts by substantially reducing the wound size and/or making it possible for the wound to more speedily heal by secondary intention. Once a wound has generated a healthy base, its margins may be partially approximated with sutures placed in the office setting and thereby reduce its volume without the need to return to the operating room. The technique complements the use of negative pressure wound therapy to facilitate the closure of the most challenging wounds. As the tissues adjust to the partial closure (the viscoelasticity effect), the sutures can be removed and new sutures placed to further the approximation. Once the wound has filled in to the surface level, it may be an easy matter to cover the defect with a split thickness skin graft, use bioengineered wound covering agents (Tables 9-8 and 9-9) or allow the defect to epithelialize spontaneously.

Amputations of Toes - Toe amputations are a third minimally invasive surgery where wound management techniques may be required. In certain situations, the amputations can be done in the office as discussed previously (Figure 16-10). There are three indications for partial or complete toe amputations: 1) gangrene, 2) open joint infections, and 3) osteomyelitis. Each has its own special features. Gangrene indicates that there is the loss of blood supply to the involved tissue. It has two presentations, dry and wet. If dry, the blood supply to the proximal margin is intact, the demarcation between the viable and non-viable tissue is sharp and the toe tissue proximal to the line of demarcation is healthy, auto-amputation (mummification) is a choice. Auto-amputation has many desirable features. It preserves the most toe tissue, since the only portion of the toe that is lost is that distal to the line of demarcation. Auto-amputation avoids a surgical procedure and post-operative convalescence. Care for the mummified toe is minimal with daily cleansing of the line of demarcation with soap and water or hydrogen peroxide and

> To establish surgical margins and sufficient flap tissue to close the amputation site, proximal bone resection with resultant toe shortening amounting to approximately the width of the toe is required.

covering with a dry gauze dressing. Periodically, the eschar at the proximal margin of the mummified toe should be debrided. Usually, the edges start to lift up from the underlying healthy tissues, and with moisture accumulation in the recesses, provide an environment for bacteria proliferation. Finally, while patients are cautioned to avoid traumatizing the mummified toe, they can carry out their activities of daily living in protective footwear. Antibiotics are not required.

Wet Gangrene of the Toes - Gangrene of the wet variety indicates that the blood supply to the edge of the gangrenous region is inadequate for sharp demarcation to occur. Typically, a scant but odorous exudate is present and tissues proximal to the obviously gangrenous tissues are profoundly ischemic. In this situation, options are limited. Immediate open amputation is required with antibiotics, non-weight bearing, wound care and possibly hyperbaric oxygen treatments. If the amputation is delayed, there is the risk that the infection, especially in association with a poor blood supply, will dissect proximally along tissue planes and/or tendon sheaths leading to abscess formation, purulent tenosynovitis, necrotizing fasciitis, or combinations of these. After the amputation and the toe tissues proximal to the level of the open amputation become healthy, closure options include healing by secondary intention, partial approximation of the flaps with placement of sutures in the office, or debridement of the open margins and delayed closure. This latter choice is best done in an operating room. However, it will further shorten the toe.

Open Toe Joint Infections - Open joint infections and osteomyelitis of the distal tuft of the toe invariably are a result of toe deformities. Management of open joint infections was discussed previously in the toe deformities section of this chapter. Once osteomyelitis of the distal tuft of the toe is present, eradication with antibiotics and wound care is usually not successful. This is because the blood supply to the tuft is end-arterial. Swelling and inflammation lead to interference with perfusion of the tenuous blood supply, ala the pathophysiology of a compartment syndrome (Chapters 2 and 12). The result is osteonecrosis of the distal tuft from the occlusion of its blood supply. Once the bone is dead and infected, debridement is required; the distal tuft, in effect, becomes a sequestrum. Since the problem arises with ulceration at the toe tip, this can be done in the office with a ronguer through the wound. It is another application of the MIS/KISS principle and is proactive, in that the expectation is elimination of the need for a more proximal toe amputation. Excision of the ulcer margins, including the toenail and its matrix, may be needed to provide sufficient access to the distal tuft. Antibiotics, wound care and protective footwear are employed post-operatively. As in similar situa-

> The pathophysiology of distal tuft bone necrosis is similar to the mechanisms that occur from a felon (deep pulp infection) of the fingertip that is not immediately incised and drained.

tions, wound closure may occur by secondary intention or sutures to partially approximate the flaps. Obviously, the toe deformity (mallet, hammer or claws) must be corrected in conjunction with managing the tuft ulceration.

Toe Amputations - When a toe amputation is required, the anatomy of the toe lends itself to doing the procedure as a MIS/KISS surgery. This is because each segment of the toe is separated by a thin joint capsule composed of fibrous connective tissue. To amputate the diseased portion of the toe, merely incise the skin and subcutaneous tissues around the joint, the flexor and extensor tendons and the joint capsule. This can be done in a few moments with a scalpel. Bone protruding beyond the soft tissues can be debrided with a ronguer either at the time of the amputation or later when wound closure options (see the previous section of this chapter) are considered. The open

> The more diseased the toe, the more likely a profound sensory neuropathy accompanies the problem. A second corollary to this is that the longer the gangrene problem has existed, the more profound the neuropathy. The reason for these observations is that in the absence of pain, the patient all too often delays seeking medical attention until late in the course of the problem.
>
> As mentioned before, the sensory neuropathy facilitates the in-office or on-the-ward amputation by obviating the need for anesthesia.
>
> The mummified toe is usually not a source of pain even in the patient with normal sensation. Regardless, the mummified toe should be protected whether or not protective sensation is present to avoid premature separation of the diseased toe.

amputation is particularly recommended when sepsis accompanies wet gangrene of the toe and the diseased toe needs to be removed expediently. Of course, judgment must be used when making a decision to do a toe amputation in a setting other than an operating room. If there is any suspicion that the infection has progressed beyond the diseased toe, the better decision is to do the toe amputation in an operating room where exploration along the tissue planes, debridement, electrocautery, tourniquet control, and anesthesia are available.

Management of Bone Extending Beyond Soft Tissues - Open ostectomy is a fourth wound management technique. Ostectomy is the generic term for the removal of a bone or a portion of a bone. When a bone is exposed in the toe or foot, it should be managed

Clinical correlations:

A 71-year-old male patient with diabetes, with minimal to moderate peripheral arterial disease and profound sensory neuropathy of his feet, is admitted on an emergency basis with sepsis (fever, elevated WBC count, unstable blood glucose) secondary to wet gangrene of his right great toe and cellulitis extending proximal to the forefoot, midfoot junction. The patient sought medical care when a neighbor visiting the patient commented about the odor emanating from the patient's foot.

Clinical assessment and X-rays indicated the gangrene was limited to the toe and gas had not dissected beyond the diseased toe.

Immediately after the exam, a scalpel was obtained and the toe excised on-the-ward through the metatarsophalangeal joint without any discomfort for the patient. Capsular, fibrous, and tendinous tissue was excised around the joint with the scalpel and a disposable forceps. Bleeding was controlled with a compression dressing.

Sepsis and cellulitis resolved rapidly with wound care and antibiotics. A few days later the patient was discharged with an open wound. Considerations presented to the patient for closure included healing by secondary intention, sutures to partially approximate the wound or negative pressure wound therapy. The patient opted for the partial approximation of flaps in the office.

Comments:

This patient's toe problem demonstrates many of the concepts presented earlier in this chapter including delay of diagnosis, absence of pain, complications of wet gangrene, merits of open amputation, rapid resolution of sepsis with elimination of the source of sepsis, healing responsiveness when perfusion is not seriously impaired and wound closure options.

The expedient removal of the toe is another example of how effective the MIS/KISS procedures are for situations like this and how cost-effective (avoidance of using an operating room and very short period of hospitalization) they are when doing them without delay.

While the amputation was not proactive in the literal sense, it was in the figurative sense in that by delaying the surgery until the patient could be prepared for the operating room (probably the next day), the infection could have extended rapidly into the foot as necrotizing soft tissue infections often do.

expediently. In many situations, it can be managed appropriately in the office setting as a MIS/KISS procedure. Two variations of ostectomies were previously discussed in this chapter, namely open joint amputations of the toe in the deformities section and distal tuft resections in this section. The term "proud" is a descriptive term that can be used when a wound is present and the bone extends beyond the surrounding soft tissues (Figure 16-14). This may occur as a result of open amputations, as a result of failed amputations, or after soft tissues begin to contract (secondary to edema reduction and control of infection) around bony elements in the wound base. A second cause of exposed bone can result from spurs, bone deformities, or bony prominences that have eroded through the soft tissues from pressure stresses over the areas. Frequent associations, especially with the latter two causes, are pre-existing foot deformities and neuropathies so that abnormal stresses, usually unnoticed, are placed on the skin overlying the protuberance. Naturally, the skin is more vulnerable to breakdown than the underlying bone element, and when this occurs, the bone appears "proud" in the wound base. Other causes of exposed bone result from skin sloughs associated with pressure sores and after debridements of necrotizing soft tissue infections.

Bone Debridement in the Office Setting - The patient with bone that is "proud" in the wound base does not always have to have this problem managed in the operating room (Figure 16-15). Judgment is required for making the decision whether to manage

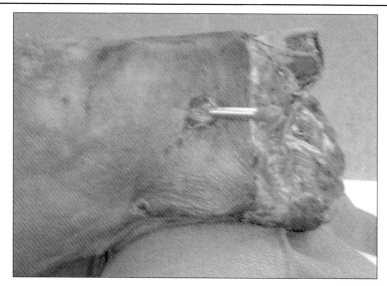

Legend: Failed, sloughed, dehisced complex below knee amputation after the patient fell and broke open the closure several days post-op.

The necrotic end of the tibia extended beyond the adjacent soft tissues (i.e is "proud" in the wound).

The knee amputation was complex due to its short length necessitated by necrotic tissue in the leg and a knee flexion contracture. Note the pin placed across the knee joint to maintain the knee in extension after the knee joint was manipulated into full extension.

Figure 16-14. "Proud" bone after a failed below-knee amputation.

the problem in the operating room or in the office setting. Factors that favor this latter choice include involvement of a single bony element, profound sensory neuropathy, and a healthy appearance of the soft tissues surrounding the bone.

Clinical correlations:

A 57-year-old female patient with diabetes and a profound sensory neuropathy of her feet develops gangrene at the tip of a mallet toe deformity. An open amputation of the toe tip is done in the office.

When the patient returns a week later, the soft tissue margins appear healthy, but the distal end of middle phalanx of the toe is "proud" in the wound. This is attributed to contraction of the soft tissues with resolution of the inflammatory process adjacent to the gangrenous toe tip.

The "proud" bone was debrided (ostectomy) with a ronguer until the bone end lay well below the skin edges. Several sutures were placed at the edges of the wound to partially approximate the margins and reduce the size of the open area. The remaining small open area was managed with Nu Gauze™ moistened with acetic acid solution wicking and healed by secondary intention over several weeks.

Comment:

This scenario shows how expediently a wound problem can be managed with MIS/KISS interventions. It also demonstrates how one MIS/KISS procedure complements another, for example partial toe amputation followed by ostectomy, which, in turn was followed by partial wound closure.

Of equal consideration is the economics of doing the procedures in the office in contrast to doing them in the operating room, which would probably have amounted to ten times or more the charges generated for the in-office procedures.

Also, if the initial surgery were done in the operating room, there would be a strong incentive to establish "surgical margins" and primarily close the wound. Likely, this would have required an amputation of the entire toe rather than just the distal tip as resulted with these MIS/KISS interventions.

When these criteria are met, then the proud bone can be debrided with a ronguer or bone cutter. Debridement is continued until the bone surface lies deep to the distal or outward portions of the soft tissues. If a question arises as to the depth, it is better to be conservative and have the patient return for a second debridement several weeks later—again espousing the MIS/KISS principle. Spicules of bone can often be seen and felt in the bases of wounds. At the minimum, these bone excrescences are colonized with bacteria (osteitis). Their removal is recommended and can be done easily as a MIS/KISS procedure using a ronguer during a clinic visit or on the ward.

Achilles Tendon Lengthening - Lengthening of the Achilles tendon is a fifth proactive wound management technique. Due to muscle imbalances secondary to neuropathy, protracted bed rest, injuries, surgeries or combinations of these, equinus contractures

Anticoagulation is not a contraindication for in-office ostectomies. If only bone is removed, bleeding is usually controlled easily with a simple compression dressing in association with these procedures. If the patient is anticoagulated, soft tissue debridement should be minimized in conjunction with the ostectomy. If bleeding of the adjacent soft tissue is not readily controlled with silver nitrate sticks, consideration for placement of a ligature around the bleeding soft tissue should be given. Suture material with swaged-on needles should be available in any office where in-office procedures are done.

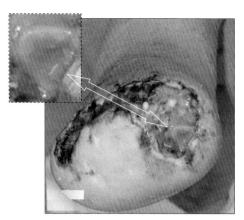
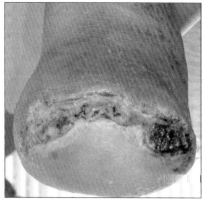

"Proud" first metatarsal after a failed, sloughed, dehisced transmetatarsal amputation

Wound appearance several weeks after in-office open ostectomy and debridement of the biofilm

Legend: The end of the first metatarsal was necrotic and infected (arrow to insert photo). The bone extended beyond the adjacent soft tissues, i.e. was "proud." Debridement with a ronguer to healthy bone allowed granulation tissue to cover the wound base and eventually complete healing of the amputation.

This avoided returning the patient to the operating room and revising the transmetatarsal amputation, which inevitably would have shortened the remaining portion of the foot.

Figure 16-15. In-office open ostectomy.

are frequently observed in the patient who has lower extremity wounds. Weight bearing in the presence of an equinus contracture concentrates forces under the metatarsal heads in the forefoot. This leads to wounds developing under the metatarsal heads, or if wounds are already present, a deterrent to healing because of concentration of forces to the soft tissues under the metatarsal heads with weight bearing.[15-18] A second concern is that after a foot amputation, the suture line and plantar flaps will receive the entire force directed to the foot with weight bearing. The consequences can be wound dehiscence, tissue slough and failed amputation. However, other factors such as foot defor-

> The shorter the foot amputation, that is from proximal transmetatarsal to Lisfranc (tarsal/metatarsal joints) to Chopart (navicular-calcaneal/cuneiform-cuboid joints) to Boyd (Talo-calcaneal/navicular joint + partial calcanectomy), the more likely an equinus contracture will occur.
>
> This occurs because each successively more proximal amputation progressively shortens the lever arm of the foot. This, in turn, magnifies the effects of the powerful calf muscles (gastrocsoleus group) against the relatively weaker ankle dorsiflexor muscles, which no longer have the full effect of the foot lever arm to counteract the strength of the calf muscles.
>
> When the equinus posture of the ankle is sustained, for example with prolonged bed rest, the calf muscles shorten. Inflammation around the ankle or the muscles lead to fibrosis and fixed contractures.
>
> Consequently, care providers must be aware of the equinus contracture complication and use appropriate orthotics, such as splints, casts or multipodus boots to prevent this from occurring in the high-risk patient.

mities, sensation, muscle weaknesses, obesity, nutrition, and gait characteristics can not be neglected in the management and prevention of forefoot plantar wounds.[19]

Considerations When Lengthening the Achilles Tendon - Whenever an equinus contracture is present and other foot surgery is performed, consideration for a percutaneous Achilles tendon lengthening (or gastrocnemius muscle recession if the soleus muscle is not contributing to the contracture, as differentiated by the Silfverskiold test) should be done. The percutaneous Achilles tendon lengthening is another example of a MIS/KISS surgery, but needs to be done in the operating room (Figure 16-16). If there are concerns about flap healing or the foot amputation markedly shortens the foot, such that maintaining the ankle in the neutral position would be difficult with casting or splinting, an axial placed pin or pins can be driven through the calcaneous and talus into the medullary canal of the distal tibia. This maintains the ankle in the neutral position until healing is completed and the soft tissues contract sufficiently to prevent an equinus deformity from occurring. At this time, the axial pins(s) would be removed. The relatively small diameter Steinmann pin (3/16" or less) transecting the articular cartilage has not been a source of ankle joint complaints after removal and the patient resumes ambulation.

With the patient in the supine position and the lower extremity maximally internally rotated, the medial and lateral edges of the tendon are identified by palpation and marked with a skin-marking pen. Percutaneous lengthening of the Achilles tendon by the tri-hemisection method is done with a #11 (or #15) scalpel.

The medial half of the tendon is released adjacent to its insertion on the calcaneous starting with a 3 mm vertical incision through the skin level only. After the skin is incised, the scalpel is rotated 90 degrees and the tip advanced until it extends through the anterior-posterior width of the tendon. The medial half of the tendon is incised by a combination of moving the knife blade medially and gently pressing the Achilles tendon onto the knife blade. The medial half of the tendon is incised first to help correct the hindfoot varus deformity, which is frequently associated with the equinus contracture.

If the hemisection is not complete, the blade tip can be withdrawn to the skin level and carefully insinuated between the skin and the Achilles tendon. Then, the blade tip is moved in a lateral direction to the midpoint of the tendon, thereby incising the remaining tendon fibers of the hemisection.

Two to three cm proximal to the distal incision, the lateral half of the tendon is incised in similar fashion as just described. The third hemisection of the tendon is again done on the medial side of the tendon two to three cm proximal to the lateral incision.

After the tri-hemisections are completed, pressure is placed on the forefoot in the dorsal-ward direction. Audible and palpable sensations signal the release of the tendon with concomitant correction of the equinus contracture. Palpation of the tendon confirms that it remains in continuity, with concavities at the tri-hemisection levels. The small incisions need not be sutured or stapled. A compression wrap controls bleeding. The ankle is splinted or casted in the neutral position. Protective weight bearing in a cast should be done for six weeks. In special circumstances a temporary pin may be placed through the ankle (see text and text box) to maintain the ankle in the neutral position.

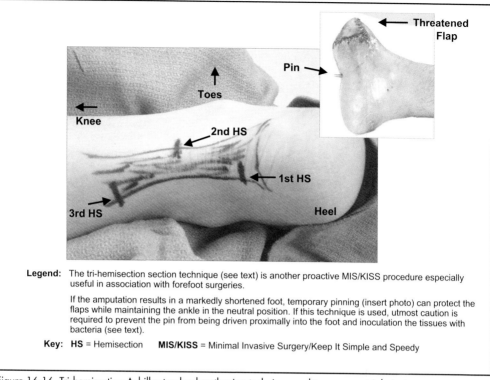

Legend: The tri-hemisection section technique (see text) is another proactive MIS/KISS procedure especially useful in association with forefoot surgeries.

If the amputation results in a markedly shortened foot, temporary pinning (insert photo) can protect the flaps while maintaining the ankle in the neutral position. If this technique is used, utmost caution is required to prevent the pin from being driven proximally into the foot and inoculation the tissues with bacteria (see text).

Key: **HS** = Hemisection   **MIS/KISS** = Minimal Invasive Surgery/Keep It Simple and Speedy

Figure 16-16. Tri-hemisection Achilles tendon lengthening technique and temporary axial pinning.

If an axial pin(s) is required to maintain the ankle in neutral position after the Achilles tendon lengthening, utmost precautions must be taken to prevent the patient from loading the pin with weight bearing. Loading the pin can drive it proximally and potentially inoculate the soft tissues and bone with bacteria.

To prevent this, maximal compliance from the patient is required. If this is not possible due to weakness, lack of patient cooperation/impaired cognitive function or significant obesity and there is a risk that the patient will weight bear through the pin, a cast with a metal stirrup attached to it can protect the pin end. If there is any question that these measures will fail, then the pin(s) should be removed before the patient is discharged from the hospital and the neutral position maintained as well as possible with casting.

CONCLUSIONS

A Stitch in Time - The essence of preventive medicine is the use of interventions that will prevent or minimize the consequences of a medical or surgical problem. Nowhere in medicine can this be better exemplified and appropriately addressed than in the foot that has risk factors (deformity, peripheral vascular disease, previous foot wound, previous amputation or neuropathy) for a wound to occur or become more complicated. This prevention concept cannot be more elegantly stated than "an ounce of prevention is worth a pound of cure" and better come to fruition than by utilizing the prevention strategies presented in this and the three preceding chapters. The information in this chapter is exemplified by the adage "a stitch in time saves nine." Many of the proactive, Minimally Invasive Surgeries/Keep It Simple and Speedy (MIS/KISS) procedures can be done appropriately in an office setting by wound care specialists without residency training in foot surgery procedures (Table 16-3). Of the three primary reasons "problem" wounds fail to heal (namely deformities, ischemia and underlying infection), correction of the deformity is the one that can be most effectively and appropriately managed by proactive surgeries. Reimbursements for these interventions are delineated in Medicare (Center for Medicare/Medicaid Services) Resource-Based/Relative Value System reimbursements (Table 7-3). Finally, the procedures described in this chapter integrate so well with the other measures to prevent recurrent or new foot wounds (Chapters 13-15) that no discussion of wound prevention measures is complete without adequate attention being given to proactive MIS/KISS procedures.

TABLE 16-3. MINIMALLY INVASIVE SURGERIES/KEEP IT SIMPLE AND SPEEDY PROCEDURES (See Table 7-3 for Medicare reimbursement codes and rates)

Procedure	Site for Doing Procedure	Instruments	Comment
Debridements			
Partial thickness skin debridement, paring of callus	In office (IO)	#10 or #21 scalpel	Any foot surgery done in the operating room should not be concluded until callused skin is debrided
Full thickness skin	IO Debridement	Same as above (SAA) with or without forceps	Same as above (SAA)
Subcutaneous tissues	IO if chronic wound; in operating room (IOR) if patient septic	Scalpel, forceps, curettes, ronguer	Control bleeding with direct compression, silver nitrate applicators or electrocautery (if in OR)
Muscle and tendon	SAA	Scalpel, forceps, ronguer	Ligatures to control bleeding; usually in conjunction with previous levels of debridements
Bone and joint	Usually IOR; IO if bone "proud" or for an open toe amputation	Ronguer, osteotome, power saw	SAA
Specific Procedures			
Percutaneous tenotomy	IO for single tendon; IOR for multiple tendons	#11 scalpel if percutaneous; Scalpel and hemostat if IOR (plus sutures or staples)	Use peri-operative prophylactic antibiotics
Toe amputation	IO if isolated problem; IOR if associated sepsis	#10 or #21 scalpel; ronguer for debridement of bone and articular cartilage	Leave open if infection present; closure with more proximal debridement if in OR
Partial wound approximations	IO	Suture material, needle holder or hemostat	Almost always done in conjunction with debridement
Excision of ulcer; debridement of underlying tissues	IOR	Scalpel, forceps, ronguer, power saw, osteotome and rasp	OR counterpart of debridements; may involve all layers of tissues
Ostectomy	IO if bone is "proud"	Ronguer, bone cutter	Almost always done with associated debridements; see bone and joint in this table
Metatarsal head realignment	IOR	Mini-fluoroscopy; drill	For Stage 3 malperforans ulcer (see figure 16-12)
Partial ray amputation	IOR	Same equipment as for excision of ulcer	May require complex skin flaps to close primarily
Achilles tendon lengthening	IOR	#11 scalpel	If percutaneous, no closure needed

Abbreviations: IO = In office (in clinic, on the ward), **IOR** = In operating room, **SAA** = Same as above, **#** = number

QUESTIONS

1. What are the main risk factors for developing foot wounds?

2. What are the differences between proactive and reactive surgeries for managing foot problems?

3. What are conditions that predispose callus/hyperkeratosis formation?

4. How should calluses/hyperkeratosis be managed?

5. What is the pathophysiology of the development of toe deformities?

6. What are the stages of the malperforans ulcer under the metatarsal head and what are the appropriate interventions?

7. What are the main indications for toe amputations?

8. Compare and contrast the management of malperforans ulcers with total contact casting versus MIS/KISS surgeries?

9. What are the benefits of percutaneous Achilles tendon lengthening?

REFERENCES

1. Strauss MB. The orthpaedic surgeon's role in the strategies for treatment and prevention of diabetic foot wounds. Foot & Ankle International, 2005; 26(1):5-14

2. Strauss MB. Surgical treatment of problem foot wounds in patients with diabetes. Clinical Orthopaedics and Related Research, 2005; 439:91-96

3. Apelqvist J, Larsson J. What is the most effective way to reduce incidence of amputation in the diabetic foot. Diabetes/Metabolism, Research and Reviews, 2000; 16(Suppl 1):S75-S83

4. Brem H, Stojadinovic O, Diegelmann RF, et al. Molecular markers in patients with chronic wounds to guide surgical debridement. Mol Med. 2007 Jan-Feb; 13(1-2):30-9

5. Attinger CE, Bulan EJ. Debridement: the key initial first step in wound healing. Foot Ankle Clin N Amer., 2001:627-660

6. Sargent RL. Management of blisters in the partial-thickness burn: an integrative research review J Burn Care Res., 2006 Jan-Feb; 27(1):66-81

7. Ono I, Gunji H, Zhang JZ, et al. A study of cytokines in burn blister fluid related to wound healing. Burns, 1995 Aug; 21(5):352-5

8. Swain AH, Azadian BS, Wakeley CJ, Shakespeare PG. Management of blisters in minor burns. Br Med J., 1987 Jul 18; 295(6591):181

9. Uchinuma E, Koganei Y, Shioya N, Yoshizato K. Biological evaluation of burn blister fluid. Ann Plast Surg., 1988 Mar; 20(3):225-30

10. Nektarios L, Parenti J, Cush G, et al. Percutaneous flexor tenotomy—office procedure for diabetic toe ulcerations. Wounds, 2007; 19(3):64-68

11. Stephens HM. Technique Tip, The diabetic plantar hallux ulcer: A curative soft tissue procedure. Foot & Ankle International, 2000; 21(4):954-955

12. Shuttleworth RD. Amputation of gangrenous toes: effect of sepsis, blood supply and debridement on healing rates, S Afr Med J., 1983; 63:973-975

13. Costerton, JW, Stewart, PS, Greenberg, EP. Bacterial biofilms: a common cause of persistent infections. Science, 1999; 284:1318-1322

14. Qi X, Gao J, Sun D, et al. Biofilm formation of the pathogens of fatal bacterial granuloma after trauma: potential mechanism underlying the failure of traditional antibiotic treatments. Scand J Infect Dis., 2008; 40(3):221-8

15. Nishimoto G, Attinger C, Cooper P. Lengthening the Achilles tendon for the treatment of diabetic plantar forefoot ulceration. Surgical Clinics of North America, 2003; 83(3), 707-726

16. Armstrong DG, Stacpoole-Shea S, Nguyen H, Harkless LB. Lengthening of the Achilles tendon in diabetic patients who are at high risk for ulceration of the foot. J Bone Joint Surg Am., 1999, 81-A(4):535-538

17. Holstein P, Lohmann M, Bitsch M, Jorgensen B. Achilles tendon lengthening, the panacea for plantar forefoot ulceration? Diabetes/Metabolism Research and Reviews, 2004; 20 (Suppl 1):S37-240

18. Mueller MJ, Sinacore SDR, Hastings MK, et al. Effect of Achilles tendon lengthening on nueropathic plantar ulcers: A randomized clinical trial. J Bone Joint Surg Am., 2003; 85-A(8):1436-1445

19. Orendurff MS, Rohr ES, Sangeorzan BJ, et al. An equinus deformity of the ankle accounts for only a small amount of the increased forefoot plantar pressure in patients with diabetes. J Bone Joint Surg Br., 2006; 88-B(1):65-68

NOTES

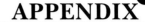

APPENDIX A

MASTERMINDING WOUNDS FROM A TO Z

INTRODUCTION 485

FROM A TO Z. 485

INTRODUCTION

This reference is an easy way to quickly review the subjects mentioned in this text. It is not designed to be all-inclusive or to fully summarize the information on a subject. The topics under each letter of the alphabet are limited to eight or less. One or more chapters that include further information on the subject(s) are included in parentheses.

In some ways, this appendix supplements the questions listed at the end of each chapter. The questions at the ends of the chapters were designed with two purposes: first, to help the reader recall the most important concepts in the chapter, and second to provide ideas and subject topics for discussions, presentations, and topics for research projects (for those in academic settings and/or educational programs). This appendix was generated with the same goals as the second purpose, i.e. to provide ideas for further discussions and inquiries.

FROM A TO Z

A = Assessments i.e. 0-to-2 grades based on objective, easily recognizable criteria that are typically summated with four other assessments to generate a score (Chapters 1, 2, 5, 7, 13, and 14)

- Components of the **Wound Score**
- Components of the **Host-Function Score**
- Components of the **Goal-Aspiration Score**
- Sensory assessment of the patient with a wound, callus, and/or deformity
- Skin condition
- Toenail condition

B = Biofilms; relatively impervious protein-carbohydrate complexes generated by microorganisms that often cover implants, wound bases, and infected bone. They act as barriers to antibiotic penetration and host responses to infection (Chapters 7 and 11)

- Presentations
- Role in "problem" and "end-stage" wounds
- Antibiotic interactions
- Surgical management

C = Coverage/closure of wounds (Chapters 7, 9, and 16)

- Options
- Hierarchy of oxygen requirements for coverage/closure options
- Partial wound approximations
- Use of bioengineered wound covering agents
- Negative pressure wound therapy/sub-atmospheric wound dressings

D = Debridements (Chapters 7, 11, 12, 14, and 16)

- Goals
- Types
- Techniques
- In-clinic limitations versus in-operating room challenges

E = "End-stage" hypoxic wounds (Chapters 1, 2, 5, and 11)

- Definitions with and without using the **Wound Score**
- Role of the **Host-Function** and **Goal-Aspiration Score**
- Management
- Predicted outcomes

F = Failed, sloughed, dehisced (FSD) wounds (Chapters 1, 2, 5, 10, 11, and 12)

- Predictors of failure based on the **Wound Score** and transcutaneous oxygen measurements
- Decision-making regarding salvage versus lower limb amputation
- Management
- Stages of healing
- Outcome expectations

G = Grading systems for wounds; their merits and their deficiencies (Chapters 3, 4, and 5)

- Criteria used to evaluate wound grading systems
- The **Wound Score**
- Diabetic foot wound grading systems
- Pressure ulcers/indolent wound grading systems

H = Hyperbaric oxygen (Chapters 2, 10, and 11)

- Mechanisms
- Quantifying the effects of hyperoxygenation
- Oxygen tension requirements for wound healing and controlling infection
- Indications for wound healing
- Side effects

I = Indications for proactive surgeries (Chapters 7 and 16)

- Contractures and deformities attenuating skin coverage associated with these problems
- Adjunct to wound management
- Prevention of new and recurrent wounds
- Improved function
- Cosmesis

J = Judging patients' desires with respect to their wounds (Chapters 1, 11, 13, and 14)

- **Goal-Aspiration Score**
- Measures to assess compliance
- The roles of family and/or caregivers
- Usefulness in making decisions whether to salvage or recommend amputation for "end-stage" wounds

K = Keeping wounds from recurring (Chapters 13, 14, 15, and 16)

- Wound prevention strategies
- Grading and managing foot/leg skin and toenail findings
- Decision-making regarding protective footwear
- The role and indications for proactive surgeries (see "I" above)

L = Limiting factors that prevent wound healing (Chapters 2, 5, 6, 7, 8, 11, and 12)

- Ischemia and hypoxia
- Infected, non-perfused tissue—especially bone
- Significant deformities; inadequately managed pressure concentrations on skin over deformities
- Uncontrolled shear stresses
- Multiple drug resistant organisms/uncontrolled sepsis
- Malnutrition
- Inadequately managed edema in the lower extremities
- Patient compliance

M = Master Algorithm (Chapters 5-16)

- Scoring of wounds into "healthy," "problem," or "futile" types
- Management of wounds
- Decision-making regarding salvage, lower limb amputation, or comfort care measures only for managing "end-stage" wounds
- Prevention of new and recurrent wounds

N = Nutrition (Chapters 6 and 11)

- Function in wound healing, infection management, and repair processes of the body
- Clinical markers of nutrition status
- Biochemical (albumin, prealbumin) markers of nutrition status
- Importance of the CRP (C-reactive protein) inflammatory marker in interpreting biochemical markers
- Management of malnutrition
- Use of clinical and biochemical markers to assess progress

O = Oxygen requirements for wound healing (Chapters 2, 5, 10, and 11)

- Regulation of perfusion (oxygen delivery) with considerations for blood volume versus the potential capacity of the vascular system
- Oxygen requirements for "critical" versus "non-critical" tissues
- The magnitude oxygen requirements change in "non-critical" tissues from resting states to conditions necessary for wound healing and infection control
- Assessment of wound oxygenation: palpation of pulses, skin temperature, skin coloration, capillary refill, Doppler testing, transcutaneous oxygen measurements, and indirectly through imaging techniques using a 0-to-2 grading system
- Clinical outcomes of wounds where oxygenation is adequate as in "healthy" wounds, marginal as is often observed in "problem" wounds, and (usually) inadequate as in "futile" wounds

P = "Problem" wounds (Chapters 1, 2, 5, 6, 7, 8, 9, and 10)

- Wounds that have the potential to heal with adequate management
- Clinical appraisal
- Use of the **Wound Score** to objectively define
- Use of the **Wound Score** to quantify progress
- Anticipated healing outcomes with appropriate management
- Considerations for dealing with "problem" wounds that fail to improve with strategic management

Q = Quantifying the seriousness of wounds, the patient's capacity to heal, and his/her aspirations using 0-to-10 scores (with 10 being best). Each score is generated by summating five 0-to-2 point assessments (see A = assessments and Chapters 1, 2, 5, and 11)

- **Host-Function Score**
- **Goal-Aspiration Score**
- **Wound Score**

R = Risk factors for generating new or recurrent wounds and the need for extra vigilance when one or more of these factors are observed in a patient (Chapters 7, 13, 14, 15, and 16)

- Peripheral artery disease
- Deformity
- History of a previous wound
- Previous amputation
- Sensory neuropathy
- Other considerations in addition to the five "gold standards" above include obesity, smoking, diabetes, malnutrition, immobility, older age, incontinence, chronic venous insufficiency, deficits in cognitive function, etc.

S = Strategic management, the five interventions that need to be addressed for the management of every "problem" wound and every "end-stage" wound where the decision is made to salvage the extremity (Chapters 6, 7, 8, 9, 10, 11, and 12)

- Medical management interventions
- Preparation (debridements) of the wound base
- Protection and stabilization of the wound
- Selection of wound dressing agents
- Wound oxygenation and hyperbaric oxygen therapy

T = Toenail and skin care (Chapters 7, 8, and 14)

- Toenail and skin evaluation and management
- Using toenail and skin condition as a measure of compliance
- Who should do toenail management
- Surgical versus medical management of the dystrophic, fungus-infected toenail

U = Utilization of resources and the multidisciplinary approach to wound care (Chapters 6-15 and 16)

- Physicians including foot surgeons, plastic surgeons, vascular surgeons, primary care doctors, hyperbaric medicine specialists, infectious disease consultants, nephrologists, etc.
- Nurses with special expertise including wound care, enterostomal therapy, diabetic education, epidemiology, discharge planning, home health care, and hyperbaric medicine
- Clinical pharmacists
- Clinical nutritionists
- Physical therapists
- Social workers
- Clergy

V = Vascular evaluation (Chapters 5, 10, and 11)

- As a component of the **Wound Score**
- Primary, secondary, and tertiary measures of perfusion/oxygenation; see "O" (oxygen requirements for wound healing)
- Angioplasty, stenting, and revascularization
- Options when revascularization, stenting, and/or angioplasty are not feasible or have been done but perfusion is still inadequate

W = Wound dressings/covering agents (Chapters 9, 11, 12, and 16)

- Number of options/choices
- Categories of agents
- Use of combination agents
- Roles of bioengineered dressings and negative pressure wound therapy
- Cost considerations
- Switching agents as the wound improves—i.e. the hierarchy of selection choices

X= X-rays and other imaging techniques (Chapters 7, 10, 11, and 12)

- Roles in evaluating osteomyelitis
- Roles and techniques for evaluating perfusion
- Differentiation of bone inflammation from osteomyelitis
- Magnetic resonance imaging
- Uses of ultrasound for wound evaluation

Y = "Why" salvage limbs and avoid amputations? (Chapters 1, 2, and 11-16)

- Cost considerations
- Challenges of using prostheses
- Loss of independence after a lower limb amputation in the presence of other comorbidities
- Psychological perspectives and mental health
- Allowing patients to choose their own options

Z = Zero tolerances (Chapters 5, 7, 8, and 13-16)

- Inadequate wound evaluation and documentation
- Lack of properly timed follow-up care
- Insufficient protection and stabilization of "problem" wounds
- Failure to utilize methods to improve wound oxygenation
- Smoking
- Failure to proactively address and manage precursors/risk factors for wound development; see "R" (Risk factors for wounds)

APPENDIX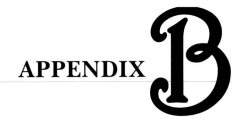

AIDS FOR MASTERMINDING WOUNDS

INTRODUCTION 493

B-1: ALGORITHMS 493

B-2: ASSESSMENTS 496

B-3: SCORES 499

B-4: FORMS 502

INTRODUCTION

A compendium of algorithms, assessments (0-to-2 point grades), scoring systems (summation of 5 assessments adding up to a 0-to-10 point score), and data acquisition forms used in this text.

Algorithms Assessments

Aids to facilitate evaluation, management, and prevention of "problem" wounds

Scores Forms

The aim of this appendix is to make the text as user-friendly as possible. The following sources of information are interspersed throughout the text, and often the information they contain are mentioned in chapters after their original appearance. By including these sources of information in an appendix, sans their legends, the reader can readily find the information referred to in the text.

In addition, for those who desire to use portions or all of these sources of information for their wound evaluation, management, and prevention programs, all the information is available in this appendix.

APPENDIX B-1: ALGORITHMS

Algorithms

Illustrations or figures that serve as a guide or provide information in a step-wise and/or chart-like pattern for problem solving or working through challenging situations

- Master Algorithm

- Evaluation component of the **Master Algorithm**

- Management component of the **Master Algorithm**

- Decision-making and management of the "end-stage" wound

- Prevention component of the **Master Algorithm**

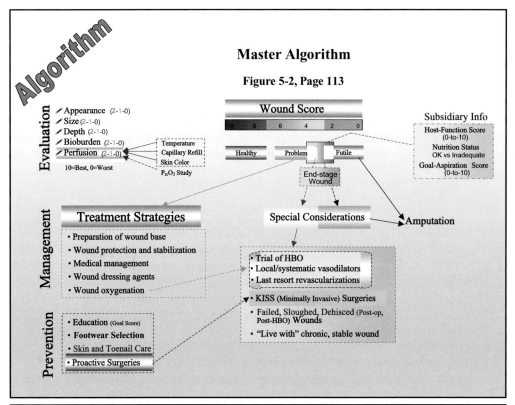

Master Algorithm

Figure 5-2, Page 113

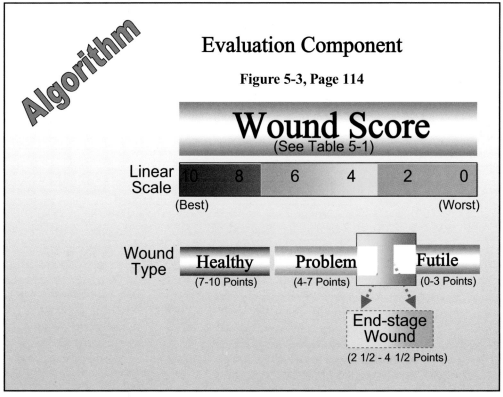

Evaluation Component

Figure 5-3, Page 114

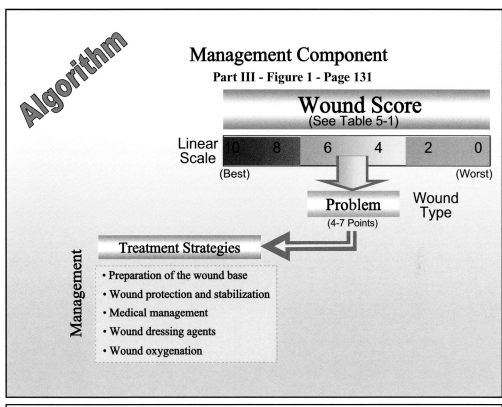

Management Component
Part III - Figure 1 - Page 131

Decision-Making and Management of the "End-Stage" Wound Component
Part IV - Figure 1 - Page 290

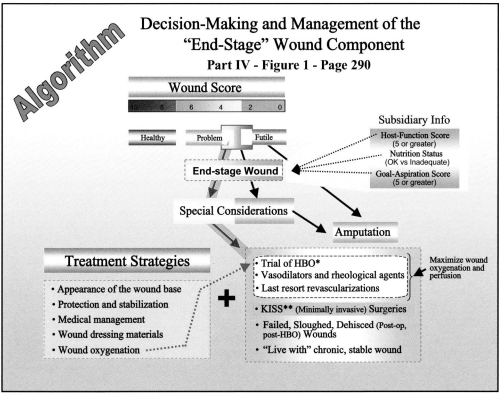

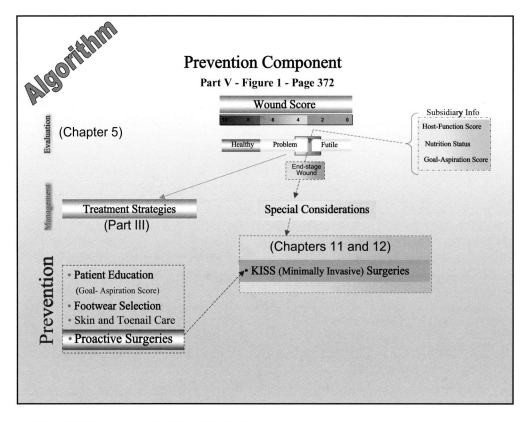

APPENDIX B-2: ASSESSMENTS

Assessments

Assessments are numerical grades from 2 points (best) to 0 points (worst). The summation of 5 assessments generates a **Score**. However, some assessments are not integrated into **Scores** such as those for the skin and toenail.

Although findings to determine a point grade are selected for their objectivity as well as importance, they grade a continuum of responses. Consequently, half points are used in the grading when findings are mixed or intermediate between two grade points.

- Assessing sensation

- Secondary and tertiary assessments of perfusion

- Grading progress/outcomes

- Skin assessment

- Toenail assessment

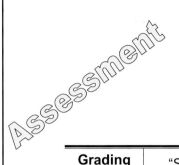

Assessing Sensation

Table 2-5, Page 46

Grading (Use half points if mixed or intermediate between 2 grades)	"See, Touch, and Go" (No Wound)	Wound "Manipulation" (Wound Present)	Anesthesia Required for Surgeries
2 Points	• No deformities • Sensation: Feet = hands	Normal pain perception	Full
1 Point	• Palpable discomfort of deformities, calluses, etc. • Sensation: Feet = about 50% of hand feeling	Discomfort; able to do procedure(s) with minimal anesthesia	Surface or local with patient awake
0 Points	• No palpable discomfort of deformities, calluses • Anesthetic feet	Able to do procedure(s) without anesthesia	None

Secondary and Tertiary Assessments of Perfusion

Table 5-4, Page 121

Method	2 Points	1 Point	0 Points
Secondary Methods			
Color (Of surrounding skin)	Pink	Pale/Dusky	Cyanotic/Purplish
Temperature (Of surrounding skin)	Warm	Cool	Cold
Capillary Refill (Adjacent to wound)	< 2 Seconds	2 to 5 Seconds	> 5 Seconds
Tertiary Methods			
Room Air $P_{tc}O_2$	>40 mmHg	30-40 mmHg	< 30 mmHg
$P_{tc}O_2$ with HBO	>200 mmHg	50-200 mmHg	< 50 mmHg

Grading Progress/Outcomes
Figure 5-5, Page 124

Observation	Grade (Points)	Management
Healed	2	Initiate wound prevention measures
Improving	1 1/2	Continue present management. If wound transitions from "problem" to "healthy," use less complicated dressings
No Change	1	Re-evaluate management and initiate changes
Worsening	1/2	Reassess options and if revascularization/angioplasty is not feasible, consider lower limb amputation or comfort care only
Major amputation or death	0	

Skin Assessment
Figure 14-2, Page 409

Grade (If mixed findings or intermediate between two findings, use half points)	Findings	Management
2 (Optimal, normal)	Soft, pliable, well-moisturized, clean skin; Free of scaling and plaques	Compliment patient and/or caregivers; Continue the same management as before
1 (Sub-optimal, marginally satisfactory)	Dry, scaly skin; Skin in need of cleansing and lubrication	Instruct and demonstrate to patients and/or caregivers skin care measures (see text)
0 (Unsatisfactory, in need of immediate attention)	Crusts, plaques, eschars, scaling desquamated skin, debris and/or maceration	Debride in-office or hospital; Skin moisturization and cleansing; Skin lubrication

Assessment

Toenail Assessment
Figure 14-6, Page 414

Grade (If mixed findings or intermediate between two findings, use half points)	Findings	Management
2 (Optimal, normal)	Healthy appearing, appropriate length toenails	Compliment patient and/or caregivers Continue the same management as before
1 (Sub-optimal, marginally satisfactory)	Long and/or irregular ends of trimmed toenails	Trim toenails with sterilized surgical quality nail clippers in the office/clinic Instruct patients in trimming techniques including use of nail file to contour and shape toenail ends
0 (Unsatisfactory, in need of immediate attention)	Diseased toenails (Figure 14-5) in need of immediate management	Debride, debulk with sterilized surgical quality nail clippers File and contour with a nail file or rotating sanding drum Teach patient and/or caregivers toenail filing techniques

APPENDIX B-3: SCORES

Scores

Scores are numerical values from 0 (worst) to 10 (best) derived from the summation of five objective, easy to measure assessments each graded from 2 points (best) to 0 points (worst). Scores provide quantitative information to make decisions, guide treatments, evaluate progress and document outcome

- Rational decision making

- **Goal-Aspiration Score**

- **Host-Function Score**

- **Wound Score**

- **Risk assessments for PU/IW** (pressure ulcer/indolent wounds)

Score

Rational Decision Making
Table 1-2, Page 13

Elements	Comments, Further Elaboration	Grading Criteria[1] (For each Element)
Clinical Judgment	Based on personal experiences, reports of other's experiences and review studies	**2 Points** Overwhelming information or experiences support the element
Mechanisms	How the mechanisms of the intervention modify the pathophysiology of the condition	
Laboratory Studies	Provides objective indications, e.g. selection of antibiotics from C and S's and use of HBO based on $P_{tc} O_2$ studies	**1 Point** Information is consistent with the element
Need for other Treatment Options	Failure to improve and/or poor outcomes with current or usual management(s)	**0 Points** No data, no benefit, or possible harm from information regarding the element
Evidence-based Clinical Reports	Randomized control trial(s) and/or other high quality studies, e.g. cohort, head-to-head, etc.	

1) Use half points if information is mixed or found to be between two grading criteria

Treatment Choice: Summate the grades for each of the five elements and if equal to or
(Rational Approach)   greater than 5, justification exists for the treatment choice

Score

Goal-Aspiration Score
Table 1-3, Page 14

Assessments	Comments, Further Elaboration	Full	Some	None
		Use half points if the information is mixed or intermediate between 2 of the grading criteria		
Comprehension	Awareness of the problems and the options for management	2 Points	1 Point	0 Points
Motivation	To heal the wounds and/or avoid lower limb amputations			
Compliance	Attention to diabetes management, weight control, skin and toenail care, diet, non-smoking, etc.			
Family/Caregiver Support	Degree and quality of care provided			
Level of Independence	Ability for patient to perform			

Goal-Aspiration Score: Summate the points for each of the five assessments

Interpretation: Scores of 5 or greater support the decision for limb salvage and/or surgeries to facilitate wound healing such as contracture releases and major debridements. This score (5 or greater) indicates the patient, family, and/or caregivers are able and willing to take an active part in wound care

Host-Function Score
Table 2-4, Page 43

Assessment	2- Points	1 Point	0-Points
	Use half points if mixed or intermediate between 2 grades		
Age	< 40	40-60	>60
	◄-----Subtract 1/2 point if diabetes or collagen-----► vascular disease present		
Ambulation	Community	Household	None
	◄------------------- Subtract 1/2 point if ambulation aids are used -------------------►		
CV/Renal (Whichever gives the lower score)	Normal	Impaired	Decompensated
Smoke/Steroid (Whichever gives the lower score)	None	Past	Current
Neurological Deficits	None	Some	Severe

Host-Function Score Interpretation (Summation of the grades of the 5 assessments)

   8-10 = **Healthy**
   4-7 = **Impaired** (May subcategorize as mildly to severely impaired)
   0-3 = **Decompensated**

Wound Score
Table 5-2, Page 114

Assessment	2 Points	1 Point	0 Points
	Use half points if mixed or intermediate between 2 grades		
Appearance (Of the wound base)	Red	White/Yellow	Black
Size (Include undermining)	< Thumb Print	Thumb Print-to-Fist	> Fist Area
Depth (Depth of probe)	Skin/SC Tissue	Muscle/Tendon	Bone/Joint
Infection (Bioburden)	Colonization	Cellulitis/ Maceration	Sepsis (↑WBC, bacteremia, fever, malaise, dysglycemia)
Perfusion*	Palpable Pulses (Warm, pink, normal capillary refill)	Doppler (Cool, dusky-pale, sluggish capillary refill)	No Pulses (Cold, purplish-cyanotic, capillary refill > 5 seconds)

Note: *Use secondary assessments (in parentheses) such as skin temperature, skin color and/or capillary refill to assess perfusion when edema, wounds or scar tissue interfere with assessment of pulses. SC = Subcutaneous, WBC = White Blood Cell

Score

Risk Assessments for PU/IW*
Table 4-3, Page 92

Assessment	2 Points	1 Point	0 Points	Interpretation
	Use half points if findings intermediate between to grade points			(Summation of grades from the 5 assessments)
Deformity (Usually associated with neurological deficit)	None	Minimal to moderate (Minimal interference with function)	Severe (Severely interferes with function)	**8 to 10 Points** Minimal to no risk to generate a PU/IW*
Forces (Pressure, shear or tension)	None Apparent	Apparent, but no problems have arisen or are anticipated	Present with visible problems	
Ischemia	None (Palpable pulses, skin coloration, temperature and capillary refill OK)	Mild to moderate (Doppler pulses, poor skin coloration, temperature & capillary refill)	Severe (Necrotic tissue in wound)	**4 to 7 Points** At risk for generation of a PU/IW*
Malnutrition	None	Mild to moderate (Depressed visceral proteins)	Severe (Markedly abnormal visceral proteins)	**0 to 3 Points** Severe risk and/or a PU/IW* is already present
Moisture Retention	No Problems	Adequately controlled	Inadequately controlled	

Key: * PU/IW = Pressure ulcer/indolent wound

APPENDIX B-4: FORMS

Forms

These are instruments designed by the authors to record information obtained from patient evaluations. They integrate information from the scoring systems and assessments used in this text to make as much of the information objective (and quantifiable) as possible. These forms are not included in the chapters, and were added to this appendix for the reader's convenience.

Squares are used for recording numerical information (large ones for **Scores** and smaller dotted-ones for assessments) and for selecting alternative choices (the smallest boxes).

The two forms can be "cut and pasted" into single sheets of paper or converted to formats for electronic medical records (EMRs).

- • Initial evaluation
  - • History portion
  - • Examination portion
  - • Management portion
- • Follow-up evaluation
  - • Upper half
  - • Bottom half

Forms

Initial Evaluation (History portion)

Wound Evaluation, Management and Prevention
(Initial Encounter)

| Day | Month | Year |

Identification Age, race, sex, co-morbidities contributing to wound problem, reason for consultation with its duration, and referring physician

History Patient's presenting complaints, etiology, course of the problem (improving, no changes, worsening) and management (dressing agents, cultures and antibiotics, names/specialties of other physicians-care providers who have managed problem, pain level, surgeries, etc.

Past Medical History Other co-morbidities & diagnoses

Medications ☐ Include
☐ See list in EMR/Chart

Allergies ☐ None ☐ Include
Other Surgeries

See Table 2-4   Pg. 43

Host-Function Score

Age <40 = 2 points   40-to-60 =1 point   > 60 = 0 pts
Ambulation Community= 2   House =1   None = 0
CV/Renal OK = 2   Impaired =1   Decompensated = 0
Smoke/Steroids None = 2   Past =1   Current = 0
Neuro Deficit None = 2   Some =1   Severe = 0
☐ 8-10 = Healthy
☐ 4-7 = Impaired
☐ 0-3 = Decompensated   **Score =** [Points]

Goal-Aspirations Score

Motivation
Comprehension
Compliance   Full = 2
Family Support   Some = 1
Ability to do ADL's   None = 0
ADL's = Activities of daily living
☐ >4 = Understands options, can make decisions and aid in own care   **Score =** [Points]
☐ 4 or less = deficient in above

See Table 1-3   Pg. 14

Comments: This portion of the **Wound Evaluation, Management and Prevention** form (i.e. its first third) assists in obtaining and recalling the essential elements of the <u>history portion</u> of the initial encounter with a patient who has a wound problem.

Note how it includes and integrates the information from the **Host-Function** and **Goal-Aspirations Scores.**

Each third of this form (see the next 2 pages) can be combined onto a chart-sized (8 1/2" X 11") sheet of paper; then, all the **Evaluation, Management, and Prevention** information of the initial encounter is assessable on one side of a piece of paper. For those using electronic medical records (EMRs) the information in these forms can be generated into a template.

Forms

Initial Evaluation (Exam portion)

◆ Examination ◆

Ht.
Wt.   **Build** Light ☐
             Medium ☐
Contractures   Heavy ☐

Deformities

Sensation [Points]
OK = 2   Impaired = 1   None = 0
Skin [Points]
OK = 2   Scaly =1   Crusts = 0
Nails [Points]
OK =2   Long = 1   Abnormal = 0

See assessments from Tables 2-5, 14-2 & 14-6

☐ = Left side **Wound Description** Right side = ☐
Diagram with labels or describe including, site, area and depth, exudate, type of wound base, odor, biofilm, surrounding skin appearance (edema, erythema, induration, maceration), etc.

Wound Score

Appearance (Wound base)
Red = 2   White/Yellow = 1   Black = 0
Size (Including recesses)
<Thumb print = 2   Thumb-to-fist =1
>Fist area = 0
Depth (To tip of probe)
Healed skin= 2   Sub-cutaneous =1 1/2
Muscle/ tendon = 1   Bone/ Joint =0
Infection/Bioburden
Colonized = 2   Cellulitic =1   Septic = 0
Perfusion
Palpable/pink = 2   Doppler/ pale= 1
Nonel purplish = 0

See Table 5-2   Pg. 114

Impression(s)
Wound Problem(s)

Comorbidities
Contributing to wound problems
Incidental Diagnoses

☐ 8-10 = Healthy   **W.S. =** [Points]
☐ 4-7 = Problem   1 1/2- 4 1/2=
☐ 0-3 = Futile   ☐ End-stage
                  ☐ Salvage ☐ Amputate

Comments: This portion of the **Wound Evaluation, Management, and Prevention** form (i.e. its second third) assists in obtaining and recalling the essential elements of the <u>examination portion</u> of the initial encounter with a patient who has a wound problem.

Note how it includes and integrates the information from the **Wound Score** and the sensation, skin and toenail assessments.

Also note how the **Impression(s)** portion is divided into three components to facilitate management (next section) as well as coding and billing.

Initial Evaluation (Management Portion)

▶ Management ◀

Preparation of Wound Base
Debridements, surgeries/biopsies, hydrotherapy

Protection/Stabilization
Dressings, wraps, splints, casts, orthotics

Medical Interventions
Cultures, antibiotics, nutrition, lab, referrals

Dressing Agents
Moistened gauze, impervious, absorptive ,ointments

Wound Oxygenation
Meds, edema reduction, surgery, HBO, TCOMS

The subjects for Chapters 6-10

Management Strategies

Skin/Toenails
☐ Continue present management
☐ In-clinic skin care and instruction; continuation at home
☐ Toenail care; # of toenails____

Additional Activities/weight
Bearing; schedule surgery; consultations; special studies, etc.

Management Algorithm
Return____Week(s)

Better	No Change	Worse

Signature _____
Revised: 24 November 2009

Name
MR #

Comments: This portion of the **Wound Evaluation, Management, and Prevention** form (i.e. its third third) assists in recalling and initiation of the essential elements of the <u>management</u> interventions for the initial encounter with a patient who has a wound problem.

Note how it includes the **Management Strategies** (Chapters 6-10) to ensure that no strategy is overlooked.

The **Management Algorithm** is included to give the patient the possible outcome permutations for his/her wound, what will be done for each permutation (depending on which one occurs) at the time of the return visit and as a concluding comment for the medical records as well as the information sent to the referring physician.

Follow-up Evaluation (Upper half)

Wound Follow-up and Continuing Care

Day	Month	Year

Status Recapitulation including age, sex, co-morbidities contributing to wound, interval since hospital discharge or last wound clinic evaluation, wound location and mini-description, changes in wound since previous exam, pain level and past surgeries for wound problem

New Information New intercurrent problems, new laboratory and/or imaging information, changes in activity level/ travels, changes in medications, changes in severity of pain, etc.

▶ Examination ◀

Wound Description
(Diagram with labels or describe including, site, area and depth, exudate, type of wound base, odor, biofilm, surrounding skin—including edema, erythema, induration, maceration, etc.)

Skin = ☐ Points
OK = 2/Dry = 1/Crusts = 0

Toenails = ☐ Points
OK = 2/Long = 1/Abnormal = 0

Wound Score

Appearance (Wound base)
Red = 2 White/Yellow = 1 Black = 0 ☐

Size (include recesses)
<Thumb print = 2   Thumb-to-fist =1
>Fist area = 0 ☐

Depth (To tip of probe)
Skin = 2   Sub-Q = 1   Muscle/
Tendon=1   Bone/ Joint =0 ☐

Infection/Bioburden
Colonized = 2   Cellulitic/
Macerated = 1   Septic = 0 ☐

Perfusion Palpable/pink/warm = 2
Doppler/pale/cool=1   No pulses/
purplish/black/cyanotic/cold = 0 ☐

See Table 5-2   Pg. 114

☐ 8-10 = Healthy   **W.S. =** ☐ Points
☐ 4-7 = Problem   ☐ 2 1/2-4 1/2 =
☐ 0-3 = Futile   End-stage
                               ☐ Salvage ☐ Amputate

Interval Changes Describe changes if improved or worsened
☐ **Healed** (2 points)
☐ **Improved** (1 1/2 points)
☐ **No Change** (1 point)
☐ **Worsened** (1/2 point)
☐ **Major amputation/Death** (0 points)

Previous Wound Score ☐ Points

Date | | | | | | |
Day   Month   Year

Forms

Follow-up Evaluation (Bottom half))

Remaining Wound Challenges

The subjects for Chapters 6-10

◆◆◆ Management ◆◆◆

Management Strategies

Preparation of Wound Base ☐ None needed ☐ Interventions
Debridements, surgeries/biopsies, hydro therapy

Protection/Stabilization ☐ No change ☐ Changes
Dressings, wraps, splints, casts. orthotics

Medical Interventions ☐ No change ☐ Changes
Cultures, antibiotics, nutrition, lab/imaging

Dressing Agents ☐ No change ☐ Changes
Moistened gauze, impervious, absorptive, medicinal

Wound Oxygenation ☐ No change ☐ Changes
Meds, edema reduction, surgery, HBO, TCOMS

Skin/ Toenails
☐ Continue present management
☐ In-clinic instruction and care; continue at home
☐ Toenail care; Number of Toenails____

Additional Activity/weight bearing, scheduling surgery, consultations, discharge follow-up
_____
_____
_____

Return _____ ☐ **Discharge**

Name

MR #

Signature _____
Revised: 25 November 2009

Comments : Each portion of this **Follow-up Documentation** form (see the previous page) can be combined onto a chart-sized (8 1/2 X 11) sheet of paper so all information is assessable on one side of a piece of paper. For those using electronic medical records (EMRs), the information in these forms can be generated into a template.

The **Status** section of the form should concisely summarize the patient's wound problem, significant comorbidities and changes since the previous exam; it should negate the need to review the patient's chart for succeeding evaluations.

The **Interval Changes** section uses word descriptions, but also includes corresponding numbers ala an assessment (i.e. 0-to-2 point grading). For "benchmarking" outcomes or research purposes, quantification of outcomes will expedite the review process.

This form also integrates the **Wound Score** and skin and toenail assessments identical to the initial evaluation form.

The **Management Strategies** are likewise analogous to those of the initial evaluation; note boxes are used to indicate choices for each strategy, but the actual interventions should be reiterated.

APPENDIX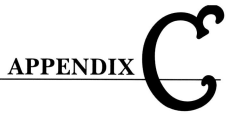

ADDITIONAL SOURCES OF INFORMATION ON PROBLEM WOUNDS AND RELATED SUBJECTS

INTRODUCTION 509
C-1: GUIDELINES AND POSITION PAPERS. 509
C-2: TEXTBOOKS 513
C-3: WOUND JOURNALS. 518
C-4: AUTHORS' RECENT PUBLICATIONS ON
      WOUND-RELATED SUBJECTS. 521
C-5: AUTHORS' RECENT PUBLISHED
      ABSTRACTS/POSTER PRESENTATIONS 530

INTRODUCTION

An enormous body of literature is available on diabetic foot wounds, other problem wounds, pressure ulcers/indolent wounds, and related subjects. Sources include guidelines, textbooks, journals dedicated to or which frequently include articles related to wounds, and the authors' own presentations/publications.

This appendix, while not intended to include every citation available from the above four categories of information, does provide a starting point for the reader of *MasterMinding Wounds* who may want to inquire further on these subjects.

An important objective of *MasterMinding Wounds*, as stated in the preface, is the synthesis of information from the variety of sources mentioned above and then integrating it with the authors' experiences to generate a coherent, organized approach to the evaluation, management, and prevention of problem wounds.

APPENDIX C-1: GUIDELINES AND POSITION PAPERS

Guidelines and position papers are very extensive reviews done by one or more recognized authorities on the titled subject. Essentially, each is a "white paper" (i.e. detailed or authoritative account) on the titled subject. Some of those included in this appendix were generated by ten or more recognized experts.

Because of their focused objectives, they tend to be narrow in scope; hence, the rationale for consolidating their information (with other sources) into a logically organized text as our goal has been in generating *MasterMinding Wounds*. Consider the following, listed alphabetically by the first listed author's surname.

1. **Practical Guidelines on the Management and Prevention of the Diabetic Foot,** APELVIST, J, K Bakker, WH van Houtum, NC Shaper, *Diabetes/Metabolism. Research and Reviews,* 2008; 24(S1): S181-187

   Comment: Excellent, relatively brief summary using bulleted format and numerical lists to minimize verbiage.

2. **Evidence-Based Protocol for Diabetic Foot Ulcers,** BREM, H, P Sheehan, HJ Rosenberg, et al. X-2, *Plastic and Reconstructive Surgery,* 2006; 117(S):193S-209S

   Comment: The authors elaborate on a protocol they developed that rests on six items of information obtained at the initial visit; 161 references.

3. **The Basic Science of Wound Healing,** BROUGHTON, G, JE Jeffrey, C Attinger, *Plastic and Reconstructive Surgery,* 2006; 117(&S):12S-34S

   Comment: Excellent, coherent, and lucid review of a complex and an ever-increasing body of information on this subject; 125 references.

4. **The Effectiveness of Footwear and Offloading Interventions to Prevent and Heal Foot Wounds and Reduce Plantar Pressure in Diabetes: A Systematic Review,** BUS, SA, GD Valk, RW van Derursen, et al. X-5, *Diabetes/Metabolism Research and Reviews, 2008*; 24(S1):S162-S-180

   Comment: A companion paper that elaborates on subjects mentioned in reference #1. The authors' Appendix A is "Literature Search Strings for Each Database" and Appendix B consists of "Evidence Tables;" 116 references.

5. **Consensus Development Conference on Diabetic Foot Wound Care,** CAVANAUGH, PR, JB Buse, RG Frykberg, et al. X-4, *Diabetes Care*, 1999; 22(8):1354-1360

> Comment: Consensus panel's comments to 6 questions relevant to diabetic foot wound care following talks by 25 presenters; 8 references.

6. **International Guidelines. Pressure Ulcer Prevention, Prevalence and Incidence in Context,** HARDING, K, M Baharestani, J Black, M Clark, et al. X-11, Medical Education Partnership Ltd (www.mepltd.co.uk), London , 2009,

> Comment: Consensus opinion of an international group of experts in pressure ulcer prevention and treatment. Includes information about both the NPUAP (National Pressure Ulcer Advisory Panel) and EPUAP (European Pressure Ulcer Advisory Panel) staging systems. The document's goals are to contribute to accurate, standardized data collection and valid interpretation to reduce rates of pressure ulceration worldwide.

7. **Guidelines for the Treatment of Arterial Insufficiency Ulcers,** Hopf, HW, C Ueno, A Rummana, et al. X-12, *Wound Repair and Regeneration*, 2006, 14:693-710

> Comment: Provides guidelines each with their levels of evidence for 1) diagnosis, 91 references; 2) surgery, 20 references; 3) infection control, 41 references; 4) wound bed preparation, 52 references; 5) dressings, 10 references; 6) adjuvant therapy, 62 references; and 7) long term maintenance; 18 references.

8. **Economic Cost of Diabetes in the U.S. in 2002,** HOGAN, P, T Dall, *Diabetes Care*, 2003; 26(3):917-932

> Comment: The authors estimated that the direct costs of diabetes care was 132 billion dollars in 2002. They felt that this "underestimates the true burden of care provided." Included in indirect cost is the care provided by non-paid caregivers, lost work time, and the greater need for ancillary medical services such as dental, optometry, and dietetic. This report was prepared by authors for the Lewin Group, Inc., Falls Church, Virginia.

9. **Diagnosis and Treatment of Diabetic Foot Infections,** LIPSKY, BA, AR Berendt, HG Deery, et al., X-8, **Plastic and Reconstructive Surgery**, 2006; 117(7S): 212S-238S

> **Comments:** Designed as a guideline for managing the diabetic patient with suspected or evident foot infection. Algorithms for diabetic patient with a foot wound, hospitalization considerations, poor response to treatment, established foot infection, and suspected osteomyelitis are somewhat confusing and not well-integrated. Heavy emphasis on infections disease/bacteriological considerations; 290 references.

10. **Chronic Wound Pathogenesis and Current Treatment Strategies: A Unifying Hypothesis,** MUSTOE, TA, K O'Shaughnessy, O Kloeters, **Plastic and Reconstructive Surgery**, 2006; 117S:35S-41S

   Comment: Classification of chronic wounds into three major types: pressure ulcers, venous ulcers, and diabetic ulcers. Much discussion of the ischemia-reperfusion injury; 60 references.

11. **Guidelines for Diabetic Foot Care: Recommendations Endorsed by the Diabetes Committee of the American Orthopaedic Foot and Ankle Society,** PINZUR, MS, MP Slovenkai, E Trepman, NN Shields, **Foot and Ankle International**, 2005, 26(1):113-119

   Comment: The authors emphasize prophylactic foot care for the diabetic with emphasis on the screening examination, patient education, and treatment based on the risk level.

12. **Guidelines for the Treatment of Venous Ulcers,** ROBSON, MC, DM Cooper, A. Rummana, et al. X-10, **Wound Repair and Regeneration**, 2006, 14: 649-662

   Comment: Guidelines with level of evidence for 1) diagnosis, 23 references; 2) compression treatment, 9 references; 3) infection control, 40 references; 4) wound bed preparation, 42 references; 5) dressings, 38 references; 6) surgery, 21 references; 7) adjuvant agents, 63 references; and 8) long term maintenance, 7 references.

13. **Guidelines for the Best Care of Chronic Wounds,** ROBSON, MC, A Barbul, *Wound Repair and Regeneration*, 2006; 14:647-648

   Comment: Defines a chronic wound and then describes the process that evolved in the Wound Healing Society's generation of panels charged to develop guidelines for evaluation and management of 1) arterial insufficiency ulcers, 2) venous ulcers, 3) diabetic ulcers, and 4) pressure sores. A short editorial precedes this article and explains the genesis of the project (pages 645-646). The four guidelines are cited in this appendix (Nos. 7, 12, 14, and 17); 2 references.

14. **Guidelines for the Treatment of Diabetic Ulcers,** STEED, DL, C Attinger, T Colaizzi, et al. X-11, **Wound Repair and Regeneration**, 2006; 14:680-692

   Comment: Guidelines with levels of evidence for 1) diagnosis, 17 references; 2) offloading, 15 references; 3) infection control, 52 references; 4) wound bed preparation, 58 references; 5) dressings, 19 references, 6) surgery, 11 references; 7) adjuvant agents, 44 references; and 8) prevention of recurrences; 14 references.

15. **Practice Guidelines for the Diagnosis and Management of Skin and Soft-Tissue Infections,** STEVENS, DL, AL Bisno, HF Chambers, et al. X-8, *Clinical Infectious Diseases,* 2005; 41-1373, 1406

   Comment: A comprehensive review of skin and soft-tissue infections from an infectious disease perspective with antibiotic recommendations. An algorithm describes the management and treatment of surgical site infections; 236 references.

16. **Consensus Recommendations on Advancing the Standard of Care for Threatening Neuropathic Foot Ulcers in Patients with Diabetes,** SYNDER, RJ, RS Kirsner, RA III Warriner, et al., Wounds, 2010, 22(4 Suppl):S1-S25

   Comment: The end of this consensus report provides a concise summary of recommendations for assessment and treatment of neuropathic diabetic foot ulcers. The article omits information about surgical management of these problems. For example, Figure 2 in the article shows pictures of six diabetic foot wounds and the off-loading options. For almost all of the problems, minimally invasive surgical interventions (which were not mentioned) would effectively manage the problems. Of all the consensus articles in this section, this article provides the most supporting information for using hyperbaric oxygen treatments as an adjunct to management; 111 references.

17. **Using Physiology to Improve Surgical Wound Outcomes,** UENO, C, TK Hunt, HW Hopf, *Plastic and Reconstructive Surgery*, 2006; 117(S):59S-71S

   Comment: Wound healing and prevention of infection can be enhanced in moderate to high risk surgical patients with appropriate antibiotic use, warming to prevent vasoconstriction, maintenance of high oxygen tensions, pain relief, and adequate fluid volume; 89 references.

18. **Guidelines for the Treatment of Pressure Ulcers,** WHITNEY, JA, L Phillips, R Aslam, et al. X-7, *Wound Repair and Regeneration*, 2006; 14:663-679

   Comment: Guidelines with levels of evidence for 1) methods, 12 references; 2) classification of evidence, 5 references; and 3) results (7 subsections): 1-positioning and support surfaces, 13 references; 2-nutrition, 47 references; 3-infection, 50 references; 4-wound bed preparation, 79 references; 5-dressings, 40 references; 6 surgery, 47 references; and 7-adjuvant agents; 23 references.

19. **Current Concepts Review: Diabetic Foot Ulcers,** WUKICH, DK, *Foot & Ankle International,* 2010: 31(5): 460-467

   Comment: A well-referenced review article that addresses evaluation and management of diabetic foot ulcers from Level of Evidence and Grades of Recommendations perspectives. The author states that surgical treatment is indicated for patients who have failed to respond to nonoperative methods or in high risk patients who are subject to recurrences. The author concludes his summary by stating the evidence to support the use of hyperbaric oxygen for diabetic foot ulcers is insufficient at this time, although this adjunctive therapy appears to reduce the incidence of major amputations; 85 references.

APPENDIX C-2: TEXTBOOKS

There are many books dedicated to wound management. An even larger number of books are written on related subjects such as diabetes, foot surgery, vascular insufficiency, hyperbaric oxygen therapy, nutrition, etc., that include information on wound problems. Many of the texts or chapters in them are directed to special audiences such as primary care physicians, nurses, surgeons, podiatrists, wound care specialists, hyperbaric medicine specialists, endocrinologists, etc.

The following is an alphabetical listing of some of the textbooks that are available on wound subjects or have chapters that include information dedicated to wounds. Further information and reviews from readers about these texts can be found on the internet.

1. *Acute & Chronic Wounds: Nursing Management*, 2nd edition, 2000, Ruth Bryant, Mosby, 558 pages

    Comment: Well presented information on anatomy and physiology as well as a comprehensive review of nursing management; reported as a good reference to prepare for nursing wound care board examinations.

2. *Care of Wounds: A Guide for Nurses*, 3rd edition, 2005, Carol Dealey, Oxford, UK, Blackwell Science Inc., 248 pages, paperback

    Comment: A holistic approach to wound management with information about the increasingly important roles of nurses in wound clinics and other venues of wound management.

3. *Chronic Wound Care: A Clinical Source Book for Health Care Professionals*, 3rd edition, Diane Krasner, George Rodeheaver, Gary Sibbald, 2001, HMP Communications, Inc., 760 pages

    Comment: A highly regarded, comprehensive source book for all aspects of wound care. New 4th edition became available in 2007 with 20 new chapters and 135 contributors.

4. *Chronic Wound Care: A Problem-based Learning Approach*, 2004, Edited by Moya Morison, Liza Ovington, Kay Wilkie, Edinburgh; New York, Mosby, 352 pages

    Comment: A similar titled book to the previous citation, but using a problem based learning approach. Paperback book; well illustrated, divided into three sections: approaches (to the subject), case studies, and wound management principles.

5. *Clinical Care of the Diabetic Foot*, 2005, David Armstrong, Lawrence Lavery, American Diabetes Association, 124 pages

    Comment: Contemporary information on diabetes as related to foot care; provides guidelines for evaluation and risk factors.

6. *Clinical Guide to Wound Care,* 4th edition, 2002, Cathy Hess, Lippincott, Williams and Wilkins, 487 pages

    Comment: Minimal wound care information and management, but a good source and description of wound care products; spiral bound.

7. ***Comprehensive Wound Management,*** 2002, Glen Irion, Delmar Learning, 320 pages; 2nd edition scheduled for publication in November 2009 (Slack Incorporated)

   Comment: Single authorship adds continuity to the information presented, but lacks comprehensiveness. Four sections include anatomy, physiology and pathology, establishing a data base (i.e. evaluation), characteristics of wounds, and treatment interventions.

8. ***Cutaneous Wound Healing,*** 2001, Vincent Falanga, T & F STM, Informa Health Care, 520 pages

   Comment: Written by experts in research and clinical practice; discusses state of the art and emerging therapies for cutaneous wound healing; excellent figures.

9. ***Diabetic Foot,*** 7th edition, 2007, Marvin Levin, Lawrence O'Neil, Mosby, 648 pages

   Comment: Well organized with 60 contributors; describes general pathologies and mechanisms of the diabetic and their feet.

10. ***Diabetic Foot (Contemporary Diabetes),*** 2nd edition, 2006, Histidis Veves, John Giurini, Frank Logerfo, Humana Press, 576 pages

    Comment: Written from a surgical perspective; multiple authors; topics range from preventive strategies to cutting edge wound care.

11. ***Epidermis in Wound Healing (Dermatology: Clinical and Basic Science),*** 2003, David Rovee, Howard Maibach, Informa Health Care, 408 pages

    Comment: Multi-authored, current information with the latest research developments.

12. ***Foot in Diabetics,*** 3rd edition, 2000, Andrew Bolton, Henry Connor, Peter Cavanaugh, Wiley-Blackwell, 388 pages

    Comment: Comprehensive and contemporary reviews of diabetic foot disease; vascular surgery perspectives.

13. ***Hyperbaric Medicine Practice,*** 3rd edition, 2008, Eric Kindwall, Harry Whelan, Best Publishing Company, 2008, 1076 pages

    Comment: Written from a hyperbaric medicine focus with chapters on wound healing, chronic wound management, soft tissue infections, refractory osteomyelitis, crush injuries, and burns; multiple contributors.

14. ***Leg and Foot Ulcers:*** A Clinicians Guide, 1995, Vincent Falanga, William Eaglstein, Martin Dunitz, LTD, 192 pages

    Comment: Sections on systemic diseases, peri-wound skin, the wound bed, wound coverage and dressings.

15. ***Management of Diabetic Foot Problems***, 2nd edition, 1995, GP Kozak, DR
    Campbell, RG Frykberg, GM Habershaw, WB Saunders, 308 pages

    Comment: Reviews and guides management of the majority of foot problems
    encountered in diabetic patients. Well illustrated with photos and user
    friendly tables; multiple contributors.

16. ***Molecular and Cell Biology of Wound Repair***, 1996, Richard Clark, Plenum Press,
    611 pages

    Comment: Multiple contributors; the text focuses, as the title indicates, on the
    fundamental biochemistry and cell physiology of wound repair.

17. ***Pressure Ulcers: Guidelines for Prevention and Management***, 2002, 3rd (sub)
    edition, Joann Maklebust, Mary Sieggreen, Lippencott, Williams and Wilkins, 322
    pages

    Comment: Current knowledge on the prevention and treatment of pressure
    ulcers; includes assessment scales, algorithms, and care maps;
    paperback.

18. ***Quick Reference to Wound Care, 2nd edition***, 2005, Pamela Brown, Julie Maloy,
    Jones and Bartlett Publishers, Inc., 300 pages

    Comment: Easy-to-use information for efficient and cost-effective wound care;
    algorithms aid in decision making.

19. ***Scottsdale Wound Management Guide***, 2009, Matthew Livingston, Tom Wolvos,
    HMP Communications Limited, 160 pages

    Comment: A comprehensive guide in an outline format; includes chapters on
    wound assessment, wound etiologies, treatment guidelines,
    products, procedures, studies (assessment), and references
    including indications for hyperbaric oxygen. For those involved
    with wound care, the information is probably too fundamental; for
    others, the outline format could be overwhelming.

20. ***Surgery of the Foot and Ankle***, 8th edition, 2006, Michael Coughlin, Roger Mann,
    Charles Saltzman, Mosby, 2 volumes, 2,400 pages

    Comment: Multi-authored; includes an 87 page chapter with 345 references
    (James Brodsky) on the diabetic foot; written from an orthopaedic
    perspective.

21. ***Surgical Reconstruction of the Diabetic Foot and Ankle***, 2009, Thomas Zgonis,
    Lippincott, Williams and Wilkins, 488 pages

    Comment: Describes surgical management of diabetic limb salvage especially
    from plastic, orthopaedic, and podiatric perspectives; 1200 illustra-
    tions, multi-authored.

22. ***The Wound Care Handbook***, 2nd Edition, 2008, Mona Baharestani, Anne Blackett, Teresa Conner-Kerr, et al; X-22, Medline Industries, Inc., Mundelein, Illinois, 522 pages

> Comment: An excellent reference source from a nursing perspective on almost all aspects of wound care including chapters on guidelines and codes. Information laden tables and test boxes make the text "user friendly." A wound care product list tabulated by product categories includes almost 700 entries. A CD with wound images accompanies the text.

23. ***Text Atlas of Wound Management***, 2001, Vincent Falanga, Tania Phillips, Keith Harding, et al. X-2, Informa Health Care, 320 pages

> Comment: A pictorial guide to wound management; photos used to describe alternatives for diagnosis and treatment of wounds; paperback.

24. ***Wound Care***, 1986, Stephen Westaby, Mosby, 205 pages

> Comment: Information presented from a surgical perspective; excellent illustrations; paperback.

25. ***Wound Care: A Collaborative Practice Manual for Physical Therapists and Nurses***, 2nd edition, 2006, Carrie Sussman, Barbara Bates-Jensen, Lippincott, Williams and Wilkins, 720 pages

> Comment: Very comprehensive dual authorship text that discusses almost every possible consideration for the evaluation and management of wounds; this new edition has added chapters on pain and negative pressure wound therapy.

26. ***Wound Care Essentials: Practice Principles***, 2004, Sharon Baranoski, Elizabeth Ayello, Lippincott, Williams and Wilkins, 432 pages

> Comment: Thorough coverage of wound assessments and management with focus on pressure ulcers from a nursing perspective.

27. ***Wound Care Facts Made Incredibly Quick!***, 2006, Springhouse and Springhouse Corporation, Lippincott, Williams and Wilkins, 128 pages

> Comment: One third of the "incredible" series wound book collection; pocket size (3 ½ by 6 square inches) paperback book with assessment tools, wound coverage products, and algorithms on how to manage different types of wounds.

28. **Wound Care Made Incredibly Easy!**, 2nd edition, 2006, Springhouse and Springhouse Corporation, Lippincott, Williams and Wilkins, 288 pages

> Comment: Basic principles for wound evaluation and management; uses memory aids, illustrations, logos, and algorithms to convey the information in a simplified, easy to assimilate fashion; paperback.

29. ***Wound Care Made Incredibly Visual!***, 2007, Springhouse and Springhouse Corporation, Lippincott, Williams and Wilkins, 192 pages

> **Comments:** Effectively employs hundreds of full-color graphics to demonstrate anatomy, physiology, and wound evaluation and management; uses mnemonics and quizzes as learning aids.

30. *Wound Care Practice*, 2nd edition, 2007, Paul Sheffield, Caroline Fife, Best Publishing Company, 1312 pages (2 volumes)

    Comments: Comprehensive resource on wounds with 65 contributors, with some repetition of information; the second edition expands information on pain management, nutrition, wounds in the young and elderly, and ethics and legal medicine; illustrated with over 500 photos, graphs and figures; more a collection of monographs than a textbook on wound practice.

31. *Wound Healing: Alternatives in Management (Contemporary Perspectives in Rehabilitation)*, 3rd edition, 2001, Luther Kloth, Joseph McCulloch, F.A. Davis, 568 pages

    Comment: Information presented from a physical therapy and rehabilitation perspective; the 3rd edition has improved illustrations and added chapters on electrical stimulation and alternative interventions, 18 contributors.

32. *Wound Healing (Basic and Clinical Dermatology)*, 2005, 08 & 09, Anna Falabella, Robert Kirsner, Taylor & Francis Group, 723 pages

    Comment: Comprehensive review and recent developments from basic sciences to treatment strategies; analyses of the newest wound care research; information is presented from a dermatology perspective; multiple contributors.

33. *Wound Healing Methods and Protocols*, 2003, LA DiPietro, AL Burns, Humana Press, 467 pages

    Comment: Totally science/research oriented with animal models for wound studies and wound repair; 78 contributors.

34. *Wound Management*, 2nd edition, 2007, Betsy Hall, Prentice Hall, 504 pages

    Comment: A comprehensive, holistic approach with emphasis on the patient rather than the wound; learning aids include key terms and objectives at the beginnings of chapters, case studies, and review questions at the ends of chapters.

APPENDIX C-3: WOUND JOURNALS

The nine journals described in this section are fully dedicated to wound subjects. Because of their periodicity, journals offer more up-to-date information than textbooks. However, even though most of the journals are peer reviewed, the information that is published in them often can not be directly and/or immediately applied to wound care practice because of its investigative and/or anecdotal nature. This contrasts to textbooks where the authors, editors, and contributors typically present their information as "state of the art" so it can be directly applied to managing and preventing wounds.

Many other journals publish articles on wound related subjects such as wound problems in diabetes (e.g. *Diabetes Care*), Charcot arthropathy (e.g. *American Journal of Foot Surgery, Foot & Ankle International*), orthotics (e.g. *BioMechanics*), wound coverage/closure (e.g. *Journal of Plastic and Reconstructive Surgery*), peripheral vascular disease (e.g. *Journal of Vascular Surgery*), wound repair and biochemistry (e.g. *Journal of Investigative Dermatology*), wound infections (e.g. *Journal of Infectious Diseases*), etc. Wound related articles occasionally even appear in such renowned journals as the *Journal of the American Medical Association, Lancet,* and the *New England Journal of Medicine*. It is difficult to keep informed of all the new information that appears on wounds from such diverse sources. Wound review articles, sections in the dedicated wound journals with published abstracts from other journals (such as those mentioned above), and internet searches can help mitigate this challenge.

1. *Advances in Skin and Wound Care* (Lippincott, Williams and Wilkins)

Focus:	Multidisciplinary; cutting edge original research and practical clinical management
Review Process:	Peer review
Associations:	Professional Wound Care Association and National Alliance of Wound Care
Miscellaneous:	Continuing medical education/continuing education credit for physicians and nurses
Contact:	http://www.woundcarejournal.com

2. *International Wound Journal* (Wiley-Blackwell)

Focus:	Clinically relevant and focused research; fostering of partnerships between industry, clinicians, and researchers
Review Process:	Peer review
Miscellaneous:	Strategic partners include: 1) Medical Help Lines.Com, Inc (3M), 2) Smith & Nephew, 3) KCI, and 4) ConvaTec
Contact:	http://www.iwjregister.com; Box 2394, Cardiff DF239WQ, United Kingdom

3. *Journal of Wound Care* (MA Health care)

Focus:	A leading source of tissue viability research and clinical information; cutting edge and state-of-the-art research and practice articles
Review Process:	Peer review
Contact:	http://www.journal ofwoundcare.com; MA Health care Ltd., St Jude's Church, Dulwich Road, London, SE24OPB, United Kingdom

4. *Ostomy Wound Management* (HMP Communications, LLC)

Focus: Contemporary and comprehensive review and research papers that are practical, clinically oriented, and cutting edge

Review Process: Peer review, blinded by both an editorial advisory board and an ad-hoc peer review panel

Associations: Official publication of the Advanced Wound Care Society

Miscellaneous: Editorial philosophy: 1) advance the science and art of skin, wound, ostomy, and incontinence care, 2) help authors clearly express and share their findings and ideas, and 3) improve the quality of patient care and protect the public by monitoring the scientific integrity of information published in the journal

Contact: http://www.o-wm.com; 83 General Warren Blvd., Suite 100, Malvern, Pennsylvania 19355

5. *Wound Ostomy Continence Nursing* (Lippincott, Williams and Wilkins)

Focus: Wound, ostomy, and continence care from a nursing perspective with examination of topics such as abdominal stomas, wounds, pressure sores, etc., from in-hospital, home, and long term care settings

Review Process: Peer review

Associations: Wound, Ostomy, and Continence Nurses Society

Miscellaneous: Continuing medical education for the entire scope of nursing practice of wound, ostomy, and continence care

Contact: http://journals.lww.com; 530 Walnut street, Philadelphia, Pennsylvania 19106

6. *World Wide Wounds* (Joint publication of Surgical Materials Testing Laboratory and the Medical Education Partnership)

Focus: An online resource for information on dressing materials that provides guidance on all aspects of wound management

Review Process: Peer review

Associations: Wound, Ostomy, and Continence Nurses Society

Miscellaneous: Information varies in complexity from those nurses in training on to experts in the field

Contact: http://www.worldwidewounds.com

7. *Wound Care Canada*

Focus: Dedicated to the advancement of wound care in Canada; coordinates collaborative interdisciplinary effort among individuals and organizations involved with wounds

Review Process: Not specified

Associations: Canadian Association of Wound Care

Miscellaneous: Programs: 1) public policy, clinical practice, 2) education research and 3) connecting with international wound care committees

Contact: http://www.cacw.net/os/open/wcc/index.html; 2171 Avenue Road, Suite 102, Toronto, Ontario, Canada M5M 4B4

8. *Wound Repair and Regeneration* (Wiley-Blackwell)

Focus: Extensive international coverage of cellular and molecular biology, connective tissue, and biological mediator studies in the field of tissue repair and regeneration

Review Process: Peer reviewed

Associations: Wound Healing Society, European Tissue Repair Society, The Japanese Society for Wound Healing, and the Australian Wound Management Association

Miscellaneous: For diverse audience including plastic surgeons, dematologists, biochemists, cell biologists, and others

Contact: http://www.wiley.com/bw/journal.asp?ref=1067-1927; John Wiley & Sons, Inc., 350 Main Street, Malden, Massachusetts 02148

9. *Wounds* (HMP Communications, LLC)

Focus: Wound care and wound research; information includes research commentaries on wound repair and regeneration, biology and biochemistry of wound healing, and clinical managements of wounds that have a variety of etiologies

Review Process: Peer reviewed

Associations: Advanced Wound Care Society

Miscellaneous: "Sister" publication of the other HMP Communications publication ***Ostomy Wound Management;*** reported to be the most widely read peer reviewed wound journal; it has a multidisciplinary readership that includes surgeons (general, plastic, vascular, orthopaedic), dermatologists, internists/family medicine/infectious disease practioners, gerontologists, podiatrists, research scientists, nurse practioners/wound care specialists, and physician assistants

Contact: http://www.woundresearch.com; 83 General Warren Blvd, Suite 100, Malvern, Pennsylvania 19355

APPENDIX C-4: AUTHORS' RECENT PUBLICATIONS ON WOUND-RELATED SUBJECTS

The following is a chronological listing of articles, book chapters, and letters to the editors that we have authored during the past decade. They have appeared in a variety of publications, some peer reviewed, some editor reviewed, and others as invited experts on the subject. A couple of the later articles are updated versions requested by journal editors of articles written earlier in the decade.

The attentive reader will note that there is some repetition of information among the publications, but probably no more so than would be expected from any other author's oeuvre on a focused subject such as wounds.

Regardless, the connection between the information in all of our publications is that each has links in one form or another to our **Master Algorithm** (Chapters 5-16 and Appendix C-2) for the evaluation, management, and prevention of problem wounds. Again, the attentive reader will notice that as the list of articles progresses, the information builds on itself, and becomes more organized and better defined. The result is the generation of a "final product," that has become our text, *MasterMinding Wounds*.

1. *Wound Scoring System Streamlines Decision-Making*, Strauss, MB & WG Strauss, *BioMechanics*, 1999; VI (8):37-43

    Comment: This article introduces our new simplified scoring systems based on summating 5 assessments, each graded from 2 points (best) to 0 points (worst) to generate 0 to 10 point scores. **The Wound Score**, **Host-Function Score,** and **Goal-Aspiration Score** evolved from this system. From these scores it became possible to make objective decisions with quantifying information for wound management.

2. **Problem Wounds, Practical Solutions, MB Strauss**, J Musculoskeletal, 2000; May: 267-283

    Comment: The **Wound Score** makes it possible to quantify wound types, i.e. "healthy," "problem," and "futile" based on the five assessment 0 to 10 scoring system. From this information, rational decisions are made for wound management.

3. **Problem Wounds: How to Promote Healing, Prevent Recurrence**, Strauss, MB, *Consultant*; 2000; 40(13):2259-2273

    Comment: The **Wound Score** is used to differentiate "problem" from "futile" wounds. Comprehensive management is required for healing of "problem" wounds and includes optimizing the host status and making the wound environment as healthy as possible. Amputation is typically required for "futile" wounds. Measures to prevent wound recurrences include appropriate skin and toenail care, immediate attention to skin sites that show pressure concentrations, and rehabilitation maximized for each patient's potential.

4. **Treatment Strategies for Managing Problem Diabetic Foot Wounds**, Strauss, MB & Pinzar, MS, *68th Annual Meeting Proceedings of the American Academy of Orthopaedic Surgeons*, 2001, 2:675-676

> Comment: This summary accompanied our first scientific exhibit on diabetic foot wounds presented at the American Academy of Orthopaedic Surgeons and the American College of Surgeons (2002) meetings. This and three succeeding scientific exhibits (2002, 2003 and 2005) were generated as a project of the Diabetic Foot Committee of the American Orthopaedic Foot and Ankle Society. Four treatment strategies are discussed, namely: 1) wound base preparation, 2) wound protection, 3) dressing selection, and 4) wound oxygenation. These were the four predecessors to our five treatment strategies (Part III) of our **Master Algorithm**. The strategies complement one another and need to be used in order to achieve optimal results for healing diabetic foot wounds. Surgeons contribute primarily to the wound base preparation and wound protection strategies.

5. **Diabetic Foot and Leg Wounds, Principles, Management and Prevention**, Strauss, MB, *Primary Care Reports*, 2001; 7(22):187-197

> Comment: This article begins with a discussion of three factors that must be addressed for healing of "problem wounds," namely: 1) perfusion/oxygen requirements, 2) stages of healing, and 3) the metabolic demands of wound healing and infection control. In addition, strategies for healing and prevention of diabetic foot wounds are described.

6. **Diabetic Foot Problems: Keys to Prompt, Aggressive Prevention**, Strauss, MB, *Consultant*, 2001; 41:1693-1705

> Comment: Direct (e.g. hypoxia and mechanical problems) and indirect (neuropathy) causes of diabetic foot wounds are put into perspective and used as a basis for detailing prevention strategies.

7. **Diabetic Foot Problems: Keys to Prompt, Aggressive Therapy,** Strauss, MB, *Consultant*; 42(1): 81-93

> Comment: This article is a sequel to the previous article and focuses on the four strategies for managing "problem" wounds including 1) preparation of the wound base, 2) protection and stabilization of the wound, 3) selection of dressing agents, and 4) proactive surgeries.

8. **Management Strategies for Preventing New or Recurrent Diabetic Foot Wounds.** Strauss, MB & MS Pinzur, *69th Annual Meeting Proceedings of the American Academy of Orthopaedic Surgeons*, 2002, 3:752

> Comment: This summary accompanied our second scientific exhibit presented at the American Academy of Orthopaedic Surgeons annual meeting. Four prevention strategies including 1) patient education, 2) foot/leg skin and toenail care, 3) protective footwear, and 4) proactive surgeries effectively prevent new or recurrent diabetic foot wounds.

9. **Hyperbaric Oxygen, The Cutting Edge**, Strauss, MB, BJ Bryant, *Orthopaedics*, 2002; 25(3):303-310

> Comment: Orthopaedic related, Medicare approved indications for hyperbaric oxygen (HBO) are discussed. Not surprisingly, all these approved conditions, which range from gas gangrene to crush injuries to diabetic foot problems, are associated with wounds. Criteria are offered to objectify the use of HBO for these indications.

10. **Forefoot Narrowing with External Fixation for Problem Cleft Wounds**, Strauss, MB & BJ Bryant, *Foot & Ankle International*, 2002, 23(5):433-439

> Comment: This article describes the application of mini external fixators to narrow ischemic forefoot cleft wounds in over 20 patients who would have otherwise required transmetatarsal or higher amputation.

11. **Transcutaneous Oxygen Measurements under Hyperbaric Oxygen Conditions as a Predictor for Healing of Problem Wounds**, Strauss, MB, BJ Bryant & GB Hart, *Foot & Ankle International*, 2002; 23(5):433-439

> Comment: If juxta-wound transcutaneous oxygen (HBO) measurements increase to over 200 mmHg during a hyperbaric oxygen exposure, the positive predictive value for wound healing is 0.87 if HBO is used as an adjunct to management regardless of the room air transcutaneous oxygen measurements.

12. **Pressure Ulcers**, Strauss, MB, *Hospital Physician*, 38(6): 18-19

> Comments: This letter to the editor was written in response to Drs. Daharmarajan and Ugalino's article (*Hospital Physician*, 2002; 38(3):64-71) about prevention and management of pressure ulcers. Concerns were expressed about the failure of the authors to address the "end-stage" pressure sore where surgical release of lower extremity contractures may be the only method for managing the problems short of major lower limb amputations.

13. **The Role of Hyperbaric Oxygen in the Surgical Management of Chronic Refractory Osteomyelitis**, Strauss, MB, *Hyperbaric Surgery*, 2002, ed D Bakker & F Cramer, Chapter 3, pp 37-62

> Comment: The chapter presents justification for the use of hyperbaric oxygen in the management of refractory osteomyelitis. It includes 21 illustrations all in color, except those of x-rays.

14. **Hyperbaric Oxygen for Crush Injuries and Compartment Syndromes: Surgical considerations**, Strauss, MB, *Hyperbaric Surgery*, 2002, ed D Bakker & F Cramer, Chapter 13, pp 341-360

> Comment: This chapter provides objective indications for using hyperbaric oxygen as an adjunct for management of crush injuries and compartment syndromes based on contemporary classifications systems, natural history, and outcomes for these conditions.

15. **Hyperbaric Oxygen as an Adjunct to Surgical Management of the Problem Wound**, Strauss, MB, *Hyperbaric Surgery*, 2002, ed D Bakker & F Cramer, Chapter 15, pp 383-396

> Comment: The "problem" wound is defined quantitatively using the **Wound Score**. The specific diagnoses for using hyperbaric oxygen as an adjunct for managing "problem" wounds are listed by acuity. The precursor of the **Master Algorithm** is introduced and includes a section on "pushing the envelope" for managing the particularly difficult wound. Surgical interventions, both in-office and in the operating room, are summarized

16. **A Simplified Neurological Assessment for Management of Problem Wounds,** Strauss, MB, JD Hart & P Aslmand, *Proceedings of the Fourteenth International Congress on Hyperbaric Medicine, ed.* D Bakker & F Cramer, 2003, Best Publishing Company, Flagstaff, Arizona, pp 214-217

> Comment: Sensory neuropathy associated with diabetic foot wounds obviates the need to use the time consuming Semmes-Weinstein monofilament testing protocol. Our wound directed sensory evaluation system is a function of how much pain the patient experiences with wound manipulation (e.g. palpation/probing, dressing changes, discomfort with walking, etc.). From this information, the practioner can readily determine how much, if any, anesthesia is needed for wound debridements and other surgical interventions.

17. **Keep it Simple Management for the Malperforans Ulcer,** Strauss, MB, *Proceedings of the Fourteenth International Congress on Hyperbaric Medicine,* ed. D Bakker & F Cramer, 2003, Best Publishing Company, Flagstaff, Arizona, pp 210-213

> Comment: This brief article introduces the four-stage approach to evaluation and management of the impending and fully manifested malperforans ulcer. A minimally invasive, keep it simple and speedy (MIS/KISS) surgery is described where the metatarsal neck of the depressed metatarsal head (which leads to the pressure concentration occurring with weight bearing and generation of the ulcer) is scored with a 0.62 mm Kirshner wire through a single drill hole. Then, an osteoclasis is performed to elevate the metatarsal head. Immediate weight bearing is encouraged to allow the fractured metatarsal head to balance itself with the adjacent metatarsals.

18. **Hyperbaric Oxygen for the Management of Muscle-Compartment Syndrome,** Strauss, MB**,** *Proceedings of the Fourteenth International Congress on Hyperbaric Medicine,* ed. D Bakker & F Cramer, 2003, Best Publishing Company, Flagstaff, Arizona, pp 157-160

> Comment: The progression of the skeletal muscle compartment syndrome from suspected to impending to manifested ("full blown" requiring a fasciotomy) is described. Previously published laboratory studies and clinical reports strongly support the use of hyperbaric oxygen (HBO) during the impending stage where no other treatment interventions exist. In addition, HBO should be used for wound healing and recovery purposes after a fasciotomy for the manifested syndrome when residual problems such as ischemic muscle, marked edema, threatened flaps, neuropathy, etc. are observed.

19. KISS (Keep It Simple and Speedy) Surgical Strategies for Diabetic Foot Problems, Strauss, MB & MS Pinzur, 70th *Annual Meeting Proceedings of the American Academy of Orthopaedic Surgeons*, 2003, 4:668-669

> Comment: This summary accompanied our third scientific exhibit presented at the American Academy of Orthopaedic Surgeons annual meeting. Proactive surgical procedures, both in-office and in the operating room, including debridements, tenotomies, toe and partial ray amputations, ostectomies, controlled osteoclases, and forefoot narrowing effectively prevent limb threatening complications arising from diabetic foot problems. The thesis of the exhibit is exemplified by the maxim "an ounce of prevention is worth a pound of cure."

20. TCC Substitutes, MB Strauss, *BioMechanics*, 2003; X(9):9-10

> Comments: This letter to the editor in the Contact Point of the journal was written in response to Dr. Gregory Guyton's article (*BioMechanics*, 2003; X(5):55-66) and expresses concerns about using total contact casting (TCC) for management of diabetic foot wounds. TCC concerns include: 1) interference with optimal wound care by preventing access to wounds, 2) overlooking surgically remedial deformities that underlie the wound, 3) its very limited applications (i.e. superficial wounds with minimal exudate and peripheral erythema), and 4) risks of developing limb threatening sepsis from the wound in the enclosed cast. The letter takes exception to Dr. Guyton's statement that "No truly adequate substitute either exists or is likely to be developed in the near future [for the TCC]" for management of the neuropathic wound of the lower extremity.

21. Hyperbaric Oxygen, Aksenov, IV, *New England Journal of Medicine*, 2004, 35:1694

> Comments: This letter to the editor in the journal was written in response to Drs. AJM Bolton, RS Kirsner, and L Vileikyte's article (*New Eng J Med*, 2004, 351:48-55) which discussed evaluation and management of diabetic foot ulcers. The authors considered the use of hyperbaric oxygen (HBO) as an area of uncertainty with lack of supporting data. The letter refutes this statement with evidence from randomized control trials, transcutaneous oxygen measurements, specific clinical indications for using HBO, and authorization of reimbursement by insurance carriers including Medicare when using HBO for diabetic foot ulcers.

22. **Management of Charcot Arthropathy,** Strauss, MB& NN Shields, 72nd *Annual Meeting Proceedings of the American Academy of Orthopaedic Surgeons*, 2005, 6:469

> Comment: This summary accompanied our fourth scientific exhibit presented at the American Academy of Orthopaedic Surgeons annual meeting. Decision making for management of Charcot arthropathy is simplified by using a two question algorithm based on acuity and whether or not a wound is present. Inherent in the decision making process is the need to establish the patient's functional status and aspirations which are quantified by using the **Host-Function** and **Goal-Aspiration Score.**

23. **The Orthopaedic Surgeon's Role in the Strategies for Treatment and Prevention of Diabetic Foot Wounds**, Strauss, MB, *Foot & Ankle International*, 2005; 26(1):5-14

> Comment: This article describes the roles of the orthopaedic surgeon in the management of problem diabetic foot wounds with special emphasis on the wound base preparation and protection-immobilization strategies.

24. **Hyperbaric Oxygen as an Intervention for Managing Wound Hypoxia; Its Role and Usefulness on Diabetic Foot Wounds**, Strauss, MB, *Foot & Ankle International,* 2005, 26 (1):15-18

> Comment: This position paper succinctly defines the indications and the supporting data for using hyperbaric oxygen for hypoxic, problem diabetic foot wounds.

25. **Consideration of Motor Neuropathy for Managing the Neuropathic Foot,** Sussman, C, MB Strauss, DD Barry & E Ayyapa, *Journal of Prosthetics and Orthotics,* 2005; 17(2) Suppl:528-531

> Comment: The latter half of this article discusses the pathomechanics of foot wounds in patients with motor neuropathies, the importance of medical management, and the in-office procedures that can be used for managing these problems.

26. **Vascular Assessment of the Neuropathic Foot,** Strauss, MB & DD Barry, *Journal of Prosthetics and Orthotics*, 2005; 17(2) Suppl:535-537

> Comment: This article concisely describes the importance of and methods for doing the vascular assessment of the diabetic foot as well as other conditions which may be associated with peripheral artery disease. The vascular assessment is considered in the context of the comprehensive wound evaluation.

27. **Evaluation of Diabetic Wound Classifications and a New Wound Score**, Strauss, MB & IV Aksenov, *Clinical Orthopaedics and Related Research, 2005, 439:79-86*

> Comment: Seven published diabetic foot wound scoring systems are evaluated from ten perspectives. The **Wound Score** is then evaluated from the same perspectives to confirm the value of this paradigm for assessing, managing, and quantifying healing responses of "problem" wounds.

28. **Surgical Treatment of Problem Foot Wounds in Patients with Diabetes**, Strauss, MB, *Clinical Orthopaedics and Related Research*, 2005, 439:91-96

    Comment: This paper summarizes the "art" of surgical management of foot wounds in patients with diabetes. Minimally invasive surgical techniques for five types of wounds are described. Misconceptions regarding functional outcomes and durability of wound healing are addressed.

29. **Problem Wounds, Practical Solutions**, MB Strauss, *Journal of Musculoskeletal Medicine*, 2006; 23(4):251-262

    Comment: This is an updated version of the 2000 article with the same title generated at the request of the journal's editors. It "fine tunes" the **Wound**, **Host-Function** and **Goal-Aspiration Score**, and discusses nutrition and wound covering dressing agents. Algorithms for decision-making in wound management are included.

30. **Diabetic Foot Problems: Keys to Effective, Aggressive Prevention,** Strauss, MB & SS Miller, *Consultant*, 2007, 47)3):245-252

    Comment: This totally rewritten article at the editor's request utilizes the title of the 2001 article (see citation 6). It further updates and refines the four strategies (i.e. patient education, skin and toenail care, selection of appropriate protective footwear, and proactive surgeries) for prevention of new and/or recurrent diabetic foot wounds.

31. **Addressing Foot Skin and Toenail Concerns in Diabetics,** Strauss, MB & SS Miller, *Journal of Musculoskeletal Medicine*, 2007; 24(8):348-351

    Comment: "Tools" are introduced for the objective evaluation and management of foot skin and toenail concerns in diabetics. "Quick and Easy" scoring systems in table formats are provided to assess patient goals, perfusion, sensation, skin condition, ambulation, and toenail conditions.

32. **Diabetic Foot Skin and Toenail Care: Debunking the Myths**, Strauss, MB & SS Miller, *Journal of Musculoskeletal Medicine*, 2007; 24(8):348-351

    Comment: Five myths regarding diabetic foot skin and toenail problems are presented, and the "realities" of the situations explained. Advice accompanies each debunked myth.

33. **Practitioners Face Facts in Foot Care Treatment**, Strauss, MB & SS Miller, *BioMechanics, 2007*; XIV(11):49-53

    Comments: This article, requested by the journal's editor, presents information from the previous article in a different perspective. While myths persist, especially for the management of diabetic foot problems, quality patient care calls for practical solutions. It includes information that explains why neuropathy is not a direct cause of diabetic foot wounds, and if present, usually does not interfere with wound healing. Likewise, peripheral artery disease may slow healing, but in most situations healing will occur with proper wound management.

34. **Crush Injuries: Justification of and Indications for Hyperbaric Oxygen Therapy,** Strauss, MB & L Garcia-Covarrubias, *Physiology and Medicine of Hyperbaric Oxygen*, 2008; ed T Neuman & S Thom, Saunders, Elsevier, Philadelphia, Pennsylvania,, Chapter 20, pp 427-429

   Comment: This chapter presents the most evidence-based and up-to-date biochemical information available for justifying the use of hyperbaric oxygen in the management of crush injuries and skeletal muscle compartment syndromes.

35. **The Role of Hyperbaric Oxygen in the Management of Chronic Refractory Osteomyelitis,** Strauss, MB & SS Miller, *Hyperbaric Medicine Practice*, 3rd edition, 2008, ed. E Kindwall & H Wheelan, Best Publishing Company, Flagstaff, Arizona, Chapter 25, pp 677-709

   Comment: This entirely new chapter (different author from previous editions) for the 3rd edition explains the pathophysiology of refractory osteomyelitis and updates the laboratory and clinical literature. The authors provide their own definition of refractory osteomyelitis and its presentations and use the **Host-Function** and **Goal-Aspiration Score** to justify decisions regarding treating the infection or proceeding directly to a limb amputation. Management strategies are described including the use of hyperbaric oxygen (HBO). The authors use their "Rational-based, Evidence-Appropriate" 0 to 10 point scoring system to further justify the use of HBO for this condition. Finally, ten salient observations about using HBO for refractory osteomyelitis are elaborated.

36. **The Role of Hyperbaric Oxygen in Crush Injury, Skeletal Muscle-compartment Syndrome and other Acute Traumatic Peripheral Ischemias,** Strauss, MB & SS Miller, *Hyperbaric Medicine Practice,* 3rd edition, 2008, ed. E Kindwall & H Whelan, Best Publishing Company, Flagstaff, Arizona, Chapter 28, pp 755-790

   Comment: This chapter is the authors' updated version from the previous two editions. Major changes include all new figures and tables (totaling 22) and the utilization of text boxes to highlight information or add historical tidbits. The chapter remains the definitive source of information for the clinical application of hyperbaric oxygen (HBO) for crush injuries and compartment syndromes. Again, the fundamental concepts of trauma plus ischemia as the initiating problem, a gradient of injury and a self perpetuating hypoxia-edema vicious circle are utilized to explain the pathophysiology of these conditions. Criteria using clinical findings and manometrics to establish the diagnosis and document the stage (e.g. suspected, impending, or manifested—that is "full blown" requiring a fasciotomy) of skeletal muscle-compartment syndrome have been further refined. The "Rational-based, Evidence-Appropriate" scoring system is utilized to justify the decision for using HBO for these conditions.

37. Crush Injury, Compartment Syndrome and Other Acute Traumatic Ischemias, Strauss, MB, *Hyperbaric Oxygen Therapy Indications*, 12th edition, 2008, ed. LB Gesell, Undersea and Hyperbaric Medical Society, Durham, North Carolina, pp 39-50

Comments: The brief section of the Hyperbaric Oxygen Therapy Committee Report of the Undersea and Hyperbaric Medical Society is designed to be a position paper for the use of hyperbaric oxygen (HBO) for the conditions titled above. It has six components including: 1) rationale, 2) patient selection criteria, 3) clinical management, 4) supporting literature 5) utilization review, and 6) cost impact. Four tables and two figures similar to those used in the preceding citation supplement 6 ¼ pages of prose. The Food and Drug Administration recognizes the report as an original source document and uses it to answer inquiries it receives about approved indications (from the report) and off-label uses of HBO. Most medical insurance payors use the Committee Report as a guide for reimbursements of HBO treatments.

APPENDIX C-5: AUTHORS' RECENT PUBLISHED ABSTRACTS/ POSTER PRESENTATIONS

To complete this section of Appendix C, we list our recently (1997-2009) published abstracts with their conclusions produced during the past decade. Each abstract was the precursor to a poster presentation. Like our publications, they confirm our broad interest in problem wound related matters and show the refinement of our thinking about this subject with succeeding generations of posters.

Often the information in published abstracts is not appreciated, not readily available, nor considered substantial enough to be included as a reference. For this reason, we rarely include a published abstract as a reference in the chapters of our text. However, the perusal of the following abstracts will add to the appreciation of our algorithmic and ten-point scoring approaches to the evaluation, management and prevention of problem wounds. More importantly, for those who are interested, they may become a stimulus to further validate or refute the conclusions given in the abstracts.

In our situation, the published abstracts/poster presentations became a valuable learning experience. Not only did they require us to organize our information concisely, but it gave us the chance to generate graphics which ultimately evolved to the quality that could be used in *MasterMinding Wounds*. The constructive criticisms and provocative questions the viewers of our posters (and in some cases associated podium presentations) rendered stimulated us to resolve the conflicts and streamline our thinking on challenging and perplexing wound matters.

Because of the Undersea and Hyperbaric Medical Society's (UHMS) widespread interest in wound healing and hyperbaric oxygen, almost all of these posters were initially presented at their annual meetings. However, some of them were subsequently presented at other meetings, such as the American Academy of Orthopaedic Surgeons, the American Foot and Ankle Society, The American College of Chest Physicians, Advanced Society of Wound Care, and the Pacific Chapter of the UHMS meetings.

Below are the titles of our recently published abstracts along with their conclusions. To view the complete abstracts, please go online to http://archive.rubicon-foundation.org/ and enter the abstract title in the search box.

1. **Undersea and Hyperbaric Medical Society Annual Meeting, 15-22 June 1997, Cozumel, Mexico, *Undersea and Hyperbaric Medicine*, Volume 24, 1997 Supplement**

- **Use of Transcutaneous Oxygen Measurements to Predict Healing in Foot Wounds,** Strauss MB. JW Breedlove & GB Hart #40, p15

  Transcutaneous oxygen measurements (TCOM) under hyperbaric oxygen conditions in our study group have clearly separated out two patient groups with respect to healing of foot wounds. Healing of foot wounds can be anticipated (98% likelihood) if TCOM's adjacent to the wound during a HBO treatment are equal to or greater than 200 mmHg. If they are less than 100 mmHg, healing is unlikely.

- **Management of Infected Charcot Arthropathies of Foot and Ankle Wounds,** Strauss MB. P. Weinstein #109, p27

  Comprehensive management of infected Charcot arthropathies of the foot and ankle has resulted in acceptable limb salvage and function in 72% of the patients (excellent or good results) in our series of 21. Hyperbaric oxygen was a useful adjunct in controlling infection and achieving healing in all of the foot and ankle wounds. We feel that the results from our series provide an acceptable alternative to amputation, the traditional management of infected Charcot arthropathies of the foot and ankle.

- **Effect of Smoking Cessation on Transcutaneous Oxygen Measurements—A Case Report and Review,** Strauss AG, GB Hart & MB Strauss, #166, p 36

  This report quantifies the benefits smoking cessation has on tissue oxygenation. A 220% improvement in transcutaneous oxygen with room air (breathing) and a 144% improvement with hyperbaric oxygen were recorded at identical measurement sites immediately after smoking was stopped in our study group.

- **Use of the One-Two-Three Protocol to Augment HBO Management of Dysvascular Foot Wounds,** Strauss MB. P. Chase, N Kustich & P Nation, # 167, p37

  The 1-2-3 Protocol (augmenting tissue oxygenation by pharmacological means using nitroglycerin patches locally, nifedipine systemically or combinations) appears to be a useful intervention in managing dysvascular wounds where hyperbaric oxygen alone does not elevate transcutaneous oxygen (levels) sufficiently for wound healing to occur. Further observations with this protocol are needed in order to fully establish its efficacy.

2. **Undersea and Hyperbaric Medical Society Annual Meeting, 19-26 May 1998, Seattle, Washington,** *Undersea and Hyperbaric Medicine*, **Volume 25, 1998 Supplement**

   - **The Memorial (Strauss) Wound Grading Score,** Strauss MB. DM Winant & MB Symes, #28, p16

     Our new wound grading system corrects the deficiencies of the other currently used scores. It is objective enough that correlations with other wound predicting factors (e.g. $PtcO_2$'s, nutrition, host status) are easy to calculate. It is dynamic enough that interval scoring can accurately measure progress. Finally, it is simple enough that it only takes a few seconds to generate a score.

   - **The Predictability of Transcutaneous Oxygen Measurements for Wound Healing,** Strauss, MB, DM Winant, JW Breedlove, et al. X-2 #58, p24

     Transcutaneous oxygen measures with hyperbaric oxygen (HBO) define a responder group, which have a high predictive value for healing of hypoxic (in room air) problem wounds. The information helps to objectify the indications for HBO in the problem wound.

- **Predicting Outcomes in Problem Wounds with the Memorial (Strauss) Wound Grading Score,** Strauss, MB, DM Winant & MB Symes, #74, p 29

  A trial evaluation of our Wound Grading System (WGS) found that it was user friendly and predicted clinical outcomes. Our data suggests that wound scores < 4 (Group 1) will not likely heal even with adjunctive hyperbaric oxygen (HBO). **Wound Scores** of 4-7 (Group 2) will likely heal with adjunctive HBO and in Group 3 with **Wound Scores**, >7 healing will occur without HBO. This simple WGS provides useful information for decision making and management of problem wounds as well as quantifying wound progress. Further clinical validation of the WGS is in progress.

- **Healing in Post-hyperbaric Oxygen, Post-operative Failed, Sloughed, Dehisced Foot Wounds,** Strauss, MB, CE Futenma, JD Hart, #78, p 30

  Our surprisingly good results in what otherwise would be considered treatment failures are attributed to optimal wound management and compliant, highly motivated patients. Hyperbaric oxygen appears to initiate the neovascularization process in these dysvascular patients which continues, albeit slowly, through the four phases of healing in these failed, sloughed, dehisced wounds. Awareness of these healing stages allows the wound healing team to provide sound, realistic, and predictable advice.

- **Pharmacologic Augmentaton of Blood Flow to Dysvascular Foot Wounds Using the 1-2-3 Protocol with Hyperbaric Oxygen Therapy,** Strauss, MB, DM Winant & P Nation, #151, p 50

  In patients with wound hypoxia, a responder group to hyperbaric oxygen (HBO) augmented their transcutaneous oxygen measurements with the use of nitroglycerin patches, Nifedipine orally, and combinations of the two agents. A non-responder group to HBO did not show similar responses. The combined use of these two agents resulted in over a 200% improvement in the responder group's transcutaneous oxygen measurements.

3. **Undersea and Hyperbaric Medical Society Annual Meeting, 18-20 June 2000, Stockholm Sweden,** *Undersea and Hyperbaric Medicine,* **Volume 27, 2000 Supplement**

- **Prospective Evaluation of a Clinical Wound Score to Identify Lower Extremity Wounds for Comprehensive Wound Management,** Borer, KM, RC Borer & MB Strauss, #81, p 34

  Our prospective data indicate that a simple wound score performed on initial examination of lower extremity problem wounds can be useful in selecting wounds appropriate for comprehensive management that results in wound healing.

- **An Algorithm Approach to Decision Making in Problem Wounds,** Strauss, MB, RC Borer & KM Borer #84, p 35

  Our algorithm approach was predictive of healing in 41/50 (82%) of patients with [initial] wound scores greater than 3. When wound scores are 3 or less, supplemental scores help decide which patients are candidates for amputation or for "special considerations" such as revascularization, a trial of ten HBO treatments, pharmacological augmentation of wound oxygenation, and/or special surgical techniques for wound coverage.

- **Nutrition Assessment in Management of Problem Wounds,** Strauss, MB, MB Syms, KM Borer & WG Strauss, # 85 p 35

  The Nutrition Score supplements the clinical assessment of a patient with a problem wound. Nutrition scores respond, albeit slowly, to interventions. Healing and infection control are incompatible with low nutrition scores. In cases where the wound does not improve (due to peripheral artery disease), nutrition scores may improve. Improvement in nutrition scores parallel the improvements observed in the wound.

- **Prospective Serial Transcutaneous Hyperbaric Oxygen Challenge Measures in Problem Lower Extremity Wounds,** RC Borer, KM Borer & MB Strauss, #100, p 40

  Our prospective data indicate that a HBO challenge transcutaneous oxygen threshold equal to or greater that 200 mmHg can be useful in predicting a favorable response to HBO therapy in selected lower extremity wounds.

- **Do Transcutaneous Carbon Dioxide Measurements Predict Healing of Problem Wounds?** Strauss, MB, AG Strauss, KM Borer. #101, 40

  Transcutaneous carbon dioxide (CO_2) values should be used to supplement the information gained from the transcutaneous oxygen (O_2) values when making predictions about outcomes for problem wounds. Our observations suggest that the "target" group of problem wounds for using hyperbaric oxygen (HBO) are those in which transcutaneous CO_2 values are normal (44 mmHg or less) and transcutaneous O_2s increase to over 200 mmHg with HBO. If transcutaneous CO_2s are elevated and transcutaneous O_2s do not increase to over 200 mmHg with HBO, angioplasty and/or revascularization will probably need to be done if wound healing is to occur. These preliminary observations warrant additional studies to verify the usefulness of transcutaneous CO_2s for problem wound management.

4. Undersea and Hyperbaric Medical Society Annual Meeting, 14-16 June 2000, San Antonio, Texas, *Undersea and Hyperbaric Medicine*, Volume 28, 2001 Supplement

- **Evidence Review of HBO for Crush Injury, Compartment Syndrome and Other Traumatic Ischemias, Wounds,** MB Strauss, #50, p 35
  Hyperbaric oxygen (HBO) qualifies as an evidence-based indication for the acute traumatic peripheral ischemias (ATPI's) on three different evaluation systems. HBO is recommended as an adjunct for managing ATPI's.

- **Augmenting Transcutaneous Oxygen Tensions in Dysvascular Feet with the 1-2-3 Protocol,** Appel, M, P Nation, N Kustich, et al. X-3, # 107, p 60

  Oral nifedipine and local cutaneous nitroglycerin delivery both improve tissue oxygen concentration in patients undergoing hyperbaric oxygen therapy. Oral nifedipine is more effective than local cutaneous nitroglycerin alone or in combination. Its superiority to combination therapy may be due to relative decrease in systemic blood pressure or cardiac output with the combination therapy.

- **Transcutaneous Oximetry as a Predictor of Healing Lower-Extremity Wounds Managed with Hyperbaric Oxygen,** Hartman, LA, MB Strauss & GB Hart, # 109, p 61

  The ultimate criterion for the usefulness of a diagnostic test is whether it adds information that leads to a change in management that is beneficial to the patient. Transcutaneous oxygen tests have likelihood ratios that result in only minor changes in the predictive value (probability) of healing or failing when compared to the known pretest probability. These changes are not of sufficient magnitude to determine which patients should be included or excluded from hyperbaric oxygen therapy.

- **Delayed Healing of Failed Flaps in Problem Wounds after Hyperbaric Oxygen and Surgery,** Strauss, MB & JD Hart, #117, p 65

  Initial failure of healing in problem wounds does not always indicate a major amputation will be necessary. Hyperbaric oxygen (HBO) appears to "jump start" the healing process so gradual sustained wound closure occurs even though HBO may not have provided enough supplemental oxygen to avoid initial wound sloughs or dehiscence. Awareness of this healing potential and stages of healing allows the wound healing team to provide sound, realistic, and predictable advice for their patients.

- **Management of the Skeletal Muscle-Compartment Syndrome, the Role of Hyperbaric Oxygen,** Strauss, MB, #122, p 68

  Knowledge of the stages of the skeletal muscle-compartment syndrome and when hyperbaric oxygen is indicated can lessen the morbidity associated with this problem.

- **The Goal Score as an Aid to Decision Making in Foot Salvage vs. Leg Amputation,** Strauss, MB & LV Smith, #123, p 68

  The **Goal-Aspiration Score** is an adjunct to the clinical assessment of a patient and his/her wound. When wound scores are 4 or greater, there is justification to continue with comprehensive wound management including revascularization, hyperbaric oxygen, pharmacological augmentation of local oxygenations, and innovative surgeries. Low **Goal-Aspiration Scores** (3 or less) support the decision to amputate.

- **Treatment Strategies for Problem Diabetic Foot Wounds,** Strauss, MB & MS Pinzur, #124, p 69

  Major amputation cannot be prevented in all diabetic foot wounds. In the motivated, functional patient, utilization of the 4 strategies described above (wound protection, wound base management, wound dressings and wound oxygenation) can be expected to prevent transtibial or higher amputations in 80% of the patients with problem foot wounds.

- **KISS (Keep It Simple and Speedy) Procedures for Problem Foot Wounds** Strauss, MB & JD Hart #125, p 69

  The KISS approach helps achieve optimal outcomes in the special patient group who have problem wounds associated with host compromising factors. The wound care center needs to be familiar with in-office/in-clinic KISS procedures, while their surgical consultants (orthopaedists, vascular surgeons, plastic surgeons, podiatrists, etc.) with the in-operating room KISS procedures.

5. **Undersea and Hyperbaric Medical Society Annual Meeting, 25-29 May 2004, Sydney, Australia,** *Undersea and Hyperbaric Medicine,* **Volume 31(3), 2004`**

    - **Establishment of Normal Values for Transcutaneous Oxygen and Carbon Dioxide Comparing a Multiplace Exposure with a Monoplace Exposure, Hart, GB & MB Strauss,** #194, p 373

      No statistical significant differences exist between the two protocols' transcutaneous oxygen (TCOM) tensions at the foot (level) or the chest (level). The foot TCOMs, however, are significantly lower than the chest TCOM at all levels when breathing oxygen. The chest transcutaneous carbon dioxide tension in Protocol B (multiplace) increases (it) approximately 8-10 mmHg and is significantly different from Protocol A (monoplace). The foot transcutaneous carbon dioxide tensions decline significantly during the oxygen exposure in both protocols.

6. Undersea and Hyperbaric Medical Society Annual Meeting, 16-18 June 2005, Las Vegas, Nevada, *Undersea and Hyperbaric Medicine*, **Volume 32(4), 2005**

- **The Spectrum and Significance of Medical Problems in Patients with Problem Wounds,** Strauss, AG, IV Aksenov & MB Strauss, #135, p 285
  All patients with problem wounds had one or more medical problems. Those with five or more that interfered with healing (i.e. grade = 0) had poor outcomes (death or major amputation), while those with less than five did not. Since most medical problems are remedial, their management is essential for wound healing.

- **Evaluation of Seven Diabetic Wound Classifications and the Genesis of a New Paradigm for Wound Scoring,** Strauss, MB, IV Aksenov, AG Strauss & EV France, #136, p 285

  Analysis of seven published wound classification systems showed that none meet all the requirements of an optimal wound scoring system. From this review, a new paradigm for wound evaluation evolved which stands up well to the scrutiny of the ten perspectives used to evaluate the published diabetic foot scoring systems.

7. Undersea and Hyperbaric Medical Society Annual Meeting, 16-18 June 2006, Orlando, Florida, *Undersea and Hyperbaric Medicine*, **Volume 33(5), 2006**

- **Classification of Wound Types Using an Objective Scoring System,** Strauss, MB, IV Aksenov & SS Miller, # K9, p 380

  Management of wounds requires the recognition of their severity. This is easy and quickly accomplished using 5 assessments that generate a **Wound Score**. From this information, the severity type, that is, healthy, problem, or futile is established using objective criteria. Management then becomes obvious and outcomes highly predictable.

- **The Goal-Aspiration Score as an Aid in Decision Making for Management of "End-stage" Wounds, Using an Objective Scoring System,** Strauss, MB, IV Aksenov & SS Miller, # K10, p 380

  The **Goal-Aspiration Score** validates the wisdom of William Osler who said it is "better to know the patient than the disease." It (the **Goal-Aspiration Score**) provides another instrument in making a decision to salvage an "end-stage" wound.

- **The Wagner Score: A Boon or Bane,** Strauss, MB, IV Aksenov, SS Miller & EV France # K11, p 380

  Use of the Wagner Grading System for making decisions to justify hyperbaric oxygen (HBO) as an adjunct for managing diabetic foot wounds is a matter of concern. Use of this archaic system may become a liability and a reason diabetic foot wounds (Wagner Grade 3 or higher) may be downgraded to an investigational use of HBO. A more objective approach is the measurement of juxta-wound hypoxia in problem wounds and confirming its resolution with HBO.

8. Undersea and Hyperbaric Medical Society Annual Meeting, 25-28 June 2008, Salt Lake City, Utah, *Undersea and Hyperbaric Medicine,* **Volume 35(4), 2008**

- **Tools for the Objective Management of Diabetic Patients' Foot & Ankle Skin and Toenails,** Strauss, MB, SS Miller & IV Aksenov # D65, p 271

  Our 0-2 point assessment system provides an expedient evaluation of foot ankle skin and toenails (FASTN) conditions and what management is needed. It behooves the wound care specialist, as well as the foot and ankle surgeon, to optimize FASTN care of all diabetic patients being managed for wound or other problems in these structures.

- **The "Quick & Easy" Neurological Assessment of the Diabetic Foot,** Strauss, MB, SS Miller & IV Aksenov # D71, p 274

  The "Quick and Easy" sensory evaluation system of the neuropathic foot makes it possible to do an assessment almost instantaneously, yet is uniformly accurate in predicting the level of anesthesia needed for wound debridements or other surgical procedures.

- **New Roles of Hyperbaric Oxygen in Sepsis** Aksenov, IV, Strauss, MB, SS Miller, et al. X-2, # E-91, p 283

  At this time, insufficient data is available to justify the routine use of hyperbaric oxygen (HBO) in sepsis based on the subcellular mechanisms listed above (in results section). We feel that there is a potential role for HBO in severe sepsis and septic shock when tissue oxygenation is severely impaired

9. Undersea and Hyperbaric Medical Society Annual Meeting, 24-28 June 2009, Las Vegas, Nevada, *Undersea and Hyperbaric Medicine,* **Volume 36, 2009**

- **The Art and Science of Wound Debridement,** Strauss, MB, SS Miller & IV Aksenov # C14, pg 280

  The "science of debridement" is mastered by didactics and training. The "art of debridement" reflects the experiences and judgment garnered by working with wounds. Debridements in the operating room are driven by the goal of establishing healthy surgical margins even at the cost of sacrificing possibly viable and/or healthy tissues or more proximal lower limb amputations. Clinic debridements obviate the need for establishing surgical margins at a single visit. By doing serial debridements of only obviously non-viable tissue, there is maximal conservation of tissue. Questionably, viable tissues must establish their own lines of demarcation. This maxim is achieved through appropriate debridement, optimal wound care, optimizing oxygen delivery to the wound and attention to nutrition needs as is required for dealing with the "problem" and "end-stage" wound.

- **Decision Making for Closure/Coverage of Problem Wounds,** Strauss, MB, GA Wirth, SS Miller, et al. X-2 # C17, pg 283

  For wounds to heal and infection to be controlled, oxygen/perfusion (O/P) need to increase about 20-fold. There is a continuum of O/P and metabolic requirements for the closure/coverage (C/C) choices for "problem" wounds. Do not overlook the use of O/P enhancing methods to improve C/C outcomes of "problem" wounds; often, more than one O/P improving technique is used. Always choose the "best fit" of the C/C techniques with the potential of the wound to increase its O/P and metabolic activity.

- **Hyperbaric O$_2$ Indications for the Salvage of Limb Threatening Wounds: An Algorithmic Approach,** Strauss, MB, SS Miller, GB Hart & IV Aksenov #C18. pg 283

  When wound healing concerns arise due to oxygen/perfusion deficits, juxta-wound transcutaneous oxygen measurements (TCOMS) should be obtained. If over 40 mmHg in room air, primary healing is likely without hyperbaric oxygen (HBO). If less than 40 mmHg, then TCOMS should be obtained with HBO. If over 200 mmHg, healing with adjunctive HBO is likely. If less than 50 mmHg, amputation will likely be required. If between 50 and 200 mmHg, 50% of post-operative wounds heal primarily while 90% of those that fail initially, eventually heal passing through 4 stages with wound care and HBO.

- **Strategies for the Pevention of Diabetic Foot Wounds,** Strauss, MB, SS Miller & IV Aksenov #C15, pg 281

  Most diabetic foot wounds are preventable; feet at risk are identifiable by having one or more primary risk factors. Four strategies provide the essential evaluation and management interventions to prevent diabetic foot wounds. **The Goal-Aspiration Score** reflects the patient's desire to keep his/her feet and provide guidelines for the frequency of return visits.

- **Staging the Healing of Failed, Sloughed, Dehisced (FSD) "End-stage" Wounds,** Strauss, MB, SS Miller, AJ Lewis & IV Aksenov # C16, pg 282

  The "end-stage" wound is defined by healing observations/expectations and quantified by transcutaneous oxygen measurements and the **Wound Score.** The decision to "salvage" the "end-stage" wound requires ancillary information (in addition to the description of the wound) that includes the patient's **Host-Function** and **Goal-Aspiration Score** plus nutrition status. In addition to the five strategic management interventions, five additional special considerations must be utilized to obtain the best possible outcomes for the "end-stage" wound. Once an "end-stage" wound heals, the results are durable when the patient follows wound prevention strategies.

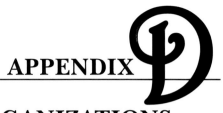

APPENDIX

WOUND CARE ORGANIZATIONS, SOCIETIES, AND ASSOCIATIONS

INTRODUCTION 541

AMERICAN ACADEMY OF WOUND MANAGEMENT (AAWM) 541

AMERICAN COLLEGE OF CERTIFIED WOUND SPECIALISTS (CCWS) 542

AMERICAN PROFESSIONAL WOUND CARE ASSOCIATION (APWCA) 542

ASSOCIATION FOR THE ADVANCEMENT OF WOUND CARE (AAWC) 542

CANADIAN ASSOCIATION OF WOUND CARE (CAWC) 543

NATIONAL ALLIANCE OF WOUND CARE (NAWC) 543

WOUND CARE SOCIETY (WCS) 543

WOUND HEALING SOCIETY (WHS) 544

THE WOUND, OSTOMY, AND CONTINENCE NURSES SOCIETY (WOCN) . 544

INTRODUCTION

The following is a listing of nine organizations devoted to wound care. Each has different perspectives. For example, the Wound Healing Society is heavily weighted towards clinical and basic sciences from physicians, scientists, and academician perspectives, while the Wound, Ostomy, and Continence Nurses Society leans towards clinical wound care from nursing perspectives.

The common goal of all wound caregivers (and wound organizations) is to optimize the care of their patient's wounds. Buzz words like advanced wound care, standards of care, cutting edge technology, multi-disciplinary approaches, excellence in care, etc. should not be used to differentiate one society from another since wound care knowledge is assumed to be (and should be) fundamental to all these organizations.

Another challenge of these wound care organizations is to balance economic realities with the organizations' recommendations for best practice interventions. Is a bioengineered dressing that costs 100 times more than a hydrogel one hundred times more effective? Many new technologies are received with incredible enthusiasm and unrestrained usage, only to be put in proper perspective with the test of time. A recent example is that of the cutaneous applied growth factor preparations. Now, negative pressure wound therapy seems to be the answer for every challenging wound problem. However, fundamentals such as maintaining a moist wound environment, managing sepsis, correction of deformities, and maximizing wound perfusion/oxygenation must not be overlooked when using the new technologies.

A third challenge for wound care organizations is that of fostering a multi-disciplinary approach where the caregivers "in the trenches" (those who do the day to day wound care) have the support of and immediate availability of surgeons who may be required to do deep tissue debridement, surgical wound closure/coverage, revascularization, and amputations. A good approach and a great philosophy for all wound care providers is to adhere to the five treatment strategies presented in Part III of this text.

1. American Academy of Wound Management (AAWM)

The American Academy of Wound Management is a voluntary, non-profit organization established for the purpose of credentialing interdisciplinary practitioners on the field of wound management. The Board of Advisors is an interdisciplinary panel of experts in wound care consisting of practitioners, academicians and researchers. The American Academy of Wound Management is a full voting member of the National Organization for Competency Assurance (NOCA).

```
Contact:  1155 15th Street. NW
          Suite 500
          Washington, DC 20005
  Phone:  202.457.8408
  Email:  jmargeson@aawm.org
Website:  www.aawn.org
```

2. American College of Certified Wound Specialists (CCWS)

The American College of Certified Wound Specialists was incorporated in January 2005. The American Academy of Wound Management had grown to the point that the formation of CCWS was a natural progression in the development of its goal to promote advanced wound care and set the standard of care in wound management in the wound community.

Contact: 1155 15th Street, NW, Suite 500
Washington, DC 20005
Phone: 202.457.8409
Fax: 202.530.0659
Email: dabts@theccws.org
Website: www.theccws.org

3. American Professional Wound Care Association (APWCA)

The American Professional Wound Care Association represents all wound care medical disciplines. The association sponsors multidisciplinary conferences and seminars, provides cutting-edge education, and is legislatively active on wound care issues.

Member benefits include:
- Insurance company representation
- Discounted registration for conferences and seminars
- A Medline-indexed journal, *Advances in Skin and Wound Care*
- Newsletters
- Regular email updates regarding wound care products
- Research updates
- Legislative representation.

Contact: 853 Second Street Pike # A-1
Richboro, PA 18954
Phone: 215.364.4100
Fax: 215.364.1146
Email: wounds@apwca.org
Website: www.apwca/org

4. Association for the Advancement of Wound Care (AAWC)

The Association for the Advancement of Wound Care (AAWC) is the leading society for medical professionals and industry members. It promotes excellence in education, clinical practice, public policy, and research, and is dedicated to the advancement of wound care.

The AAWC gives its members the opportunity to build a collaborative community to facilitate optimal care for wound sufferers. This community encourages an equal partnership among all who care for patients.

Contact: 83 General Warren Blvd., Suite 100
Malvern, PA 19355
Phone: 866.AAWC.999
Fax: 610.560.0501
Email: info@aawconline.org
Website: www.aawconline.org

5. Canadian Association of Wound Care (CAWC)

The Canadian Association of Wound Care is a nonprofit organization of health care professionals, industry participants, patients, and caregivers dedicated to the advancement of wound care in Canada. The CAWC was formed in 1995, and its official meeting is the CAWC held in Canada each year.

        Contact: 2171 Avenue Road, Suite 102
                  Toronto, Ontario, Canada
                  M5M 4B4
          Phone: 416.485.2292
            Fax: 416.485.2291
          Email: info@cawc.net
        Website: www.cawc/net

6. National Alliance of Wound Care (NAWC)

The National Alliance of Wound Care (a NCCA accredited program) is a professional wound care certification and membership organization with over 6,000 Wound Care Certified (WCC) practitioners and members nationwide. The aspiration of the NAWC is to unify wound care providers and practitioners from different professional backgrounds along the health care continuum in an effort to facilitate the delivery of quality wound care. The NAWC is a member of the National Organization for Competency Assurance, American Board of Nursing Specialties, American, Health Care Association, and the National Pressure Ulcer Advisory Panel.

        Contact: 5464 N Port Washington Rd #134
                  Glendale, WI 53217
          Phone: 877.WCC.NAWC
            Fax: 800.352.8339
          Email: editor@nawccb.org

7. Wound Care Society (WCS)

The Wound Care Society is a charitable organization concerned with all aspects of wound care. It aims to improve the care and treatment of persons with wounds through the provision of education to nurses interested or working in the field of wound management. The WCS aims to assist nurses to provide wound management based on sound research, while emphasizing the importance of providing total care for the patient.

        Contact: P.O. Box 170
                  Hartford Huntingdon
                  Cambridge, UK
                  PE 29 1PL
          Phone: 01480.434401
            Fax: 01480.434401
          Email: wound.care.society@talk21.com
        Website: www.woundcaresociety.com

8. Wound Healing Society (WHS)

The Wound Healing Society is composed of clinician and basic scientists and provides a forum for scientists, physicians, practitioners, industrial representatives, and government agencies. The WHS is open to individuals interested in wound healing. The WHS is a leading scientific organization in wound healing. Its membership consists of physicians, residents, practitioners, students, and researchers. The WHS also publishes the journal *Wound Repair and Regeneration*.

          Contact: 341 N. Maitland Ave., Suite 130
                    Maitland, FL 32751
            Phone: 407.647.8839
              Fax: 407.629.2502
            Email: member@woundheal.org
          Website: www.woundheal.org

9. The Wound, Ostomy, and Continence Nurses Society (WOCN)

The Wound, Ostomy, and Continence Nurses Society is a professional nursing society that supports its members by promoting educational, clinical, and research opportunities to advance the practice and guide the delivery of expert health care to individuals with wounds, ostomies, and incontinence.

          Contact: WOCN National Office
                    15000 Commerce Parkway, Suite C
                    Mount Laurel, NJ 08054
            Phone: 888.224.9626 (WOCN)
              Fax: 856.39.0525
            Email: wocn_info@wocn.org
          Website: www.wocn.org

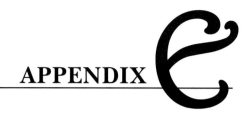

APPENDIX

PARTING COMMENTARIES

INTRODUCTION 547

GROWTH OF WOUND CLINICS 547

WOUND CLINIC BY-LINES 547

WOUND CLINIC ECONOMICS 547

IN-HOSPITAL VERSUS WOUND CLINIC PROVIDERS 548

PUTTING WOUND CARE IN PERSPECTIVE 548

THE WOUND TEAM 549

PATIENT/FAMILY PARTICIPATION 551

DECISION-MAKING CHALLENGES 552

SYNERGY 553

MULTIDISCIPLINARY WOUND CARE ROUNDS AND
    PATIENT CARE CONFERENCES 555

"PET PEEVES" ABOUT CONTEMPORARY MANAGEMENTS
    AND SOME PROPOSED SOLUTIONS 557

INTRODUCTION

To complete the appendices and send the reader on to "masterminding" wounds, we include information about wound centers, reimbursement considerations, who should be included in the wound team, the challenges of new technologies, and the integration of wound team participants activities.

GROWTH OF WOUND CLINICS

In the United States there has been rapid growth in the number of and services provided by wound clinics. Conversely, the treatment of these problems in the private office setting has markedly declined. Many reasons account for this, such as the fact that wound science has advanced to the point that specially trained and dedicated practitiononers are needed to manage the complex wound. Also, clinicians want to keep patients with multiple drug resistant organism out of their offices, optimal wound care such as debridements and skin and toenail care can be time-consuming, stocking of wound supplies for only a small percentage of the private office patients is not cost-effective, and arranging home health care can be time-consuming.

WOUND CLINIC BY-LINES

Perusal of the internet approximates more than 700 wound center listings. The centers are marketed by very compelling descriptors/tag lines. The following table includes descriptors found in the initial four pages alone of the internet listings.

Descriptors/Tag Lines for Some of the Wound Centers Listed on the Internet		
• Aggressive treatment	• Exceptional outpatient program	• One of the most successful
• Caring for wounds that have resisted traditional means of healing	• Exceptional outpatient services	• Premier provider
• Center for advanced wound care	• Full range of services	• Specialized care
• Center of excellence	• Full service wound care	• Specialists in the latest therapeutic methods
• Center of the year	• Heals thousands of patients with chronic wounds	• Specialize treatment of chronic wounds
• Clinically proven treatment methods	• Industry leader	• Specialized wound care faculty
• Comprehensive care	• Intensive therapies	• State of the art
• Comprehensive and compassionate care	• Latest in clinical research and practice	• The right treatment to heal
• Comprehensive treatment	• Latest technology	• Top notch treatment options
• Enhanced service	• Leading provider of wound and disease management solutions	• Unique team
• Evidence-based approaches	• Major commitment	• We can find out why a wound won't heal
	• Most advanced techniques	

WOUND CLINIC ECONOMICS

The proliferation of outpatient wound services is "driven" by economic realities as well as the goal to provide the best possible care to the patient. Due to DRG's (diagnostic related groups) implemented by Medicare/CMS (Center for Medicare/Medicaid Services), in addition to per diem rates for hospital days and included hospital services that are contracted between insurance payors and medical centers, it is much more cost-effective for hospitals to discharge patients with wounds as early as possible—or not admit them at all (see ED wound evaluation algorithm in this appendix), and have their wound care performed in the outpatient setting.

> The ramifications of Diagnostic Related Groups are that CMS provides a fixed payment for a hospital admission diagnosis. The fees are based on formulations as to what would be "fair and reasonable" for usual services and hospital stays for patients admitted with similar conditions. All services needed to evaluate and manage the diagnosis are included in the fixed fee.
>
> If fewer services or hospital days are needed, the hospital will "make money" on the DRG; if more, then the hospital will "lose money" on the patient. Wound care—as well as hyperbaric oxygen treatments—is included in the hospital service.
>
> The bottom line is that there is no additional income generation for providing wound care and/or hyperbaric oxygen treatments for patients who have comorbidities that require these services in addition to the patient's admitting DRG diagnosis. There are some provisions for outliers and complications, but the disallowment of reimbursements for "never events" (i.e. complications deemed preventable by CMS) tend to negate additional income that might be generated from outliers.

Reimbursements for outpatient wound care services typically include income generation for a facility use fee, for equipment and supplies utilized, and for procedures performed by clinic staff other than physicians. Physicians can be reimbursed for outpatient wound care services as if performed in the private office, i.e. identical RB/RVS (resource based/relative value system) codes.

Another disincentive for the management of wounds in the private office is the exclusion of "facility use" charges as is typically done for wound centers.

IN-HOSPITAL VERSUS WOUND CLINIC PROVIDERS

Unfortunately, there appears to be another dichotomy, and that is between the practitioners who manage the wounds that are so serious that they require hospitalization and those that are managed in wound healing clinics.

For the former, surgeons almost always make the major wound care management decisions, since surgeries are often necessary if the wound problem requires hospitalization. For the outpatient wound clinics, other caregivers including dermatologists, emergency medicine physicians, hyperbaricists, nurse practitioners, and nurse wound care specialists are usually responsible for managing their patients' wounds. Podiatrists are becoming increasingly involved as serving in both capacities.

PUTTING WOUND CARE IN PERSPECTIVE

The next challenge is to define "state of the art" of wound care—as is so heavily marketed by wound clinics. There are two considerations for this. First is the buzz word "cutting-edge technology." This phrase implies using relatively recent inclusions in the wound care armamentarium that have some theoretical, laboratory-based, and/or clinical support for their effectiveness (e.g. silver impregnated dressings, bioengineered wound covering agents, negative pressure wound therapy, autologous platelet rich plasma, genetically produced growth factors, etc. [see Chapter 9]), and automatically qualifies the wound center as a "state of the art" facility.

This must be tempered with what is "tried and true." Often less expensive interventions are equally effective and have proven their efficacy by the "test of time." Finally, the underlying causes—namely deformities, uncontrolled infection/osteomyelitis, and wound ischemia/hypoxia—that account for 90% or more of the reasons problem wounds fail to heal must be addressed before labeling the wound as non-healing to justify the use of newer technologies. This concept is what we have tried to express in Part III of *MasterMinding Wounds*, i.e. the five treatment strategies, and really reflects the philosophy of "getting back to fundamentals."

Although evidence-based indications (EBI) are important when making decisions about wound care, rational decisions for treatment need to be based on more than EBI (Table 1-2). The following figure modifies the information expressed in Table 1-2.

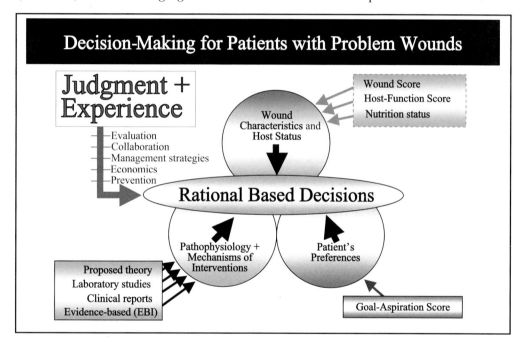

THE WOUND TEAM

The more complicated the wound problem, the greater the need for the multidisciplinary wound team approach. There are three main care provider divisions, and each has their special roles.

Physicians are responsible for decision-making and performing procedures. Nurses are responsible for executing physicians' orders and patient management. Allied health care members provide supportive and information services. However, there are overlapping functions between groups. For example, nurses perform evaluations such as staging pressure ulcers and debridements (within their defined scope of practice guidelines). Physical therapists not only rehab patients, but also perform hydrotherapy and wound debridements. Below is a list of possible wound team participants for each caregiver division.

Possible Participants in the Wound Team

Physicians Decisions /Procedures	Nurses Management	Allied Health Care Support / Information
• Endocrinologist • Dermatologist (typically outpatient clinics) • **Emergency medicine physician** • **Hyperbaric medicine physician** • Infectious disease specialists • **Orthopaedic surgeon** • Nephrologist • Physiatrist • **Plastic surgeon** • **Podiatrist** • **Primary care physician** • Psychiatrist • Radiologist • **Vascular surgeon**	• **Case managers/discharge planner** • **Diabetes educator** • Dialysis service • **Epidemiologist** • Home health care provider • Enterostomal therapist • **Hyperbaric nurse specialist** • **Program director** • Skilled and long term acute care nursing facility liaison • **Wound care specialist**	• Cast technician • Chaplain • **Clinical nutritionist** • **Clinical pharmacist** • Hyperbaric medicine technician • Medical photographer • Orthotist/prosthetist • **Physical therapist** • Transport orderlies (especially for hyperbaric O_2 treatments) • Clinical social worker • **Negative pressure therapy wound collaboration** • **Specialty bed liaison**

Note: Bolded entries indicate frequent participants in the evaluation, management, and prevention of patients' wounds and is ideally executed through multidisciplinary rounds on hospital inpatients or patient care conference settings for inpatients as well as outpatients.

Wielding a Partnership in Care

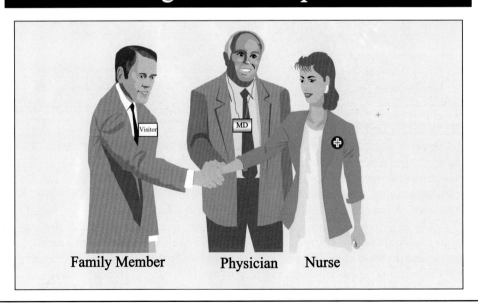

Family Member   Physician   Nurse

PATIENT/FAMILY PARTICIPATION

Not to be forgotten—and perhaps the most important of all the care providers, especially once the patient leaves the hospital setting, is the patient and/or his/her family. Some of the most resounding wound healing success stories are those of patients or their families who take over the daily wound care of the patient after hospital discharge. This often becomes a necessity if home health insurance provisions are exhausted or not available.

In addition to dressing changes, the family members help assure that doctors' orders are followed such as extremity elevation, edema control, weight bearing restrictions, skin care diabetes monitoring, nutrition management, etc. Whereas a home health nurse may spend thirty minutes a day with the patient for dressing changes, the family members are often there for the patient 24/7.

The **Goal-Aspiration Score** (Chapter 1) provides guidance as to how much cooperation by the patient and support by family members can be expected.

Regardless of the complexity of the wound, optimal management requires directing attention to both the host factors and the wound environment. The goals are to make the host as competent as possible paired with making the wound environment as conducive for healing as possible. If one thesis could be used to express the philosophy of *MasterMinding Wounds*, it would be the above statement. The following figure summarizes this concept.

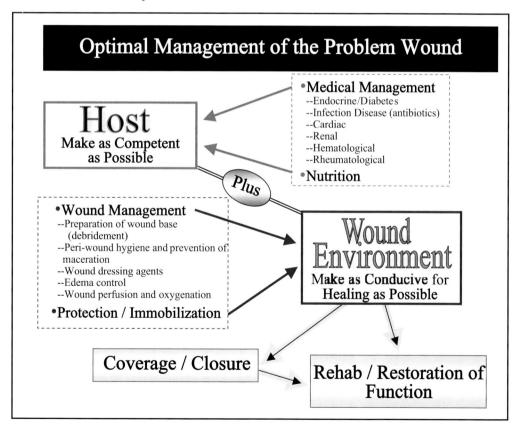

DECISION-MAKING CHALLENGES

There are two difficult decision-making challenges when patients' wounds are initially evaluated. First, does the patient with a wound who presents at the emergency department (or wound clinic) require immediate hospitalization, and second, if the patient is hospitalized, who should assume responsibility for the management? This

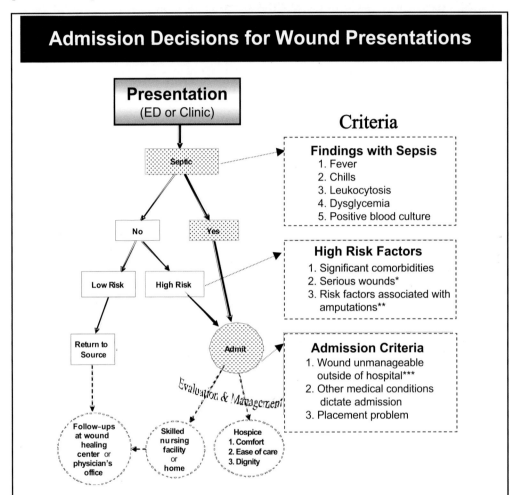

Admission Decisions for Wound Presentations

Presentation
(ED or Clinic)

Criteria

Septic

No **Yes**

Low Risk **High Risk**

Return to Source

Admit

Evaluation & Management

Follow-ups at wound healing center or **physician's office**

Skilled nursing facility or **home**

Hospice
1. Comfort
2. Ease of care
3. Dignity

Findings with Sepsis
1. Fever
2. Chills
3. Leukocytosis
4. Dysglycemia
5. Positive blood culture

High Risk Factors
1. Significant comorbidities
2. Serious wounds*
3. Risk factors associated with amputations**

Admission Criteria
1. Wound unmanageable outside of hospital***
2. Other medical conditions dictate admission
3. Placement problem

*Serious wounds are those that may result in loss of life or limb. They can be quantified by using the Wound Score (Chapter 5 and Appendix B). Serious wounds have scores of 4 ½ or less (i.e. the "end-stage" and "futile" wound types).

**Risk factors associated with amputations include: 1) Deformity, 2) Peripheral artery disease, 3) Previous wound, 4) Prior amputation and 5) Neuropathy.

***Findings associated with unmanageable wounds include: 1) Continuing deterioration, 2) Large size, 3) Wet gangrene with odor and drainage, 4) Lower extremity contractures, and/or 5) Location that makes wound care all but impossible for the caregivers.

Solid arrows and enclosures indicate decisions by the (ED) emergency department or clinic physicians; dotted arrows and enclosures are decisions and management by other caregivers.

latter situation arises when the wound care/continence-entostomal therapy nurse is requested by the admitting physician to manage a co-existing wound and the reason for admission is something other than the wound itself. The following two algorithms provides solutions to these challenges.

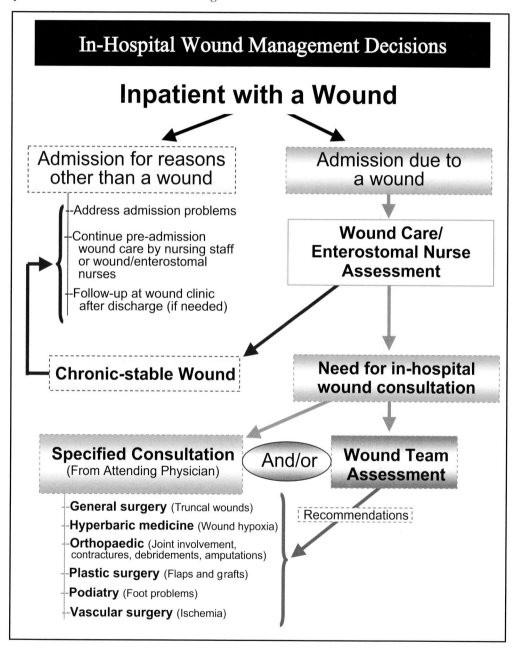

SYNERGY

The ideal wound program is one where there is synergy between in-hospital wound management, the outpatient wound center and the hyperbaric medicine program. The synergy works best when the three divisions are within a hospital setting, a single manager administers all three programs, there are medical directors for the wound and hyperbaric programs, the physicians that participate in the in-hospital wound care also follow the patients in the clinic setting, and weekly multidisciplinary rounds are made on the inpatients.

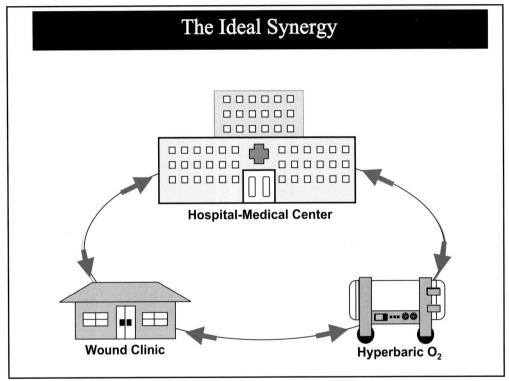

There is no disputing the fact that the wounds that require management that "really make a difference" are so serious that the patient requires hospitalization. These include patients who are septic from their wounds; necrotizing fasciitis; clostridial myonecrosis; wounds with underlying deformities that obviate any chance for healing; wounds secondary to severe lower extremity contractures; major burns; wounds associated with severe crush injuries; wounds that require revascularization, flaps or grafts; wounds or amputations that were initially closed and then failed, sloughed and/or dehisced; and wounds so severe that lower limb amputations are necessary. In the majority of these wounds, hyperbaric oxygen treatments are an indicated adjunct and surgical interventions in the operating room are required.

The wounds should be stabilized as rapidly as possible so the patients can be discharged to lower levels of care and followed in the wound clinic (preferably by the same physicians who managed their wounds in the hospital, i.e. the epitome of continuity of care). If hyperbaric oxygen treatments are indicated, they can be continued as an outpatient once the patient is discharged. The expedited discharge from in-hospital care is driven by economic considerations and facilitated by newer technologies such as composite (e.g. absorptive + antimicrobial +/- occlusive) dressing materials, negative pressure wound therapy, and bioengineered dressings that reduce the need for day-to-day or more frequent wound management.

For the chronic non-healing wound, the wound clinic is the place to initiate wound evaluation and management. The decision makers in the clinic must be sure that the five management strategies (Part III of *MasterMinding Wounds*) required for optimal wound management are followed. Especially not to be neglected are the wound protection/ stabilization and wound oxygenation strategies. For the latter when revascularization, stenting and/or angioplasty is not feasible and/or perfusion is insufficient to heal the wound after these procedures are done, hyperbaric oxygen treatments must not be overlooked.

MULTIDISCIPLINARY WOUND CARE ROUNDS AND PATIENT CARE CONFERENCES

Wound programs that include these components help qualify them as "Centers of Excellence." Optimally, multidisciplinary in-hospital wound care rounds should be done on a weekly basis and include as many wound team participants as possible. The goal is to evaluate/re-evaluate every patient in the hospital who has a wound that requires specialized care (see previous figure).

Wound Care Rounds
Case Presentation Format: **New Patient**

Name: Date:

1. Identification
1. Age _____
2. Sex _____
3. Hospital days _____ Date of admission _____
4. Referring physician _____

2. Wound Problem
1. Site _____
2. Duration/Management _____
3. Why admitted _____

3. Comorbidities
1. _____   5. _____
2. _____   6. _____
3. _____   7. _____
4. _____   8 _____

4. Functional Capacity and Type of Host

Host-Function Score
(0-10 scale with 10 being best)

Type of Host
☐ **Non-compromised--Healthy** (8-10 Points)
☐ **Impaired** (4-7 Points)
☐ **Severely compromised** (0-3 points)

5. Wound Score and Type

Wound Score
(0-10 scale with 10 being best)

Wound Type
(Scoring on back)
☐ **Healthy** (8-10 points)
☐ **Problem** (4-7 points)
◇ "End-stage" (2 1/2 to 4 1/2 points with good Host-Function nd Goal-Aspiration Score
☐ **Futile** (0-3 points)

Wound Care Rounds

Continuation of the New Patient Evaluation Form

6. Laboratory and Imaging Information

1. WBC _____ HCT _____ Albumin/Prealbumin_____

2. C and S _____

3. Other (BUN, BNP, K+, X-RAYS, Scans, $P_{tc}O_2$ Study with HBO, etc)_____
_____

7. Management

1. Wound _____   5. Bed Type _____

2. Nutrition _____   6. Physical Therapy _____

3. Antibiotics _____   7. HBO _____

4. Surgery _____   8. Other _____

8. Problems to Resolve
(In order of importance)

1. _____

2. _____

3. _____

Wound Care Rounds

Case Presentation Format: **Follow-up Patient**

Name: _____   Date: _____

1. Identification

1. Age _____

2. Sex _____

3. Reason for Wound Care Unit admission_____
_____

4. Hospital days _____

2. Status

☐ **Improved**

☐ **No Change**

☐ **Worse**

Reason/Justification (Use **WoundScore** to quantify-see below changes; also include wound appearance, lab studies, function, etc.)

_____
_____
_____

3. Changes in Management
(Since last week)

1. Wound Care_____

2. Surgery_____

3. Other (Nutrition, bed selection, antibiotic, activity, physical therapy, etc.) _____
_____

4. Goals
(Previous and new problems to resolve)

1. _____

2. _____

3. _____

An added feature of rounds is the opportunity to present new information to the attendees in the form of a mini-talk that is brief and concise. Examples include the presentation of an algorithm analogous to those seen in this section, review of a pertinent article from the wound literature, or discussion of a new product. These "academic" presentations help to justify multidisciplinary rounds as a continuing medical education activity.

Each participant contributes information with which he/she is most familiar. For example, the nurse epidemiologist updates wound culture information and what isolation techniques are required, while the clinical nutritionist updates the patient's nutrition status and what interventions should be done. The clinical pharmacist provides information on antibiotic selection, other medication usage, and drug allergies/ undesirable drug interactions. Because of time limitations, any information presented needs to be brief and concise. The forms depict formats devised to present the essential information on a new admission wound problem and for follow-up multidisciplinary rounds visits concisely and without omissions. Note that forms include **Host-Function** and **Wound Scores**. The wound team participants should be briefed on these scores, and they can also be printed on the back of each form.

Patient care conferences are appropriate for the wound clinic. Although several participants such as the physician, the wound care nurse, the case worker, and the patient's family may be present, at the time evaluation and management of the patient are done, typically the wound care nurse documents what orders need to done and insures that the treatment plan is executed. This may require faxing copies to the patient's home health care provider, the referring physician, the skilled nursing facility, and/or writing out the wound care instructions so there will be no ambiguity as to what the patient and/or his family need to do regarding the wound care.

"PET PEEVES" ABOUT CONTEMPORARY MANAGEMENTS AND SOME PROPOSED SOLUTIONS

We complete this appendix (and the *MasterMinding Wounds* text) with some concerns we have about the contemporary management of wounds and related problems. Information how to address them is provided. Please consider the following:

1. **Failure to recognize and address the fact that the majority (>than 90%) of chronic, non-healing wounds have underlying deformities, unresolved infection/osteomyelitis, ischemia/hypoxia, or combinations of these.** In the majority of patients, these problems are remedial.

2. **Failure to address wound base hygiene and the hygiene of the skin surrounding the wound and the rest of the foot and leg.** This can usually be resolved with appropriate debridements of the wound base, application of desiccating ointments around macerated skin margins, and moisturization plus lubrication of the remaining skin of the foot and leg.

3. **Failure to appreciate that most intractable wounds associated with severe lower extremity contractures occur because the contractures make off-loading of the wound sites impossible** or tension over the sites (e.g. hip adduction contractures over the greater trochanters) attenuates the soft tissues to prevent healing. This problem requires surgical release of the contractures. Many times the "impossible" wounds heal spontaneously once the contractures are released.

4. **Failure to recognize that protection and immobilization of a wound site is a primary strategy for managing wounds.** The more serious the wound, the more this strategy must be followed. For example, in the severest Charcot arthropathy wounds of the foot, the deformities must be corrected and the foot and ankle stabilized with intramedullary rodding or temporary external fixation. In most other situations, casts or orthotics can satisfactorily immobilize the foot wound.

5. **Failure to manage edema.** Edema not only contributes to venous stasis ulcers, but oozes through the skin in the dependent portions of the extremity wound to delay healing, macerates the skin surrounding the wound, increases the diffusion distance from the capillary to the healing which contributes to tissue hypoxia, and leads to compartment syndromes. Edema is managed by elevation and compression dressings. However, malnutrition and heart failure must not be overlooked as causes of edema; both are remedial problems.

6. **Failure to use an objective grading system of wound severity (such as the Wound Score)** to evaluate new wound products. It is difficult to justify the use of new, costly products where studies report relatively small percentage reductions in wound surface area in somewhat briefer healing times using the new product versus the controls and for what all appearances (photo examples in brochures) look like healthy, vascular based wounds.

7. **The use of hyperbaric oxygen (HBO) for diabetic foot wounds that have persisted for greater than 30 days when remedial problems such as deformity and uncontrolled infection/osteomyelitis co-exist and can be controlled.** To use HBO, juxta-wound transcutaneous oxygen studies should be done to confirm that hypoxia is a reason the wound is not healing.

8. **The treatment of malperforans ulcers (especially of the toes and forefoot) when osteomyelitis is not present by total contact casting, bone resection or transmetatarsal amputation** rather than correction of the underlying deformity. In most instances, deformities in the forefoot can be corrected by simple tenotomies or realigning the metatarsal head with scoring the bone and osteoclasis.

9. **Assumption that antibiotics alone will cure a sub-acute or chronic diabetic foot infection** when infected bone, cicatrix, infected bursa, foreign material (sutures, implants, grafts, etc.) remain in the wound.

10. **Failure to use hyperbaric oxygen as continuity of care** for diabetic foot wounds after hospitalization was required because of their severity and concerns remain about wound healing.

11. **Failure to realize that most failed amputations at the transmetatarsal and higher levels will eventually heal with strategic management** (including hyperbaric oxygen) of the wound and thereby obviate the need for doing a more proximal amputation.

12. **Labeling a patient as non-compliant for not doing foot hygiene, not using elastic support hose, or not elevating the legs** when problems such arthritis, obesity, back pain, and/or peripheral artery disease (the patient keeps the leg in the dependent position for pain relief) make it impossible for the patient to do such.

13. **Using costly imaging studies to demonstrate osteomyelitis** when the wound tracks to bone, induration is present around the wound margins, and plain x-rays have changes consistent with osteomyelitis.

14. **Failure to appreciate that anemia in patients with chronic diabetic foot infections is often resolved with eradication of the infection.**
15. **Failure to recognize that malnutrition may be one of the most important co-morbidites** when chronic wounds fail to improve, overwhelming infection is present, wounds are very large, or combinations of these even if the patient is morbidly obese.
16. **Failure to optimize glycemic control with appropriate monitoring and medications.**

INDEX

ABI 60, 61
abscess 40
Achilles tendon lengthening.......475, 476, 477
acrosclerosis 408
activities 394
activity level 395
activity recommendations 394
acute decubitus ulcer 88
adenosine triphosphate (ATP) content 28
AFOs 428
Agency for Health Care
    Policy and Research........................ 99
aggravated infections 38
albumin 487
allodynia 45
alteration of the blood-brain barrier ..276
ambulation assessment 394
amputation 315, 373, 430, 554, 558
amputations of toes 470
anemia 559
angiogenesis 32, 272
angiogenesis stage 181
ankle foot orthosis (AFO) 209, 428
ankle wounds 188
ankle-brachial index (ABI) .. 60, 122, 295
anticoagulation 146
antimicrobial agents 242
Apgar scoring system 112
appearance of wound base 117
appreciation that the healing of the
    problem wound represents a
    continuum of responses 19
Armstrong 72
arterial-venous (A-V)
    oxygen extraction 266
arteriosclerosis 34
assessing sensation 497
assessments 485, 496
atherosclerosis 402
auto-amputation 470
autonomic 45
autonomic nerve injury 44
avascular 37
avascular soft tissues 28
B-Jensen.....................................103, 125
barefoot 390
Bates-Jensen Pressure Sore
    Status Tool (PSST) 93, 94

bioburden 224
bioengineered dressings 9, 489, 554
bioengineered wound covering
    agents 485
biofilm 120, 467, 468, 485
black based wound 173
blister 42, 403, 453
blister formation 453
blood rheology 300
blood transfusion 145
body mass index 389
bone resorption 273
bone spurs 39, 40
bony prominences 38
Boyd 430
Boyd amputations 432
Boyle's law 269
Braden scale 90
Brodsky Depth-Ischemia Classification 72
Brodsky system 70, 71, 73
Brodsky's classification 70
bubble reduction 269
Buerger's disease 35
bunion deformities 424
bunions 393, 405
bunionettes 187
burns 47
bursa 38, 44, 404, 558
C-reactive protein 487
calciphylaxis 408
callus 39, 391, 404, 449, 451, 463
capillaries 8
cardiovascular problems 136
cast complications 203
casts 203
cellulitis 40
"centers of excellence"........................ 555
central motor neuropathies 46
cerebral vascular accident 46
cessation of toxin formation 274
challenges 19
Charcot arthropathy 39, 40, 41, 341, 428, 436
Charcot restraint orthotic
    walkers (CROW boot) 422
chronic ulcer 88
chronic venous insufficiency 9
chronic wounds 375
cicatrix 36, 37, 44, 167, 558

cigarette 393
circular wrap 198
classification of wounds 27
classification system 67
clawed toes 405, 424, 436, 461, 463
clinical applications of
    hyperbaric oxygen 260
clinical judgment 14
clinical significance 13
closed space foot infections
    and ascending tenosynovitis 186
closed spaced abscesses 38
clostridial myonecrosis 554
coagulopathies 47
combinations 39, 40
comfort care 333
comparisons and contrasts between
    monoplace and multiplace
    chambers 259
compartment syndromes respectively . 35
compassionate care for the
    "end-stage" wound 333
complex regional pain syndrome 45
compliance 16, 382
compliance assessment 401
complications from protection
    and immobilization devices 212
comprehension 16
comprehension assessment 396
compression dressings 558
compression stockings 424
compressive 46
concurrent..64
conditions causing other
    "end-stage" extremity wounds 362
connective tissue diseases 406
construct...64
contractures 39, 40, 44, 404, 434,
                                          554, 557
content...64
coverage/closure 485
coverage/closure stage 182
creative casts 204
criterion-related...................................64
CROW (Charcot restraint orthotic
    walker) boot 432
crush injury 42, 554
crusts 453, 455
cushioned plantar inserts 422

custom molded diabetic shoes 422
custom molded orthotics 437
custom prescribed orthotics 439
customized molded protective
    footwear 430
cytokines 31
Dalton's Law 265
debridement 38, 455, 466, 468
decubitus ulcer 87, 88
definition of hyperbaric oxygen 257
deformities 28, 39, 46, 47, 313, 403,
                                          436, 449
deformities from malunited fractures ..43
demyelinating conditions 46
"DEPA" score.................................. 77, 79
dermatomyositis 406
diabetes 18, 46, 405
diabetes mellitus 139
diabetic shoes 422, 426, 428
distal toe tuft wounds 184
donut pad 437
Doppler blood pressure 59
dosing of hyperbaric oxygen 274
dress the wound base 19
dressing agent selection 221
drop foot 405, 428
drying agents 244
dynamic problems 42
dysmorphic toenail changes 413
dystrophic toenail changes 413
dysvascularity 46, 47
eburnations 404
economic impact attributable to a
    newly diagnosed diabetic foot 18
edema 35, 42, 137, 402, 558
elephantiasis 47
"end-stage" 486
"end-stage" wound 14, 295, 493, 495
endocrine 139
energy metabolism 28
enzymatic debridement agents 244
epithelialization 455
equinus contracture ... 405, 436, 475, 476
equinus deformities 423
erosion...88
erythralgia 47
eschars 453, 455
etiological-associated reasons 27
evidence-based clinical reports 14

evidence-based indications 14
exercise 389, 395
exostoses 404
extent and costs of all problem wounds 17
external skeletal fixation 212
face 64
failed below knee amputation 346
failed, sloughed, dehisced
    post-op, post-HBO wound 320
failed surgeries 47
family and/or care givers' support 16
features of hyperoxygenation 267
features of other (than hypoxic)
    "end-stage" wounds 334
fiberglass (or plaster) splint 201
fibroblast 31, 32
fibroblast activity 32
fibrosis 36
fillers 422
five components of the
    Wound Score 117
flaps or grafts 554
flat feet 437
flexible fiberglass cast (FFC) 205
foot deformities 435
foot skin care 410
footwear 419
forefoot adductus 436
Forrest and Gamborg-Nilsen 66
Forrest System 66
Foster and Edmonds 76
fracture 28
fracture healing 29
"frustrated" granulation tissue 172
FSD post-op wounds 325
fungicidal 410
fungicidal agents 415
fungus infected (onychomycosis) 413
futile 115
futile wounds 116
gangrene 470
gas gangrene 38
gel inserts 437
gels 241
glycemic control 559
Goal-Aspiration Score 14, 15, 43, 45,
    64, 116, 123, 384, 485, 488, 500, 551
gradient of injury 42
grading systems 7

growth factors 9, 31, 245
hallux valgus 393, 405, 424
hammer toes 405
Harkless 72
healing stages 31
healing stages of the "problem"
    wound 178
healthy 115
healthy and problem wounds 115
heat exposures 391
heating pads 391
hematological problems 143
Henry's law 263
hereditary conditions............................40
heredity factors 39
hind foot wounds 187
hindfoot varus 436
hip, ischial, and presacral
    pressure sores 189
hospital admissions 18
Host Factors 270
Host-Function Score ...14, 27, 43, 64, 116,
           123, 135, 485, 488, 501
host status 42
hygiene 388
hyperbaric oxygen 486, 554, 555, 558
hyperbaric oxygen physiology 263
hypercholesterolemia 35
hyperkeratosis 39
hyperoxygenation 263
hyperpathia 45
hypertropic bursa 41
hypesthesia 45
hypoxia 42, 402
hypoxic encephalopathy 46
hypoxic wound 295
imaging studies 558
imaging techniques 489
immobilization 558
immunosuppression 47
immunosuppressors 408
impairment of motor function 405
in-grown toenails 391
in-toeing 437
indirect effects of edema 35
indolent ulcer......................................88
indolent wound subtypes in patients
    with critical comorbidities 181
indolent wounds 88

infected bone 37
infected soft tissues 37
infection 42, 46, 146
infection/bioburden 120
inflammatory response 31
inflammatory stage 31
inflatable waffle air cushion boot 202
ingenious risk measurement scale
    for pressure ulcers 90
ingrown toenail 413, 415
ischemia 35
ischemia/hypoxia 47, 557
ischemia index 61
Jeffcoate 74
joint collapse...................................... 39
joint contracture 436
keratinization 449
Klenzak (double upright) brace   209, 428
knee immobilizers 201
Knighton 67
Knighton system 68
Knighton's classification 68
Krasner 101, 103
laboratory studies 14
lamb's wool 438
last resort distal arterial bypass
    surgery 304
latency stage 178
Lavery.. 72
leg ulcers 188
leukocytes 31
level of evidence................................. 12
"Life without Blood" 263
lifts 422
ligament insufficiency 39, 40
limb amputation 43
living with a chronic, stable
    non-healing wound 325
logical decision making based
    on an objective scoring system 19
loss of sensation 405
lupus 406
macerated 404
Macfarlane.. 74
Macfarlane and Jeffcoate
    classification adds 75
magnetic resonance imaging 489
major burns 554
mallet toe deformities 461

mallet toes 405
malnutrition 46, 47, 558, 559
malperforans ulcer 404, 436, 463, 465,
                                558
malperforans ulcers under
    metatarsal heads 186
malunited fractures 43
massive bursa 41
Master Algorithm   113, 123, 487, 493, 494
medical management strategies 19
Medicare..103
Medicare approved wound
    uses of hyperbaric oxygen 278
Medicare classification of
    decubitus ulcers 104
Medicare therapeutic footwear
    benefits 439
Medicare Therapeutic
    Shoe Bill 425, 426, 428
medications 47
meta-analysis 11
metabolic requirements 28
metatarsal pad 428, 437
metatarsus adductus 423
microangiopathy 35
microbiological effects 274
Minimally Invasive "Keep it Simple
    and Speedy" surgeries 308
minimally invasive procedures 319
minimally invasive surgeries 448
mixed connective tissue disorders 406
mobility assessment 395
moist wound healing 8, 175, 224
moistened gauze dressings 229
moisture retention 46, 47
moisturization 408
moisturizing agents 245
monofilament 405
monoplace hyperbaric chamber 257
motivation 16
motor 45
motor nerve 44
motor neuropathies 405
multidisciplinary approach 131
multidisciplinary wound care 555
multipodus boot 201
mummification 470
mummified toe 470, 471
muscle imbalances 39, 434

myths, misconceptions and fallacies
about wound dressing agents 247
National Pressure Ulcer Advisory
Panel (NPUAP) 97
necrotizing fasciitis 38, 40, 471, 554
necrotizing soft tissue wound
subtype 181
need for other treatment options 14
negative pressure wound
therapy 485, 489, 554
neurodegenerative diseases 46
neurological problems 150
neuropathy 27, 39, 44, 374, 404
neuropathy induced 40
neutrophil oxidative killing 273
neutrophils 28
new medical products 10
nicotine 393
non-compliant 558
non-healing of the fracture 42
non-healing wound subtype 180
non-planar 436
Norton 89
NPUAP Staging System for
Pressure Ulcerations 99, 101, 103
nutrition 152, 487
odds ratios 11
off-loading 44
Ohura 90
Ohura system 90
Ohura-Hotta system 91
ointments and solutions 241
One-Two-Three Protocol 300, 302
onychomycosis 415
open joint infections 471
open toe joint infections 471
ortho wedge shoe (OWS) 210
orthoses 209
orthotics 419, 422, 433, 435, 436,
437, 439, 441
orthotist 425
ostectomy 473, 474
osteitis 120
osteoclasis 465, 558
osteoclast 273
osteomyelitis 28, 37, 42, 453, 489,
557, 558
osteophytes 404
outcomes 325

oxidative burst 28
oxygen gradient 272
oxygen requirements 31
oxygen requirements for wound
healing 487
oxygen reserves 29
oxygen tensions and
wound healing 255
oxygen transfer from the capillary
to tissue fluids 265
padded inserts 437
panniculitis 40
paronychia 391, 413
partial approximations 470
partial wound approximations 485
partial wound closure 470
Patella Tendon-Bearing (PTB) cast ... 208
pathological bursae 41
pathological calluses 40
pathophysiologic mechanisms 14
patient compliance 381, 382
Pecoraro and Reinber 69
pedorthotist 425, 439, 442
percutaneous tenotomy 456, 459
perfusion 28, 33, 121
periostitis 404
peripheral artery disease 33, 488
peripheral motor neuropathies 46
peripheral neuropathies 404
peroneal nerve palsy 428
persistence of deformities 27
pharmacological methods to
increase perfusion 300
pillow splints 201
planar 436
plantar inserts 426
plasma transported oxygen 263
post-HBO (hyperbaric oxygen)
treated wound 321
post-infection 35
post-op shoe 210
post-traumatic 40
post-traumatic cicatrix formation 35
post-traumatic tissue damaged beyond
all repair 27
post-traumatic wound 44, 350
prealbumin 487
predictive 64
prefabricated plastic shell splints 202

preparation of the wound base 19
prescription footwear 428
pressure sore risk scale 89
Pressure Sore Status Tool (PSST) 93
pressure sores 42, 47
Pressure Ulcer Scale for
    Healing (PUSH) 96, 97
pressure ulcer/indolent wound
    prediction tool-strauss 92
pressure ulcers 87
pressure ulcers/indolent wounds . 89, 335
prevention 381
prevention of wounds 396
proactive surgeries 445, 486, 496
problem 115
"problem" type 116
"problem" wound 7, 488
products for wound management 9
protection and stabilization of the
    wound environment 19
protective footwear 389, 392, 419,
            421, 424, 441, 442, 451
protective sensation 44, 405
PSST 95
psychiatric conditions 157
pulmonary problems 158
pumice stone 391
purpura fulminans.............................. 47
PUSH score 98, 103
PUSH tool 99
pyoderma gangrenosum 47
pyogenic granuloma 413
radiation injury 47
randomized control trials (RCT) 11
Raynaud's phenomenon 35, 402, 408
recurrences 385
red based wound 172
red blood cell deformability 275
refractory osteomyelitis 42, 148
regional control of blood flow 29
remodeling stage................................. 33
removable walker boot 210
renal disease 158
repair stage 32
revascularization 489, 554, 555
rheumatological conditions 159
rigid foot deformities 432
risk assessment instrument 89
risk factors 46, 382

rocker bottom 424
salves 241
Salzberg 90
San Antonio system 72, 73, 74
scale to predict pressure ulcers 90
scleroderma 406
scoring systems 111
scoring systems 89
Seattle Wound Classification
    System (Pecoraro/Reiber) 70
secondary mechanisms of
    hyperbaric oxygen 270
secretion producing wounds 237
selection of agents to cover 19
Semmes-Weinstein monofilament
    testing 45
sensory 45
sensory neuropathy 390, 405, 449, 488
serial casts 205
Sessing...103
Sessing Scale 95, 96, 97
Sessing Scale Pressure Ulcer Healing . 94
severe burns 361
Shea...103
Shea Grading System 91, 93
Shea system 92, 95, 96
shear 46
side effects and contraindication
    of hyperbaric oxygen 276
Simple Staging System 76, 77
size of the deformity 39
skin and toenail problems 402
skin assessment 498
skin care 399
skin hygiene 408
sloughed, dehisced (FSD) post-op 321
smoking 393
smoking, ergotamine poisoning 35
soaking 391
socks 392
soft compression dressing 196
sore..88
splayed forefoot 432
splints 200
spurring 404
stabilization of joints with pinnings ... 211
stages of healing are identifiable
    for the failed 321
stains on socks 388

static problems 39
statistical significance 13
steroids and naturopathic additives .. 246
"Strategic Management" approach 28
strategic management of the
    problem wound 19
Strauss (Wound Score)......................125
suction-irrigation 313
support hose 392
surgical debridement 174
surgical stabilization 210
surgical wound management 466
Sussman Wound Healing
    Tool (SWHT) 97, 98, 102, 103
techniques to improve
    wound oxygenation 256
tender loving care 410
tendon 39
tenosynovitis 38, 40, 463, 471
tenotomy 459
tensile 46
"terrible triad" of pressure
    ulcer/indolent wound evolution ... 337
Therapeutic Shoe Bill 421, 439, 440
Thomas heels 423
thrombotic events 35
tissue and transcutaneous oxygen
    tensions 29
tissue oxygen tensions 29
tobacco 393
toe amputations 461, 470, 471
toe boxes 424
toe deformities 456
toe walking 437
toenail assessment 499
toenail care 388, 401
toenail evaluation 410
toenail management 399
toenail polish 392
toenail problems 402
toenails 391
topox 260
total contact casting (TCC) 206, 466, 558
transcutaneous oxygen
    measurements 295
transcutaneous oxygen studies 558
transforming growth factor-1 36
transmetatarsal amputation 558
trauma 28, 39, 46

trial of hyperbaric oxygen 296
trophic ulcer..88
types of neuropathies 45
ulcerations along the medial side
    of the great toe 185
ulcer.. 88, 310
ultrasound 489
uncontrolled forces 46, 47
uncontrolled infection 27, 47
underlying deformities 557
use of objective parameters to
    measure outcomes 19
valgus 436
validity measures 64
various agents 9
varus 436
vascular evaluation 489
vasculitis 406
vasculitities 35
venous stasis disease 35
venous stasis ulcers 47, 356, 558
Virchow's triad 357
Wagner based 59
Wagner Grades 60
Wagner score 65
Waterlow 89
wear patterns 437
wedges 422
wet gangrene 470
white or yellow based wound 173
WHS alphabetic modifiers 102
wound 88
wound base 169
wound clinic 547, 554, 555
wound depth 119
wound depth grade 120
wound descriptors 111
wound dressings 489
wound grading system....................... 55
Wound Healing Scale (WHS) 101
wound ischemia/hypoxia 27
wound oxygenation 19
wound prevention 385
Wound Score 14, 19, 55, 112, 113, 114,
    115, 116, 118, 121, 122, 123, 124, 485,
              488, 494, 501, 558
wound severity 115
wound size 117, 118
wound team 549

wounds 313
wounds associated with midfoot
    hyperpronation and dropout 187
wounds over the apices
    of interphalangeal joints 185
x-rays 489, 558
Yarkony-Kirk 93
Younes, et al. 77
Younes' DEPA score 123, 125